Coding for Pediatrics 2018

A Manual for Pediatric Documentation and Payment

For Use With AMA CPT® 2018

23rd Edition

Author
Committee on Coding and Nomenclature (COCN)
American Academy of Pediatrics

Edward A. Liechty, MD, Editor

Cindy Hughes, CPC, CFPC, Consulting Editor
Becky Dolan, MPH, CPC, CPEDC, Staff Editor

American Academy of Pediatrics
DEDICATED TO THE HEALTH OF ALL CHILDREN®

American Academy of Pediatrics Publishing Staff

Mark Grimes, *Director, Department of Publishing*

Barrett Winston, *Senior Editor, Professional/Clinical Publishing*

Leesa Levin-Doroba, *Production Manager, Practice Management*

Jason Crase, *Manager, Editorial Services*

Peg Mulcahy, *Manager, Art Direction and Production*

Mary Lou White, *Chief Product and Services Officer/SVP, Membership, Marketing, and Publishing*

Mary Jo Reynolds, *Marketing Manager, Practice Publications*

Published by the American Academy of Pediatrics

141 Northwest Point Blvd

Elk Grove Village, IL 60007-1019

Telephone: 847/434-4000

Facsimile: 847/434-8000

www.aap.org

The recommendations in this publication do not indicate an exclusive course of treatment or serve as a standard of medical care. Variations, taking into account individual circumstances, may be appropriate. Vignettes are provided to illustrate correct coding applications and are not intended to offer advice on the practice of medicine.

Products are included for informational purposes only. Inclusion in this publication does not imply endorsement. The American Academy of Pediatrics does not recommend any specific brand of products or services.

This publication has been developed by the American Academy of Pediatrics. The contributors are expert authorities in the field of pediatrics. No commercial involvement of any kind has been solicited or accepted in development of the content of this publication.

Quantity prices on request. Address all inquiries to American Academy of Pediatrics Department of Membership Engagement, Marketing, and Sales, 141 Northwest Point Blvd, Elk Grove Village, IL 60007-1019

Printed in the United States of America

CPT® copyright 2017 American Medical Association (AMA). All rights reserved.

Fee schedules, relative value units, conversion factors, and/or related components are not assigned by the AMA, are not part of *CPT*, and the AMA is not recommending their use. The AMA does not directly or indirectly practice medicine or dispense medical services. The AMA assumes no liability for data contained or not contained herein.

CPT® is a registered trademark of the AMA.

This publication has prior approval of the American Academy of Professional Coders (AAPC) for 4.0 continuing education units. Granting of this approval in no way constitutes endorsement by AAPC of the publication content or publication sponsor.

11-35M   1 2 3 4 5 6 7 8 9 10

MA0832

ISBN: 978-1-61002-102-9

eBook: 978-1-61002-108-1

ISSN: 1537-324X

Disclaimer

||||||||||

Every effort has been made to include the new and revised 2018 *Current Procedural Terminology (CPT®)*; *International Classification of Diseases, 10th Revision, Clinical Modification (ICD-10-CM)*; and Healthcare Common Procedure Coding System (HCPCS) codes, their respective guidelines, and other revisions that might have been made. Due to our publishing deadlines and the publication date of the American Medical Association *CPT*, additional revisions and/or additional codes may have been published subsequent to the date of this printing. It is the responsibility of the reader to use this manual as a companion to the *CPT*, *ICD-10-CM*, and HCPCS publications. Vignettes are provided throughout this publication to illustrate correct coding applications. They are not intended to offer medical advice on the practice of medicine. Further, it is the reader's responsibility to access the American Academy of Pediatrics Web site (www.aap.org/cfp) routinely to find any corrections due to errata in the published version.

Copyright Acknowledgment

In Memoriam

This edition of *Coding for Pediatrics* is dedicated to the life and memory of Edward Zimmerman, former Director of the Department of Pediatrics at the American Academy of Pediatrics. He supported this work as a director and also brought his insight to the manual by contributing to the ongoing evolution of content, particularly The Business of Medicine chapter. Ed was an advocate for children and pediatricians. Those who knew him remember him as a well-dressed gentleman who also was well-read. A voracious bookworm, he often would gift books to others and urge them to "read it forward." He will be missed.

Contents

Foreword

||||||||||

The American Academy of Pediatrics (AAP) is pleased to publish this, the 23rd edition of *Coding for Pediatrics*—an instructional manual and reference tool for use by primary care pediatricians, pediatric sub-specialists, and others involved in the provision of care to children. The purpose of this manual is to support the delivery of quality care to children by providing the pediatric practitioner with the knowledge to best support appropriate business practices. Many changes have been made to this edition, including updating the 2018 *Current Procedural Terminology* (*CPT*®) codes and update of *International Classification of Diseases, 10th Revision, Clinical Modification* (*ICD-10-CM*) codes with guidelines for their application. New features are the addition of a chapter addressing telemedicine and new chapters separately addressing common surgical procedures and sedation and common testing and therapeutic services. Readers will also find several chapters reorganized and enhanced with more detail on appropriate coding and documentation. In addition, the AAP is pleased to continue to offer *Coding for Pediatrics 2018* as an eBook.

Any corrections that may be necessary subsequent to the publication of the manual will be available to readers of *Coding for Pediatrics 2018* by accessing www.aap.org/cfp. *Coding for Pediatrics 2018* does not replace *CPT*, *ICD-10-CM*, or Healthcare Common Procedure Coding System; rather, it supplements those manuals. Every effort has been made to include the 2018 codes and their respective guidelines; however, revised codes and/ or guidelines may have been published subsequent to the date of this printing. Updates to this manual will be posted as appropriate on the *Coding for Pediatrics* Web site (www.aap.org/cfp).

The AAP actively works with the American Medical Association (AMA) *CPT* Editorial Panel and the AMA/ Specialty Society Relative Value Scale Update Committee (RUC) to develop pediatric specialty codes and assign them appropriate relative value units. Since 1995, the AAP has contributed to the process that evaluates and reviews changes to the Medicare Resource-Based Relative Value Scale (RBRVS). Pediatricians have been actively involved in the AMA RUC Practice Expense Review Committee to review direct practice expenses for all existing codes. As importantly, the AAP is represented on the AMA *CPT* Editorial Advisory Panel and on the *ICD-10-CM* Editorial Advisory Board. The AAP continues to be involved in all areas of payment. The AAP Committee on Coding and Nomenclature oversees all areas of coding as they relate to pediatrics, including *CPT* procedure coding, *ICD-10-CM* diagnosis coding, and the valuation of *CPT* services through the Medicare RBRVS.

The AAP will continue to request new code changes and attempt to expeditiously notify membership of changes through various means. *AAP Pediatric Coding Newsletter*™—a monthly newsletter available in print and online—provides members and their office personnel with up-to-date coding and payment information. The newsletter and other online resources can be accessed through the AAP newsletter Web site (http://coding. aap.org). Other resources include coding seminars presented at the AAP National Conference & Exhibition; webinars sponsored by the AAP (www.aap.org/webinars/coding); instructional materials in *AAP News*, including the Coding Corner; *Pediatric ICD-10-CM: A Manual for Provider-Based Coding*; and various quick reference cards. The use of these resources should provide the membership with the skills needed to report their services appropriately. The Division of Health Care Finance at the AAP headquarters stands ready to assist with problem areas not adequately covered in this manual. The AAP Coding Hotline can be accessed through e-mail at aapcodinghotline@aap.org.

Acknowledgments

||||||||||

Coding for Pediatrics, 23rd Edition, is the product of the efforts of many dedicated individuals. My work has been made immeasurably easier and the final edition dramatically improved by the dedicated work of my collaborators. First and foremost, I must thank Cindy Hughes, CPC, CFPC, consulting editor, for her professional input. Additionally, I must thank the Committee on Coding and Nomenclature (COCN) support staff at the American Academy of Pediatrics (AAP), particularly Becky Dolan, MPH, CPC, CPEDC, staff editor, for her many excellent suggestions as well as for reviewing major portions of the project. Thank you also to Teri Salus, MPA, CPC, CPEDC, for her review of new *Current Procedural Terminology* (*CPT*®) codes and suggestions for changes to content. I would also like to thank the members of COCN and the AAP Coding Publications Editorial Advisory Board. The members of these committees have each contributed extensive time in reviewing and updating content of the manual. We want to especially thank the following reviewers:

Jamie Calabrese, MD, CPC, FAAP

David M. Kanter, MD, MBA, CPC, FAAP

Steven E. Krug, MD, FAAP

Jeffrey F. Linzer Sr, MD, FAAP

Jeanne Marconi, MD, FAAP

Linda Parsi, MD, MBA, CPEDC, CMOM, CMC, FAAP

Renee F. Slade, MD, FAAP

Sanjeev Y. Tuli, MD, FAAP

I would like to particularly acknowledge those current and past COCN members who have devoted their time and expertise to providing a breadth of knowledge not otherwise possible: Lynn Wegner, MD, FAAP, former COCN member and advocate for developmental and behavioral health issues; Margie C. Andreae, MD, AAP representative to the American Medical Association/Specialty Society Relative Value Scale Update Committee (RUC); Eileen D. Brewer, MD, AAP alternate RUC representative; Steven E. Krug, MD, AAP RUC advisor; Joel F. Bradley, MD, AAP *CPT* advisor and former *CPT* Editorial Panel member; David M. Kanter, MD, MBA, CPC, AAP alternate *CPT* advisor; Julia M. Pillsbury, DO, *CPT* Editorial Panel member; Jeffrey F. Linzer Sr, MD, AAP *International Classification of Diseases, 10th Revision, Clinical Modification* Editorial Advisory Board representative and *ICD-11* Pediatrics Topic Advisory Group chairperson; and Richard A. Molteni, MD, COCN chair, former AAP *CPT* advisor, and former *CPT* Editorial Panel member.

I am most grateful to the invaluable input of the following AAP committees and individuals: the Committee on Medical Liability and Risk Management, specifically James P. Scibilia, MD, FAAP, and AAP staff Julie Ake, senior health policy analyst; the Private Payer Advocacy Advisory Committee, specifically Sue Kressly, MD, FAAP, and AAP staff Lou Terranova, senior health policy analyst; Samuel D. Smith, MD, liaison for the American Pediatric Surgical Association; the Section on Telehealth Care, specifically Peter Dehnel, MD, FAAP; and the Section on Neonatal-Perinatal Medicine coding trainers.

This project would not have been completed were it not for the outstanding work of AAP staff. In the departments of Publishing and Membership Engagement, Marketing, and Sales, Barrett Winston, senior editor, professional/clinical publishing; Jason Crase, manager, editorial services; Peg Mulcahy, manager, art direction and production; Leesa Levin-Doroba, production manager, practice management; and Mary Jo Reynolds, marketing manager, practice publications, deserve special recognition for their outstanding skill and dedication to this project. In the Division of Health Care Finance, I am especially appreciative of the support and professional expertise of Linda Walsh, MAB, division director, and AAP staff support to the AAP COCN, dedicated advocates for all of us who provide medical care to children.

Edward A. Liechty, MD
Editor

New and Revised *CPT®* Codes for 2018

Contents

Chapter 1: New and Revised *CPT*® Codes for 2018

Current Procedural Terminology (*CPT*®) is published annually by the American Medical Association. It is used by national carriers and is designated as the official procedure code set under the Health Insurance Portability and Accountability Act of 1996. *Current Procedural Terminology* codes are known as Level I codes of the broader-based Healthcare Common Procedure Coding System, termed HCPCS. The HCPCS coding system includes Level I codes (*CPT-4*), Level II codes (Centers for Medicare & Medicaid Services national codes), and Level III codes (local codes assigned and used by Medicare carriers).

    Current Procedural Terminology Category I codes are updated annually. New or revised codes are effective on January 1 of each year. The symbols on page 4 are used to assist physicians in recognizing the annual revisions made in *CPT*. Exceptions are the vaccine product and Category III (emerging technology) codes, which are updated twice annually (January and July) and, in the case of vaccine products, may be released earlier when specific criteria for rapid release are met.

    Current Procedural Terminology includes specific guidelines that are located at the beginning of each section and throughout the *CPT* manual. Always read the applicable instructions and guidelines before selecting a code.

New, Revised, and Deleted *CPT* Codes for 2018

The following new codes, revisions, and code deletions are effective with services provided on or after January 1, 2018. We have made every effort to include those procedures and services that are applicable to pediatric practices. However, revisions and/or additional codes may have been published subsequent to the date of this printing. This list does not include all changes made to *CPT 2018*. Please note that in the interest of efficiency, we will follow the established format of the *CPT* Editorial Panel meeting minutes; therefore, sections without any revisions will include only the first few italicized words of the section followed by an ellipsis (eg, *In the instance where a physician is on call…*). This represents the sections that were unchanged in the *CPT 2018* manual to more easily direct you toward the revised text within the guidelines. Always refer to *CPT 2018* for a complete listing of new codes, complete descriptions, and revisions.

    New text is underlined, deleted text is indicated with a ~~strikethrough~~, new codes are identified with the bullet (●) symbol, and revised codes are identified with the triangle (▲) symbol.

    A few of the changes presented in this chapter include

- Revisions to the prefatory instructions for critical care services instruct that physicians of the same or different group practice but different specialty from a physician reporting neonatal or pediatric critical care may report hourly critical care services (**99291, 99292**).
- New codes **99492–99494** describe psychiatric collaborative care management (PCCM) services provided under the supervision of a treating physician or other qualified health care professional by a behavioral care manager and in collaboration with a psychiatric consultant, and code **99484**, for general behavioral health integration care management services, is reported for models of integrated behavioral health care management other than PCCM.
- 2017 codes for view-specific radiographs of the chest and abdomen are deleted and replaced with new codes that are reported based on the number of views obtained.
- Code **94620** (simple pulmonary stress testing) is deleted and new codes **94617** (exercise test for bronchospasm) and **94618** (pulmonary stress testing) are added. Code **94621** (complex cardiopulmonary exercise testing) is revised to include measurement of minute ventilation.

Symbols	Description
●	A bullet at the beginning of a code means the code is a new code for the current year. For example, ●**71045** Radiologic examination, chest; single view
▲	A triangle means the code descriptor has been revised. For example, ▲**38220** <u>Diagnostic</u> bone marrow; aspiration(<u>s</u>) only Within revised codes, the deleted language appears with a ~~strikethrough~~, while new text appears <u>underlined.</u>
✚	A plus sign means the code is an add-on code. For example, ●✚**99494** **Initial or subsequent psychiatric collaborative care management,** each additional 30 minutes in a calendar month of behavioral health care manager activities, in consultation with a psychiatric consultant, and directed by the treating physician or other qualified health care professional (List separately in addition to code for primary procedure)
Ø	A null sign means the code is a "modifier **51** exempt" code and, therefore, does not require modifier **51** (multiple procedures) even when reported with other procedures. For example, Ø**31500** Intubation, endotracheal, emergency procedure
►◄	Arrows enclose new or revised text in the current edition of *CPT.* For example, ►<u>For Psychiatric Collaborative Care Management Services, see 99492, 99493, 99494.</u>◄
⚡	The lightning bolt identifies codes for vaccines that are pending US Food and Drug Administration approval. For example, ⚡**90587** Dengue vaccine, quadrivalent, live, 3 dose schedule, for subcutaneous use
#	The pound symbol is used to identify re-sequenced codes that are out of numerical sequence. This allows related codes to be placed in an appropriate location, making it easier to locate a procedure or service.
O	The **O** symbol precedes codes that are recycled or reinstated.
★	A star means the service represented by the code is included in Appendix P as a code to which modifier **95** may be appended to indicate the service was rendered via real-time telemedicine services.

Category I
Evaluation and Management

Observation Care Discharge Services

▲**99217**   Observation care discharge day management (This code is to be utilized to report all services provided to a patient on discharge from <u>outpatient hospital</u> "observation status" if the discharge is on other than the initial date of "observation status." To report services to a patient designated as "observation status" or "inpatient status" and discharged on the same date, use the codes for Observation or Inpatient Care Services [including Admission and Discharge Services, **99234–99236** as appropriate].)

Initial Observation Care

New or Established Patient Guidelines

►The following codes are used to report the encounter(s) by the supervising physician or other qualified health care professional with the patient when designated as <u>outpatient hospital</u> "observation status." This refers to the initiation of observation status…◄

▲99218   Initial observation care, per day, for the evaluation and management of a patient which requires these 3 key components:

- A detailed or comprehensive history;
- A detailed or comprehensive examination; and
- Medical decision making that is straightforward or of low complexity.

Counseling and/or coordination of care with other physicians, other qualified health care professionals, or agencies are provided consistent with the nature of the problem(s) and the patient's and/or family's needs.

Usually, the problem(s) requiring admission to <u>outpatient hospital</u> "observation status" are of low severity. Typically, 30 minutes are spent at the bedside and on the patient's hospital floor or unit.

▲99219   Initial observation care, per day, for the evaluation and management of a patient, which requires these 3 key components:

- A comprehensive history;
- A comprehensive examination; and
- Medical decision making of moderate complexity.

Counseling and/or coordination of care with other physicians, other qualified health care professionals, or agencies are provided consistent with the nature of the problem(s) and the patient's and/or family's needs.

Usually, the problem(s) requiring admission to <u>outpatient hospital</u> "observation status" are of moderate severity. Typically, 50 minutes are spent at the bedside and on the patient's hospital floor or unit.

▲99220   Initial observation care, per day, for the evaluation and management of a patient, which requires these 3 key components:

- A comprehensive history;
- A comprehensive examination; and
- Medical decision-making of high complexity.

Counseling and/or coordination of care with other physicians, other qualified health care professionals, or agencies are provided consistent with the nature of the problem(s) and the patient's and/or family's needs.

Usually, the problem(s) requiring admission to <u>outpatient hospital</u> "observation status" are of high severity. Typically, 70 minutes are spent at the bedside and on the patient's hospital floor or unit.

Domiciliary, Rest Home (eg, Boarding Home), or Custodial Care Services

▶The following codes are used to report evaluation and management services in a facility which provides room, board, and other personal assistance services, generally on a long-term basis. <u>These codes include</u> ~~Also used to report~~ evaluation and management services <u>provided</u> in an assisted living facility<u>, group home, custodial care, and intermediate care facilities</u>. The facility's services do not include a medical component.

99324   *Domiciliary or rest home visit for the evaluation and management of a new patient, which requires these 3 key components:...*◀

Critical Care Services

The prefatory text for critical care services is affected by changes to the codes for radiologic examination of the chest. New codes for single view **71045** and **71046** are bundled into critical care in 2018. See new codes under the Radiology section later in this chapter for radiologic examination of the chest.

Critical Care Services

Critical care is the direct delivery by a physician(s) or...
Providing medical care to a critically ill...
Inpatient critical care services provided to infants 29 days...
Services for a patient who is not critically ill...
Critical care and other E/M services may be provided...

▶*For reporting by professionals, the following services are included in critical care when performed during the critical period by the physician(s) providing critical care: the interpretation of cardiac output measurements (*93561*, *93562*), chest X-rays (*71010, 71015, 71020 71045, 71046*), pulse oximetry…*◀

Coding Tip

Services Included in Critical Care Services
▶*For reporting by professionals, the following services are included in critical care when performed during the critical period by the physician(s) providing critical care: the interpretation of cardiac output measurements (93561, 93562), chest X-rays (71010, 71015, 71020 71045, 71046), pulse oximetry…. Facilities may report the above services separately.*◀

Inpatient Neonatal Intensive Care Services and Pediatric and Neonatal Critical Care Services

Pediatric Critical Care Patient Transport

Codes **99466**, **99467** *are used to report the…*
Codes **99485**, **99486** *are used…*
For the definition of the critically…
The non-face-to-face direction of emergency…
*Emergency department services (***99281–99285***), initial…*
▶*The following services are included when performed during the pediatric patient transport by the physician providing critical care and may not be reported separately: routine monitoring evaluations (eg, heart rate, respiratory rate, blood pressure, and pulse oximetry), the interpretation of cardiac output measurements (***93562***), chest X-rays (***71010, 71015, 71020 71045, 71046***), pulse oximetry…*◀

Changes were also made to the prefatory text for inpatient neonatal and pediatric critical care to emphasize that time-based evaluation and management (E/M) services may be reported by an individual of a different specialty on the same date that another physician or qualified health care professional (QHP) reports neonatal or pediatric critical care services.

Inpatient Neonatal and Pediatric Critical Care

The same definitions for critical care services apply for the adult, child, and neonate.
Codes **99468**, **99469** *are used to report…*
The initial day neonatal critical care code…
When a neonate, infant, or child requires…
▶*Time-based critical care services (***99291***, ***99292***) are not reportable by the same individual or different individual within of the* <u>same specialty and same</u> *group when neonatal or pediatric critical care services (***99468–99476***) may be reported for the same patient on the same day.* <u>Time-based critical care services (</u>**99291, 99292**<u>) may be reported by an individual of a different specialty from either the same or different group on the same day that neonatal or pediatric critical care services are reported. Critical care interfacility transport face-to-face (</u>**99466, 99467**<u>) or supervisory (</u>**99485, 99486**<u>) services may be reported by the same or different individual of the same specialty and same group when neonatal or pediatric critical care services (</u>**99468–99476**<u>) are reported for the same patient on the same day.</u>◀

Psychiatric Collaborative Care Management Services

<u>Psychiatric collaborative care services are provided under the direction of a treating physician or other qualified health care professional (see definitions below) during a calendar month. These services are provided when a patient has a diagnosed psychiatric disorder that requires a behavioral health care assessment; establishing, implementing, revising, or monitoring a care plan; and provision of brief interventions. These services are reported by the treating physician or other qualified health care professional and include the services of the treating physician or other qualified health care professional, the behavioral health care manager (see definition below), and the psychiatric consultant (see definition below) who has contracted directly with the treating physician or other qualified health care professional, to provide consultation.</u>

Patients directed to the behavioral health care manager typically have newly diagnosed conditions, may need help in engaging in treatment, have not responded to standard care delivered in a non-psychiatric setting, or require further assessment and engagement, prior to consideration of referral to a psychiatric care setting.

The following definitions apply to this section:

Episode of Care

Patients are treated for an episode of care, defined as beginning when the patient is directed by the treating physician or other qualified health care professional to the behavioral health care manager and ending with:

* the attainment of targeted treatment goals, which typically results in the discontinuation of care management services and continuation of usual follow-up with the treating physician or other qualified healthcare professional; or
* failure to attain targeted treatment goals culminating in referral to a psychiatric care provider for ongoing treatment; or
* lack of continued engagement with no psychiatric collaborative care management services provided over a consecutive six month calendar period (break in episode).

A new episode of care starts after a break in episode of six calendar months or more.

Health Care Professionals

Treating Physician or Other Qualified Health Care Professional

The treating physician or other qualified health care professional directs the behavioral health care manager and continues to oversee the patient's care, including prescribing medications, providing treatments for medical conditions, and making referrals to specialty care when needed. Evaluation and management (E/M) and other services may be reported separately by the same physician or other qualified health care professional during the same calendar month.

Behavioral Health Care Manager

The behavioral health care manager refers to clinical staff with a masters/doctoral-level education or specialized training in behavioral health who provides care management services as well as an assessment of needs, including the administration of validated rating scales, the development of a care plan, provision of brief interventions, ongoing collaboration with the treating physician or qualified health care professional, maintenance of a registry, all in consultation with a psychiatric consultant. Services are provided both face-to-face and non face-to-face and psychiatric consultation is provided minimally on a weekly basis, typically non face-to-face.

The behavioral health care manager providing other services in the same calendar month, such as psychiatric evaluation (**90791, 90792**), psychotherapy (**90832, 90833, 90834, 90836, 90837, 90838**), psychotherapy for crisis (**90839, 90840**), family psychotherapy (**90846, 90847**), multiple family group psychotherapy (**90849**), group psychotherapy (**90853**), smoking and tobacco use cessation counseling (**99406, 90407**), and alcohol and/or substance abuse structured screening and brief intervention services (**99408, 99409**), may report these services separately. Activities for services reported separately are not included in the time applied to **99492, 99493, 99494**.

Psychiatric Consultant

The psychiatric consultant refers to a medical professional trained in psychiatry or behavioral health and qualified to prescribe the full range of medications. The psychiatric consultant advises and makes recommendations, as needed, for psychiatric and other medical care, including psychiatric and other medical differential diagnosis, treatment strategies regarding appropriate therapies, medication management, medical management of complications associated with treatment of psychiatric disorders, and referral for specialty services; which are communicated to the treating physician or other qualified health care professional typically through the behavioral health care manager. The psychiatric consultant does not typically see the patient nor prescribe medications, except in rare circumstances.

The psychiatric consultant may provide services in the calendar month described by other codes, such as evaluation and management (E/M) services and psychiatric evaluation (**90791, 90792**). These services may be reported separately by the psychiatric consultant. Activities for services reported separately are not included in the services reported using **99492, 99493, 99494**.

Chapter 1: New and Revised *CPT*® Codes for 2018

Code Selection

Do not report **99492** and **99493** in the same calendar month.

Selection of Psychiatric Collaborative Care Management Codes

Type of Service	Total Duration of Collaborative Care Management Over Calendar Month	Code(s)
	Less than 36 minutes	Not reported separately
Initial – 70 minutes	36-85 minutes (36 minutes – 1 hr. 25 minutes)	**99492**
Initial plus each additional increment up to 30 minutes	86-116 minutes (1 hr. 26 minutes – 1 hr. 54 minutes)	**99492 X 1 AND 99494 X 1**
	Less than 31 minutes	Not reported separately
Subsequent – 60 minutes	31-75 minutes (31 minutes – 1 hr. 15 minutes)	**99493**
Subsequent plus each additional increment up to 30 minutes	76-105 minutes (1 hr. 16 minutes – 1 hr. 45 minutes)	**99493 X 1 AND 99494 X 1**

●**99492**   **Initial psychiatric collaborative care management**, first 70 minutes in the first calendar month of behavioral health care manager activities, in consultation with a psychiatric consultant, and directed by the treating physician or other qualified health care professional, with the following required elements:
   ⦿ outreach to and engagement in treatment of a patient directed by the treating physician or other qualified health care professional;
   ⦿ initial assessment of the patient, including administration of validated rating scales, with the development of an individualized treatment plan;
   ⦿ review by the psychiatric consultant with modifications of the plan if recommended;
   ⦿ entering patient in a registry and tracking patient follow-up and progress using the registry, with appropriate documentation, and participation in weekly caseload consultation with the psychiatric consultant; and
   ⦿ provision of brief interventions using evidence-based techniques such as behavioral activation, motivational interviewing, and other focused treatment strategies.

●**99493**   **Subsequent psychiatric collaborative care management**, first 60 minutes in a subsequent month of behavioral health care manager activities, in consultation with a psychiatric consultant, and directed by the treating physician or other qualified health care professional, with the following required elements:
   ⦿ tracking patient follow-up and progress using the registry, with appropriate documentation;
   ⦿ participation in weekly caseload consultation with the psychiatric consultant;
   ⦿ ongoing collaboration with and coordination of the patient's mental health care with the treating physician or other qualified health care professional and any other treating mental health providers;
   ⦿ additional review of progress and recommendations for changes in treatment, as indicated, including medications, based on recommendations provided by the psychiatric consultant;
   ⦿ provision of brief interventions using evidence-based techniques such as behavioral activation, motivational interviewing, and other focused treatment strategies;
   ⦿ monitoring of patient outcomes using validated rating scales; and
   ⦿ relapse prevention planning with patients as they achieve remission of symptoms and/or other treatment goals and are prepared for discharge from active treatment.

●+**99494**   **Initial or subsequent psychiatric collaborative care management,** each additional 30 minutes in a calendar month of behavioral health care manager activities, in consultation with a psychiatric consultant, and directed by the treating physician or other qualified health care professional (List separately in addition to code for primary procedure)
(Use **99494** in conjunction with **99492, 99493**)

Coding Tip

If the treating physician or other qualified health care professional personally performs behavioral health care manager activities and those activities are not used to meet criteria for a separately reported code, his or her time may be counted toward the required behavioral health care manager time to meet the elements of codes **99492, 99493, 99494.**

Behavioral health care manager time spent coordinating care with the emergency department may be reported using **99492, 99493, 99494,** but time while the patient is inpatient or admitted to observation status may not be reported using **99492, 99493, 99494.**

General Behavioral Health Integration Care Management

General Behavioral Health Integration Care Management services **99484** are reported by the supervising physician or other qualified health care professional. The services are performed by clinical staff for a patient with a behavioral health (including substance use) condition that requires care management services (face-to-face or non face-to-face) of 20 or more minutes in a calendar month. A treatment plan is required as well as the specified elements of the service description. The assessment and treatment plan is not required to be comprehensive and the office/practice is not required to have all the functions of chronic care management (**99487, 99489, 99490**). **99484** may be used in any outpatient setting, as long as the reporting professional has an ongoing relationship with the patient and clinical staff and as long as the clinical staff is available for face-to-face services with the patient. The reporting professional must be able to perform the Evaluation and Management (E/M) services of an initiating visit. General behavioral integration care management (**99484**) and chronic care management services may be reported by the same professional in the same month as long as distinct care management services are performed. Behavioral health integration care management (**99484**) and psychiatric collaborative care management (**99492, 99493, 99494**) may not be reported by the same professional in the same month. Behavioral health care integration clinical staff are not required to have qualifications that would permit them to separately report services (eg, psychotherapy), but, if qualified and they perform such services, they may report such services separately, as long as the time of the service is not used in reporting **99484.**

●**99484**   Care management services for behavioral health conditions, at least 20 minutes of clinical staff time, directed by a physician or other qualified health care professional, per calendar month, with the following required elements:
  ❖ Initial assessment or follow-up monitoring, including the use of applicable validated rating scales;
  ❖ Behavioral health care planning in relation to behavioral/psychiatric health problems, including revision for patients who are not progressing or whose status changes;
  ❖ Facilitating and coordinating treatment such as psychotherapy, pharmacotherapy, counseling and/or psychiatric consultation; and
  ❖ Continuity of care with a designated member of the care team
  (Do not use **99484** in conjunction with **99492, 99493, 99494** in the same calendar month)

▶(E/M services, including care management services [**99487, 99489, 99490, 99495, 99496**], and psychiatric services [**90785–90899**] may be reported separately by the same physician or other qualified health care professional on the same day or during the same calendar month, but activities used to meet criteria for another reported service do not count toward meeting criteria for **99484**).◀

Coding Tip

If the treating physician or other qualified health care professional personally performs behavioral health care manager activities and those activities are not used to meet criteria for a separately reported code, his or her time may be counted toward the required behavioral health care manager time to meet the elements of **99484, 99492, 99493, 99494.**

Behavioral health care manager time spent coordinating care with the emergency department may be reported using **99484, 99492, 99493, 99494,** but time while the patient is inpatient or admitted to observation status may not be reported using **99484, 99492, 99493, 99494.**

Clinical staff time spent coordinating care with the emergency department may be reported using **99484,** but time while the patient is inpatient or admitted to observation status may not be reported using **99484.**

Surgery

The code for chemical cauterization of granulation tissue is revised to remove reference to sinus or fistula and to direct that use of chemical cauterization to achieve wound hemostasis is not reported with code **17250.** Cauterization to achieve hemostasis is included in the code for wound care, excision, or repair.

Integumentary System

Destruction, Benign or Premalignant Lesions

▲17250   Chemical cauterization of granulation tissue (ie, proud flesh, sinus or fistula)
(Do not report **17250** is not to be used with removal or excision codes for the same lesion)
(Do not report **17250** when chemical cauterization is used to achieve wound hemostasis)
(Do not report **17250** in conjunction with active wound care management **97597, 97598, 97602** for the same lesion)

Medicine

Physical Medicine and Rehabilitation

Active Wound Care Management
Active wound care procedures are performed to remove devitalized and/or necrotic tissue and promote healing. Chemical cauterization (**17250**) to achieve wound hemostasis is included in active wound care procedures (**97597, 97598, 97602**) and should not be separately reported for the same lesion. Services require direct (one-on-one) contact with the patient.

Digestive System

A new parenthetic instruction follows code **44300** to prohibit reporting of this code when tube placement is for intraoperative colonic lavage. In addition, the instruction below code **44701** (intraoperative colonic lavage) is revised to allow reporting of codes **44300** and **44701** except in instances when the tube placement is for intraoperative colonic lavage.

Intestines (Except Rectum)

Enterostomy—External Fistulization of Intestines
44300   Placement, enterostomy or cecostomy, tube open (eg, for feeding or decompression) (separate procedure)
(Do not report **44300** in conjunction with **44701** for cannulation of the colon for intraoperative colonic lavage)
(*For percutaneous placement of duodenostomy, jejunostomy, gastro-jejunostomy or cecostomy [or other colonic] tube including fluoroscopic imaging guidance, see* **49441–49442**)

Other Procedures

+44701   Intraoperative colonic lavage (List separately in addition to code for primary procedure)
(*Use* **44701** *in conjunction with* **44140, 44145, 44150,** *or* **44604** *as appropriate*)
(Do not report **44701** in conjunction with **44300, 44950–44960**)

Musculoskeletal System

Codes **38220** and **38221** (bone marrow aspiration and biopsy) are revised in 2018 to clarify that they represent diagnostic services. In addition, new code **38222** is added for reporting biopsy and aspiration at the same encounter. Parenthetic instructions are revised and/or added following all codes for diagnostic and therapeutic biopsy or aspiration to direct to appropriate codes for each.

General

Excision

20150   *Excision of epiphyseal bar, with or without autogenous soft tissue graft obtained through same fascial incision*

~~(For aspiration of bone marrow, use 38220)~~

20220   *Biopsy, bone, trocar, or needle; superficial (eg, ilium, sternum, spinous process, ribs)*

20225   *deep (eg, vertebral body, femur)*

(*Do not report* **20225** *in conjunction with* **22510, 22511, 22512, 22513, 22514, 22515, 0200T, 0201T** *when performed at the same level*)

(For bone marrow biopsy(ies) and/or aspiration(s), ~~use~~ see **38220, 38221**, **38222**)

(*For radiologic supervision and interpretation, see* **77002, 77012, 77021**)

Grafts (or Implants)

Codes for obtaining autogenous bone, cartilage, tendon, fascia lata grafts, <u>bone marrow</u> or other tissues through separate skin/fascial incisions should be reported separately unless the code descriptor references the harvesting of the graft or implant (eg, includes obtaining graft).

+20936   *Autograft for spine surgery only (includes harvesting the graft); local (eg, ribs, spinous process, or laminar fragments) obtained from same incision (List separately in addition to code for primary procedure)*

+20938   *structural, bicortical or tricortical (through separate skin or fascial incision) (List separately in addition to code for primary procedure)*

(*Use* **20938** *in conjunction with* **22319, 22532, 22533, 22548–22558, 22590–22612, 22630, 22633, 22634, 22800–22812**)

~~(For needle aspiration of bone marrow for the purpose of bone grafting, use 38220–20999. Do not report 38220–38230 for bone marrow aspiration for platelet rich stem cell injection. For bone marrow aspiration for platelet rich stem cell injection, use 0232T)~~

<u>(For aspiration of bone marrow for bone grafting, spine surgery only, use **20939**)</u>

●**+20939**   Bone marrow aspiration for bone grafting, spine surgery only, through separate skin or fascial incision (List separately in addition to code for primary procedure)

<u>(Use **20939** in conjunction with **22319, 22532, 22533, 22534, 22548, 22551, 22552, 22554, 22556, 22558, 22590, 22595, 22600, 22610, 22612, 22630, 22633, 22634, 22800, 22802, 22804, 22808, 22810, 22812**)</u>

<u>(For bilateral procedure, use **20939** with modifier **50**)</u>

<u>(For diagnostic bone marrow aspiration(s), see **38220, 38222**)</u>

<u>(For aspiration of bone marrow for the purpose of bone grafting other than spine surgery and other therapeutic musculoskeletal applications, use **20999**)</u>

<u>(For bone marrow aspiration(s) for platelet rich stem cell injection, use **0232T**)</u>

Hemic and Lymphatic Systems

General

Bone Marrow or Stem Cell Services/Procedures

▲**38220**   <u>Diagnostic B</u>bone marrow; aspiration<u>(s)</u> only

~~(For needle aspiration of bone marrow for the purpose of bone grafting, use 38220)~~

<u>(Do not report **38220** in conjunction with **38221**)</u>

<u>(For diagnostic bone marrow biopsy(ies) and aspiration(s) performed at the same session, use **38222**)</u>

(Do not report 38220–38230 for bone marrow aspiration for platelet rich stem cell injection or for therapeutic musculoskeletal applications. For bone marrow aspiration(s) for platelet rich stem cell injection, use 0232T.)

(For aspiration of bone marrow for bone graft, spine surgery only, use 20939)

(For bone marrow aspiration(s) for platelet rich stem cell injection, use 0232T)

▲38221   biopsy(ies), needle or trocar

(Do not report 38221 in conjunction with 38220)

(For diagnostic bone marrow biopsy(ies) and aspiration(s) performed at the same session, use 38222)

(For bone marrow biopsy interpretation, use 88305)

●38222   biopsy(ies) and aspiration(s)

(Do not report 38222 in conjunction with 38220 and 38221)

(For bilateral procedure, report 38220, 38221, 38222 with modifier 50)

(For bone marrow biopsy interpretation, use 88305)

38230   *Bone marrow harvesting for transplantation; allogeneic*

38232   *autologous*

(For autologous and allogeneic blood-derived peripheral stem cell harvesting for transplantation, see 38205,–38206)

(For diagnostic bone marrow aspiration(s), use see 38220, 38222)

(For aspiration of bone marrow for bone graft, spine surgery only, use 20939)

(For bone marrow aspiration(s) for platelet rich stem cell injection, use 0232T.)

Transplantation and Post-Transplantation Cellular Infusions

38242   *Allogeneic lymphocyte infusions*

(For diagnostic bone marrow aspiration(s), use see 38220, 38222)

(For aspiration of bone marrow for bone graft, spine surgery only, use 20939)

(For bone marrow aspiration(s) for platelet rich stem cell injection, use 0232T.)

Radiology

Nine codes for reporting chest radiographs have been deleted and replaced with 4 new codes that specify only the number of views. In addition, cross-references in other sections of *CPT* have been updated to reflect the new codes. Also deleted are codes for view-specific abdominal radiographs, with 3 new codes specifying the number of views.

Diagnostic Radiology (Diagnostic Imaging)

Chest

71010   Radiologic examination, chest; single view, frontal

(71010 has been deleted. To report, use 71045)

71015   stereo, frontal

(71015 has been deleted. To report, use 71045)

71020   Radiologic examination, chest, 2 views, frontal and lateral;

(71020 has been deleted. To report, use 71046)

71021   with apical lordotic procedure

(71021 has been deleted. To report, use 71047)

71022   with oblique projections

(71022 has been deleted. To report, see 71047, 71048)

71023   with fluoroscopy

(71023 has been deleted. To report, see 71046, 76000, 76001)

71030   Radiologic examination, chest, complete, minimum of 4 views;

(71030 has been deleted. To report, use 71048)

71034   with fluoroscopy

(**71034** has been deleted. To report, see **71048, 76000, 76001**)

(For separate chest fluoroscopy, use 76000)

71035   Radiologic examination, chest, special views (eg, lateral decubitus, Bucky studies)

(**71035** has been deleted. To report, see **71046, 71047, 71048**)

▲76000   Fluoroscopy (separate procedure), up to 1 hour physician or other qualified health care professional time, other than 71023 or 71034 **71048** (eg, cardiac fluoroscopy)

●71045   Radiologic examination, chest; single view

●71046   2 views

●71047   3 views

●71048   4 or more views

(For acute abdomen series that includes a single view of the chest and one or more views of the abdomen, see **74022**)

(For concurrent computer-aided detection [CAD] performed in addition to codes **71045, 71046, 71047, 71048**, use **0174T**. Do not report **71045, 71046, 71047, 71048** in conjunction with **0175T** for CAD performed remotely from the primary interpretation)

Abdomen

74000   Radiologic examination, abdomen; single anteroposterior views

(**74000** has been deleted. To report, use **74018**)

74010   anteroposterior and additional oblique and cone views

(**74010** has been deleted. To report, see **74019, 74021**)

74020   complete, including decubitus and/or erect views

(**74020** has been deleted. To report, see **74019, 74021**)

●74018   Radiologic examination, abdomen; 1 view

●74019   2 views

●74021   3 or more views

74022   *complete acute abdomen series, including supine, erect, and/or decubitus views, single view chest*

Gynecological and Obstetrical

(For abdomen and pelvis, see **72170–72190, 74000–74019, 74021, 74022, 74150, 74160, 74170**)

74710   *Pelvimetry, with or without placental localization*

Category III

+0174T   *Computer-aided detection (CAD) (computer algorithm analysis of digital image data for lesion detection) with further physician review for interpretation and report, with or without digitization of film radiographic images, chest radiograph(s), performed concurrent with primary interpretation (List separately in addition to code for primary procedure)*

▶(Use **0174T** in conjunction with 71010, 71020, 71021, 71022, 71030 **71045, 71046, 71047, 71048**)◀

0175T   *Computer-aided detection (CAD) (computer algorithm analysis of digital image data for lesion detection) with further physician review for interpretation and report, with or without digitization of film radiographic images, chest radiograph(s), performed remote from primary interpretation*

▶(Do not report **0175T** in conjunction with 71010, 71020, 71021, 71022, 71030 **71045, 71046, 71047, 71048**)◀

Pathology and Laboratory

Two new codes (**86794** and **87662**) are added to identify exposure to Zika virus. Codes are selected based on time since exposure—if immediately following potential exposure (less than 2 weeks: **87662**) and for individuals with antibodies to the virus (2 weeks or more: **86794**).

A new code (**87634**) is added for reporting nucleic acid detection of respiratory syncytial virus.

Immunology

86710   *Antibody; influenza virus*

86793   *Yersinia*

●86794   Zika virus, IgM

Microbiology

87633   *Infectious agent detection by nucleic acid (DNA or RNA); respiratory virus (eg, adenovirus, influenza virus, coronavirus, metapneumovirus, parainfluenza virus, respiratory syncytial virus, rhinovirus), includes multiplex reverse transcription, when performed, and multiplex amplified probe technique, multiple types or subtypes, 12-25 targets*

●**87634**   Infectious agent detection by nucleic acid (DNA or RNA); respiratory syncytial virus, amplified probe technique

(For assays that include respiratory syncytial virus with additional respiratory viruses, see **87631, 87632, 87633**)

87660   *Trichomonas vaginalis, direct probe technique*

●**87662**   Zika virus, amplified probe technique

Medicine

Pulmonary

Pulmonary Diagnostic Testing and Therapies

94060   *Bronchodilation responsiveness, spirometry as in* **94010**, *pre- and post-bronchodilator administration*

(Do not report **94060** in conjunction with **94150, 94200, 94375, 94640, 94728**)

(Report bronchodilator supply separately with **99070** or appropriate supply code)

▶(For ~~prolonged~~ exercise test for bronchospasm with pre- and post-spirometry, use ~~94620~~94617)◀

94250   *Expired gas collection, quantitative, single procedure (separate procedure)*

▶(Do not report **94250** in conjunction with **94621**)◀

●**94617**   Exercise test for bronchospasm, including pre- and post-spirometry, electrocardiographic recording(s), and pulse oximetry

94620   ~~Pulmonary stress testing; simple (eg, 6-minute walk test, prolonged exercise test for bronchospasm with pre- and post-spirometry and oximetry)~~

(**94620** has been deleted. To report pulmonary stress testing, use **94618**)

●**94618**   Pulmonary stress testing (eg, 6-minute walk test), including measurement of heart rate, oximetry and oxygen titration, when performed

▲**94621**   Cardiopulmonary exercise testing, complex (including measurements of minute ventilation, CO_2 production, O_2 uptake, and electrocardiographic recordings)

▶Do not report **94617, 94621** in conjunction with **93000, 93005, 93010, 93040, 93041, 93042** for ECG monitoring performed during the same session◀

(Do not report **94621** in conjunction with **94250, 94680, 94681** and **94690**)

(Do not report **94617, 94618, 94621** in conjunction with **94760, 94761**)

94760   *Noninvasive ear or pulse oximetry for oxygen saturation; single determination*

(For blood gases, see **82803–82810**)

94761   *multiple determinations (eg, during exercise)*

(Do not report **94760, 94761** in conjunction with **94617, 94618, 94621**)

94680   *Oxygen uptake, expired gas analysis; rest and exercise, direct, simple*

94681   *including CO_2 output, percentage oxygen extracted*

94690   *rest, indirect (separate procedure)*

(For single arterial puncture, use **36600**)

(Do not report **94680, 94681, 94690** in conjunction with **94621**)

Vaccines, Toxoids

The following codes were effective on January 1, 2017, and are included in *CPT*® 2018. Code **90682** was previously published to the American Medical Association (AMA) *CPT* Category I Vaccine Web page (https://www.ama-assn.org/practice-management/cpt-category-i-vaccine-codes) with the lightning bolt symbol (⚡) indicating that approval by the US Food and Drug Administration (FDA) was pending. Approval was granted by the FDA in October 2016, so the lightning bolt symbol is no longer applied.

●90682　Influenza virus vaccine, quadrivalent (RIV4), derived from recombinant DNA, hemagglutinin (HA) protein only, preservative and antibiotic free, for intramuscular use

The following code changes were effective on July 1, 2017, following publication to the AMA *CPT* Category I Vaccine Web page on January 1, 2017. These codes are included in *CPT 2018*. Codes **90621** and **90651** are revised due to addition of a 2-dose schedule for vaccines described by these codes.

●⚡90587　Dengue vaccine, quadrivalent, live, 3 dose schedule, for subcutaneous use

#▲90620　Meningococcal recombinant protein and outer membrane vesicle vaccine, serogroup B (MenB-4C), 2 dose schedule, for intramuscular use

#▲90621　Meningococcal recombinant lipoprotein vaccine, serogroup B (MenB-FHbp), 2 or 3 dose schedule, for intramuscular use

▲90651　Human Papillomavirus vaccine types 6, 11, 16, 18, 31, 33, 45, 52, 58, nonavalent (9vHPV), 2 or 3 dose schedule, for intramuscular use

Appendix A

Modifiers

Modifiers **96** and **97** are added to *CPT 2018* for use in reporting that a service was either habilitative or rehabilitative. Differentiation of habilitative and rehabilitative services is necessary when services are rendered to a patient whose health plan is subject to the Patient Protection and Affordable Care Act provision that certain health plans must provide equal coverage for habilitative and rehabilitative services and count the rehabilitative and habilitative visits separately. See further discussion of modifiers in Chapter 3, Modifiers and Coding Edits.

▶96　**Habilitative services:** When a procedure that may be either habilitative or rehabilitative in nature is provided for habilitative purposes, the physician or qualified healthcare provider may add Modifier **96** Habilitative services to the procedure code to indicate that the procedure provided was a habilitative service. Habilitative services help an individual learn skills and functioning for daily living that the individual has not yet developed, and then keep and/or improve those learned skills. Habilitative services also help an individual keep, learn, or improve skills and functioning for daily living.

97　**Rehabilitative services:** When a procedure that may be either habilitative or rehabilitative in nature is provided for rehabilitative purposes, the physician or qualified healthcare provider may add Modifier **97** Rehabilitative services to the procedure code to indicate that the procedure provided was a rehabilitative service. Rehabilitative services help an individual keep, get back, or improve skills and functioning for daily living that have been lost or impaired because the individual was sick, hurt, or disabled.◀

Category III Emerging Technology

Category III *CPT*® codes are temporary codes used for data collection purposes to substantiate the usage of emerging technologies, services, and procedures. Assignment of a Category III code to a service is not a statement of support, or lack thereof, for the efficacy of, use of, or payment for the service. Category III *CPT* codes are not assigned relative value units, and payment for these services is based strictly on payer policies. If you are performing any procedure or service identified with a Category III *CPT* code, work with your payers to determine their coverage and payment policies.

Category III codes are released biannually with an implementation date 6 months following the release date. For instance, code **0333T** was released on July 1, 2016; implemented January 1, 2017; and published in *CPT 2018*. The most recent Category III code listing is found online at https://www.ama-assn.org/practice-management/cpt-category-iii-codes.

In general, Category III codes must be replaced for reporting by Category I codes or approved for continued Category III status within 5 years following the Category III code assignment. Category III codes that are not renewed for continued utilization are archived and the codes are not reused.

Current Category III codes and 2018 changes include

●**0479T**   Fractional ablative laser fenestration of burn and traumatic scars for functional improvement; first 100 cm² or part thereof, or 1% of body surface area of infants and children

●+**0480T**   each additional 100 cm², or each additional 1% of body surface area of infants and children, or part thereof (List separately in addition to code for primary procedure)

(Use **0480T** in conjunction with **0479T**)

0188T, +**0189T**   Remote real-time interactive video-conferenced critical care, E/M of the critically ill or critically injured patient

(See Chapter 13, Telemedicine, for specific *CPT* reporting guidelines when reporting remote critical care.)

0208T   Pure tone audiometry (threshold), automated; air only
0209T   air and bone

0210T   Speech audiometry threshold, automated
0211T   with speech recognition

0212T   Comprehensive audiometry threshold evaluation and speech recognition (**0209T**, **0211T** combined), automated

(For audiometric testing using audiometers performed manually by a qualified health care professional, see **92551–92557**.)

▲**0333T**   Visual evoked potential, screening of visual acuity, automated, with report

(For visual evoked potential testing for glaucoma, use **0464T**)

(See Chapter 6, Preventive Services, for more information on screening of visual acuity by automated visual evoked potential.)

0341T   Quantitative pupillometry with interpretation and report, unilateral or bilateral

0359T   Behavior identification assessment, by the physician or other qualified health care professional, face-to-face with patient and caregiver(s), includes administration of standardized and non-standardized tests, detailed behavioral history, patient observation and caregiver interview, interpretation of test results, discussion of findings and recommendations with the primary guardian(s)/caregiver(s), and preparation of report

0360T   Observational behavioral follow-up assessment, includes physician or other qualified health care professional direction with interpretation and report, administered by one technician; first 30 minutes of technician time, face-to-face with the patient

0361T   each additional 30 minutes of technician time, face-to-face with the patient (List separately in addition to code for primary service.)

0362T   Exposure behavioral follow-up assessment, includes physician or other qualified health care professional direction with interpretation and report, administered by physician or other qualified health care professional with the assistance of one or more technicians; first 30 minutes of technician(s) time, face-to-face with the patient

+**0363T**   each additional 30 minutes of technician(s) time, face-to-face with the patient (List separately in addition to code for primary procedure.)

0364T   Adaptive behavior treatment by protocol, administered by technician, face-to-face with one patient; first 30 minutes of technician time

+**0365T**   each additional 30 minutes of technician time (List separately in addition to code for primary procedure.)

0366T   Group adaptive behavior treatment by protocol, administered by technician, face-to-face with two or more patients; first 30 minutes of technician time

+**0367T**   each additional 30 minutes of technician time (List separately in addition to code for primary procedure.)

0368T Adaptive behavior treatment with protocol modification administered by physician or other quali-fied health care professional with one patient; first 30 minutes of patient face-to-face time

+0369T each additional 30 minutes of patient face-to-face time (List separately in addition to code for primary procedure.)

0370T Family adaptive behavior treatment guidance, administered by physician or other qualified health care professional (without the patient present)

0371T Multiple-family group adaptive behavior treatment guidance, administered by physician or other qualified health care professional (without the patient present)

0372T Adaptive behavior treatment social skills group, administered by physician or other qualified health care professional face-to-face with multiple patients

0373T Exposure adaptive behavior treatment with protocol modification requiring two or more techni-cians for severe maladaptive behavior(s); first 60 minutes of technicians' time, face-to-face with patient

+0374T each additional 30 minutes of technicians' time face-to-face with patient (List separately in addition to code for primary procedure.)

0381T External heart rate and 3-axis accelerometer data recording up to 14 days to assess changes in heart rate and to monitor motion analysis for the purposes of diagnosing nocturnal epilepsy seizure events; includes report, scanning analysis with report, review and interpretation by a physician or other qualified health care professional

0382T review and interpretation only

(Do not report **0381T**, **0382T** in conjunction with **0383T**, **0384T**, **0385T**, **0386T**)

0383T External heart rate and 3-axis accelerometer data recording from 15 to 30 days to assess changes in heart rate to monitor motion analysis for the purposes of diagnosing nocturnal epilepsy seizure events; includes report, scanning analysis with report, review and interpretation by a physician or other qualified health care professional

0384T review and interpretation only

(Do not report **0383T**, **0384T** in conjunction with **0381T**, **0382T**, **0385T**, **0386T**)

0385T External heart rate and 3-axis accelerometer data recording more than 30 days to assess changes in heart rate to monitor motion analysis for the purposes of diagnosing nocturnal epilepsy seizure events; includes report, scanning analysis with report, review and interpretation by a physician or other qualified health care professional

0386T review and interpretation only

(Do not report **0385T**, **0386T** in conjunction with **0381T**, **0382T**, **0383T**, **0384T**)

0403T Preventive behavior change, intensive program of prevention of diabetes using a standardized diabetes prevention program curriculum, provided to individuals in a group setting, minimum 60 minutes, per day

(Note: This service is provided only by trained coaches using a standardized curriculum. This service is typically provided in a community setting rather than a physician practice or health care facility.)

0446T Creation of subcutaneous pocket with insertion of implantable interstitial glucose sensor, including system activation and patient training

(Do not report **0446T** in conjunction with **95251**, **0447T**, **0448T**)

0447T Removal of implantable interstitial glucose sensor from subcutaneous pocket via incision

0448T Removal of implantable interstitial glucose sensor with creation of subcutaneous pocket at different anatomic site and insertion of new implantable sensor, including system activation

(Do not report **0448T** in conjunction with **0446T** or **0447T**)

(For placement of non-implantable interstitial glucose sensor without pocket, use **95250**)

●**0469T**   Retinal polarization scan, ocular screening with on-site automated results, bilateral

(Do not report **0469T** in conjunction with **92002**, **92004**, **92012**, **92014**)

(For ocular photoscreening, see **99174**, **99177**)

●**0485T**   Optical coherence tomography (OCT) of middle ear, with interpretation and report; unilateral

●**0486T**   bilateral

Diagnosis Coding: *ICD-10-CM*

Contents

International Classification of Diseases (ICD)

The *International Classification of Diseases (ICD)* is published by the World Health Organization (WHO) for epidemiologic tracking and collection of mortality statistical data worldwide. The *ICD* is currently in its 10th revision. The United States adopted a clinical modification of *ICD-10, International Classification of Diseases, 10th Revision, Clinical Modification (ICD-10-CM)*, on October 1, 2015. The World Health Organization is currently working on the next revision, *International Classification of Diseases, 11th Revision (ICD-11)*, which has had multiple delays and is currently expected to be presented to the World Health Assembly for approval in May 2018.

The current US version is the official system for reporting morbidity and mortality associated with health care data. The clinical modifications in the US version are generally proposed by specialty medical societies to improve injury and illness tracking and are reviewed by the *ICD-10* Coordination and Maintenance Committee. For diagnosis codes, this process is coordinated by the National Center for Health Statistics (NCHS) of the Centers for Disease Control and Prevention, which then publishes new and revised codes in the public domain after approval by the Secretary of the US Department of Health and Human Services (HHS). Oversight and resolution of coding questions related to the US version of *ICD* is performed by the *Coding Clinic* Editorial Advisory Board and the public-private "cooperating parties": the Centers for Medicare & Medicaid Services (CMS), NCHS, American Hospital Association (AHA), and American Health Information Management Association. The increased granularity and specificity in *ICD-10-CM* are also at the specific request of certain medical societies. No clinical diagnosis codes are added for payment purposes.

The American Academy of Pediatrics (AAP) holds a seat on the editorial advisory board. Findings are published quarterly by the AHA in *Coding Clinic*. *ICD-10-CM* codes and accompanying guidelines and findings by the editorial advisory board are part of the standard transaction code sets under the Health Insurance Portability and Accountability Act of 1996 (HIPAA) and must be recognized by all payers. For *ICD-10-CM*, the hierarchy of official coding guidelines and instructions is as follows:

* *ICD-10-CM* alphabetic index and tabular list
* *Official Guidelines for Coding and Reporting*
* AHA *Coding Clinic* advice

Another code set, *ICD-10-Procedure Coding System,* is only used to show hospital inpatient resource utilization and is not intended to show physician or other outpatient services. Physicians continue to report services and resources provided through use of *Current Procedural Terminology (CPT®)* and Healthcare Common Procedure Coding System codes.

Is ICD-11-CM Coming Soon?

With the implementation of *ICD-10-CM* still young and many other changes occurring in health care delivery and payment, concerns have been expressed about the future implementation of *ICD-11* in the United States. However, as was the case with *ICD-10-CM*, it is expected to take 5 to 6 years for development and testing of a clinical modification for use in the United States following WHO release of *ICD-11*. In its 2009 final rule adopting *ICD-10-CM* as a replacement of *International Classification of Diseases, Ninth Revision, Clinical Modification (ICD-9-CM)* for diagnosis coding, the HHS noted that had *ICD-11* been released by WHO in 2014, the earliest projected date to begin rulemaking for implementation of a US clinical modification of *ICD-11* would be 2020. At the time of this publication, the WHO Web site indicates development of *ICD-11* is expected to be completed in 2018. Given this, physicians may expect to report *ICD-10-CM* codes well beyond 2020.

ICD-10-CM

ICD-10-CM Terminology

To correctly select codes in *ICD-10-CM*, it is important to know how the reference is structured and the terminology used in the code set. The following terms describe the structure and some of the key conventions used in this code set as listed in the *ICD-10-CM Official Guidelines for Coding and Reporting:*

Code: A code is a complete set of alphanumeric characters for which there are no further subdivisions, 3 to 7 characters long, describing a condition or reason for an encounter or related factors, such as external causes. The first character of each code is a letter ranging from A to T or V to Z. The second through seventh characters may be letters or numbers.

Alphabetic index: Code selection in *ICD-10-CM* begins in the alphabetic index. The main portion of the alphabetic index consists of an alphabetic list of terms for diseases, injuries, and other reasons for encounters with their corresponding codes or code categories. The alphabetic index also includes an index to external causes of injuries, a table of neoplasms, and a table of drugs and chemicals.

Tabular list: The tabular list is the end point for code selection. It is an alphanumeric list of *ICD-10-CM* codes structured as an indented list of 21 chapters with further divisions, including blocks, categories, subcategories, and codes. Chapters are based on condition, body system, consequences of external causes, external causes, and other factors influencing health status or contact with health services.

Character: A letter or number that serves as the building block of *ICD-10-CM* codes, sometimes referred to as "digits" as a holdover of the term used in *ICD-9-CM*.

Category: A 3-character unit that may be a complete code when no further subcategories exist but often serves as the base for building a 4- to 7-character code. Categories are the main entries of the tabular list.

> When a seventh character is required to complete a code that has fewer than 6 characters, the placeholder **X** must be used to complete the undefined characters. See example in the *ICD-10-CM* Code Structure section later in this chapter.

Subcategory: A further defined category of 4 to 6 characters that may or may not be a complete code.

Placeholder: *ICD-10-CM* uses the letter **X** as a placeholder. When a subcategory of fewer than 6 characters requires 7 characters for a complete code, an **X** must be used as a placeholder to fill in for any undefined characters.

And: Means *and/or* in *ICD-10-CM*.

NEC: Not elsewhere classifiable. Indicates a code for other specified conditions that is reported when the medical record provides detail that is not captured in a specific code.

NOS: Not otherwise specified. Indicates a code for an unspecified condition that is reported when the medical record does not provide sufficient detail for assignment of a more specific code.

With: Means *with* or *due to* in *ICD-10-CM*.

First-listed diagnosis: For reporting of professional services, the diagnosis, condition, problem, or other reason for the encounter or visit shown in the medical record to be chiefly responsible for the services provided.

Combination code: A single code that represents multiple conditions or a single condition with an associated secondary process or complication.

Sequela: A late effect of an illness or injury that is no longer in the acute phase.

These terms are used throughout the *ICD-10-CM* code set and are further defined in the guidelines for its use.

ICD-10-CM *Code Structure*

As indicated by the previously given definition, codes in *ICD-10-CM* begin with a letter. All alphabetic characters are used except for the letter U. For codes that extend beyond 3 characters, the first 3 characters are found to the left of a decimal with the remaining characters to the right.

Pattern: XXX.XXXX

Although typically illustrated in capital letters, the alphabetic characters are not case sensitive. Each 3-character code category may then be further expanded with etiology, severity, site, manifestations, or intent within the fourth through sixth characters. When required, a seventh character is an extension to further define the episode of care, status of fracture healing, number of the fetus in obstetric conditions, or site of recording of the Glasgow Coma Scale.

Examples of complete codes include

R05	Cough
J06.9	Acute upper respiratory infection
H65.04	Acute recurrent serous otitis media, right ear
Z00.129	Encounter routine child health examination without abnormal findings
W07.XXXA	Fall from chair, initial encounter

Note the letter **X** is used as a placeholder in code **W07.XXXA**. The tabular listing for this code is **W07** with no further subcategories but with an instruction that the appropriate seventh character **A**, **D**, or **S** must be added to code **W07** to indicate the initial encounter, subsequent encounter, or encounter for a sequela of the fall from chair. The placeholder must be used to complete the code so the seventh character is in the appropriate position. If **W07.A** were submitted, the associated claim would likely be rejected because this is not a valid *ICD-10-CM* code. The letter **X** is also embedded in some codes to provide for future expansion of a code category (eg, **H60.8X1**, other otitis externa of the right ear).

ICD-10-CM *Guidelines*

The official conventions found in the *ICD-10-CM Official Guidelines for Coding and Reporting* are outlined in sections that include descriptions of symbols, abbreviations, and other instructional notes. The guidelines are organized into 4 sections. Only sections I and IV pertain to physicians reporting services. Sections II and III relate to hospital or facility technical services and are not discussed here. *ICD-10-CM* guidelines can be found in *ICD-10-CM* manuals or at www.cdc.gov/nchs/icd/icd10cm.htm.

The following Table provides an overview of the information pertinent to pediatric care as provided in each section of the guidelines:

> **~ More From the AAP ~**
>
> For more information on *ICD-10-CM* guidelines, see the *AAP Pediatric Coding Newsletter™* Transitioning to 10 Collection at http://coding.aap.org (subscription required).

ICD-10-CM Guidelines
Section I—Conventions, General Coding Guidelines, and Chapter-Specific Guidelines
A. Conventions   **Punctuation**   [ ] In the alphabetic index, brackets identify manifestation codes. Brackets are used in the tabular list to enclose synonyms, alternative wording, or explanatory phrases.   ( ) Parentheses are used in the alphabetic index and tabular list to enclose supplementary words (ie, non-essential modifiers) that may be included in the medical record but do not affect code selection. If a non-essential modifier is mutually exclusive to a sub-term of the main term, the sub-term is given priority.   **Notes**   ◉ **Includes:** Further defines or gives examples of the content of a category.   ◉ **Excludes1:** Not coded here—used to indicate codes for conditions that would not occur in conjunction with the code category where the note is found. An exception to the Excludes1 definition is the circumstance when the 2 conditions are unrelated to each other. If it is not clear whether the 2 conditions involving an Excludes1 note are related, coders are instructed to query the provider.   ◉ **Excludes2:** Not included here—used to indicate codes for conditions not included in the code category where the note is found but that may be additionally reported when both conditions are present.   ◉ **Code first:** A sequencing rule in the tabular list to report first a code for an underlying cause or origin of a disease (etiology).   ◉ **Code also:** An instruction that another code may be necessary to fully describe a condition.   ◉ **See:** In the alphabetic index, this instructs that another term should be referenced to find the appropriate code.   ◉ **See also:** In the alphabetic index, this instructs that another term may provide additional entries that may be useful.   ◉ **Use an additional code:** A sequencing rule often found at the listing of an etiology code, this instruction directs to also report a code for the manifestation.

ICD-10-CM Guidelines (*continued*)

Section I—Conventions, General Coding Guidelines, and Chapter-Specific Guidelines (*continued*)

B. General Coding Guidelines

- First and foremost, begin by finding a term in the alphabetic index, and then turn to the tabular list to be sure you are selecting a complete code and follow code instructions for that chapter and code category.
- Assign a code for signs and symptoms when no definitive diagnosis has been reached at an encounter.
- Do not report additional codes for conditions that are integral or routinely associated with a disease process (eg, wheezing in asthma).
- When the same condition is documented as acute and chronic, codes for both conditions are reported if the alphabetic index lists the conditions at the same indentation level. The acute condition is sequenced first.
- When a combination code describes 2 diagnoses, or a diagnosis and its associated manifestation or complication, report only the combination code. If a manifestation or complication is not identified in a combination code, it may be separately reported.
- When reporting a sequela (late effect) of an injury or illness, report first the current condition and then the sequela code.
- If both sides are affected by a condition and the code category does not include a code for the bilateral condition, assign codes for right and left. When a patient has a bilateral condition and each side is treated during separate encounters, assign the bilateral code for each encounter where the condition exists on both sides. Do not assign a bilateral code if the condition no longer exists bilaterally.
- Coders generally may not assume a complication of care without documentation of the cause-and-effect relationship (eg, infection in a patient with a central venous line).
- Unspecified codes are appropriately selected when information to support a more specific code was not available at the time of the encounter (eg, type of pneumonia is not known). Unspecified codes are not appropriate when information to support a more specific code would generally be known (eg, laterality, type of attention-deficit/hyperactivity disorder). See the Appropriate Use of Unspecified Codes box later in this chapter for more information.

C. Chapter-Specific Guidelines

- See these guidelines for specific diagnoses and/or conditions found in each chapter.
- When selecting electronic coding applications, look for inclusion of chapter-specific guidelines when using the code search functionality.
- Chapter 16, Certain Conditions Originating in the Perinatal Period (**P00–P96**)
  For conditions that originate in the perinatal or neonatal period, the provider selects diagnostic codes from Chapter 16 in *ICD-10-CM*, **P00–P96**. For coding and reporting purposes, the *perinatal period* is defined as before birth through the 28th day following birth. Should a condition originate in the perinatal period and continue to have health care implications throughout the life of the patient, the Chapter 16 code should continue to be used regardless of the patient's age. If the reason for a particular encounter is a perinatal or neonatal condition (ie, originated in the perinatal or neonatal period), the Chapter 16 code may be sequenced first (exception: the **Z38** series type of delivery code ranks as primary for care by the attending physician during the admission that began with the neonate's birth). *ICD* coding guidelines allow for exclusive use of perinatal or neonatal period codes to characterize a patient's clinical condition on an encounter claim so long as the condition(s) originated in the perinatal or neonatal period and so long as the condition(s) continues to have clinical implications for the care of the patient. Typical scenarios that may require exclusive use of perinatal or neonatal codes beyond the perinatal period are often found in neonatal intensive care unit settings where early gestational ages and evolving maturation extend diagnostic effect, such as in drug withdrawal syndrome of infant of dependent mother (**P96.1**), chronic respiratory disease arising in the perinatal period (**P27.-**), necrotizing enterocolitis (**P77.-**), and prematurity (**P07.-**). (Note that these codes are not reported for conditions with onset after the patient is 28 days old. For example, necrotizing enterocolitis with onset after the neonatal period is reported with codes **K55.30–K55.33**.)

ICD-10-CM Guidelines (*continued*)

Section I–Conventions, General Coding Guidelines, and Chapter-Specific Guidelines (*continued*)

- Chapter 19: Injury, Poisoning and Certain Other Consequences of External Causes (**S00–T88**)
  Most categories in Chapter 19 have a seventh character requirement for each applicable code. Most categories in this chapter have 3 seventh character values (with the exception of fractures): **A,** initial encounter; **D,** subsequent encounter; and **S,** sequela. Categories for traumatic fractures have additional seventh character values. While the patient may be seen by a new or different provider over the course of treatment for an injury, assignment of the seventh character is based on whether the patient is undergoing active treatment (services to establish a pattern of healing) and not whether the provider is seeing the patient for the first time.

Section IV–Diagnostic Coding and Reporting Guidelines for Outpatient Services

Selecting a code
- The coding conventions and guidelines of Section I take precedence over these outpatient guidelines.
- Never assign a code for a condition that is unconfirmed (eg, probable obstruction). Instead, assign codes for signs and symptoms.
- Use codes in categories **Z00–Z99** when circumstances other than a disease or injury are recorded as the reason for encounter.

Sequencing of diagnosis codes
- Physicians and other providers of professional services should list first the condition, symptom, or other reason for encounter that is chiefly responsible for the services provided. List also any coexisting conditions. (Note: Some codes and chapters have specific guidelines with regard to sequencing.)

Reporting previously treated conditions
- Do not code conditions that have been previously treated but no longer exist. History codes **Z80–Z87** may be used to identify historical conditions or family history that affects current care.
- Report codes for chronic or recurring conditions as many times as the patient receives care for each condition.

Reporting diagnoses for diagnostic examinations
- The condition, symptoms, or other reason for a diagnostic examination or test should be linked to the service. For laboratory or radiology testing in the absence of related conditions, signs, or symptoms, report code **Z01.89**, encounter for other specified special examinations.
- When diagnostic tests have been interpreted by a physician and the final report is available at the time of coding, code any confirmed or definitive diagnosis(es) documented in the interpretation. Do not code related signs and symptoms as additional diagnoses.

Reporting preoperative evaluations
- When the reason for an encounter is a preoperative evaluation, a code from subcategory **Z01.81-,** encounter for pre-procedural examinations, is reported first, followed by codes for the condition that is the reason for surgery and codes for any findings of the preoperative evaluation.

Reporting health examinations (preventive care)
- Codes for pediatric health examinations are found in subcategory **Z00.1-**. Encounters for routine child health examinations are reported based on findings—with or without new abnormal findings. Abnormal findings in the context of a routine examination are new (not previously diagnosed) or exacerbated conditions. When reporting an encounter with abnormal findings, report also codes to describe the findings. When a previously diagnosed condition is stable but managed at the same encounter as a routine child health examination, this is not reported as an abnormal finding of the routine child examination. Codes for conditions managed may be assigned in addition to the code for a routine child health examination without abnormal findings (**Z00.129**).

Application of the Guidelines and Conventions of *ICD-10-CM*

Formatting and Reporting Instructions for ICD-10-CM

It is important to recognize and follow instructions found in the alphabetic index and tabular list. These are the prevailing instructions for reporting that are supplemented by the guidelines and guidance published in *AHA Coding Clinic for ICD-10-CM*. The indentation and instructions in the alphabetic index guide the user to the correct chapter and category of the tabular list. The alphabetic index may include many sub-terms for a single main entry. The indentation of each term directs to the appropriate listing.

Example

Otitis (acute) **H66.90**
… (entries omitted)
- media (hemorrhagic) (staphylococcal) (streptococcal) **H66.9-**
… (entries omitted)
- - nonsuppurative **H65.9-**
- - - acute or subacute NEC **H65.19-**
- - - - allergic **H65.11-**
- - - - - recurrent **H65.11-**
- - - - recurrent **H65.19-**
- - - - secretory—*see* Otitis, media, nonsuppurative, serous
- - - - serous **H65.0-**
- - - - - recurrent **H65.0-**
- - - chronic **H65.49-**
- - - - allergic **H65.41-**
- - - - mucoid **H65.3-**
- - - - serous **H65.2-**
- - post-measles **B05.3**
- - purulent—*see* Otitis, media, suppurative

Notes

1. Attention to the level of indentation is necessary for accurate selection. The 4 hyphens that precede "recurrent **H65.19-**" indicate the pathway to this entry is otitis, -media, --nonsuppurative, ---acute, ----recurrent.
2. Note how the index listings for otitis media start with an unspecified code category (**H66.9-**). This is the default entry that is followed only if no further specification is provided in the medical record.
3. The alphabetic index uses a dash (**H66.9-**) to indicate code subcategories and incomplete codes. Although subcategory **H66.9-** represents an unspecified type of otitis media, the tabular list will provide additional specificity, such as laterality. In contrast, the alphabetic list entry for otitis, -media, --post-measles directs to a complete code, **B05.3**, and the tabular list is consulted to verify the code selection and any additional coding instruction.
4. A *see* note is also illustrated for the diagnosis of acute secretary otitis media directing to otitis, -media, --nonsuppurative, ---acute, ----serous.

In the tabular list, instructions are found at many levels, starting with chapter instructions and following down through the block, category, and subcategory levels. These instructions provide important details on the use of the codes that follow each instruction. For instance, the following notes are found in Chapter 16:

Example of Chapter-Level Note

Chapter 16
Certain conditions originating in the perinatal period (**P00–P96**)

Note: Codes from this chapter are for use on newborn records only, never on maternal records.

Appropriate Use of Unspecified Codes

Unspecified codes are valid *ICD-10-CM* codes used to report conditions for which a more specific diagnosis has not yet been determined and/or testing to determine a more specific diagnosis would not be medically necessary. However, misuse of unspecified codes may result in claim denials and unnecessary delays in receiving prior authorizations for testing or procedures.

Do not report the default code (first code listed in the alphabetic index) when more detail about the patient's conditions should be documented to support another, more specific code. For example, do not report **J45.909** for unspecified asthma, uncomplicated, for reevaluation of asthma, which includes clinical classification of intermittent, mild persistent, moderate persistent, or severe persistent asthma. The diagnosis code reported should reflect what is known at the end of the current encounter.

The following examples of unspecified codes that should be acceptable are provided by Jeffrey F. Linzer Sr, MD, American Academy of Pediatrics representative to the Editorial Advisory Board for the American Hospital Association *Coding Clinic for ICD-10-CM* and *ICD-10-PCS*:

- Viral intestinal infection, unspecified (**A08.4**)
- Infectious gastroenteritis and colitis, unspecified (**A09**)
- Hb-SS disease with crisis, unspecified (**D57.00**)
- Acute pharyngitis, unspecified (**J02.9**)
- Pneumonia, unspecified organism (**J18.9**)
- Sprain of unspecified site of right knee (**S83.91X-**)
- Sprain of unspecified ligament of right ankle (**S93.401-**)

Dr Linzer also provides the following examples of unspecified codes that indicate inappropriate coding due to failure to document information that would typically be known at the time of the encounter and/or inappropriate code selection:

- Acute suppurative otitis media without spontaneous rupture of ear drum, unspecified ear (**H66.009**)
- Otitis media, unspecified, unspecified ear (**H66.90**)
- Cutaneous abscess of limb, unspecified (**L02.419**)
- Extremely low birth weight newborn, unspecified weight (**P07.00**)
- Abrasion of unspecified finger (**S60.419-**)
- Sprain of unspecified ligament of unspecified ankle (**S93.409-**)

In short, unspecified codes are necessary and should be reported when appropriate. However, physicians must document in sufficient detail to capture what is known at the time of the encounter and codes selected must reflect the documented diagnosis(es). If, at the time of code selection, documentation does not appear to include information that would be known at the time of the encounter, it is appropriate for coders to query the physician for more information and/or request an addendum to the documentation to more fully describe the conditions addressed at the encounter.

Includes: conditions that have their origin in the fetal or perinatal period (before birth through the first 28 days after birth) even if morbidity occurs later

Excludes2: congenital malformations, deformations, and chromosomal abnormalities (**Q00–Q99**)

    endocrine, nutritional, and metabolic diseases (**E00–E88**)

    injury, poisoning, and certain other consequences of external causes (**S00–T88**)

    neoplasms (**C00–D49**)

    tetanus neonatorum (**A33**)

Notes

1. The first note advises that codes from Chapter 16 are never used on the maternal record.
2. The inclusion note further defines that codes in this chapter represent conditions that originate in the newborn period but may be reported even if morbidity occurs later.
3. The *Excludes2* note provides information on potentially coexisting conditions that may be separately reported but are not included in this chapter.

 Coding Pearl |||||||||||

Excludes2 notes in *ICD-10-CM* mean the code and the excluded code can both be reported when appropriate.

Chapter 2: Diagnosis Coding: *ICD-10-CM*

Example of Block-Level Note

Newborn affected by maternal factors and by complications of pregnancy, labor, and delivery (P00–P04)

Note: These codes are for use when the listed maternal conditions are specified as the cause of confirmed morbidity or potential morbidity which have their origin in the perinatal period (before birth through the first 28 days after birth).

Example of Category-Level Note: Asthma

J45   Asthma

Includes: allergic (predominantly) asthma

allergic bronchitis NOS

allergic rhinitis with asthma

atopic asthma

extrinsic allergic asthma

hay fever with asthma

idiosyncratic asthma

intrinsic nonallergic asthma

nonallergic asthma

Use additional code to identify

exposure to environmental tobacco smoke (**Z77.22**)

exposure to tobacco smoke in the perinatal period (**P96.81**)

history of tobacco use (**Z87.891**)

occupational exposure to environmental tobacco smoke (**Z57.31**)

tobacco dependence (**F17.-**)

tobacco use (**Z72.0**)

Excludes1:   detergent asthma (**J69.8**)

eosinophilic asthma (**J82**)

miners' asthma (**J60**)

wheezing NOS (**R06.2**)

wood asthma (**J67.8**)

Excludes2:   asthma with chronic obstructive pulmonary disease (**J44.9**)

chronic asthmatic (obstructive) bronchitis (**J44.9**)

chronic obstructive asthma (**J44.9**)

J45.2   Mild intermittent asthma

J45.20   Mild intermittent asthma, uncomplicated

Mild intermittent asthma NOS

J45.21   Mild intermittent asthma with (acute) exacerbation

J45.22   Mild intermittent asthma with status asthmaticus

J45.3   Mild persistent asthma

J45.30   Mild persistent asthma, uncomplicated

Mild persistent asthma NOS

J45.31   Mild persistent asthma with (acute) exacerbation

J45.32   Mild persistent asthma with status asthmaticus

J45.4   Moderate persistent asthma

J45.40   Moderate persistent asthma, uncomplicated

Moderate persistent asthma NOS

J45.41   Moderate persistent asthma with (acute) exacerbation

J45.42   Moderate persistent asthma with status asthmaticus

J45.5   Severe persistent asthma

      J45.50 Severe persistent asthma, uncomplicated

            Severe persistent asthma NOS

      J45.51 Severe persistent asthma with (acute) exacerbation

      J45.52 Severe persistent asthma with status asthmaticus

J45.9   Other and unspecified asthma

      J45.90 Unspecified asthma

            Asthmatic bronchitis NOS

            Childhood asthma NOS

            Late-onset asthma

            J45.901   Unspecified asthma with (acute) exacerbation

            J45.902   Unspecified asthma with status asthmaticus

            J45.909   Unspecified asthma, uncomplicated

Excludes2:   lung diseases due to external agents (**J60–J70**)

      J45.99 Other asthma

            J45.990   Exercise induced bronchospasm

            J45.991   Cough variant asthma

            J45.998   Other asthma

Notes

1. Format: The indented format directs the coder to the more specific code.
2. *Excludes1* notes: Indicate the code excluded should never be used at the same time as codes in the category that includes the *Excludes1* note. Used when 2 conditions cannot occur together.
3. *Excludes2* notes: Indicate the condition excluded is not part of the condition represented by the code, but a patient may have both conditions at the same time. The code and excluded code can be reported when appropriate.
4. Abbreviations: The designation of NOS means the information available does not allow a more specific code.
5. Use additional code: Used to show sequencing for certain codes that are not part of an etiology/manifestation combination. Note that the instructions to use additional codes for tobacco use or exposure apply to all codes in categories **H66** and **J45** when use or exposure is documented.

Examples of Subcategory-Level Note

R06.1   Stridor

        Excludes1: congenital laryngeal stridor (**P28.89**)

          laryngismus (stridulus) (**J38.5**)

R06.2   Wheezing

        Excludes1: asthma (**J45.-**)

Notes

1. Note that these subcategories of category **R06** include exclusion notes to direct to an appropriate code or category for conditions that are not reported at the same encounter as the codes for stridor and wheezing. The exclusion notes indicate stridor and wheezing may occur in the excluded conditions but are not separately reported (eg, wheezing is considered integral to asthma).
2. Each of the subcategories is also a complete code with no further subdivisions.

Who Assigns the Codes?

The clinician (pediatrician, pediatric nurse practitioner, or physician assistant) should assign a principal (primary) diagnosis that best explains the reason with the highest risk of morbidity or mortality for the patient encounter unless the tabular instructions direct to "code first" a specific condition (eg, code first cystic fibrosis [**E84.-**] in a patient with secondary diabetes [**E08.-**] due to cystic fibrosis). Assignment of the specific diagnosis code by a nonphysician provider or administrative staff should be done under the physician's or reporting provider's supervision. For those practices using a printed encounter form, including 50 to 100 of the most commonly used diagnoses *and* their respective codes on the outpatient encounter form allows the physician or health care professional to mark the appropriate code(s), indicating which is primary. All contributing (secondary) diagnoses that help explain the medical necessity for the episode of care should also be listed. Only those conditions that specifically affect the patient's encounter should be listed. If a specific diagnosis code is not included on your form, write it in! Do not select a diagnosis code that is "closest to" your diagnosis. The AAP has developed an encounter form including *ICD-10-CM* codes. For a copy, go to www.aap.org/cfp (access code AAPCFP23). Refer to Chapter 19, The Business of Medicine: Working With Current and Emerging Payment Systems, for tips on designing an encounter form.

Linking the Diagnosis

❋ Every encounter and physician service must be linked to the appropriate *ICD-10-CM* code.

❋ Physicians and qualified nonphysician professionals should clearly designate the primary diagnosis on the encounter form (superbill) or use another method that easily sequences the diagnoses and links them to the appropriate service or procedure. For example, when using an electronic health record (EHR), physicians should list the primary diagnosis in the EHR first and make certain the software knows that it should be reported as the first listed. In addition, the EHR should be able to link diagnosis codes to the appropriate services.

❋ The diagnosis code may be the same for each service performed. For example, if a child is diagnosed with a urinary tract infection (UTI), the code for a UTI (*ICD-10-CM* code **N39.0**) should be linked to the evaluation and management (E/M) service (eg, **99213**) and a dipstick urinalysis without microscopy (**81002**) performed.

  ❖ Linking of the *ICD-10-CM* code to the service on the billing form is illustrated in **Claim Form Example 1 for Linking *ICD-10-CM* Code to Service** in the context of a paper claim (1500 claim form) on which each *ICD-10-CM* code is placed in diagnosis fields labeled 21A–L. A diagnosis pointer in field 24E indicates which diagnosis code relates to each service line by indicating the letter of the related diagnosis field.

Claim Form Example 1 for Linking ICD-10-CM Code to Service

21. Diagnosis or nature of illness or injury (Relate A–L to service line below 24E)				ICD Ind. 0					
A. **N39.0**	B.	C.	D.						
E.	F.	G.	H.						
I.	J.	K.	L.						

24. A. Dates of service	B. Place of service	C. EMG	D. Procedures, services or supplies CPT/HCPCS	Modifier	E. Diagnosis Pointer	F. Charges	G. Days or units	H. EPSDT	I. ID Qual	J. Rendering Provider #
1/1/2017–1/1/2017	11		**99213** (E/M)		A	$$$	1		NPI	123456789
1/1/2017–1/1/2017	11		**81002** (dipstick urinalysis)		A	$$$	1		NPI	123456789

Abbreviations: CPT, Current Procedural Terminology; *E/M, evaluation and management; EMG, emergency; EPSDT, Early and Periodic Screening, Diagnosis, and Treatment; HCPCS, Healthcare Common Procedure Coding System;* ICD, International Classification of Diseases; *NPI, National Provider Identifier.*

The diagnoses may differ for each service or procedure. For example, when the physician reports a significant, separately identifiable problem-oriented (sick) visit and a preventive medicine visit during the same encounter, he or she must link the appropriate diagnosis codes to each service. *ICD-10-CM* code **Z00.110** (health examination for newborn under 8 days old), **Z00.111** (health examination for newborn 8 to 28 days old), **Z00.121** (routine child health examination with abnormal findings), or **Z00.129** (routine child health examination without abnormal findings) would be linked to the preventive medicine visit, and the appropriate abnormal finding or "sick" diagnosis code would be linked to the sick visit (**Claim Form Example 2 for Linking *ICD-10-CM* Code to Service**).

Claim Form Example 2 for Linking ICD-10-CM Code to Service

21. Diagnosis or nature of illness or injury (Relate A–L to service line below 24E)				ICD Ind. 0				
A. **Z00.121**	B. **H65.196**	C.	D.					
E.	F.	G.	H.					
I.	J.	K.	L.					

24. A. Dates of service	B. Place of service	C. EMG	D. Procedures, services or supplies CPT/HCPCS	Modifier	E. Diagnosis Pointer	F. Charges	G. Days or units	H. EPSDT	I. ID Qual	J. Rendering Provider #
1/1/2017– 1/1/2017	11		**99392** (preventive service)		A, B	$$$	1		NPI	123456789
1/1/2017– 1/1/2017	11		**99213** (E/M)	**25**	B	$$$	1		NPI	123456789

Abbreviations: CPT, Current Procedural Terminology; *E/M, evaluation and management; EMG, emergency; EPSDT, Early and Periodic Screening, Diagnosis, and Treatment; HCPCS, Healthcare Common Procedure Coding System; ICD, International Classification of Diseases; NPI, National Provider Identifier.*

- Appropriate information should be documented in the medical record to support the principal and contributing diagnoses. Just listing them in a problem list is not sufficient.
- Diagnosis code assignment by a non-clinician should be done only by trained personnel and with clinician supervision. Remember that coders are not medical professionals and cannot make presumptions as to a diagnosis if the documentation is unclear to them. Coding professionals are instructed to "query the physician" whenever there is a question as to a diagnosis. Ultimately, the clinician in whose name the service is reported is responsible for the code assignment and linkage.
- The primary diagnosis code should best identify the condition carrying the highest risk or that is the main reason for the encounter (procedure, service, or visit) unless otherwise instructed by the coding guidelines or tabular instructions.

Examples

➤ **A child who had an incision and drainage of a leg abscess on the left calf 2 days ago is seen in the pediatrician's office for a wound check.** The pediatrician reviews the emergency department record and current medication and inspects the wound for signs of improvement. The culture report shows the patient has methicillin-resistant *Staphylococcus aureus* (MRSA) that is sensitive to the current antibiotic. The plan is to continue the current antibiotic and have the child return at the end of therapy. You would report the service and diagnosis as

ICD-10-CM		CPT®	
L02.416	(cutaneous abscess left lower limb)	**9921X**	(E/M)
Z48.817	(aftercare following surgery of the skin and subcutaneous tissue)		
B95.62	(MRSA)		

Chapter 2: Diagnosis Coding: *ICD-10-CM*

➤ **During a recheck for otitis media (resolved), the physician recommends the influenza vaccine to a patient who is accompanied by the nanny.** The nanny is unsure whether the parent would really want the child to receive the vaccine so refuses the administration until such time that the parent can consent. You would report the service and diagnoses as

ICD-10-CM		*CPT*	
Z09	(follow-up examination after completed treatment for conditions other than malignant neoplasm)	**9921X**	(E/M)
Z86.69	(personal history of other diseases of the nervous system and sense organs)		
Z23	(encounter for immunization)		
Z28.82	(immunization not carried out because of caregiver refusal)		

Additional examples of *ICD-10-CM* code assignment are included in each chapter of this manual with specific documentation elements and code-reporting instructions highlighted in coding tips.

New Pediatric *ICD-10-CM* Codes Effective October 1, 2017

The *ICD-10-CM* Coordination and Maintenance Committee issued the annual update to *ICD-10-CM* effective on October 1, 2017 (fiscal year 2018). This update to *ICD-10-CM* includes 363 new codes, 226 revised codes, and deletion of 142 codes. Changes implemented on October 1, 2017, are published to the NCHS Web site at www.cdc.gov/nchs/icd/icd10cm.htm.

Notable changes for pediatrics are included in **Table 2-1**. Please see your *ICD-10-CM* coding reference for coding instructions.

Information about *ICD-10-CM* changes can also be obtained by contacting the AAP Coding Hotline at aapcodinghotline@aap.org and reading articles in *AAP Pediatric Coding Newsletter*™ at http://coding.aap.org (subscription required).

> **~ More From the AAP ~**
>
> For more information on specific *ICD-10-CM* coding topics, see the *AAP Pediatric Coding Newsletter*™ Transitioning to 10 Collection at http://coding.aap.org (subscription required).

Requesting New *ICD-10-CM* Codes

The *ICD-10-CM* Coordination and Maintenance Committee typically meets in March and September of each year to consider proposals for new codes or revisions to existing codes or instructions. Annual updates of *ICD-10-CM* are implemented on October 1 each year.

Pediatricians with suggestions for new or changes to existing *ICD-10-CM* codes related to pediatric care are encouraged to forward their suggestions to coding staff at the AAP headquarters. The AAP staff and advisor who are involved in the process can be of great assistance. E-mail the coding staff at aapcodinghotline@aap.org.

Resources

The AAP *Pediatric ICD-10-CM: A Manual for Provider-Based Coding* is a condensed version of the entire *ICD-10-CM* manual and provides only the guidelines and codes that are applicable and of importance to pediatric practitioners. The manual was designed for use in conjunction with the complete *ICD-10-CM* code set. The *ICD-10-CM* codes are found at www.cdc.gov/nchs/icd/icd10cm.htm.

AAP Pediatric Coding Newsletter™ will continue to provide articles on diagnosis coding for pediatric conditions.

Table 2-1. New *ICD-10-CM* Codes	
F50.82	Avoidant/restrictive food intake disorder
M33.03	Juvenile dermatomyositis without myopathy
P29.30	Pulmonary hypertension of newborn
P29.38	Other persistent fetal circulation
P78.84	Gestational alloimmune liver disease
P83.81	Umbilical granuloma
P83.88	Other specified conditions of integument specific to newborn
P91.811	Neonatal encephalopathy in diseases classified elsewhere
P91.819	Neonatal encephalopathy, unspecified
P91.88	Other specified disturbances of cerebral status of newborn
Q53.111	Unilateral intraabdominal testis
Q53.112	Unilateral inguinal testis
Q53.13	Unilateral high scrotal testis
Q53.211	Bilateral intraabdominal testes
Q53.212	Bilateral inguinal testes
Q53.23	Bilateral high scrotal testes
R06.03	Acute respiratory distress
R39.83	Unilateral non-palpable testicle
R39.84	Bilateral non-palpable testicles
T07.XXX- (A, D, S)	Unspecified multiple injuries
T14.8XX- (A, D, S)	Other injury of unspecified body region
T14.90X- (A, D, S)	Injury, unspecified
T14.91X- (A, D, S)	Suicide attempt
V86.05X- (A, D, S)	Driver of 3- or 4-wheeled all-terrain vehicle (ATV) injured in traffic accident
V86.06X- (A, D, S)	Driver of dirt bike or motor/cross bike injured in traffic accident
V86.15X- (A, D, S)	Passenger of 3- or 4-wheeled all-terrain vehicle (ATV) injured in traffic accident
V86.16X- (A, D, S)	Passenger of dirt bike or motor/cross bike injured in traffic accident
V86.25X- (A, D, S)	Person on outside of 3- or 4-wheeled all-terrain vehicle (ATV) injured in traffic accident
V86.26X- (A, D, S)	Person on outside of dirt bike or motor/cross bike injured in traffic accident
V86.35X- (A, D, S)	Unspecified occupant of 3- or 4-wheeled all-terrain vehicle (ATV) injured in traffic accident
V86.36X- (A, D, S)	Unspecified occupant of dirt bike or motor/cross bike injured in traffic accident
V86.45X- (A, D, S)	Person injured while boarding or alighting from a 3- or 4-wheeled all-terrain vehicle (ATV)
V86.46X- (A, D, S)	Person injured while boarding or alighting from a dirt bike or motor/cross bike
V86.55X- (A, D, S)	Driver of 3- or 4-wheeled all-terrain vehicle (ATV) injured in nontraffic accident
V86.56X- (A, D, S)	Driver of dirt bike or motor/cross bike injured in nontraffic accident
V86.65X- (A, D, S)	Passenger of 3- or 4-wheeled all-terrain vehicle (ATV) injured in nontraffic accident
V86.66X- (A, D, S)	Passenger of dirt bike or motor/cross bike injured in nontraffic accident

Chapter 2: Diagnosis Coding: *ICD-10-CM*

Table 2-1. New *ICD-10-CM* Codes (*continued*)

V86.75X- (A, D, S)	Person on outside of 3- or 4-wheeled all-terrain vehicle (ATV) injured in nontraffic accident
V86.76X- (A, D, S)	Person on outside of dirt bike or motor/cross bike injured in nontraffic accident
V86.95X- (A, D, S)	Unspecified occupant of 3- or 4-wheeled all-terrain vehicle (ATV) injured in nontraffic accident
V86.96X- (A, D, S)	Unspecified occupant of dirt bike or motor/cross bike injured in nontraffic accident
Z71.82	Exercise counseling
Z91.841	Risk for dental caries, low
Z91.842	Risk for dental caries, moderate
Z91.843	Risk for dental caries, high
Z91.849	Unspecified risk for dental caries

Abbreviation: ICD-10-CM, International Classification of Diseases, 10th Revision, Clinical Modification.

Diagnosis Coding Tips

* Physicians and other practitioners should become familiar with the documentation elements that are captured in *ICD-10-CM* code categories for conditions commonly seen in their practice. For example, when documenting care for otitis media, key documentation elements include whether the condition affects the right, the left, or both ears; is acute, acute recurrent, or chronic; is suppurative or nonsuppurative; and is with or without spontaneous rupture of the tympanic membrane. Exposure to or use of tobacco is also reported in conjunction with otitis media.
* Pay close attention to the terminology for nonspecific diagnoses. For example, the diagnosis "reactive airways disease" is to be coded as asthma per the guidelines. In children treated for an asthma-like condition who have not been diagnosed with asthma, it may be more appropriate to report the signs or symptoms as the primary diagnosis.
* When testing is performed to rule out or confirm a suspected diagnosis or condition on a patient with a sign(s) or symptom(s), it is considered a diagnostic examination and is not screening. Therefore, the code that explains the reason for the test (ie, sign or symptom) should be reported. Screening codes may be reported as the primary code if the reason for the visit is specifically for the screening examination or test.
* Codes for routine examinations that include "with abnormal findings" in the code descriptor are reported only when there are new abnormal findings at the time of the preventive encounter (ie, new problem or exacerbation of previously managed problem). If preexisting (ie, known) conditions are stable but addressed at the preventive encounter but there are no new abnormal findings, report first the code for routine examination without abnormal findings (eg, **Z00.129**) and then the code(s) appropriate for the conditions addressed.
* When routine vision, developmental, and/or hearing screening services are performed in conjunction with a preventive medicine visit, the diagnosis code for a routine infant or child health check should be linked to the appropriate screening service.
* Codes for reporting live-born neonates according to type of birth (*ICD-10-CM* codes **Z38.0–Z38.8**) are reported by the attending physician as the first-listed diagnosis for a newborn at the time of birth and for the duration of the birth admission as long as the baby is consuming health care (ie, crib or bassinet occupancy). This includes reporting for a neonate kept in the normal newborn nursery (eg, awaiting adoption) or mother's room (awaiting a mother's discharge) and those neonates who stay in the birth hospital for a prolonged time.

Diagnosis Coding Tips (*continued*)

- Codes in Chapter 16, Certain Conditions Originating in the Perinatal Period (**P00–P99**), are used when the diagnosis is made on a fetus or a neonate who is 28 days or younger. The World Health Organization defines the day of birth as day of life 0 (zero). A baby reaches 28 days of life on day 29 of age. These codes are only to be reported when the condition originates in this time but can be reported beyond the perinatal period if the condition(s) causes morbidity or is the primary reason for or contributing to why the patient is receiving health care.

- If, after evaluation and study of a suspected condition, there is no diagnosis or signs or symptoms that are appropriate, report the codes for observation and evaluation for suspected conditions not found. Codes for observation and evaluation for suspected conditions not found in a neonate (*ICD-10-CM* codes **Z05.0–Z05.9**) are distinct from those for reporting suspected conditions not found in older children and adults (*ICD-10-CM* code **Z03.89**).

- Disorders of newborn related to slow fetal growth and fetal malnutrition are reported with codes in category **P05**. Codes in subcategory **P05.0-** are reported for newborn light for gestational age. The World Health Organization defines *light for gestational age* as usually referring to weight below but length above the 10th percentile for gestational age (may be referenced as asymmetrical). In contrast, codes in subcategory **P05.1** are reported for newborn small for gestational age, including the newborn who is small and light for dates. This usually refers both to weight and length below the 10th percentile (often called symmetrical). Note that head circumference is NOT considered in choosing *light* versus *small*.

- Use aftercare codes (**Z42–Z49, Z51**) for patients who are receiving care to consolidate treatment or managing residual conditions.

- Conditions that were previously treated and no longer exist cannot be reported. Therefore, it is correct coding to report care following completed treatment with *ICD-10-CM* code **Z09**, encounter for follow-up examination after completed treatment for conditions other than malignant neoplasm. Personal history codes (**Z86.-, Z87.-**) may be used to provide additional information on follow-up care. If a payer does not accept follow-up care codes as primary and requires that the service be reported with the diagnosis code that reflects the condition that had been treated, report the follow-up care codes as secondary. However, get the payer's policy in writing and inquire why it is not following coding guidelines.

- Do not select a diagnosis code that is "closest to" the diagnosis or condition documented in the medical record. If a specific diagnosis code is not included on your encounter form, write it in. For example, do not report unspecified joint pain (**M25.50**) if the diagnosis is right knee pain (**M25.561**).

- Pay attention to age factors within certain code descriptors. For example, *ICD-10-CM* code **R10.83** is used to report infantile colic. Colic in the child older than 12 months is reported with *ICD-10-CM* code **R10.84**.

- There is no limit to the number of diagnosis codes that can be reported. Although space is only allotted for up to 12 codes on the CMS-1500 claim form and each service line may be connected to 1 to 4 of the included codes, you may submit as many claim forms as necessary to report the diagnoses. Electronic claims in HIPAA version 5010 may also include up to 12 diagnosis codes.

- "Unspecified" codes can still be reported if, at the time of the encounter, more information cannot be obtained. However, it will be important to not report "unspecified" for conditions or information that should be documented, such as laterality.

- "Recurrent" is not defined by *ICD*. Therefore, to use a recurrent code, the documentation should reflect that a practitioner believes it to be a recurrence.

- "Confirmed" influenza or other conditions do not require a positive laboratory test result or other test. What is required is that the practitioner, through training and experience, believes the patient has the condition based on clinical assessment and documents the condition in the chart.

Modifiers and Coding Edits

Contents

CPT® Modifiers

Current Procedural Terminology (*CPT®*) defines a *modifier* as a means to indicate that a service or procedure has been altered by some specific circumstance but not changed in its basic code definition. Because a modifier is used to report a service or procedure that was altered, medical record documentation must always support the use of the modifier.

In addition to *CPT* modifiers, the Centers for Medicare & Medicaid Services (CMS) maintain a list of modifiers for use with Healthcare Common Procedure Coding System (HCPCS) and *CPT* codes. Most state Medicaid programs and many commercial payers follow CMS guidelines and may recognize HCPCS modifiers as well.

When are modifiers needed? In brief, a modifier or combination of modifiers is appended to a procedure code when it is necessary to add context of how or when the service was provided. Context often affects payment, such as when a procedure for which the code does not indicate unilateral or bilateral is performed bilaterally. By appending modifier **50** (bilateral procedure), the claim for services provides context allowing claims adjudication systems to process for payment at a higher rate (typically 150% of the allowable amount for the unilateral service). Examples of information provided by modifiers include

- A service provided on the same date or within the global period of a previous service is unrelated, more extensive, performed on a different body area, or performed at separate encounters.
- A face-to-face service was provided via telemedicine using real-time, interactive communication technology.
- The same service was repeated on the same date.
- An evaluation and management (E/M) service that might otherwise be considered part of another service is significantly beyond the typical preservice and/or post-service components of the other service.
- The units of services provided were medically necessary but exceed the payer's unit of service edits.
- A service that may be provided for diagnostic or preventive purposes was provided for preventive purposes.

Some modifiers are used exclusively with E/M services, and others are reported only with surgical or other procedures. Refer to the Modifiers and E/M Services Table to review modifiers used with E/M service codes and those used only for other services. Multiple modifiers can be appended to a single *CPT* or HCPCS code.

Payers use coding edits (paired codes and/or unit of service limitations) to aid in automated claims adjudication. Modifiers play an important role in this process. When a modifier is appropriately applied to one code in a pair or to a code for services that exceed the units of service typically allowed by payer edits, the payer may allow charges that would otherwise be denied as bundled or non-covered. Further illustration of the use of modifiers in relation to payer edits is discussed in the Coding Edits section later in this chapter.

The Health Insurance Portability and Accountability Act of 1996 requires recognition of all *CPT* modifiers, but payers may have their own payment and billing policies for the use of modifiers that can vary from *CPT* guidelines. Know and understand their policies. When payment is denied inappropriately because of nonrecognition or the incorrect application of a modifier, appeal the denied services. For more information, contact the American Academy of Pediatrics (AAP) Coding Hotline (aapcodinghotline@aap.org).

Modifiers and E/M Services	
24, 25, 57	E/M-only modifiers
22, 26, 47, 50, 51, 52, 53, 54, 55, 56, 58, 59, 62, 63, 66, 76, 77, 78, 79, 80, 81, 82, 91	Procedure-only (non-E/M service) modifiers
32, 33, 95, 99, EP	Either E/M or procedures

22–Increased Procedural Services

- Modifier **22** is used to report procedures when the work required to provide a service is substantially greater than typically required.
- Modifier **22** is only appended to anesthesia, surgery, radiology, laboratory, pathology, and medicine codes.
- Documentation must support the substantial additional work and the reason for the additional work (eg, increased intensity, time, technical difficulty of procedure, severity of patient's condition, physical and mental effort required).

- Most payers will require that a copy of the medical record documentation be sent with the claim when modifier **22** is reported. Make certain the procedure or progress note clearly reflects the complexity of the procedure and/or the increased time that was required. Report additional diagnoses that contributed to the increased work.
- For an electronic claim, indicate "additional documentation available on request" in the claim level loop (2300 NTE) or in the line level loop (2400 NTE) segment. If the payer allows electronic claim attachments, follow the payer's instructions to submit the procedure note and, if necessary, a physician statement about the increased difficulty of the procedure.

Examples—Modifier 22

➤ The physician required 45 minutes to perform a simple repair of a 1-cm laceration on a 2-year-old because the child was combative and several stops and starts were necessary.

  12011 22 (simple repair superficial wound of face; ≤2.5 cm)

➤ An appendectomy is performed on a morbidly obese 12-year-old. The surgery is complicated and requires additional time because of the obesity.

  44950 22 (appendectomy)

24—Unrelated E/M Service by the Same Physician or Other Qualified Health Care Professional During a Postoperative Period

- Modifier **24** is appended to an E/M code when the physician or other qualified health care professional (QHP) who performed a procedure provides an unrelated E/M service during the postoperative period.
- The CMS has its own system for definition of global periods, and some payers will follow those guidelines or assign a specific number of follow-up days for surgical procedures. (See Chapter 15, Common Surgical Procedures and Sedation, for information on global surgery guidelines.)

  Link the appropriate *International Classification of Diseases, 10th Revision, Clinical Modification (ICD-10-CM)* code to the E/M visit to support that the service was unrelated to the surgical procedure. Do not report the surgical diagnosis code if it was not the reason for the encounter.

> ### ~ More From the AAP ~
>
> For more information on reporting evaluation and management or procedural services in the global period of another service, see the article "Subspecialty Corner: Surgery—The Package Deal" in the February 2014 *AAP Pediatric Coding Newsletter*™ online at http://coding.aap.org (subscription required).

Example—Modifier 24

➤ The physician sees a 6-year-old established patient for swimmer's ear (right ear) and performs a problem-focused history and physical examination. Eight days prior to this visit, the physician had performed a removal of a subcutaneous foreign body (by incision) not involving the fascia from the foot. The CMS has assigned a 10-day global postoperative period to code **10120** (removal foreign body subcutaneous tissues, simple), indicating that payment for all follow-up visits within that period related to that surgical service are included under the code. Many payers will follow the CMS global period.

ICD-10-CM	CPT®
H60.331 (acute swimmer's ear, right ear)	**99212 24** (established office/outpatient E/M)

25—Significant, Separately Identifiable E/M Service by the Same Physician or Other Qualified Health Care Professional on the Same Day of the Procedure or Other Service

- Modifier **25** is used when a procedure or service identified by a *CPT*® code is performed by the same physician or other QHP, or physician or other health care professional of the same specialty and group, and the patient's condition requires a significant, separately identifiable E/M service (**99201–99499**) above and beyond the other service provided or beyond the usual preoperative and post-operative care associated with the procedure that was performed.

- Different diagnoses are not required for reporting of the E/M service on the same date.

- Separate documentation is required for the E/M service and the procedure or other service. Documentation for both services may be on one progress note. The performed and documented E/M components must support the level of service reported and be separately identifiable from the procedure or other service documentation.

- *Current Procedural Terminology* procedure codes include evaluation services routinely performed prior to the procedure and the routine postoperative care. An assessment of the problem with an explanation of the procedure to be performed is considered inherent to the procedure and should not be reported separately with an E/M service code. (See Chapter 15, Common Surgical Procedures and Sedation, for information on global surgery guidelines.)

- When appropriate, modifier **25** may be reported on more than one E/M service for a single encounter. An example would be if a physician performed and reported a preventive medicine service (eg, **99393 25**) along with a problem-oriented service (eg, **99212 25**) in addition to giving the patient vaccines with counseling (eg, **90460**).

- **DO *NOT* USE MODIFIER 25 WHEN**

  - The medical record does not support both services.
  - A problem encountered during a preventive medicine visit is insignificant or incidental (eg, minor diaper rash, renewal of prescription medications, minor cold, stable chronic problem) or did not require additional work to perform the key components (history, physical examination, medical decision-making [MDM], or time) of the E/M service.
  - The E/M service is a routine part of the usual preoperative and postoperative care.
  - Modifier **57** (decision for surgery) is more appropriate. The ultimate decision on whether to use modifier **25** or **57** requires knowledge of payer policies. (See modifier **57** later in this chapter.)

> **~ More From the AAP ~**
>
> For more information on reporting modifier **25**, see the article "Revisiting Modifier **25**: Still Confused After All These Years" in the February 2016 *AAP Pediatric Coding Newsletter*™ online at http://coding.aap.org (subscription required).

Examples—Modifier 25

> A 2-year-old established patient is seen in the office for a preventive medicine visit. The mother reports that he had vomiting and diarrhea since last evening. An expanded-level history and physical examination are performed and the patient is treated for acute gastroenteritis. The work performed for the illness (history, physical examination, and MDM) is documented in addition to the preventive medicine service.

ICD-10-CM	CPT
Z00.121 (routine child health examination with abnormal findings)	**99392** (preventive medicine visit, established patient, 1–4 years of age)
K52.9 (unspecified noninfective gastroenteritis and colitis)	**99213 25** (established office/outpatient E/M)

Teaching Point: See Chapter 5, Time-Based Coding, for additional examples and guidelines for reporting a preventive medicine visit and a problem-oriented visit on the same day of service. Be aware of certain circumstances in which there is no patient co-payment for preventive medicine visits, yet there is for office visits. Non-preventive services are often subject to coinsurance or co-payment and deductible amounts even when provided on the same date as a preventive service.

➤ **A patient is scheduled for an office encounter for excision of ingrown toenail.** The physician takes a problem-focused history from the patient, who has no other complaints; examines the affected nail; and agrees with excision, explaining the procedure, risks, and benefits. The ingrown nail is corrected by wedge excision of the nail fold.

ICD-10-CM	CPT®
L60.0 (ingrowing nail)	**11765** (wedge excision of skin of nail fold)

Teaching Point: An E/M service with modifier **25** is *not* reported. A separate charge for an E/M service is reported only when the E/M service is significant and separately identifiable from the preservice work of a procedure reported on the same date.

➤ **An established patient is seen for evaluation after falling from a tree in her backyard.** An expanded history and physical examination are performed to evaluate the extent of injuries. She has a 1-cm laceration (repaired) on the left forearm and abrasions on her right elbow and right hand.

ICD-10-CM	CPT
S50.311A (abrasion right elbow, initial encounter) **S60.511A** (abrasion right hand, initial encounter) **S51.812A** (laceration without foreign body, left forearm, initial encounter) **W14.XXXA** (fall from tree, initial encounter) **Y92.017** (injury occurred in the yard of a private residence) **Y93.39** (injury occurred while climbing)	**99213 25** (established patient office visit) **12001** (simple repair superficial wound of forearm; ≤2.5 cm)

Teaching Point: Because the patient required E/M significantly beyond the typical preservice work of a minor laceration repair (eg, evaluation of all apparent and potential injuries), a separate E/M service is reported. Place of occurrence (category **Y92**) and activity (category **Y93**) codes are used only once, at the initial encounter for treatment. These codes do not require seventh characters.

➤ **An E/M service is performed on a 6-year-old established patient.** He is given 600,000 units of Bicillin (penicillin G benzathine) by intramuscular injection for strep throat.

ICD-10-CM	CPT
J02.0 (streptococcal pharyngitis)	**99212–99215 25** (established patient E/M visit, office) **J0561** × 6 units (injection penicillin G benzathine, 100,000 units) **96372** (administration therapeutic injection)

Teaching Point: *Current Procedural Terminology* requires that modifier **25** be appended to a significant and separately identifiable E/M service when also reporting the administration of a therapeutic injection.

➤ **A 12-year-old established patient is seen for his preventive medicine visit.** The patient complains of an increasingly severe itchy rash on his hands, arms, and legs for 3 days. A problem-focused history related to the complaint is performed. He is diagnosed and treated for a moderately severe case of poison ivy, requiring a prescription for a topical steroid. He has not yet received his tetanus, diphtheria, and acellular pertussis (Tdap) or meningococcal (MenACWY, intramuscular) vaccines. The physician counsels the parents on the risks and protection from each of the diseases. The Centers for Disease Control and Prevention (CDC) Vaccine Information Statements are given to the parents and the nurse administers the vaccines.

ICD-10-CM	*CPT*®
Z00.121 (well-child check with abnormal findings) **Z23** (encounter for immunization)	**99394 25** (preventive medicine visit, established patient, age 12 through 17 years) **90715** (Tdap, 7 years or older, intramuscular) **90734** (MenACWY) **90460** × 2 units **90461** × 2 units
L23.7 (allergic contact dermatitis due to plants, except food)	**99212 25** (office/outpatient E/M, established patient)

Teaching Point: Medical record documentation supports that a significant, separately identifiable E/M service was provided and is reported in addition to the preventive medicine service. Modifier **25** is appended to code **99212** to signify it is significant and separately identifiable from the preventive medicine service. Modifier **25** is also appended to code **99394** to signify it is significant and separately identifiable from immunization administration (required by payers that have adopted Medicare and Medicaid bundling edits).

CMS Versus *CPT* Guidelines: Reporting a Significant, Separately Identifiable E/M Service and Minor Procedures

The CMS allows modifier **25** to be used when a significant, separately identifiable E/M service is provided by the same physician or other QHP on the same day as a minor procedure (eg, suturing, removal of foreign bodies, endoscopy) but not with a major procedure. (See modifier **57**.) The CMS defines a *minor procedure* as one with a 0- to 10-day Medicare global period.

Current Procedural Terminology does not define global periods, but most commercial payers will assign their own definition of a global service period for minor procedures. Medical record documentation must clearly support the care as distinct or over and above the usual preoperative care associated with the procedure.

26–Professional Component

✷ Certain procedures (eg, electrocardiograms [ECGs], radiographs, surgical diagnostic tests, laboratory tests) include a professional and technical component. The professional component includes the physician work (eg, interpretation of the test, written report). Modifier **26** is used to indicate that only the physician or other QHP component (supervision and interpretation) is being reported on a procedure that includes technical and professional (physician) components.

✷ When reporting the professional component of diagnostic tests, interpretation should be documented in a report similar to that which is typical for the physicians that predominantly provide the service and should include indication(s) for testing, description of test, findings, limitations (when applicable), and impression or conclusion.

✷ If the report of a physician's interpretation is included in the documentation of another service (eg, office visit), it is important that the report is distinct and complete.

CPT copyright 2017 American Medical Association. All rights reserved.

- The professional component is not reported when a physician reviews a test and notes agreement with the interpreting physician or when only a quick read without formal interpretation is provided.
- Some codes were developed to distinguish between technical and professional components (eg, routine ECG codes **93000–93010**). Modifier **26** is not appropriate when reporting codes that distinguish professional and technical components.

Examples—Modifier 26

➤ A physician interprets a radiograph of the foot that was taken at the outpatient department of the hospital and creates a report of the findings.

73620 26 (x-ray foot, 2 views)

The physician reports modifier **26** indicating professional component only because the hospital provided the technical component.

➤ A physician reviews a radiograph of the foot that was taken at the outpatient department of the hospital and interpreted by a radiologist at that facility. The physician notes agreement with the interpretation.

The review of the radiograph is not separately reported. The physician did not perform the medically necessary interpretation and report that constitutes the professional component of the foot radiograph. However, the physician's review of the image increases the level of MDM in a related E/M service.

➤ A surgeon reprograms a cerebrospinal fluid shunt in the radiology department of the hospital.

The surgeon would report code **62252 26** (reprogramming of programmable cerebrospinal shunt) and the hospital would report code **62252 TC**.

Reporting Procedures With Modifier TC

Current Procedural Terminology® does not have a modifier for reporting only the technical component. However, most payers recognize HCPCS modifier **TC** (technical component only). If a service includes a professional and technical component and the physician owns the equipment, employs the staff to perform the service, and interprets the test, the procedure is reported without a modifier. The physician who does not own the equipment but performs the written interpretation and report should report the service with modifier **26** appended to the appropriate *CPT* code. The facility or provider who owns the equipment and is responsible for the overhead and associated costs would report the same procedure code with modifier **TC** appended.

32—Mandated Services

- Modifier **32** is appended to services (eg, second opinion) that are mandated by a third-party payer or governmental, legislative, or regulatory requirements.
- The modifier is not limited to E/M services.
- Modifier **32** would be used when, for example, radiologic services are requested from a worker's compensation carrier, laboratory testing (eg, drug tests) is requested by a court system, or a physical therapy assessment is requested by an insurer.

Example—Modifier 32

➤ A developmental pediatrician is asked by a managed care organization (MCO) to provide a second opinion on a family physician's patient for selected treatment services for autism spectrum disorder (ASD). A comprehensive history and physical examination with high MDM are performed and documented and a report with recommendations is sent back to the MCO.

ICD-10-CM	CPT
F84.0 (autistic disorder)	**99245 32** (office/outpatient consultation)

33—Preventive Services

Current Procedural Terminology® modifier **33** is used to communicate to payers that a preventive medicine service (defined by the Patient Protection and Affordable Care Act [PPACA] provisions listed as follows) was performed on a patient enrolled in a health care plan subject to the preventive service coverage requirements of PPACA and, therefore, should not be subject to cost sharing.

- The appropriate use of modifier **33** will reduce claim adjustments related to preventive services and corresponding payments to members.
- Modifier **33** should only be appended to codes represented in one or more of the following 4 categories:
  - ❖ Services rated A or B by the US Preventive Services Task Force
  - ❖ Immunizations for routine use in children, adolescents, and adults as recommended by the Advisory Committee on Immunization Practices of the CDC
  - ❖ Preventive care and screenings for children as recommended by Bright Futures (AAP) and newborn testing (American College of Medical Genetics and Genomics)
  - ❖ Preventive care and screenings provided for women supported by the Health Resources and Services Administration
- **DO *NOT* USE MODIFIER 33**
  - ❖ When the *CPT* code(s) is identified as inherently preventive (eg, preventive medicine counseling)
  - ❖ When the service(s) is not indicated in the categories noted previously
  - ❖ With an insurance plan that continues to implement the cost-sharing policy on preventive medicine services
- Check with your payers before reporting modifier **33** to verify any variations in reporting requirements.

Example—Modifier 33

➤ **A 17-year-old established patient is seen for an office visit on Monday for missed period and suspected pregnancy.** The physician provides an E/M service with a problem-focused history and physical examination and straightforward MDM. The physician determines the patient is not pregnant and does not want to become pregnant but has been sexually active with multiple partners. The physician then spends approximately 10 minutes discussing contraception and risks of sexually transmitted infection (STI) with the patient. Point-of-care HIV-1 and HIV-2 testing is conducted with negative results. Specimen is collected for chlamydia and gonorrhea screening by an outside laboratory. The patient chooses to adopt barrier contraception methods and acknowledges understanding of risks and benefits.

ICD-10-CM	CPT
Z32.02 (encounter for pregnancy test, result negative)	Problem-oriented **99212 25** (office visit) **81025** (urine pregnancy test)
Z30.09 (encounter for other general counseling and advice on contraception) **Z11.4** (encounter for screening for HIV) **Z11.3** (encounter for screening for STI)	Preventive **99401** (preventive counseling approximately 15 minutes) **86703 33 92** (antibody; HIV-1 and HIV-2; single assay)

    Teaching Point: Append modifier **33** to code **86703** to indicate the test was performed as a preventive service because, although recommended as a preventive service, the test is also used for diagnostic purposes. Modifier **92** is reported to indicate use of the HIV test kit (not all payers recognize modifier **92**).

47—Anesthesia by Surgeon

- Modifier **47** is used when a physician performing a procedure also personally performs the regional and/or general anesthesia. The physician may report regional nerve blocks but may not report anesthesia codes **00100–01999**.

Chapter 3: Modifiers and Coding Edits

- ⚙ Modifier **47** is considered informational by many payers and does not affect payment.
  - ❖ Medicaid considers all anesthesia (other than moderate conscious sedation) provided by the same physician performing a procedure to be included in the procedure.
  - ❖ Other payers may restrict use of modifier **47** to specific procedure codes and provide specific reporting instructions. Be sure to verify payer policy prior to reporting.
- ⚙ **DO *NOT* USE MODIFIER 47 WHEN**
  - ❖ Administering local anesthesia because that is considered inherent to the procedure
  - ❖ Performing moderate (conscious) sedation (See Chapter 15, Common Surgical Procedures and Sedation, for information on reporting moderate sedation.)

Example—Modifier 47

➤ The surgeon performs a nerve block on the brachial plexus (**64415**) and removal of a ganglion cyst on the wrist (**25111**).

  25111 47 and **64415**

  The regional anesthesia is separate from the procedure.

50—Bilateral Procedure

- ⚙ Modifier **50** is used to identify bilateral procedures that are performed at the same session.
- ⚙ It is used only when the services and/or procedures are performed on identical anatomic sites, aspects, or organs.
- ⚙ Modifier **50** is not appended to any code with a descriptor that indicates the procedure includes "one or both" or "unilateral or bilateral."
- ⚙ The Medicare Physician Fee Schedule (Resource-Based Relative Value Scale [RBRVS]) includes a column (Column Z, BILAT SURG) that identifies codes that may be reported with modifier **50**. Procedures with a 1 indicator can be reported with modifier **50**. Many private payers also publish lists of codes that may be reported as bilateral procedures.
- ⚙ When the *CPT*® code descriptor indicates a bilateral procedure and only a unilateral procedure is performed, modifier **52** (reduced services) should be appended to the procedure code.
- ⚙ For Medicaid claims that require use of modifier **50**, only report one unit of service on the line item for the bilateral procedure.

Examples—Modifier 50

➤ A physician performs an incision and drainage of abscesses on both legs.

  10060 50 (incision and drainage of abscess; simple or single)

  Report based on payer guidelines. (See Coding Conundrum: Modifier **50** box.)

➤ A physician performs bilateral computerized corneal topography.

  Modifier **50** would not be appended to code **92025** (computerized corneal topography, unilateral or bilateral, with interpretation and report) because the code descriptor indicates a unilateral or bilateral procedure. (Modifier **52** is also not required for reporting a unilateral service when the code descriptor includes unilateral or bilateral.)

Coding Conundrum: Modifier 50

Current Procedural Terminology® guidelines and Medicaid National Correct Coding Initiative (NCCI) edits require that bilateral procedures be reported with modifier **50** and 1 unit of service. Some payers may require that the procedure be reported with modifier **50** appended to the second code. Other payers may require that HCPCS modifiers **RT** (right) and **LT** (left) be appended to the code.

   For example: Foreign bodies are removed from both ears.

   Report with code **69200 50** with 1 unit, or

   69200 50 with 2 units, or

   69200 and **69200 50**, or

   69200 RT and **69200 LT**

Know payer guidelines and report services accordingly.

51—Multiple Procedures

* Modifier **51** is appended to additional procedures(s) or service(s) when multiple procedures are performed at the same session by the same individual or individuals in the same group practice. The primary procedure or service is reported first without a modifier.

* When multiple procedures or services are reported, payers usually reduce the payment for the second code by 50% because there is some resource cost duplication when both are done at the same visit or session. Medicare and some state Medicaid programs follow this policy.

   ❖ The Medicare Physician Fee Schedule (RBRVS) includes a column (Column S, MULT PROC) that identifies codes that are subject to multiple procedure payment adjustment. The numerical indicators for multiple procedures are

      — 0 Procedure is not subject to multiple procedure payment adjustment.

      — 2 Procedure is subject to standard multiple procedure payment adjustment if reported on the same date as other procedures with indicators of 2 or 3.

      — 3 Procedure is subject to special rules for endoscopy when reported on the same date as another procedure in the same endoscopy family.

      — 4 Procedure is subject to special rules for diagnostic imaging when reported on the same date as another procedure in the same diagnostic imaging family (affects technical component only).

      — 5 The practice expense component for certain therapy services is subject to 50% reduction.

      — 6 The technical component of a diagnostic cardiovascular service is subject to 25% reduction.

      — 7 The technical component of a diagnostic ophthalmology service is subject to 25% reduction.

      — 9 Concept does not apply.

   For more information on multiple surgery indicators and adjustments, see Chapter 12, Section 40.6, of the *Medicare Claims Processing Manual* at www.cms.gov/Regulations-and-Guidance/Guidance/Manuals/Downloads/clm104c12.pdf.

* **DO *NOT* USE MODIFIER 51 WHEN**

   ❖ Reporting add-on procedures (codes identified with the + symbol are exempt from the need to report this modifier because the services are performed in addition to a primary procedure or service).

   ❖ Reporting *CPT* codes identified with the symbol Ø (exempt from modifier **51**) because they have no associated or already reduced work relative value units (RVUs) (see Appendix E in *CPT* for a list of these codes).

   ❖ Different providers perform the procedures.

   ❖ Two or more physicians perform different and unrelated procedures (eg, multiple trauma) on the same patient on the same day (unless one of the physicians performs multiple procedures).

   ❖ Reporting E/M services, physical medicine and rehabilitation services, or provision of supplies (eg, vaccines).

- Most payers identify those procedures that are eligible for modifier **51** and, therefore, are subject to multiple procedure or service payment reductions. Although many claims adjudication systems now automatically identify the primary procedure, it is advisable that the first-reported service is that with the highest relative value, followed by additional services appended with modifier **51**, when applicable.
- Some payers, including some Medicare administrative contractors, have advised against reporting this modifier because their systems automatically assign multiple service reductions to the appropriate services. In these cases, the system ignores modifier **51**. Check payer policies prior to reporting services with this modifier.

Examples—Modifier 51

➤ A simple repair of a 1.5-cm laceration on the left forearm and an intermediate repair of a 2.0-cm laceration on the head are performed on a child who has fallen while in-line skating at the local park.

ICD-10-CM	CPT®
S01.01XA (laceration without foreign body of scalp, initial encounter) **S51.812A** (laceration without foreign body of left forearm, initial encounter) **V00.111A** (fall from in-line roller skates, initial encounter) **Y93.51** (injury occurred while in-line skating) **Y92.830** (place of occurrence, public park)	**12031** (layer closure of wound of scalp; ≤2.5 cm) **12001 51** (simple repair of superficial wound of extremity; ≤2.5 cm)

Teaching Point: Code **12031** is reported without the modifier because it carries the highest relative value (6.74 non-facility total RVUs vs 2.54 for code **12001**).

➤ Incision and removal of a foreign body of the left foot in the fascia and cryotherapy wart removal for common warts were performed at an office visit.

ICD-10-CM	CPT
S90.852A (superficial foreign body, left foot, initial encounter) **B07.8** (other viral warts)	**28190** (removal foreign body, foot, subcutaneous) **17110 51** (destruction of benign lesions other than skin tags or cutaneous vascular proliferative lesions; up to 14 lesions)

Teaching Point: Code **28190** is reported without the modifier because it carries the highest relative value (7.42 non-facility total RVUs vs 3.14 for code **17110**).

52—Reduced Services

- Modifier **52** is used when a service or procedure is partially reduced or eliminated (ie, procedure started but discontinued) at the discretion of the physician or other QHP.
- Modifier **52** is not used when a procedure is canceled prior to the induction of anesthesia and/or surgical preparation in the operating room.
- A payer may require that a letter of explanation and/or copy of the procedure or operative report be submitted with the claim.
- The diagnosis code linked to the procedure reported with modifier **52** should reflect why the procedure was reduced.
- When reporting a reduced service or a procedure code with modifier **52**, do not reduce your normal fee. Let the payer reduce the payment based on its policy and review of the submitted progress note.

Examples—Modifier 52

➤ Evoked otoacoustic emissions; limited test is performed on one ear due to a congenital deformity.

ICD-10-CM	CPT®
Q16.9 (congenital malformation of ear causing impairment of hearing, unspecified)	**92587 52** (distortion product evoked otoacoustic emissions; limited)

Teaching Point: Code **92587** includes testing of both ears. Therefore, modifier **52** would be appended for the unilateral service.

➤ Polysomnography with sleep staging and 4 or more additional parameters of sleep, with attendance by a sleep technologist, is performed on a 7-year-old patient. The study is discontinued after 4 hours of recording.

ICD-10-CM	CPT
R06.83 (snoring)	**95810 52** (polysomnography; age 6 or older, sleep staging with 4 or more additional parameters of sleep, attended by a technologist)

Teaching Point: Instructions for reporting polysomnography include appending of modifier **52** when there is less than 6 hours of recording for code **95800**, **95801**, **95806**, **95807**, **95810**, or **95811**.

Coding Conundrum: Modifier 52 or 53?

The main distinction between modifiers **52** (reduced services—service was started but the physician elected to reduce the scope or even eliminate the procedure or service) and **53** (discontinued procedure—reason for terminating the procedure is due to extenuating circumstances or because complications arise that place the patient at risk) is the basis for the decision to alter the procedure. Modifier **52** is often used when the physician plans to reduce the scope or extent of the procedure as noted, whereas modifier **53** is used for situations such as unexpected events that occur in the course of the procedure (eg, cardiac arrest, profuse bleeding, arrhythmia). The following examples demonstrate the appropriate application of these modifiers when a physician performs a routine circumcision:

52: A physician begins a circumcision (**54150**) on a 3-day-old boy. The physician elects to perform the circumcision without a dorsal penile or ring block. In this circumstance, modifier **52** would be reported with code **54150** to indicate the service was reduced from its full descriptor based on the physician's discretion.

53: A physician begins a circumcision (**54150**) on a 3-day-old boy. During the procedure, the physician notices the neonate is showing signs of respiratory distress. The physician determines that the procedure needs to be discontinued to assess the neonate. Due to the severity of the situation, the physician decides not to continue with the procedure. In this circumstance, the physician would append modifier **53** to code **54150**, linking it to *ICD-10-CM* codes **Z41.2** (encounter for routine and ritual male circumcision) and **P22.9** (respiratory distress, newborn) to indicate why the procedure was discontinued. When reporting a procedure with modifier **53**, it is important to indicate why the procedure was discontinued.

53–Discontinued Procedure

✦ Modifier **53** signifies that a procedure was terminated (ie, started but discontinued) due to extenuating circumstances or circumstances in which the well-being of the patient was threatened (eg, patient is at risk or has unexpected, serious complications, such as excessive bleeding, hypotension) during a procedure.
✦ It is not used to report the elective cancellation of a procedure prior to the patient's anesthesia induction and/or surgical preparation in the operating suite.
✦ The diagnosis code should reflect the reason for the termination of the procedure.
✦ Most payers will require that operative or procedure reports be submitted with the claim.

Examples—Modifier 53

➤ **An unsuccessful attempt is made to place a central line in the right subclavian vein.** The line is successfully placed in the left subclavian vein.

> **36555 53 RT** (insertion non-tunneled centrally inserted central venous catheter; younger than 5 years)
>
> **36555 LT**
>
> *Note:* Some payers do not recognize modifiers **RT** and **LT**. See the descriptions and use of these modifiers in the HCPCS Modifiers section later in this chapter.

➤ **During catheterization of the right side of the heart, the child experiences ventricular arrhythmia and the procedure is discontinued.**

> **93451 53** (right heart catheterization)

54—Surgical Care Only

◉ Modifier **54** is appended to the surgery procedure code when the physician does the procedure but another physician or other QHP (not of the same group practice) accepts a transfer of care and provides preoperative and/or postoperative management.

55—Postoperative Management Only

◉ Modifier **55** is appended to the surgical code to report that only postoperative care is performed because another physician or other QHP of another group practice has performed the surgical procedure and transferred the patient for postoperative care.

56—Preoperative Management Only

◉ Modifier **56** is appended to the surgical code when only the preoperative care and evaluation are performed because another physician or other QHP of another group practice has performed the surgical procedure.

Examples—Modifiers 54, 55, and 56

➤ **An infant undergoes a repair of tetralogy of Fallot.** The patient's pediatric cardiologist provides the postoperative management.

> The surgeon reports code **33692** (complete repair tetralogy of Fallot without pulmonary atresia) with modifier **54** appended, and the cardiologist reports code **33692 55** for postoperative care services.
>
> These split care arrangements will usually require a manual review by payers, with some variable amount of the global fee being carved out for the 2 physicians. Check with your payers for their payment policy if this is typical for your practice.

➤ **A child is admitted to the hospital by the pediatrician for intravenous antibiotics for a deep abscess on the right leg.** On the second day of the hospital stay, a surgeon is called in and performs an incision and drainage of the abscess. The child is discharged on day 3 and seen in follow-up by the pediatrician. Surgeon reports

ICD-10-CM	CPT®
L02.415 (cutaneous abscess of right lower limb)	**27603 54** (incision and drainage with surgical care only)

Pediatrician reports

ICD-10-CM	CPT®
L02.415	**27603 55** (incision and drainage with postoperative management only)

Coding Conundrum: Modifiers 54, 55, and 56

Modifiers **54**, **55**, and **56** typically are used to report surgical procedures that have a global period of 10 to 90 days. They are not reported with procedures that have 0-day global periods. It is important to learn which guidelines are followed by your major payers. When reporting these modifiers, coordination and communication between the physicians and their billing staff is imperative.

57—Decision for Surgery

* Modifier **57** is appended to an E/M service that resulted in the initial decision to perform the surgery or procedure.
* Appending modifier **57** to the E/M service indicates to the payer that the E/M service is not part of the global period. The global period for surgical procedures is assigned by the CMS, private payers, or state Medicaid and not by the American Medical Association.
* Many payers will follow the CMS Medicare payment policy that allows reporting of modifier **57** only when the visit on the day before or day of surgery results in a decision to perform a surgical procedure that has a 90-day global period (major procedure). Know commercial and state Medicaid policies, maintain a written copy of the policy, and adhere to the policy. Refer to Chapter 15, Common Surgical Procedures and Sedation, for more detail on surgical package guidelines.

Examples—Modifier 57

➤ **A 10-year-old is seen by the pediatrician for the evaluation of pain in her foot.** Radiograph reveals a metatarsal fracture, and the decision is made to treat the closed fracture.

The appropriate E/M code (**99201–99215 57**), based on the medical necessity and performance and documentation of the required key components, would be reported in addition to code **28470** (closed treatment, metatarsal fracture; without manipulation). Code **28470** has an assigned global surgery period of 90 days.

➤ **A circumcision is performed on the day of discharge on a 2-day-old born in the hospital, delivered vaginally.**

ICD-10-CM	CPT
Z38.00 (single liveborn infant, delivered vaginally) **Z41.2** (encounter for routine male circumcision)	**99238 25** (hospital discharge management) **54150** (circumcision using clamp/device with dorsal penile or ring block)

Teaching Point: The procedure has a 0-day global period. Per CMS guidelines, modifier **25** would be appended to the E/M service instead of modifier **57**.

58–Staged or Related Procedure or Service by the Same Physician or Other Qualified Health Care Professional During the Postoperative Period

- Modifier **58** is used to indicate that a procedure or service performed during the postoperative period was planned or anticipated (ie, staged), was more extensive than the original procedure, or was for therapy following a surgical procedure.
- Modifier **58** is a recognized modifier under the NCCI. (See the Appropriate NCCI Modifiers section later in the chapter for more on NCCI edits.) Refer to the Medicaid NCCI Web site, http://bit.ly/1mvdrGj, for more details on the proper use of modifier **58** to override an edit.
- Typically, payers recognize modifier **58** only when there is a global surgical period associated with the procedure code.
- **DO *NOT* REPORT MODIFIER 58 WHEN**
  - ❖ Treatment of a problem requires a return to the operating/procedure room (eg, unanticipated clinical condition) (see modifier **78**).
  - ❖ Reporting procedures that include as part of their *CPT®* descriptor "one or more visits" or "one or more sessions."

Examples–Modifier 58

➤ An excision of a malignant lesion (1 cm) on the leg is performed. The pathology report indicates that the margins were not adequate and a re-excision is performed 1 week later. The excised diameter is less than 2 cm.

    11602 58 (excision, malignant lesion including margins, leg; excised diameter 1.1–2.0 cm) for the second excision

    Note: The first excision would be reported using code **11601** (margin diameter 0.6–1.0 cm).

➤ Closure of a perineal urethrostomy, 5 weeks post-hypospadias repair, is performed as planned.

    53520 58 (closure of urethrostomy)

59–Distinct Procedural Service

- Modifier **59** is never appended to the code for an E/M service.
- Report modifier **59** only when no other modifier better describes the reason for separately reporting a service that might otherwise be bundled with another procedural service on the same date. Never append modifier **59** to bypass payer edits without clinical justification.
- See HCPCS modifiers **XE**, **XP**, **XS**, and **XU** for potential alternatives to modifier **59**.
- Per *CPT*, modifier **59** represents one of the following conditions of a procedure:
  - ❖ The procedure was provided at a different session from another procedure.
  - ❖ The procedure was a different procedure or surgery.
  - ❖ The procedure involved a different site or organ system.
  - ❖ The procedure required a separate incision or excision.
  - ❖ The procedure was performed on a separate lesion or injury (or area of injury in extensive injuries).

||||||| *Coding Pearl* |||||||
Never use modifier **59** in place of modifier **25** or on an E/M service.

Examples—Modifier 59

➤ The mother, teacher, and nanny each complete the Parents' Evaluation of Developmental Status. The screenings are scored and interpreted.

96110 × 2 units and 96110 59 × 1 unit (developmental screen)

Medicaid Medically Unlikely Edits (MUEs) place a per-claim line limit on the units of service for **96110** at 2 units. When more than 2 units are clinically appropriate, the edit may be bypassed by reporting 2 units of service on one claim line and appending modifier **59** to additional claim lines. Remember that payers may have different reporting requirements for these services and, in addition, may have different upper limits on the number of units allowed.

➤ Influenza A and B tests (87804) were performed. In this case, the rapid influenza test provides the physician with 2 distinct results.

87804 (infectious agent antigen detection by immunoassay with direct optical observation; influenza)
87804 59

Modifier **59** would be appended to the second test to reflect that 2 distinct tests were performed.

Coding Conundrum: Modifier 51 (Multiple Procedures) or 59 (Distinct Procedural Service)?

Modifier **51** is most often used on surgical procedures that are performed during the same session and through the same incision. This modifier identifies potentially overlapping or duplicative RVUs related to the global surgical package or the technical component of certain services (eg, radiology services). Not all payers recognize or require modifier **51**.

Modifier **59** is used to identify distinct and independent procedures that are not normally reported together but are appropriate to the clinical circumstances. They are typically unrelated procedures or services performed on the same patient by the same provider on the same day on different anatomic sites or at different encounters. This is a modifier of last resort. When another modifier, such as **51**, is more appropriate, it should be reported in lieu of modifier **59**.

62—Two Surgeons

◉ Modifier **62** is used when 2 surgeons work together as primary surgeons performing a distinct part(s) of a procedure.

◉ Each surgeon should report his or her distinct operative work by adding modifier **62** to the procedure code and any associated add-on code(s) for that procedure as long as both surgeons continue to work together as primary surgeons.

◉ Each surgeon should report the co-surgery once using the same procedure code.

◉ If an additional procedure(s) (including an add-on procedure[s]) is performed during the same surgical session, a separate code(s) may also be reported without modifier **62** added.

◉ Column AB (CO SURG) of the Medicare Physician Fee Schedule (RBRVS) identifies procedures that may or may not be performed by co-surgeons. Indicator 1 is assigned to those procedures for which co-surgery is allowed under the Medicare program. See https://www.cms.gov/Medicare/Medicare-Fee-For-Service-Payment/PhysicianFeeSched/Index.html.

Example—Modifier 62

➤ A neurosurgeon and general surgeon work together to place a ventriculoperitoneal shunt.

Both physicians would report code **62223 62** with the same diagnosis code. The operative note must include the name of each surgeon, specific role of each surgeon, and necessity for 2 surgeons. Each surgeon should dictate his or her own operative report. Most payers will require authorization prior to the procedure.

Chapter 3: Modifiers and Coding Edits

63–Procedure Performed on Infants Less Than 4 kg

* Modifier **63** is used to report procedures performed on neonates and infants up to a present body weight of 4 kg that involve significantly increased complexity and physician work commonly associated with these patients.
* Unless otherwise designated, this modifier may only be appended to procedures or services listed in the **20000–69999** code series.
* Use of modifier **63** may require submission of an operative note with the claim. The operative note should include the patient's weight. It is also beneficial to report the patient's weight on the claim.
* **DO *NOT* REPORT MODIFIER 63**
    * ❖ When the code descriptor indicates the procedure is performed on young infants or neonates because the relative value for those procedures reflects the additional work (eg, code **49491** for repair initial inguinal hernia on preterm infant)
    * ❖ With any *CPT*® code listed in Appendix F of the *CPT* manual

Examples–Modifier 63

➤ A preterm neonate weighing 2.1 kg requires a physician's skill for central venous access.
   36568 63 (insertion of peripherally inserted central venous catheter without subcutaneous port or pump; <5 years of age)

➤ A repair of patent ductus arteriosus by ligation is performed on an infant weighing less than 4 kg.
   33820 63 (repair of patent ductus arteriosus; by ligation)

66–Surgical Team

* Modifier **66** is appended to the basic procedure code when highly complex procedures (requiring the concomitant services of several physicians or other QHPs, often of different specialties, plus other highly skilled, specially trained personnel and various types of complex equipment) are carried out under the surgical team concept.
* Each surgeon reports modifier **66**.
* Each surgeon should dictate his or her own operative report and it should reflect the medical necessity for team surgery.
* Column AC (TEAM SURG) of the Medicare Physician Fee Schedule (RBRVS) identifies procedures that may or may not be performed by a team of surgeons. Indicator 1 is assigned to those procedures for which team surgery is allowed under the Medicare program.
* The operative notes are usually required by the payer.
* If a surgeon is assisting another surgeon, modifier **80**, **81**, or **82** would be more applicable.

Example–Modifier 66

➤ Multiple surgeons perform different portions of an organ transplant.
   Each physician would report his or her services with modifier **66** appended to the procedure code.

76–Repeat Procedure or Service by Same Physician or Other Qualified Health Care Professional

* Modifier **76** is used when a procedure or service is repeated by the same physician or other QHP subsequent to the original procedure or service. Use of this modifier may prevent denial as a duplicate service line.
* The repeat procedure may be performed on different days. (Payer guidance may vary.)

⚬ This modifier is appended to non-E/M procedure codes only and is not reported when the code definition indicates a repeat procedure.

⚬ The use of this modifier advises the payer that this is not a duplicate service. (See modifier **91** for repeat clinical diagnostic laboratory test.)

⚬ The CMS only recognizes this modifier on ECGs and radiographs or when a procedure is performed in an operating room or other location equipped to perform procedures. State Medicaid programs or other commercial payers may follow this guideline. Check with payers to determine their policy on use of the modifier.

Examples—Modifier 76

➤ **You see a patient in your office with severe asthma and give 3 nebulized albuterol treatments and steroids over the course of the visit.**

   Report **94640** three times with modifier **76** appended to the second and third codes, or, if required by payers, report **94640 76** with 3 units.

   (The Medicare and Medicaid NCCI manuals contradict *CPT*® instruction for code **94640**, stating that *CPT* code **94640** should only be reported once during a single patient encounter regardless of the number of separate inhalation treatments that are administered.)

➤ **A repeat radiograph is performed following insertion of a chest tube by the pulmonologist in the emergency department.**

   71046 76 26 (chest x-ray, 2 views)

➤ **A physician performs incision and drainage of a cutaneous abscess of the right thigh (10060).** Within the 10-day global period of the procedure, the physician performs a repeat incision and drainage (**10060**) of the right thigh.

   First date of service: **10060**
   Second date of service: **10060 76**

77—Repeat Procedure or Service by Another Physician or Other Qualified Health Care Professional

⚬ Modifier **77** is used when a procedure or service is repeated by another physician or health care professional subsequent to the original procedure or service.

⚬ Payers may require documentation to support the medical necessity of performing the same service or procedure on the same day or during the global surgical period (if applicable).

Examples—Modifier 77

➤ **A simple repair of a 3-cm laceration of the knee is performed by the pediatrician.** Later that day, the child falls on the knee and opens the wound. A physician at the urgent care center performs another simple repair.

   The second physician should report the service with code **12002 77**.

   Remember that the diagnosis code selected must provide the medical necessity for the duplicate procedure. Payers may require a copy of the medical record.

➤ **A physician on call replaces a central venous catheter that had been put in earlier that day by the child's regular pediatrician.**

   36555 77

   Remember that the diagnosis code selected must provide the medical necessity for the duplicate procedure and, at times, documentation must be submitted.

78–Unplanned Return to the Operating/Procedure Room by the Same Physician or Other Qualified Health Care Professional Following Initial Procedure for a Related Procedure During the Postoperative Period

- Modifier **78** is used when another procedure is unplanned and related to the initial procedure, requires a return to the operating or procedure room, and is performed during the postoperative period of the initial procedure by the same physician.
- The related procedure might be performed on the same day or anytime during the postoperative period. (For repeat procedures, see modifier **76**.)
- Link the appropriate diagnosis code(s) that best explains the reason for the unplanned procedure.

Examples–Modifier 78

➤ A pediatric surgeon returns to the operating room to stop bleeding from an abdominal procedure performed earlier in the day.

35840 78 (exploration for postoperative hemorrhage, thrombosis, or infection; abdomen)

The second procedure will usually be paid only for the intraoperative service, not the preoperative or postoperative care already paid in the original procedure.

➤ An incision and drainage of a deep abscess in the pelvis area 6 days following excision of a lipoma is performed.

26990 78 (incision and drainage, pelvis area; deep abscess)

79–Unrelated Procedure or Service by the Same Physician or Other Qualified Health Care Professional During the Postoperative Period

- The physician may need to indicate that the performance of a procedure or service during the postoperative period was unrelated to the original procedure. This circumstance may be reported by using modifier **79**.
- The diagnosis must identify the reason for the new procedure. (For repeat procedures by the same physician on the same day, see modifier **76**.)

Example–Modifier 79

➤ A patient had closed treatment of a shoulder dislocation with manipulation and 2 months later requires open treatment of a humeral shaft fracture.

24515 79 (open treatment of humeral shaft fracture with plate/screws, with or without cerclage)

80–Assistant Surgeon

- Modifier **80** is used when the assistant surgeon assists the surgeon during the entire operation.
- The primary surgeon reports the appropriate *CPT®* code for the procedure and the assistant surgeon reports the same code with modifier **80** appended.
- Payers vary on payment rules. The CMS establishes guidelines for payment of assistant surgery for each procedure code. Most payers, including the CMS, will not pay for nonphysician surgery technicians in this role.
- Many payers require documentation to support the necessity of an assistant surgeon.

81–Minimum Assistant Surgeon

- Modifier **81** is used when an assistant surgeon is required for a short time and minimal assistance is provided.
- The assistant surgeon reports the same procedure code as the surgeon with modifier **81** appended.
- Many payers require documentation to support the use of an assistant surgeon for only a portion of a procedure.

82–Assistant Surgeon (When Qualified Resident Surgeon Not Available)

- Modifier **82** is used in teaching hospitals when a resident surgeon is not available to assist the primary surgeon.
- The unavailability of a qualified resident surgeon is a prerequisite for the use of modifier **82** appended to the usual procedure code number(s).

Modifiers 80, 81, and 82

- The Medicare Physician Fee Schedule includes in column AA (ASST SURG) indicators identifying procedures that may or may not be billed by an assistant surgeon. Indicator 1 is assigned to those procedures for which an assistant surgeon is allowed to bill under the Medicare program. Note that a payer may require use of HCPCS modifier **AS** (physician assistant, nurse practitioner, or clinical nurse specialist services for assistant-at-surgery) for surgical assistance performed by a nonphysician QHP.

91–Repeat Clinical Diagnostic Laboratory Test

- Modifier **91** is used to indicate it is necessary to repeat the same laboratory test on the same day to obtain subsequent test results.
- Modifier **91** is only reported when the laboratory test is performed more than once on the same patient on the same day.
- Modifier **91** cannot be reported when repeat tests are performed to confirm initial results, because of testing problems with the specimen or equipment, or for any reason when a normal one-time, reportable result is all that is required.

Example–Modifier 91

> In the course of treatment for hyperkalemia, a patient had 2 serum potassium determinations (**84132**) done on the same day in the same office. The second was performed after a series of enemas was performed to increase elimination of potassium.
>
>   **84132 91** × 2 units of service

92–Alternative Laboratory Platform Testing

Modifier **92** is used to indicate that laboratory testing was performed using a kit or transportable instrument that wholly or in part consists of a single-use, disposable analytical chamber.

- This modifier is not required or acknowledged by all payers.
- *CPT®* instructs to report this modifier with HIV test codes **86701**, **86702**, **86703**, and **87389**.

Example–Modifier 92

> A 17-year-old established patient is seen for a preventive medicine service. The physician provides an age- and gender-appropriate E/M service including discussion of contraception and risks of STI. Point-of-care HIV-1 and HIV-2 screening is conducted with negative results. Specimen is collected for chlamydia and gonorrhea screening by an outside laboratory. The patient chooses to adopt barrier contraception methods and acknowledges understanding of risks and benefits.

ICD-10-CM	CPT
Z00.129 (encounter for routine child health examination without abnormal findings)	**99394** (preventive E/M service)
Z30.09 (encounter for other general counseling and advice on contraception) **Z11.4** (encounter for screening for HIV) **Z11.3** (encounter for screening for STI)	**86703 33 92** (antibody; HIV-1 and HIV-2; single assay)

Chapter 3: Modifiers and Coding Edits

Teaching Point: Append modifier **33** to code **86703** to indicate the test was performed as a preventive service because, although recommended as a preventive service, the test is also used for diagnostic purposes. Modifier **92** is reported to indicate use of the HIV test kit (not all payers recognize modifier **92**).

95—Synchronous Telemedicine Service Rendered via a Real-time Interactive Audio and Video Telecommunications System

Modifier **95** is used to indicate a service was rendered via real-time (synchronous) interactive audio and video telecommunications system. This modifier is not applied if the communication is not real-time interactive audio and video. Codes to which modifier **95** may be applied are found in Appendix P of *CPT® 2018* and are preceded by a star symbol in the *CPT* manual.

Appendix P codes that may be of particular interest to pediatricians include

- New and established patient office or other outpatient E/M services (**99201–99205, 99212–99215**)
- Subsequent hospital care (**99231–99233**)
- Inpatient and outpatient consultations (**99241–99245, 99251–99255**)
- Subsequent nursing facility care (**99307–99310**)
- Prolonged services in the office or outpatient setting (**99354, 99355**)
- Individual behavior change interventions (**99406–99409**)
- Transitional care management services (**99495, 99496**)
- Remote real-time interactive video-conferenced critical care codes (**0188T, 0189T**)

Appendix P also includes codes for services such as psychotherapy, health and behavior assessment and intervention, medical nutrition therapy, and education and training for patient self-management, allowing for telemedicine services provided by certain qualified nonphysician health care professionals in addition to subspecialty physicians. For more information on reporting synchronous telemedicine services, see Chapter 13, Telemedicine.

For a full listing of codes that may be reported for telemedicine services, see Appendix P in your *CPT* reference.

96—Habilitative Services

When a health plan is subject to the PPACA provision for equal benefits for habilitative and rehabilitative services, it may be necessary to append a modifier to identify those services that are habilitative (ie, intended to help the patient learn and retain new skills and functioning). As equal but separate benefit limitations for habilitative and rehabilitative services may apply, use of modifiers to distinguish services may allow for appropriate claims processing and support the patient's access to the full benefits for each type of service. Not all health plans are subject to the PPACA provision for habilitative and rehabilitative benefits, and covered services may vary. Be sure to verify benefits under each individual patient's plan prior to provision of services. When necessary, append modifier **96** (habilitative services) to the procedure code to indicate that the procedure provided was a habilitative service (eg, speech therapy for a child who is a late talker) versus rehabilitative (eg, speech therapy to assist a child with regaining speech following illness or injury). Some health plans have required HCPCS modifier **SZ** for designation of habilitative services and may or may not adopt the **96** modifier. (See modifier **97** for reporting rehabilitative services. When both habilitative and rehabilitative services are rendered on the same date, append the appropriate modifier to the code for each service.)

Example—Modifier 96

➤ A physician provides 30 minutes of **adaptive behavior treatment with protocol modification for a child with ASD.** The patient's health plan requires a modifier to distinguish this habilitative service from rehabilitative services.

0368T 96 (adaptive behavior treatment with protocol modification administered by physician or other QHP with one patient; first 30 minutes of patient face-to-face time)

97—HCPCS Rehabilitative Services

Modifier **97** is appended when it is necessary to designate that a service was rehabilitative in nature rather than for habilitative purposes. Under the PPACA, certain health plans must distinguish services that are rehabilitative (eg, services to help a patient walk following an accident that caused impairment) versus habilitative (eg, services to help a child with developmental delays learn to walk for the first time). As equal but separate benefit limitations for habilitative and rehabilitative services may apply, use of modifiers to distinguish services may allow for appropriate claims processing and support the patient's access to the full benefits for each type of service. Not all health plans are subject to the PPACA provision for habilitative and rehabilitative benefits. Be sure to verify benefits under each patient's plan prior to provision of services.

> **~ More From the AAP ~**
>
> For more information on reporting modifiers, see the article "When Are Modifiers Necessary?" in the November 2016 *AAP Pediatric Coding Newsletter*™ online at http://coding.aap.org (subscription required).

Example—Modifier 97

➤ A physician provides 30 minutes of adaptive behavior treatment with protocol modification for a child with ASD.

    96116 97

HCPCS Modifiers

The HCPCS modifiers are used to report specific information not conveyed in code descriptors or by *CPT*® modifiers, such as procedural services performed at separate encounters on the same date (**XE**), performance of tests waived by Clinical Laboratory Improvement Amendments (CLIA) (**QW**), technical component only (**TC**), and anatomic sites, such as **RT** (right side) and **E1** (upper left eyelid). Medicaid programs often use a variety of HCPCS modifiers for state-defined purposes. See your state Medicaid provider manual for information on HCPCS modifiers and definitions assigned in your state (eg, modifier **SY** [persons who are in close contact with member of high-risk population] may be used with codes for certain immunizations). Be sure to review the list of HCPCS modifiers in your 2018 HCPCS reference.

Anatomic Modifiers

An anatomic modifier may be reported to identify specific sites, such as right foot, fifth digit (**T9**). The anatomic-specific modifiers are designated as appropriate modifiers under NCCI edits and are listed in the Modifiers That Can Be Used to Override NCCI Edits box later in this chapter. The Medicaid NCCI manual indicates that procedures performed on fingers should be reported with modifiers **FA** and **F1–F9**, and procedures performed on toes should be reported with modifiers **TA** and **T1–T9**. Medically Unlikely Edit values for many finger and toe procedures are 1 (one) based on use of these modifiers for clinical scenarios in which the same procedure is performed on more than one finger or toe. (See the Medically Unlikely Edits section later in this chapter for more information.)

Example—Anatomic Modifiers

➤ A physician must amputate the fourth and fifth phalanges of the left foot.

    28820 T3 (amputation, toe; metatarsophalangeal joint)
    28820 T4 (amputation, toe; metatarsophalangeal joint)
    Note: Some payers may require that modifier **59** (distinct procedural service) or **XS** (separate structure) be reported. Verify coding edits and payer policy before reporting.

X {E, P, S, U} Modifiers

In 2015, modifiers **XE**, **XP**, **XS**, and **XU** were implemented to more specifically identify reasons for separate reporting of procedures or services that may previously have been identified by *CPT* modifier **59**. However, instructions for correct use of these modifiers are still limited and may vary by payer. As the **XE**, **XP**, **XS**, and **XU** modifiers are more specific, payers may require reporting in lieu of modifier **59**. Modifiers **XE**, **XP**, **XS**, and **XU** should not be appended to an E/M code. Do not append modifier **59** and the **XE**, **XP**, **XS**, and **XU** modifiers to the same service line of a claim (ie, single code). As payer adoption and guidance on use of these modifiers may vary, it is important to verify individual payer policy before reporting.

XE   Separate encounter (different operative session)
XP   Separate practitioner
XS   Separate structure (site/organ)
XU   Unusual nonoverlapping service

While accepted by most payers, few resources are available to describe appropriate reporting of these modifiers. National Correct Coding Initiative edits are not yet updated to require modifiers **XE**, **XP**, **XS**, and **XU** in lieu of modifier **59** for specific code pairs. *AAP Pediatric Coding Newsletter*™ will include articles featuring more information on these modifiers as it becomes available.

EP—Service Provided as Part of Medicaid Early and Periodic Screening, Diagnosis, and Treatment (EPSDT) Program

Some Medicaid and private payers require the use of modifier **EP** to denote services that are provided to covered patients as part of the Early and Periodic Screening, Diagnosis, and Treatment (EPSDT) program services required in the state.

* Can be appended to the preventive medicine service (eg, **99392**) or screening services, such as developmental screening (**96110**)

Example—Modifier EP

➤ **A 9-month-old established patient presents for her routine preventive medicine service.** As part of her state EPSDT services, she receives an age-appropriate history and physical examination, preventive counseling, and anticipatory guidance. The patient's father also receives a standardized developmental screening, which is required of EPSDT services.

99391 EP (preventive medicine service, established patient <1 year)
96110 EP (developmental screening)

JW—Drug Amount Discarded/Not Administered to Any Patient

* May be used as a tool to internally track wasted drugs and vaccines.
* This modifier is reported on claims only when required by certain payers. As of January 1, 2017, Medicare required use of modifier **JW** on codes for the unused portion of a drug or biological from a single-dose vial or package when the billing unit assigned to the drug in the HCPCS code descriptor has been exceeded. Medicaid plans may also require reporting of modifier **JW**.
* When required by payer policy, report only when the full amount of a single-dose vial is not used due to patient indications. Report only when the amount of drug wasted is equal to at least 1 billing unit (ie, do not report wastage when 7 mg of a 10-mg vial is administered and the billing unit is 10 mg, as the remaining 3 mg is already accounted for in the billing unit).
* Never report for discarded amounts from a multidose vial.
* Never report modifier **JW** for overfill wastage (ie, an excess amount placed in the single-dose vial by the manufacturer to ensure that an adequate amount can be drawn into the syringe for use).

- Use for internal tracking purposes only (ie, do not report) when
  - ❖ A parent decides to forego an immunization after the vaccine had been drawn up.
  - ❖ The vial is dropped and the medication must be discarded.
  - ❖ A vaccine is discarded due to temperature out of range during storage.

QW—CLIA-Waived Tests

- The CLIA-waived tests are those commonly done in a laboratory or an office.
- One common test in the *CPT*® **80000** series that is CLIA waived is the rapid strep test (**87880**).
- Laboratories and physician offices performing waived tests may need to append modifier **QW** to the *CPT* code for CLIA-waived procedures. The use of modifier **QW** is payer specific.
- Some of the CLIA-waived tests are exempt from the use of modifier **QW** (eg, **81002**, **82272**). To review the list of CLIA-waived procedures, go to https://www.cms.gov/Regulations-and-Guidance/Legislation/CLIA/index.html.

RT, LT—Right and Left Side

- Modifiers **RT** and **LT** are used for information only and do not affect payment of a procedure unless otherwise specified by a payer.
- Used to identify procedures performed on the left or right side of the body.
- Modifiers **RT** and **LT** are not used in place of modifier **50** but may be used in association with modifier **50**.

  Some payers may require that modifier **59** (distinct procedural service) be reported in addition to or in lieu of the laterality modifiers.

Example—Modifiers RT and LT

➤ The physician removes a subcutaneous foreign body from the left elbow and a deep foreign body from the right elbow.

  24200 LT (removal of a subcutaneous foreign body from the elbow)

  24201 RT (removal of a deep foreign body from the elbow)

Coding Edits

NCCI Edits

The NCCI edits were developed for use by the CMS in adjudicating Medicare claims, but they are also used by many private payers, and all Medicaid programs use a Medicaid-specific version of the NCCI edits. The NCCI edits frequently form the basis for proprietary claims software.

  The NCCI edits

- Have been developed based on *CPT* code descriptors and instructions, coding guidelines developed by national medical societies (eg, AAP), Medicare billing history, local and national Medicare carrier policies and edits, and analysis of standard medical and surgical practice.
- Are used by payers to translate payment policies into the claims processing system for physician services as well as to promote correct coding.
- Include 2 types of edits: procedure-to-procedure (PTP) and MUEs.

  New to the Medicaid NCCI manual for 2017 was the following guidance: "Physicians should not inconvenience beneficiaries nor increase risks to beneficiaries by performing services on different dates of service to avoid MUE or NCCI PTP edits." This is likely in response to practice policies adopted by some physicians that are focused on achieving maximum payment. Delaying patient care to avoid code edits could be seen as an abusive billing practice and policies or practices to the effect should be avoided.

Procedure-to-Procedure Edits

⚬ Identify code pairs that normally should not be billed by the same physician for the same patient on the same date of service.

⚬ Include edits based on services that are mutually exclusive based on code descriptor or anatomic considerations, services that are considered to be inherent to each other, and edits based on coding instructions.

  ❖ If 2 codes of an edit are billed by the same provider for the same patient for the same date of service without an appropriate modifier, the column 1 code is paid.

  ❖ If clinical circumstances justify appending the appropriate modifier to the column 2 code, payment of both codes may be allowed.

> ||||||| **Coding Pearl** |||||||
>
> Medicaid NCCI files are published separately from Medicare files at http://bit.ly/1mvdrGj.

Appropriate NCCI Modifiers

Modifier indicators are assigned to every code pair identified in the NCCI. They dictate whether modifiers are needed or will be accepted to override the edit. These indicators are

0   Under no circumstance may a modifier be used to override the edit.

1   An appropriate modifier may be used to override the edit.

9   This edit was deleted prior to its effective date or there is, essentially, no edit.

Modifiers That Can Be Used to Override NCCI Edits

24 Unrelated E/M service by the same physician or other qualified health care professional during a postoperative period	**FA** Left hand, thumb
25 Significant, separately identifiable E/M service by the same physician or other qualified health care professional on the same day of the procedure or other service	**F1** Left hand, second digit **F2** Left hand, third digit **F3** Left hand, fourth digit **F4** Left hand, fifth digit **F5** Right hand, thumb **F6** Right hand, second digit **F7** Right hand, third digit
57 Decision for surgery	**F8** Right hand, fourth digit
58 Staged or related procedure or service by the same physician or other qualified health care professional during the postoperative period	**F9** Right hand, fifth digit **LC** Left circumflex, coronary artery **LD** Left anterior descending coronary artery **LM** Left main coronary artery
59 Distinct procedural service	**LT** Left side
78 Unplanned return to the operating/procedure room by the same physician or other qualified health care professional following initial procedure for a related procedure during the postoperative period	**RC** Right coronary artery **RI** Ramus intermedius coronary artery **RT** Right side **TA** Left foot, great toe **T1** Left foot, second digit
79 Unrelated procedure or service by the same physician or other qualified health care professional during the postoperative period	**T2** Left foot, third digit **T3** Left foot, fourth digit **T4** Left foot, fifth digit **T5** Right foot, great toe
91 Repeat clinical diagnostic laboratory test	**T6** Right foot, second digit
E1 Upper left, eyelid	**T7** Right foot, third digit
E2 Lower left, eyelid	**T8** Right foot, fourth digit
E3 Upper right, eyelid	**T9** Right foot, fifth digit
E4 Lower right, eyelid	**XE** Separate encounter (different operative session)
	XP Separate practitioner
	XS Separate structure (site/organ)
	XU Unusual nonoverlapping service

Only certain modifiers can be used to override edits when the service or procedure is clinically justified, and they may be used only on the code pairs that are assigned the 1 indicator. For overrides of mutually exclusive edits or correct coding edits, the appropriate modifier is always appended to the code that appears in column 2 because that is considered the bundled procedure. To append the appropriate modifier and override an edit, it is imperative that the conditions of that modifier are met.

Modifiers **22** (increased procedural services), **76** (repeat procedure or service by same physician or other QHP), and **77** (repeat procedure or service by another physician or other QHP) are not Medicaid NCCI-associated modifiers. Use of any of these modifiers does not bypass an NCCI PTP edit.

Examples of Medicaid NCCI Edits			
Column 1	**Column 2**	**Modifier Indicator**	**Effective Date**
99460 Initial hospital or birthing center care, per day, for evaluation and management of normal newborn infant	**99462** Subsequent hospital care, per day, for evaluation and management of normal newborn	0	4/1/2010
The NCCI edits preclude any payment for the component code because they are mutually exclusive. Each code represents all normal newborn care on a single date of service by one physician or physicians of the same specialty and group practice.			
94640 Pressurized/non-pressurized inhalation treatment	**94664** Demonstration and/or evaluation patient use of nebulizer	1	10/1/2010
The comprehensive code (**94640**) would be paid and the component code (**94664**) would be denied unless a modifier indicating a distinct procedural service (eg, **59**) is appended to the component code (**94664**). Please note that under current CMS payment policy, both services are reported only if the nebulizer treatment and demonstration utilize different devices or occurred at separate encounters. Please refer to the CMS NCCI edit site for more information (http://bit.ly/1mvdrGj).			
94060 Bronchodilation responsiveness, spirometry as in **94010**, pre- and post-bronchodilator administration	**94010** Spirometry	0	10/1/2010
The NCCI edits preclude any payment for the component code (ie, column 2 code **94010**).			
90460 Immunization administration through 18 years of age, first or only component, with counseling by physician	**99392** Preventive medicine service, established patient age 1–4	1	1/1/2013
The comprehensive code (**90460**) would be paid and the component code (**99392**) would be denied unless modifier **25** (significant, separately identifiable E/M service) is appended to the component code (**99392**).			

Medically Unlikely Edits

The *National Correct Coding Initiative Policy Manual for Medicaid Services* describes MUEs as unit of service edits that were established by the CMS to prevent payment for an inappropriate number/quantity of the same service. An MUE for a HCPCS/*CPT*® code is the maximum number of units of service, under most circumstances, allowable by the same provider for the same beneficiary on the same date of service.

Medicaid MUEs

* Are applied separately to each line of a claim. If the unit of service on a line exceeds the MUE value, the entire line is denied.

* Are coding edits rather than medical necessity edits. State Medicaid agencies may apply payment policy that is more restrictive than the MUE.

* May be established based on claims data. Claims data are also used in considering appeals of charges denied based on MUE.

- May limit units of service based on anatomic structures.
- May limit the number of units of service based on *CPT®* code descriptors/*CPT* coding instructions.
- Are published on the CMS Medicaid NCCI Web site at http://bit.ly/1mvdrGj.
- Are published with an "Edit Rationale" for each HCPCS/*CPT* code.
    - ❖ The MUE value assigned for code **96110** (developmental screening, per instrument) is 2 based on Medicare data. This rationale indicates 100% Medicare claims data from a 6-month period was the major factor in determining the MUE value.
    - ❖ The MUE value assigned to code **96127** (brief emotional/behavior assessment, per instrument) is 2 based on the nature of the service or procedure (typically determined by the amount of time required to perform a procedure/service or clinical application of a procedure/service).
- Are applied separately to each claim line for a service when modifiers (eg, **59**, **76**, **77**, anatomic) cause the same HCPCS/*CPT* code to appear on separate lines of a claim.

It is important to recognize the use of modifiers to override the MUE must be justified based on correct selection of the procedure code, correct application of the number of units reported, medical necessity and reasonableness of the number of services, and, if applicable, reason the physician's practice pattern differs from national patterns.

Keeping Up-to-date With NCCI

Medicaid and Medicare NCCI edits are updated quarterly. Each Medicare NCCI version ends with .0 (point zero), .1, .2, or .3 indicating its effective dates.
- Versions ending in .0 (point zero) are effective from January 1 through March 31 of that year.
- Versions ending in .1 are effective from April 1 through June 30 of that year.
- Versions ending in .2 are effective from July 1 through September 30 of that year.
- Versions ending in .3 are effective from October 1 through December 31 of that year.

The CMS releases the Medicare NCCI edits free of charge on its Web site (www.cms.gov/ NationalCorrectCodInitEd/NCCIEP/list.asp). Medicaid NCCI files are published separately free of charge at http://bit.ly/1mvdrGj. Although many of the Medicaid edits mirror Medicare edits, this is not always the case. The CMS has instructed that use of the appropriate NCCI file is important to correct coding. Online NCCI edits are posted in spreadsheet form, which allows users to sort by procedure code and effective date. Furthermore, there is a "Find" tool that allows users to look for a specific code. The edit files are indexed by procedure code ranges for simplified navigation. Policy manuals that explain the rationale for edits and correct use of NCCI-associated modifiers are published to the Web pages listed previously. Updated manuals for the year ahead are published annually in late fall. Changes in the manual are shown in red font for easy identification. Be sure to update your NCCI edit files quarterly and review changes to the NCCI manual each year.

Practice management and electronic health record software may also contain tools for identifying codes affected by NCCI edits.

Reviewing and Using These Edits

1. Be aware of all coding edits that are applicable to your specialty; as each update replaces the former edits, it is important to review them quarterly. Always look for new or deleted edits. Updated files can be found at www.aap.org/coding under the "Coding Resources, National Correct Coding Initiative (NCCI) Edits" tab.

2. Pay close attention to the modifier indicator because it may have changed from the last quarterly update. For example, a code set that initially would not allow override with a modifier may now subsequently allow one, or vice versa.

3. Pay attention to the effective date and deletion date of each code set. The edits are applicable only if they are effective. The effective date is based on the date of service, and not the date the claim was submitted. Sometimes a pair is retroactively terminated. If so, you may resubmit claims for payment if the date of service is within the filing time frame of the payer.

4. Use modifiers as appropriate. Modifiers should be used only when applicable based on coding standards, when medically justified or necessary, and when supported by medical record documentation (progress notes, operative notes, procedure notes, diagrams, or pictures), or, as previously mentioned, when dictated by payers. Refer to the CMS written guidelines (because they are very explicit about billing surgical procedures) or to your payer's provider manual.

5. When billing surgical procedures, you may need to look at several different codes for possible edits. Be sure to always use the code that is reflective of the total service performed.

6. If you are denied payment for services for which there is no edit, for which a reported modifier should have allowed payment, and/or for which the edit is inconsistent with *CPT®* guidelines, you need to appeal the denial. Having knowledge of how this system works is to your benefit when appealing the denial.

7. Some payers have developed or adopted coding edit programs that are different from and often more comprehensive than the NCCI. If a payer policy differs from the CMS NCCI policy and is not clearly defined in its provider manual, refer to the payer's Web site. Make sure you get policies in writing for the services you commonly perform.

8. Report the services provided correctly based on *CPT* code guidelines (unless a payer has clearly stated otherwise). Remember that these edits are based on Medicare and Medicaid guidelines, and not all private payers follow all of these edits.

> ### ~ More From the AAP ~
>
> For more information on NCCI edits, see the article "Back to Basics: The National Correct Coding Initiative" in the March 2015 *AAP Pediatric Coding Newsletter™* online at http://coding.aap.org (subscription required).

Chapter 3: Modifiers and Coding Edits

Evaluation and Management Documentation Guidelines

Contents

Evaluation and Management (E/M) Documentation and Coding Guidelines

Three versions of evaluation and management (E/M) guidelines exist, including the *Current Procedural Terminology* (*CPT®*) and the 1995 and 1997 guidelines published by the Centers for Medicare & Medicaid Services (CMS). Most Medicaid and private payers allow use of either the 1995 or 1997 CMS guidelines in E/M code selection but include elements of the *CPT* guidelines for E/M services (eg, guidelines for distinguishing between new and established patients).

Current Procedural Terminology *(CPT) Guidelines*

- The most vague of all versions; defines the components of E/M services and provides general guidance on selecting levels of history, examination, and medical decision-making (MDM).
- Includes specialty-specific clinical examples in Appendix C of the American Medical Association (AMA) *CPT 2018.*
- Provides expanded guidelines for topics such as distinguishing new patients from established patients, use of time in E/M code selection, and distinguishing between physicians and other qualified health care professionals (QHPs) and clinical staff.

The AMA clinical examples are only examples and should not be used as a basis for coding patient encounters with the same diagnosis because the selection of a code must be based on the medically necessary services performed and documented and may include clinical variations.

CMS Documentation Guidelines for Evaluation and Management Services

- Two sets of guidelines, 1995 and 1997 (see later in this chapter or online at www.aap.org/cfp, access code AAPCFP23).
- Followed by the Medicare program, most private payers, and state Medicaid programs.
- Go beyond the *CPT* definitions and guidance for selecting levels of service providing specific documentation guidance. For example,
  - ❖ The chief complaint (CC), review of systems (ROS), and past, family, and social history (PFSH) may be listed as separate elements of history, or they may be included in the description of history of present illness (HPI).
  - ❖ Specific abnormal and relevant negative findings of the examination of the affected or symptomatic body area(s) or organ system(s) should be documented. A notation of "abnormal" without elaboration is insufficient.
- The CMS documentation guidelines were based on the adult population because few children are covered under the Medicare program. However, the 1995 and 1997 guidelines state that a history and/or examination performed on a pediatric patient may vary from the adult standard and yet be appropriate when considering the selection of an E/M code. As noted in the 1997 guidelines, under Section III, Documentation of E/M Services, paragraph 5:

"These Documentation Guidelines for E/M services reflect the needs of the typical adult population. For certain groups of patients, the recorded information may vary slightly from that described here. Specifically, the medical records of infants, children, adolescents, and pregnant women may have additional or modified information recorded in each history and examination area.

"As an example, newborn records may include under history of the present illness (HPI) the details of mother's pregnancy, and the infant's status at birth; social history will focus on family structure; family history will focus on congenital anomalies and hereditary disorders in the family. In addition, the content of a pediatric examination will vary with the age and development of the child. Although not specifically defined in these documentation guidelines, these patient group variations on history and examination are appropriate."

❉ The key difference between the 1995 and 1997 E/M guidelines is the examination component. The 1997 guideline includes specific examination elements for a general multisystem examination and for single-system examinations (eg, cardiovascular, respiratory, skin). See more in the Physical Examination section later in this chapter.

Pediatric clinical vignettes are presented throughout this manual. These too are only examples, and the associated *CPT*® codes should not be used for every patient with the same diagnosis.

Coding E/M Services From a Clinical Perspective

The definitions of the levels of service and requirements for each key component (ie, history, physical examination, and MDM) are ambiguous, and the steps defined in the requirements for selection of the code are not consistent with a physician's approach to addressing and treating an illness or problem. A physician does not enter a room and perform first a history, and then a physical examination, and finally MDM. Rather, the key components of an E/M service are performed in conjunction with one another. The MDM typically supports the level of history and/or physical examination medically necessary and is derived from the following obtained information:

❉ The documented CC helps to formulate the presenting problem or nature of the patient presentation.

❉ The level of history obtained and documented is based on the nature of the patient presentation. Concurrently, the physician is forming his or her impression of the problem's severity, possible diagnoses, other factors that require consideration in patient management, and a potential plan of care.

❉ The level of the performed physical examination is based on the presenting problem(s) and history. From the moment the physician observes the patient and while obtaining the history, the physician simultaneously is starting his or her physical assessment and examination (eg, general appearance). Additional history may be obtained concurrently with the examination. While performing the examination, the physician again is determining the severity or risk, need for diagnostic testing, differential diagnosis(es), and treatment plan.

❉ The documentation of the history, physical examination, ordered and performed diagnostic studies, assessment, and plan infer and support the complexity of MDM.

> ### ~ More From the AAP ~
>
> Get a quick reference to inpatient and outpatient E/M codes and key components with the AAP *Pediatric Evaluation and Management (E/M) Coding Card* (https://shop. aap.org/pediatric-evaluation-and-management-em-coding-card-2018).

Categories of E/M Codes

There are 23 categories of E/M codes (eg, office or outpatient services, consultations, prolonged physician services, newborn care). Specific guidelines for reporting codes within these categories are described in detail in chapters 5 through 12. Most E/M codes require the performance and documentation of key components. Those E/M services that do not require the key components as the basis for code selection include those services that are

❉ Bundled as a daily care code (eg, pediatric and neonatal critical care)

❉ Bundled as a period of care (eg, transitional care management)

❉ Based on specific guidelines (eg, normal newborn care, preventive medicine visits)

❉ Based on time (eg, hourly critical care, discharge services, prolonged service)

E/M Code Components

Seven components are considered when selecting the level of E/M service code.

Overarching Component	Description	Components
Key components	Used to select a level of evaluation and management service	1. History
		2. Examination
		3. Medical decision-making
Contributory factors	May contribute to but are not required for the selection of a code. However, they usually affect the extent of the key components that are performed.	4. Counseling
		5. Coordination of care
		6. Nature of presenting problem
Explicit component	Used to select a level of evaluation and management service when time becomes the controlling factor	7. Time

Key Components

Most E/M services require performance and documentation of the key components (ie, history, physical examination, and MDM).

Contributory Factors

Current Procedural Terminology® defines a *presenting problem* as "a disease, condition, illness, injury, symptom, sign, finding, complaint or other reason for encounter, with or without a diagnosis being established at the time of the encounter." This may be better described as *patient presentation* and may include psychosocial issues or ethical considerations determined by the physician or other QHP to require consideration in patient management. The nature of the patient presentation may be more extensive or different from the patient's CC (eg, adolescent girl states her reason for visit is headaches but also presents with anxiety about possible unwanted pregnancy).

It is the nature of the presenting problem that generally determines the level of history and physical examination performed and documented and supports MDM. For example, an infant with high fever and wheezing warrants a more comprehensive history and/or examination to determine the diagnosis or condition than an infant presenting with a diaper rash. This does not mean that all elements of examination, for example, require individual justification.

 Coding Pearl

The nature of the presenting problem is defined by severity, risk, and probability of functional impairment.

Levels of presenting problems are defined as follows:

Nature of Presenting Problem		
Problem/Severity	**Risk of Morbidity or Mortality Without Treatment**	**Probability of Functional Impairment**
Minimal physician supervision required, presence not required		
Self-limited or minor	Problem runs a definite and prescribed course, is transient in nature.	Not likely to permanently alter health status Good prognosis with management/compliance
Low	Risk of morbidity or mortality without treatment is low.	Full recovery without functional impairment is expected.
Moderate	Risk of morbidity or mortality without treatment is moderate.	Uncertain prognosis or increased probability of prolonged functional impairment
High	Risk of morbidity without treatment is high to extreme. Moderate risk of mortality without treatment	High probability of severe, prolonged functional impairment

Explicit Component—Time

Time shall be used as the key or controlling factor in the selection of some E/M services (those that are assigned a typical time) when more than 50% of the physician face-to-face patient and/or family encounter is spent in counseling and/or coordination of care. (See Chapter 5, Time-Based Coding, for more information.)

Key Components Defined

The 3 key components are further defined in 4 levels of service described for history and examination as *problem focused, expanded problem focused, detailed,* and *comprehensive* and for MDM as *straightforward* or *low, moderate,* and *high complexity.* To select the proper E/M service code, the service must meet or exceed the level required for the appropriate key components.

History

The history component includes a CC, HPI, ROS, and PFSH. To meet a particular level of history, all the elements of HPI, ROS, and PFSH listed under each level must be met (ie, an expanded problem-focused history requires that a CC, 1–3 elements of the HPI, and review of one system be performed and documented). **Table 4-1** contains an at-a-glance comparison of the elements of history.

Documentation Requirements and Tips

The nature or severity of the problem(s) should determine the level of history obtained, documented, and counted. *Only the history that is pertinent* to the problem(s) addressed at that visit should be used to establish the level of history in the code selection process.

The CC, HPI, ROS, and PFSH may be documented as separate items or in a summary format.

Chief Complaint

A CC must be documented on every encounter. If the purpose of the visit is for follow-up of a previously addressed problem, the documentation should state the problem or diagnosis responsible for the visit (eg, follow-up of pneumonia).

History of Present Illness

- The HPI must be obtained and documented by the physician. Documentation guidelines do not state this; however, it is inferred. If the HPI is documented only by ancillary staff, it is not used in determining the level of history for code selection.
- If the HPI summarizes the status of chronic conditions, include information such as current medications and their effects, a description of the patient's present condition, and patient compliance with treatment plans.
- Examples of elements used to describe an HPI
  - Location: right ear, big toe, head, right lower abdomen
  - Duration: 2 days, since last night, 1 week
  - Timing: persistent, occasionally, twice a week, recurrent, daily, 15 minutes after...
  - Quality: dull, clear, cloudy, thick, throbbing
  - Severity: moderate, pain scale (1–10), low grade, progressive, improving, worsening
  - Context: occurred when awoke from nap, while playing soccer, fell from tree
  - Modifying factors: took acetaminophen without relief, improved with albuterol treatment
  - Associated signs and symptoms: blurred vision with headache, coughing with runny nose, nausea with vomiting

Table 4-1. The Elements of History

History Components	Description	Elements
Chief complaint (CC)	The stated purpose or reason for the encounter (usually a quote of the patient's or parent's words)	Although not a defined element, a CC is required as part of the history documentation for all levels.
History of present illness (HPI)	Description of the development of the present illness from the onset of the problem or symptom or from the previous encounter to the present; described with 8 specified elements or a summary of the status of 3 or more chronic or inactive conditions	○ Location (specific anatomic site) ○ Duration (period from onset of sign/symptom to present) ○ Timing (number or frequency of occurrences of sign/symptom within the time that patient has experienced the sign/symptom) ○ Quality (characterizations of sign/symptom) ○ Severity (acuteness or intensity of sign/symptom) ○ Context (circumstances or situation in which sign/symptom occurred) ○ Modifying factors (effort taken to change the sign/symptom and its effect) ○ Associated signs and symptoms (other related or additional signs/symptoms) *Alternatively,* Status of each of 3 or more chronic or inactive conditions
Review of systems (ROS)	A series of questions asked to identify signs or symptoms experienced by the patient and to more clearly define the problem to help in establishing a diagnosis(es) and management options	○ Constitutional (eg, fever, weight loss) ○ Eyes ○ Ears, nose, mouth, and throat ○ Cardiovascular ○ Respiratory ○ Gastrointestinal ○ Genitourinary ○ Musculoskeletal ○ Integumentary (skin or breast) ○ Neurologic ○ Psychiatric ○ Endocrine ○ Hematologic/lymphatic ○ Allergic/immunologic
Past, family, and social history (PFSH)	Review of medical/surgical history	Illnesses, injuries, treatments, surgeries, hospitalizations, current medications, allergies, age-appropriate immunization status, age-appropriate feeding or dietary status, pregnancy and birth history (weight, Apgar score), developmental history
	Review of medical events in the patient's family that may place a patient at risk	Health status or cause of death of family members, specific diseases of family members, hereditary disorders in the family
	Age-appropriate review of activities	Living arrangements; use of drugs, alcohol, and tobacco by patient or caregiver; education level; sexual history; domestic violence; other relevant social factors

Review of Systems

The ROS is a series of questions seeking patient and/or caregiver signs and symptoms in some of or all 14 body systems. The documentation guidelines allow this portion of the history to be documented by patients, family or other caregivers, or clinical staff. In the past, the ROS was often documented by the patient or a family member or caregiver on a paper history form. With the move to electronic health records (EHRs), ancillary staff now often enter the patient's responses to the ROS. Although the guidelines allow documentation by patients or caregivers and clinical staff, documentation must reflect the physician's review of the information by confirmation or supplemental information.

❋ See a list of the 14 systems in **Table 4-1**. Note that ears, nose, mouth, and throat (ENMT) are one system for purposes of counting systems reviewed. The ROS also combines hematologic with lymphatic and allergic with immunologic.

❋ Documentation should clarify any conflicting information between the ROS completed by patient, family, or ancillary staff and the physician's documentation of the patient presentation (eg, ROS is negative for musculoskeletal complaints, but HPI says patient has pain in right knee).

❋ The ROS must be pertinent to the problem(s), and pertinent negative and positive responses must be documented.

❋ Appropriate documentation for a complete ROS (at least 10 of 14 systems) might include a checklist with documentation of "negative" or the pertinent response for each system. If a checklist is not used, documentation might indicate pertinent responses and "otherwise negative or unremarkable for all systems," pertinent responses and "all other systems reviewed and negative," or "complete ROS unchanged from previous review dated _____." Documentation of "ROS negative" is not sufficient.

❋ An ROS does not have to be recorded again on a subsequent encounter if there is documentation that the physician reviewed or updated in a previous version. Documentation to reflect the subsequent review might be "ROS unchanged from most recent visit dated _____." (Tip: When history is pulled forward in the EHR from a previous encounter, physicians must attest that the information has been reviewed and updated. Inconsistencies between the history pulled forward and the remainder of the encounter note may fail to represent the patient presentation and level of E/M service provided.)

❋ If a separate patient history form is used (eg, new patient history), the physician must sign and date the form to reflect his or her review. Pertinent responses to the ROS or PFSH may be documented on a separate history form, a progress note, or the signed history form.

❋ If the physician is unable to obtain a history, the record must describe the circumstance that precludes obtaining the history. In that circumstance, the history may be considered as comprehensive. For example, a child is transferred to the emergency department of a children's hospital and her parents are transferred to another facility following an accident. In this circumstance, if the accepting physician documents this limitation and any history obtained from available past medical records or the medical transport team, the history is considered comprehensive.

❋ The distinction between an HPI and ROS is often confusing. The HPI and ROS are obtained for different reasons and both contribute to the level of history performed in the selection of an E/M service code.

Documentation guidelines do not directly state that a comment made under the HPI cannot be counted again in the ROS when it is repeated. However, most coders and payers will refer to this as "double-dipping."

Example: HPI: "abdominal pain for 3 days"; ROS: "abdominal pain." Think about the context in which the information was obtained. If the information was gathered as a description of the development of the problem, consider it as HPI. If the information was obtained to help further define the scope of the problem, consider the information as part of the ROS. Example: HPI: "lower abdominal pain for 3 days without nausea, vomiting, constipation"; ROS: "not associated with eating or exercise; intermittent dysuria; denies fever."

Past, Family, and Social History

Like the ROS, the PFSH may be recorded by the patient or caregiver, clinical staff, or the physician. When recorded by someone other than the physician, the physician should review and correct, clarify, or supplement the information documented as needed.

❋ The PFSH is considered a single element of the overall history.

- Notation of allergies without current complaint and current medications are counted as past history. See more examples of PFSH in **Table 4-1**.
- No PFSH is required to support the interval histories obtained in subsequent hospital care, follow-up inpatient consultations, and subsequent nursing facility care.
- There are 2 levels of PFSH: pertinent and complete.
  - ❖ A *pertinent* PFSH is a review of history area(s) directly related to the problem(s) identified in the HPI.
  - ❖ A *complete* PFSH includes 2 of or all 3 PFSH history areas.
    - — Two areas of PFSH are required for a complete PFSH when the service provided is an established patient office or other outpatient visit, emergency department service, subsequent nursing facility care, or established patient visit in a domiciliary or patient's home.
    - — An item from each of the 3 PFSH areas must be documented for a complete PFSH when the service provided is a new patient office or other outpatient visit, hospital observation service, initial inpatient service, consultation, comprehensive nursing facility assessment, or new patient visit in a domiciliary or patient's home.
- Like the ROS, the PFSH does not have to be recorded again on a subsequent encounter if there is documentation that the physician reviewed or updated a previous version. Documentation to reflect the subsequent review might be: "No hospitalizations or other changes to PFSH since visit dated _____." (Tip: When history is pulled forward in the EHR from a previous encounter, physicians must attest that the information has been reviewed and updated. The PFSH is especially subject to change between encounters, as this history can include changes in medications or encounters with other providers, new illnesses in family members, and changes in the patient's home or school environments.)
- A pertinent PFSH may be indicated for an area that is related to the problem or condition. A complete PFSH may be required when a more comprehensive assessment is indicated. (The whole-person orientation of the patient-centered medical home and quality care initiatives may lead to increased documentation of PFSH. However, physicians must distinguish the medically necessary work of addressing patient presentation at each encounter from work associated with quality initiatives when selecting a level of service for individual encounters (eg, a complete PFSH may be considered unnecessary for an otherwise healthy patient presenting with plantar warts).

Histories Obtained on Newborns and Infants

Histories obtained on newborns and infants will vary. For example, a history obtained on a newborn might include details of the mother's pregnancy, the newborn's status at birth, family and social history, and an ROS appropriate to the age of the newborn. In young children, all or part of the history is typically obtained from the parent and/or caregiver. Obtaining additional history should not be confused with summarization in the medical record, which may increase the level of MDM (ie, increased amount and complexity of data).

Establishing the Level of History Performed

The patient history may be problem focused, expanded problem focused, detailed, or comprehensive. **Table 4-2** lists required documentation elements for each level of history. To select a particular level of history, all the elements of CC, HPI, ROS, and PFSH required for that level must be met.

For example, consider a 13-year-old established patient.
- *Problem focused:* "Here for stomachache. Stomach has hurt for 2 days."
  - ❖ *CC:* stomachache
  - ❖ *HPI:* location—stomach, duration—2 days
- *Expanded problem focused:* "Here for stomachache. Stomach has hurt for 2 days. No diarrhea or constipation."
  - ❖ *CC:* stomachache
  - ❖ *HPI:* location—stomach, duration—2 days
  - ❖ *ROS:* gastrointestinal (GI)

CPT copyright 2017 American Medical Association. All rights reserved.

Table 4-2. Four Levels of History Defined

Level of History	*CPT®* Guidelines	1995 Guidelines	1997 Guidelines
Problem focused	CC Brief HPI	CC Brief HPI (1–3 elements)	Same as 1995
Expanded problem focused	CC Brief HPI Problem-pertinent system review	CC Brief HPI (1–3 elements) Problem-pertinent system review (one system)	Same as 1995
Detailed	CC Extended HPI Problem-pertinent system review to include a review of a limited number of additional systems Pertinent PFSH directly related to the patient's problems	CC Extended HPI (4 elements or status of 3 chronic conditions) Extended system review to include a review of a limited number of additional systems (2–9 systems) Pertinent PFSH directly related to the patient's problems (requires one item from past, family, or social history)	Same as 1995
Comprehensive	CC Extended HPI ROS directly related to the problem(s) identified in the HPI plus a review of all additional body systems Complete PFSH	CC Extended HPI ROS directly related to the problem(s) identified in the HPI plus a review of all additional body systems (at least 10 of 14 systems) Complete PFSH **1 item from 2 areas required** Established patient office, outpatient, domiciliary, and home visits; subsequent nursing home visits; or emergency department visits **1 item from 3 areas required** New patient office, outpatient, domiciliary, and home visits; initial nursing facility visits; observation; initial inpatient hospital visits; consultations; or comprehensive nursing facility assessments	Same as 1995

Abbreviations: CC, chief complaint; CPT, Current Procedural Terminology; HPI, history of present illness; PFSH, past, family, and social history; ROS, review of systems.

- *Detailed:* "Here for stomachache. Stomach has hurt on and off for a few months. Pain occurs primarily after eating, worsening over the last few days. No fever, diarrhea, or vomiting; last menstrual period 2 weeks ago and normal. Takes no medication; no known allergies."
  - *CC:* stomachache
  - *HPI:* location—stomach, timing—on and off, duration—few months, context—after eating, severity—worsening
  - *ROS:* constitutional, GI, genitourinary (GU)
  - *PFSH:* past medical—no medications, no allergies
- *Comprehensive:* "Here for stomachache. Stomach has hurt on and off for a few months. Pain occurs primarily after eating, worsening over the last few days. No fever, diarrhea, or vomiting; last menstrual period 2 weeks ago and normal; no rashes; no injuries; all other systems reviewed and negative. Takes no medication, no known allergies, no exposure to illness, has excellent grades and enjoys school. Family history negative for abdominal problems or headaches."

- ❖ *CC:* stomachache
- ❖ *HPI:* location—stomach, timing—on and off, duration—few months, context—after eating, severity—worsening
- ❖ *ROS:* constitutional, GI, GU, skin, all others negative
- ❖ *PFSH:* medical—no medications, no allergies, no exposure to illness; family—negative for abdominal or headache; social—excellent grades, enjoys school

Physical Examination

Most payers follow the 1995 and 1997 CMS guidelines for documentation and selection of a level of examination. The major difference between *CPT®* and the 1995 and 1997 CMS guidelines is the level of detail provided regarding documentation of the physical examination component. The extent of the examination performed depends on clinical judgment and the nature of the presenting problem(s). There are 4 levels of examination: problem focused, expanded problem focused, detailed, and comprehensive. The following documentation tips are applicable under the 1995 or 1997 guidelines:

- The medical record must clearly indicate the areas and/or systems examined.
- All body areas and organ systems examined must be documented individually with relevant positive or negative findings appropriate to that area or system.
- All abnormal findings must be documented.
- A general multisystem examination or a single organ system examination is not specialty-specific.
- Although it may be a physician's preference to perform a detailed or comprehensive examination at every visit, only the level of physical examination that is medically indicated should be used in the selection of the code.
- Use of a checklist is acceptable. If a checklist is used to document the examination, written descriptions with positive or negative findings should be documented for any area or system related to the problem or complaint.

    A checklist without any specific findings, whether negative or normal for symptomatic systems, does not truly constitute a comprehensive (eg, thorough) level examination. In the EHR, auto-completion features should be used with caution. Documentation fields for body areas or systems that were not examined must be unchecked and all positive and pertinent negative findings should be documented in free text format, as applicable.

- Documentation of "normal" or "negative" or a simple check mark denoting normal examination findings is accepted documentation for examination of an unaffected body area or asymptomatic organ system under the 1995 and 1997 CMS guidelines. However, this method of documentation is only counted as one element when following the 1997 CMS guidelines.

    Example: If a check mark is used to document a normal examination of the abdomen, it would count as one element unless further documentation indicates that, for example, the liver and spleen were normal, no masses or tenderness was noted, and there was no hernia. This more complete documentation would support the performance of 3 elements under the 1997 guidelines.

- Using a line drawn down a physical examination checklist is not sufficient unless the documentation clearly defines the exact area or system examined. Most coders and auditors will advise physicians and physician extenders not to use lines but to define the area or system examined more clearly by using individual check marks or circles.
- **Table 4-3** compares the documentation elements required for each level of examination under the *CPT*, 1995, and 1997 guidelines.

Table 4-3. Levels of Physical Examination

Level of Examination	CPT® Guidelines	1995 Guidelines	1997 Guidelines[a]
Problem focused	Limited examination of the affected area or system	Limited examination of the affected area or system	Performance and documentation of 1–5 elements identified by a bullet (●) in one or more areas or systems
Expanded problem focused	Limited examination of the affected body area or organ system and other symptomatic or related organ system(s)	Limited examination of the affected body area or organ system and other symptomatic or related organ system(s)	Performance and documentation of at least 6 elements identified by a bullet (●) in one or more areas or systems
Detailed	Extended examination of the affected body area(s) and other symptomatic or related organ system(s)	Extended examination of the affected body area(s) and other symptomatic or related organ system(s)	Multisystem examination—Performance and documentation of at least 2 elements identified by a bullet (●) in at least 6 areas or systems or at least 12 elements identified by a bullet (●) in at least 2 areas or systems. Single organ system examination—at least 12 elements identified by a bullet (●) (Eye and psychiatric examinations require only 9.)
Comprehensive	General multisystem examination or a complete examination of a single organ system	General multisystem examination (requires 8 or more organ systems) or a complete examination of a single organ system	Multisystem examination—Examination of at least 9 organ systems or body areas with performance of all elements identified by a bullet (●) in each area/system examined. Documentation is expected for at least 2 elements identified by a bullet (●) of each area(s) or system(s). Single organ system examination—Performance of all elements identified by a bullet (●) and documentation of every element in each box with a shaded border and at least one element in a box with an unshaded border

[a] These examination requirements may be different depending on the specialty.

Abbreviation: CPT, Current Procedural Terminology.

1995 Guidelines for Physical Examination

- The 1995 guidelines are easier to follow and less complex, with no bullet points, and, therefore, are perceived as more "forgiving."
- The level of examination is determined by the number and extent of examination of *either body areas or organ systems*.
  - Recognized body areas
    - Head, including the face
    - Neck
    - Chest, including breasts and axilla
    - Abdomen
    - Genitalia, groin, and buttocks
    - Back
    - Each extremity

- ❖ Recognized organ systems
  - — Constitutional (vital signs, general appearance)
  - — Eyes
  - — ENMT
  - — Cardiovascular
  - — Respiratory
  - — GI
  - — GU
  - — Musculoskeletal
  - — Skin
  - — Neurologic
  - — Psychiatric
  - — Hematologic, lymphatic, and immunologic
- ◉ Examination of 2 to 7 body areas or organ systems is required to support expanded problem-focused or detailed examination.
- ◉ Differentiation between an expanded problem-focused examination and a detailed examination is made by clinical inference of whether the examination of the affected body area or organ system and other symptomatic or related organ system(s) was limited or extended.
  - ❖ Some payers and auditors have adopted a requirement for documentation of 4 elements for 4 body areas or systems to support a detailed examination, but this *is not supported* in any of the documentation guidelines.
  - ❖ Coders will often turn to bullet points in the 1997 examination guidelines that offer examples of individual elements of examination for each body area and organ system to differentiate between limited and extended examinations. Documentation that includes most of the elements listed for more than one body area or organ system related to the reason for encounter is considered extended. Alternatively, when documentation is limited to a smaller number of elements for each body area or organ system, the examination is limited. (This is different from using the 1997 examination guidelines, which require specific numbers of bullet points in some or all body areas and organs systems for each level of examination.)
- ◉ Documentation of a comprehensive-level examination should include specific findings of at least 8 organ systems (based on the 1995 guidelines).

1997 Guidelines for Physical Examination

- ◉ The 1997 guidelines are very specific with regard to the performance of specific elements of a physical examination and documentation requirements.
  - ❖ Specific elements have been developed for general multisystem and specialty examinations. The elements are described under each body area and organ system recognized by *CPT*®. The lists of examination elements are included in the 1997 documentation guidelines (see the full 1997 documentation guidelines later in this chapter).
  - ❖ An *element* is defined as a description of the examination or assessment of a specified site or area. To "count" as part of an examination component, the documentation must be very specific (eg, examination of lymph nodes in 2 or more specific areas).
  - ❖ Pediatric subspecialists, in particular, may find the 1997 guidelines more applicable. However, the 1997 guidelines are favorable anytime an examination is mostly focused on a single organ system.
- ◉ Examination elements for infants and children may vary from those listed in the 1997 guidelines, as common elements of the examination of children (eg, examination of fontanels in infants) are not captured. As previously noted, the guidelines recognize this, and it is appropriate to substitute clinically appropriate pediatric examination elements for those listed in the 1997 guidelines.

Chapter 4: Evaluation and Management Documentation Guidelines

Examples of Physical Examination Documentation

Here are 2 examples of acceptable documentation using different styles.

1. Physical examination: sick appearing, fussy, temperature 102.8°F (39.3°C); head: normal; eyes: normal; ENMT: tympanic membranes and oropharynx normal; neck: without tenderness or masses; cardiovascular: tachycardia; lungs: tachypnea, wheezing, rhonchi bilaterally, subcostal retractions; GI: soft, non-tender; liver and spleen normal; GU: normal; skin: normal

2. Checklist format

Acceptable Documentation of Examination of a Patient With Vomiting and Fever			
System or Body Area Bullet Points	**Normal**	**Abnormal**	**Findings**
Constitutional Vital signs (3) General appearance		x	Sick appearing, fussy, temperature 102.8°F (39.3°C) (weight and height/length documented also)
Eyes Examination of pupils/irises	x		Pupils equal, round, react to light, accommodation
Head	x		
ENMT Otoscopic examination Examination oropharynx: oral mucosa, salivary glands, hard and soft palates, tongue, tonsils, and posterior pharynx	x		Tympanic membranes normal, oropharynx normal
Neck Examination of neck (eg, masses, overall appearance, symmetry, tracheal position, crepitus) Examination of thyroid (eg, enlargement, tenderness, mass)	x		Without tenderness or masses
Respiratory Assessment of respiratory effort (eg, intercostal retractions, use of accessory) Auscultation of lungs (eg, breath sounds, adventitious sounds, rubs)		x	Tachypnea, wheezing, rhonchi bilaterally, subcostal retractions
Cardiovascular Auscultation of heart with notation of abnormal sounds and murmurs		x	Tachycardia
GI/Abdomen Examination of abdomen with notation of presence of masses or tenderness Examination of liver and spleen	x		Soft, non-tender; liver and spleen normal
GU	x		
Skin	x		

What level examination is this?

⁕ 1995 guidelines: This example would be considered a comprehensive-level examination (examination of ≥8 organ systems—constitutional, eyes, ENMT, cardiovascular, respiratory, GI, GU, skin). Documentation reflects specific findings on the pertinent areas and systems.

⁕ 1997 guidelines: This example would be considered a detailed-level examination. A detailed examination in the 1997 guidelines requires documentation of at least 2 elements identified by a bullet (●) from at least 6 areas or systems or at least 12 elements identified by a bullet in at least 2 areas or systems.

This example demonstrates the importance of clear, concise, and thorough documentation. It is not meant to discourage any physician from using the 1997 guidelines because these guidelines are very beneficial for single-system examinations. Physicians may use the 1995 or 1997 documentation guidelines to justify a level of E/M coding. It's your decision.

Medical Decision-making

Medical decision-making typically determines the level of an E/M service because it supports the level of history and physical examination, medical necessity, and severity of illness. Some payers and audit contractors are now requiring MDM as one of the 2 key components supporting the level of service for established patient E/M services in response to conceived issues of overdocumentation of history and examination in EHRs.

The descriptions in the levels of MDM are vague. The ambiguity is deliberate because of the variability within and between specialties. Physicians must use their best judgment in selecting the level of MDM. Medical decision-making is based on the complexity of establishing a diagnosis and/or selecting the management or treatment plan. There are 3 elements used to determine the level of MDM.

☀ There are 4 levels of MDM: straightforward and low, moderate, and high complexity. The Examples of Levels of Medical Decision-making box provides examples of each.

Examples of Levels of Medical Decision-making
Straightforward **Presenting problem:** *one self-limited or minor problem* **Documented management options:** no treatment necessary, rest, gargle **Nature of the presenting problem/risk:** minimal or self-limited *Examples* **Diagnosis:** uninfected bug bite, wart, resolved upper respiratory infection (URI)/otitis media (OM), sore throat
Low Complexity **Presenting problem(s):** *two or more self-limited or minor problems, one stable chronic illness, acute uncomplicated illness or injury* **Documented management options:** prescription drug management versus over-the-counter drugs, rule out allergy, rhinitis versus URI **Nature of the presenting problem/risk:** low *Examples* **Diagnoses:** minor feeding problem, umbilical drainage, stable attention-deficit/hyperactivity disorder (ADHD), asthma, URI, OM, acute gastroenteritis without systemic symptoms, tonsillitis
Moderate Complexity **Presenting problem(s):** *one or more chronic illnesses with mild exacerbation progression or side effect of treatment; 2 or more stable chronic illnesses; undiagnosed new problem with uncertain prognosis; acute illness with systemic symptoms; 3 or more self-limited problems (Although not specified in the CMS Table of Risk, this would be appropriate based on the extent of problems or conditions addressed.)* **Documented management options:** prescription drug management versus over-the-counter therapy, diagnostic testing, referrals, discussion with other physicians, observation or inpatient hospital admission, rule out respiratory syncytial virus (RSV) pneumonia versus bronchiolitis, appendicitis versus pelvic inflammatory disease **Nature of the presenting problem/risk:** moderate *Examples* **Diagnoses:** exacerbation of asthma, increased behavioral issues associated with ADHD, persistent asthma, chronic eczema, cystic fibrosis or diabetes, acute gastroenteritis with mild to moderate dehydration, bronchiolitis, pyelonephritis, abdominal pain, pneumonia, chronic OM with fever

Chapter 4: Evaluation and Management Documentation Guidelines

---

Examples of Levels of Medical Decision-making (*continued*)

High Complexity
Presenting problem(s): *one or more chronic illnesses with severe exacerbation, progression, or side effects of treatment; acute or chronic illnesses or injuries that pose a threat to life or bodily function; abrupt change in neurologic status; 4 or more stable or chronic illnesses (Although not specified on the CMS Table of Risk, this would be appropriate based on the extent of problems or conditions addressed.)*
Documented management options: admission to inpatient hospital, major surgery, invasive diagnostic tests
Nature of the presenting problem/risk: high
Examples
Diagnoses: seizure, exacerbation of asthma with respiratory distress, cyanotic heart disease, RSV with respiratory distress, child abuse, meningitis, sickle cell crisis

---

Documentation Requirements and Tips

Documentation to support MDM may be found throughout a progress note in the history and physical examination portion of the encounter as well as in the assessment and plan. Documentation should include

- Specific findings on examination that support the risk (eg, increased work of breathing, rebound tenderness)
- Elements of a patient's history that support risk (eg, a newborn whose mother used drugs while pregnant)
- That a problem or condition is stable, resolving, worsening, well controlled, or not responding to treatment (eg, diabetes under control, pneumonia resolving, otitis media resolved)
- The diagnoses and/or management options being considered (eg, will determine need for ultrasound)
- An impression, differential diagnoses (eg, viral vs bacterial or differential diagnoses include…)
- The level of uncertainty and patient risk (eg, abdominal pain of unclear etiology, fever with neutropenia)
- Response to treatment (eg, resolved after antibiotics)
- Patient compliance with the treatment plan (eg, noncompliant with diet plan)
- Psychosocial or cognitive factors that increase the effort to obtain information or that affect management options (eg, access to care)
- Support for ordering tests and procedures (eg, rule out urinary tract infection, hydronephrosis on prenatal ultrasound)
- Review of test results (eg, strep test negative, urinalysis shows ++ketones)
- Initiation or revision of treatment plans (eg, renew medication, albuterol as needed)
- Instructions for prescription management, home care, and follow-up care (eg, return for follow-up in 2 weeks, over-the-counter medications)
- Need for consultations (eg, persistent otitis media—will consult otolaryngologist)
- Insight into what the thought processes were that lead to the diagnosis(es) and management options, ordering and/or review of data, and level of risk (eg, patient complains of burning on urination; examination: listless, skin turgor poor; assessment: reflux likely due to overfeeding)

> |||||||| **Coding Pearl** |||||||
>
> Physicians must document the complexity of establishing a diagnosis and selecting the management plan.

Three Elements of MDM

Number of Possible Diagnoses and/or Management Options

Management options are supported with documentation of the problems or conditions being addressed, the patient's progress and response to treatment, and the resulting plan of care.

Considerations	Circumstances That May Increase Complexity When Determining Treatment Management
☀ The number and types of problems or conditions that are addressed ☀ The number of management options that are considered in the treatment of the patient ☀ The complexity involved in establishing the diagnosis and plan (referral, prescriptions, diagnostic tests) ☀ The nature of the presenting problem	☀ There is an undiagnosed problem. ☀ A problem or condition is unresponsive to treatment. ☀ A number of problems or conditions are being addressed. ☀ One problem or condition may have several management options. ☀ The risk of morbidity without treatment is moderate or high. ☀ There is a need for advice from others. ☀ There is a need for ordering or reviewing a number of tests or medical records.

Amount and/or Complexity of Data Ordered and/or Reviewed

Support for the amount and/or complexity of data is found in documentation such as orders for testing, referenced test results, statements about personal review of images or tracings including findings, notes from review of outside records, and notes from conversations with other providers.

Considerations	Circumstances That May Increase Complexity
☀ The number of diagnostic tests ordered and/or reviewed ☀ The complexity of the tests and/or procedures and their review ☀ The nature of the presenting problem	☀ The combination of types of diagnostic tests (pulse oximetry, chest radiograph, pulmonary function test) that are required usually constitutes a higher level of complexity in this category, while performing 1 or 2 tests within a category of service (eg, hematocrit and urinalysis) usually constitutes a minimal level. ☀ Review and summarization of old medical records. ☀ Results discussed with another physician. ☀ Order or review of invasive or complex diagnostic tests (eg, lumbar puncture, magnetic resonance imaging, computed tomography, imaging studies). ☀ Obtaining additional history with summarization in the medical record. ☀ Poor historian or no history. ☀ Problems or complaints are vague. ☀ Obtaining advice from others.

Risk of Significant Complications, Morbidity, and/or Mortality

The CMS defines the assessment of risk of the presenting problem(s) based on the risk related to the disease process anticipated between the present encounter and the next one. The assessment of risk of selecting diagnostic procedures and management options is based on the risk during and immediately following any procedures or treatment. Documentation of specific concerns and circumstances that may increase risk (eg, caregiver noncompliance with care plan) may support a higher level of risk and overall complexity of MDM.

Considerations	Circumstances That May Increase Complexity
◉ The overall risk associated with the patient's presenting problem(s) (ie, comorbidities, underlying diseases or factors) ◉ Risk related to the disease process that is anticipated between the present encounter and the next one ◉ Risk during and immediately following any diagnostic tests and/or procedures ◉ Risk associated with the treatment and/or management options ◉ The nature of the presenting problem	◉ Poor patient compliance ◉ Uncertain prognosis ◉ Increased probability of functional impairment ◉ Need for invasive procedure or surgery ◉ Need for prescription drug management ◉ Need for intravenous therapy ◉ Need for intensive or critical care ◉ Surgical risk factors

◉ The level of risk can be determined by selecting the highest level of risk from any of the 3 categories in the CMS Table of Risk.

◉ Level of risk alone does not determine the complexity of MDM. It is only 1 of the 3 elements of MDM. For example, prescription drug management alone does not constitute moderate-level MDM because it is only 1 of the 3 components of MDM.

◉ While some items in the CMS Table of Risk may not necessarily focus on items relevant to infants and children, pediatricians can extrapolate and apply the relative hierarchy of principles and concepts embedded within the table to their own population of patients.

CMS Table of Risk

Level of Risk	Presenting Problem(s)	Diagnostic Procedure(s) Ordered	Management Options Selected
Minimal	◉ One self-limited or minor problem (eg, cold, insect bite, tinea corporis)	◉ Laboratory tests requiring venipuncture ◉ Chest radiographs ◉ Electrocardiogram/electroencephalogram ◉ Urinalysis ◉ Ultrasound (eg, echocardiography)	◉ Rest ◉ Gargles ◉ Elastic bandages ◉ Superficial dressings
Low	◉ Two or more self-limited or minor problems ◉ One stable chronic illness (eg, well-controlled hypertension, non–insulin-dependent diabetes, cataract, benign prostatic hyperplasia) ◉ Acute uncomplicated illness or injury (eg, cystitis, allergic rhinitis, simple sprain)	◉ Potassium hydroxide preparation ◉ Physiologic tests not under stress (eg, pulmonary function tests) ◉ Non-cardiovascular imaging studies with contrast (eg, barium enema) ◉ Superficial needle biopsies ◉ Clinical laboratory tests requiring arterial puncture ◉ Skin biopsies	◉ Over-the-counter drugs ◉ Minor surgery with no identified risk factors ◉ Physical therapy ◉ Occupational therapy ◉ Intravenous fluids without additives

CMS Table of Risk (*continued*)

Moderate	• One or more chronic illnesses with mild exacerbation, progression, or side effects of treatment • Two or more stable chronic illnesses • Undiagnosed new problem with uncertain prognosis (eg, lump in breast) • Acute illness with systemic symptoms (eg, pyelonephritis, pneumonitis, colitis) • Acute complicated injury (eg, head injury with brief loss of consciousness)	• Physiologic tests under stress (eg, cardiac stress test, fetal contraction stress test) • Diagnostic endoscopies with no identified risk factors • Deep needle or incisional biopsy • Cardiovascular imaging studies with contrast and no identified risk factors (eg, arteriogram, cardiac catheterization) • Obtain fluid from body cavity (eg, lumbar puncture, thoracentesis, culdocentesis)	• Minor surgery with identified risk factors • Elective major surgery (open, percutaneous, or endoscopic) with no identified risk factors • Prescription drug management • Therapeutic nuclear medicine • Intravenous fluids with additives • Closed treatment of fracture or dislocation without manipulation
High	• One or more chronic illnesses with severe exacerbation, progression, or side effects of treatment • Acute or chronic illnesses or injuries that pose a threat to life or body function (eg, multiple trauma, acute myocardial infarction, pulmonary embolus, severe respiratory distress, progressive severe rheumatoid arthritis, psychiatric illness with potential threat to self or others, peritonitis, acute renal failure) • An abrupt change in neurologic status (eg, seizure, transient ischemic attack, weakness, sensory loss)	• Cardiovascular imaging studies with contrast with identified risk factors • Cardiac electrophysiologic tests • Diagnostic endoscopies with identified risk factors • Discography	• Elective major surgery (open, percutaneous, or endoscopic) with identified risk factors • Emergency major surgery (open, percutaneous, or endoscopic) • Parenteral controlled substances • Drug therapy requiring intensive monitoring for toxicity • Decision not to resuscitate or to deescalate because of poor prognosis

Chapter 4: Evaluation and Management Documentation Guidelines

Establishing the Level of Medical Decision-making Performed

• To meet the level of complexity of MDM, 2 of the 3 elements described must be met (**Table 4-4**).
• The number of diagnoses or associated risk alone does not determine the level of MDM. For example, the patient with fever and no findings on examination may require an increased complexity of MDM to try to establish a differential diagnosis or manage the condition (combination of tests or diagnostic procedures, discussion with another physician).
  ❖ The descriptors listed in the CMS Table of Risk are vague and often difficult to quantify.
  ❖ There are no defined parameters for the number of diagnoses or management options that are necessary to satisfy the requirement for each level of MDM.
  ❖ A good guide to follow is to use the nature of the presenting problem in association with the examples listed under the presenting problem(s) in the CMS Table of Risk, with good supporting documentation.
• A common tool for determining the level of MDM is the Marshfield audit form developed by CMS and the Marshfield Clinic in field-testing of the E/M guidelines. Although never officially adopted into the guidelines, the Marshfield audit form has remained the most frequently referenced tool for MDM selection. Points are assigned for specific characteristics of each element of MDM and the level of MDM is that supported by the points for at least 2 of the 3 elements of MDM. The American Academy of Pediatrics (AAP) *Pediatric Evaluation and Management Coding Card* is derived from this tool.

Table 4-4. Four Levels of Medical Decision-making Defined (2 of 3 components must be met or exceeded.)

Level of Medical Decision-making	Number of Diagnoses or Management Options	Amount and/or Complexity of Data	Risk of Complications and/or Morbidity and Mortality
Straightforward	Minimal	Minimal or none	Minimal
Low complexity	Limited	Limited	Low
Moderate complexity	Multiple	Moderate	Moderate
High complexity	Extensive	Extensive	High

Medical Decision-making as a Required Component

For those E/M services that require 2 of the 3 key components to attain a level of service, *CPT*® has never stipulated which 2 key components (history, physical examination, or MDM) are required. Recently, however, certain payers have decided that to obtain medical necessity for a level of service, MDM must be 1 of the 2 key components to reach the level reported. This has been a direct result of the emergence of EHRs and the ease of documenting more extensive history and physical examination. Some payers now compare diagnoses to the level of service reported for each claim. If the payer finds the level of service questionable, it may automatically down-code and require an appeal or ask for records and determine the level of service supported by the documented level of MDM. It is important to know your payers' rules on the role of MDM and reporting the level of E/M service.

> **~ More From the AAP ~**
>
> For more information on key components, see "You Code It!" and "You Code It: Breakdown of Key Components" in the August 2016 *AAP Pediatric Coding Newsletter*™ at http://coding.aap.org (subscription required).

New Versus Established Patient

For some encounters (ie, office, home, and preventive medicine), a distinction is made between new and established patients. *Current Procedural Terminology* defines a new patient as "one who has not received any face-to-face professional services from the physician or another physician of the **exact** same specialty **and subspecialty** who belongs to the same group practice, within the past three years" (ie, if a patient's only practice contact for the past 3 years has been nonface-to-face, such as telephone or online services, the patient would be considered a new patient on return for a face-to-face service). Telehealth services are face-to-face services, even though the physician is present only by audiovisual technology.

The complexity of care required for a new patient visit does not equal the complexity of care required for an established patient visit. New patient codes require that all 3 key components be met, while established patient visit codes only require that 2 of the 3 key components be met, unless coding is based on time spent in counseling and/or coordination of care.

Examples

※ If a physician of a different specialty is covering for another physician (eg, pediatrician covering for a family physician) and has the first face-to-face contact with the other physician's established patient, the encounter is considered new. If a physician is covering for another physician of the same specialty, the patient's encounter is coded as it would have been by the physician who is not available. For example, an established patient for a pediatrician is seen by the on-call pediatrician. The on-call pediatrician should report that patient as established. When a new physician joins a group of other pediatricians, patients who follow the physician to the new practice are considered to be established patients to any of the pediatricians in the new practice because the patients were seen by a physician of the same specialty in the group within the past 3 years.

> **||||||| Coding Pearl |||||||**
>
> If a physician is covering for another physician of the same specialty, the patient's encounter is reported as it would have been by the physician who is not available.

- If the physician has moved to a different location or changed his or her tax identification number, patients would still be considered established if they were established patients before these changes took place.
- When a newborn or child is examined in the hospital (eg, in the emergency department) and is subsequently examined in the office by the same physician or member of the same group and same specialty, the newborn or child is considered an established patient.
- A QHP who may report E/M services is considered to be working in the exact same specialty and subspecialty as the supervising physician. (Medicare assigns different specialty designations to QHPs and does not consider the specialty of the physician providing supervision when determining whether a patient is new. Medicaid and private plans may follow Medicare practices.)

More Than One E/M Service on the Same Calendar Day

Current Procedural Terminology® guidelines specify that one E/M service can be reported for services provided to a patient by the same physician (or another physician of the same specialty in the same group practice with the same tax identification number) on the same day of service. However, if the problems for which the services were required are unrelated, both E/M services may be reported.

- Services are related. One E/M service is reported based on the combined services of both physicians.
- Services are unrelated.

Coding Pearl

If reporting 2 unrelated E/M services on the same day, be prepared to submit a copy of the medical record to payers.

  - ❖ Each service is reported based on the performance and documentation of the required problem-oriented key components and/or a preventive medicine E/M service.
  - ❖ Each service is reported with the diagnosis or condition that was addressed.
  - ❖ Modifier **25** is appended to the second service to indicate a significant, separately identifiable service was performed.
    - — National Correct Coding Initiative (NCCI) edits developed for the CMS Medicare program may have edits or coding pairs that will require the use of modifier **25** on a particular E/M service to override the edit. (See Chapter 6, Preventive Services, and Chapter 7, Evaluation and Management Services in the Office, Outpatient, Home, or Nursing Facility Setting, for examples.)
    - — Prior to reporting 2 E/M services on the same day of service for the same patient, check NCCI edits. (See Chapter 3, Modifiers and Coding Edits, to learn about the NCCI.)

Be prepared to submit a copy of the medical record to payers.

Split/Shared E/M Services

A split/shared E/M service is one in which a physician and a QHP from the same group practice each personally perform a medically necessary and substantive portion of one or more face-to-face E/M encounters on the same date. A portion of the key components of the service must be provided face-to-face by the physician to report under the physician's National Provider Identifier (NPI). Split/shared services were defined and implemented for services to Medicare beneficiaries. Private payers may adopt the same or a similar policy. The split/shared concept is applied differently for inpatient services than for services in the office or clinic setting.

- In the office or clinic setting, split/shared E/M services must meet incident-to requirements for the service to be reported under the physician's NPI. Incident-to services require the physician's presence in the office suite at the time of the QHP service and that the QHP provides care only in accordance with a physician's established care plan for the patient. See Chapter 14, Allied Health and Clinical Staff Services, for more information on incident-to services.

Chapter 4: Evaluation and Management Documentation Guidelines

Example

The patient history and a portion of the examination are provided in the office by a nurse practitioner for an established patient in continuation of a physician's previously documented plan of care for irritable bowel syndrome. The physician is consulted about concerns regarding increased GI symptoms, sees the patient face-to-face, performs a more detailed examination, and documents the assessment and plan of care. The total service may be reported under the physician's NPI because incident-to provisions have been met and both professionals provided face-to-face services.

❋ Split/shared services provided in the emergency department, outpatient departments, observation, or inpatient floor/unit of a facility may be reported by the physician (which may result in higher payment) or the QHP. This often occurs when the QHP and physician provide face-to-face hospital visits at different times on the same date.

　The following conditions apply to all split/shared services:

❋ The physician and QHP must document and sign their portion of the service. A physician cannot merely sign off on the documentation of the QHP's work.

❋ If the E/M service is reported based on counseling and/or coordination of care, only the physician's time is used to select the level of service. The physician must document his or her total time spent in counseling and/or coordination of care and a summary of the issues discussed or coordination of care provided. (See Chapter 5, Time-Based Coding, for more on time-based E/M services.)

❋ Critical care is never a split/shared service because critical care services reflect the work of only one individual.

❋ Split/shared billing does not apply in the nursing or skilled nursing facility settings.

More E/M Documentation and Coding Tips

❋ When using an EHR system, it is important that the documentation for each encounter is unique and reflects the purpose and activity of that encounter. Use of documentation features, such as carryforward of prior history, copy and paste, and auto-completion, may lead to inaccurate documentation and wrong code assignment. (See Coding Conundrum: Pitfalls of EHR Coding in Chapter 18, Preventing Fraud and Abuse: Compliance, Audits, and Paybacks, for more on this topic.)

❋ Ideally, physicians in a group practice should be consistent in their documentation policies. However, if documentation practices differ between physicians, have those differences documented in the practice's written policies.

❋ The code selected for a new patient will often be one level lower than for an established patient for the same amount of work. However, the Medicare relative value units are higher for new patient visits, compensating the physician for the extra work required.

❋ The AAP has developed forms that promote good documentation of office or outpatient visits. Examples can be ordered from the AAP by calling 888/227-1770 or visiting http://shop.aap.org/Pediatric-Documentation-Forms-Economy-Package.

Guidelines for Reporting E/M Services Under Teaching Physician Guidelines

❋ A teaching physician may bill for resident or fellow services if the teaching physician personally performs the key components (history, physical examination, and MDM) of the service, performs the key components jointly with a resident, or personally observes the resident performing the key or critical components.

❋ The level of service billed will be dependent on the level of work performed and documented by the resident and the teaching physician in combination or by the teaching physician if seen independent of the resident.

❋ The teaching physician must document that he or she personally performed the service or was physically present (in the same room as the patient) during the key or critical portions of the service performed by the resident and participated in the management of the patient. The selected key or critical portion of the visit is at the discretion of the physician.

* Medical students and other students (eg, physician assistants in training) are not considered or treated as interns or residents. Therefore, the only student documentation that may be used for billing purposes is the ROS and/or PFSH. Any other documentation recorded by a student cannot be used in the selection of the E/M code. The teaching physician must verify and personally document the HPI, indicate review of the ROS and PFSH, and perform and document the physical examination, assessment, and plan.

* Time-based services (eg, face-to-face prolonged services, critical care, hospital discharge management) can only be billed when the teaching physician is present for the time required by the description of service. This also applies to E/M visits when time is considered the key component in the selection of the E/M code (>50% of the total face-to-face visit was spent counseling and/or coordinating care). The total time spent by the teaching physician must be documented.

* The teaching physician must document the key or critical part of the service personally performed, link his or her documentation back to the resident's note, and document that the care plan was reviewed and approved. It is not necessary to repeat the resident's documentation. However, the teaching physician documentation must be linked to the resident's note and all exceptions to the resident's findings must be documented. A signature alone is not acceptable documentation.

* Medicare guidelines stipulate that when documenting in an EHR, the teaching physician may use a macro (eg, predetermined text) as the required personal documentation if it is personally entered by the teaching physician. The resident or teaching physician must enter customized information to support medical necessity. If the resident and teaching physician use macros, the documentation is not sufficient.

Examples

* The resident admits a 2-month-old at 10:30 pm. The teaching physician's initial visit is performed the following morning at 8:00 am. The teaching physician reports an initial hospital care service based on the work personally performed that morning. See Chapter 10 for more information on reporting inpatient teaching physician services.

* The teaching physician sees the same patient for follow-up inpatient care subsequent to the resident's visit.

* The teaching physician and resident jointly admit or perform a subsequent visit on the same patient.

* The teaching physician performs the subsequent inpatient visit jointly with the resident.

Unacceptable	Minimal Documentation Required
Countersignature	"I performed a history and physical exam of the patient. Findings are consistent with Resident's note. Discussed patient's management with Resident and agree with his documented findings and plan of care." Signature
"Agree with above." Signature "Rounded, reviewed, agree." Signature	"I saw and evaluated the patient. I agree with the findings and the plan of care as documented in Resident's note." Signature
"Patient seen with resident and evaluated." Signature "Seen and agree." Signature	"I saw the patient with Resident and agree with Resident's findings and plans as written." Signature
"Discussed with resident." Signature	"I was present with Resident during the history and exam. I discussed the case with Resident and agree with the findings and plan as documented in Resident's note." Signature

Chapter 4: Evaluation and Management Documentation Guidelines

Primary Care Exception Rule

The primary care exception rule (PCER) in the teaching physician guidelines allows teaching physicians to bill for services provided by residents under their supervision who have completed at least 6 months of approved graduate medical education (GME).

◉ To qualify for this exception, services must be provided in a teaching hospital ambulatory care center or clinic. If the services are provided outside a hospital, there must be a written agreement with the teaching hospital that includes a contract outlining the payment for the teaching services or written documentation that the services will be "donated." In general, this exception cannot be applied in a private physician's office.

◉ Preventive medicine visit codes are not included in the Medicare exception at this time. Some state Medicaid programs have granted the exemption for preventive medicine services to established patients.

◉ No more than 4 residents can be supervised at a time by a teaching physician. This may include residents with fewer than 6 months in a GME-approved residency program in the mix of 4 residents under the teaching physician's supervision. However, the teaching physician must be physically present for the critical or key portions of services furnished by the resident with fewer than 6 months in a GME-approved residency program. That is, the primary care exception does not apply in the case of the resident with fewer than 6 months in a GME-approved residency program.

◉ Patients seen should consider this practice as their primary location for health care.

◉ The teaching physician

   ❖ Must be physically present in the clinic or office and immediately available to the residents and may not have other responsibilities (including supervising other personnel or seeing patients).

   ❖ Must review the care provided (history, findings on physical examination, assessment, and treatment plan) during or immediately after each visit. The documentation must reflect the teaching physician's participation in the review and direction of the services performed.

   ❖ May only report codes **99201–99203** for new patient visits or **99211–99213** for established patient visits. If a higher-level E/M service is necessary and performed, the teaching physician must personally participate in the care of the patient as outlined in the guidelines. As always, code selection is based on the E/M code descriptions and documentation guidelines.

>
> ||||||||| **Coding Pearl** |||||||
>
> Preventive medicine visit codes are not included in the Medicare primary care exception rule at this time despite continued advocacy from the American Academy of Pediatrics.

The AAP continues to advocate for the preventive medicine service codes (**99381–99385** and **99391–99395**) to be included under the PCER. In some instances, state Medicaid plans already consider preventive medicine service codes as part of their primary care exception, so be sure to check with your payers. Look for updates in *AAP Pediatric Coding Newsletter*™.

You can access the updated guidelines addressing the PCER at www.aap.org/cfp (access code AAPCFP23) or https://www.cms.gov/Regulations-and-Guidance/Guidance/Transmittals/downloads/R2247CP.pdf.

Example

◉ **The teaching physician is supervising the resident in the clinic under the primary care exception.** A child is diagnosed with acute otitis media. An expanded-level history and physical examination are performed with MDM of low complexity.

Unacceptable	Acceptable
Countersignature	"I reviewed Resident's note and agree with Resident's findings and plans as written." Signature "I reviewed Resident's note and agree but will refer to ENT for consultation." Signature

Reporting Procedures Under Teaching Physician Guidelines

Refer to Chapter 1, New and Revised *CPT*® Codes for 2018, for the teaching physician guidelines for billing surgical, high-risk, or other complex procedures.

1995 Documentation Guidelines for Evaluation and Management Services

I. Introduction

What is documentation and why is it important?

Medical record documentation is required to record pertinent facts, findings, and observations about an individual's health history including past and present illnesses, examinations, tests, treatments, and outcomes. The medical record chronologically documents the care of the patient and is an important element contributing to high-quality care. The medical record facilitates

- The ability of the physician and other health care professionals to evaluate and plan the patient's immediate treatment, and to monitor his/her health care over time
- Communication and continuity of care among physicians and other health care professionals involved in the patient's care
- Accurate and timely claims review and payment
- Appropriate utilization review and quality of care evaluations
- Collection of data that may be useful for research and education

An appropriately documented medical record can reduce many of the "hassles" associated with claims processing and may serve as a legal document to verify the care provided, if necessary.

What do payers want and why?

Because payers have a contractual obligation to enrollees, they may require reasonable documentation that services are consistent with the insurance coverage provided. They may request information to validate

- The site of service
- The medical necessity and appropriateness of the diagnostic and/or therapeutic services provided
- That services provided have been accurately reported

II. General Principles of Medical Record Documentation

The principles of documentation listed below are applicable to all types of medical and surgical services in all settings. For E/M services, the nature and amount of physician work and documentation varies by type of service, place of service, and the patient's status. The general principles listed below may be modified to account for these variable circumstances in providing E/M services.

1. The medical record should be complete and legible.
2. The documentation of each patient encounter should include
   - Reason for the encounter and relevant history, physical examination findings, and prior diagnostic test results
   - Assessment, clinical impression, or diagnosis
   - Plan for care
   - Date and legible identity of the observer
3. If not documented, the rationale for ordering diagnostic and other ancillary services should be easily inferred.
4. Past and present diagnoses should be accessible to the treating and/or consulting physician.
5. Appropriate health risk factors should be identified.
6. The patient's progress, response to and changes in treatment, and revision of diagnosis should be documented.
7. The *CPT* and *ICD-10-CM* codes reported on the health insurance claim form or billing statement should be supported by the documentation in the medical record.

III. Documentation of E/M Services

This publication provides definitions and documentation guidelines for the three key components of E/M services and for visits that consist predominantly of counseling or coordination of care. The three key components—history, examination, and medical decision making—appear in the descriptors for office and other outpatient services, hospital observation services, hospital inpatient services, consultations, emergency department services, nursing facility services, domiciliary care services, and home services. While some of the text of *CPT* has been repeated in this publication, the reader should refer to *CPT* for the complete descriptors for E/M services and instructions for selecting a level of service. **Documentation guidelines are identified by the symbol •DG.**

The descriptors for the levels of E/M services recognize seven components that are used in defining the levels of E/M services. These components are

* History
* Examination
* Medical decision making
* Counseling
* Coordination of care
* Nature of presenting problem
* Time

The first three of these components (ie, history, examination, and medical decision making) are the **key** components in selecting the level of E/M services. An exception to this rule is the case of visits that consist predominantly of counseling or coordination of care; for these services time is the key or controlling factor to qualify for a particular level of E/M service.

For certain groups of patients, the recorded information may vary slightly from that described here. Specifically, the medical records of infants, children, adolescents, and pregnant women may have additional or modified information recorded in each history and examination area.

As an example, newborn records may include under history of the present illness (HPI) the details of mother's pregnancy and the infant's status at birth; social history will focus on family structure; family history will focus on congenital anomalies and hereditary disorders in the family. In addition, information on growth and development and/or nutrition will be recorded. Although not specifically defined in these documentation guidelines, these patient group variations on history and examination are appropriate.

A. Documentation of History

The levels of E/M services are based on four types of history (problem focused, expanded problem focused, detailed, and comprehensive.) Each type of history includes some or all of the following elements:

* Chief complaint (CC)
* History of present illness (HPI)
* Review of systems (ROS)
* Past, family, and/or social history (PFSH)

The extent of history of present illness; review of systems; and past, family, and/or social history that is obtained and documented is dependent upon clinical judgment and the nature of the presenting problem(s).

The chart below shows the progression of the elements required for each type of history. To qualify for a given type of history, **all three elements in the table must be met.** (A chief complaint is indicated at all levels.)

History of Present Illness (HPI)	Review of Systems (ROS)	Past, Family, and/or Social History (PFSH)	Type of History
Brief	N/A	N/A	Problem focused
Brief	Problem pertinent	N/A	Expanded problem focused
Extended	Extended	Pertinent	Detailed
Extended	Complete	Complete	Comprehensive

•*DG:* *The CC, ROS, and PFSH may be listed as separate elements of history, or they may be included in the description of the history of the present illness.*

•*DG:* *A ROS and/or a PFSH obtained during an earlier encounter does not need to be rerecorded if there is evidence that the physician reviewed and updated the previous information. This may occur when a physician updates his or her own record or in an institutional setting or group practice where many physicians use a common record. The review and update may be documented by*

  ● *Describing any new ROS and/or PFSH information or noting there has been no change in the information*

  ● *Noting the date and location of the earlier ROS and/or PFSH*

•*DG:* *The ROS and/or PFSH may be recorded by ancillary staff or on a form completed by the patient. To document that the physician reviewed the information, there must be a notation supplementing or confirming the information recorded by others.*

•*DG:* *If the physician is unable to obtain a history from the patient or other source, the record should describe the patient's condition or other circumstance that precludes obtaining a history.*

Definitions and specific documentation guidelines for each of the elements of history are listed below.

Chief Complaint (CC)

The CC is a concise statement describing the symptom, problem, condition, diagnosis, physician-recommended return, or other factor that is the reason for the encounter.

•*DG:* *The medical record should clearly reflect the chief complaint.*

History of Present Illness (HPI)

The HPI is a chronological description of the development of the patient's present illness from the first sign and/or symptom or from the previous encounter to the present. It includes the following elements:

● Location
● Quality
● Severity
● Duration
● Timing
● Context
● Modifying factors
● Associated signs and symptoms

Brief and **extended** HPIs are distinguished by the amount of detail needed to accurately characterize the clinical problem(s).

A **brief** HPI consists of one to three elements of the HPI.

•*DG:* *The medical record should describe one to three elements of the present illness (HPI).*

An **extended** HPI consists of four or more elements of the HPI.

•*DG:* *The medical record should describe four or more elements of the present illness (HPI) or associated co-morbidities.*

Review of Systems (ROS)

A ROS is an inventory of body systems obtained through a series of questions seeking to identify signs and/or symptoms that the patient may be experiencing or has experienced.

For purposes of ROS, the following systems are recognized:

● Constitutional symptoms (eg, fever, weight loss)
● Eyes
● Ears, nose, mouth, throat
● Cardiovascular
● Respiratory
● Gastrointestinal
● Genitourinary
● Musculoskeletal

- Integumentary (skin and/or breast)
- Neurological
- Psychiatric
- Endocrine
- Hematologic/lymphatic
- Allergic/immunologic

A **problem-pertinent** ROS inquires about the system directly related to the problem(s) identified in the HPI.

•**DG:** *The patient's positive responses and pertinent negatives for the system related to the problem should be documented.*

An **extended** ROS inquires about the system directly related to the problem(s) identified in the HPI and a limited number of additional systems.

•**DG:** *The patient's positive responses and pertinent negatives for two to nine systems should be documented.*

A **complete** ROS inquires about the system(s) directly related to the problem(s) identified in the HPI plus all additional body systems.

•**DG:** *At least 10 organ systems must be reviewed. Those systems with positive or pertinent negative responses must be individually documented. For the remaining systems, a notation indicating all other systems are negative is permissible. In the absence of such a notation, at least 10 systems must be individually documented.*

Past, Family, and/or Social History (PFSH)

The PFSH consists of a review of three areas

- Past history (the patient's past experiences with illnesses, operations, injuries, and treatments)
- Family history (a review of medical events in the patient's family, including diseases that may be hereditary or place the patient at risk)
- Social history (an age-appropriate review of past and current activities)

For the categories of subsequent hospital care, follow-up inpatient consultations and subsequent nursing facility care, *CPT* requires only an "interval" history. It is not necessary to record information about the PFSH.

A **pertinent** PFSH is a review of the history area(s) directly related to the problem(s) identified in the HPI.

•**DG:** *At least one specific item from **any** of the three history areas must be documented for a pertinent PFSH.*

A *complete* PFSH is a review of two or all three of the PFSH history areas, depending on the category of the E/M service. A review of all three history areas is required for services that by their nature include a comprehensive assessment or reassessment of the patient. A review of two of the three history areas is sufficient for other services.

•**DG:** *At least one specific item from **two** of the three history areas must be documented for a complete PFSH for the following categories of E/M services: office or other outpatient services, established patient; emergency department; subsequent nursing facility care; domiciliary care, established patient; and home care, established patient.*

•**DG:** *At least one specific item from **each** of the three history areas must be documented for a complete PFSH for the following categories of E/M services: office or other outpatient services, new patient; hospital observation services; hospital inpatient services, initial care; consultations; comprehensive nursing facility assessments; domiciliary care, new patient; and home care, new patient.*

B. Documentation of Examination

The levels of E/M services are based on four types of examination that are defined as follows:

- **Problem Focused**—a limited examination of the affected body area or organ system.
- **Expanded Problem Focused**—a limited examination of the affected body area or organ system and other symptomatic or related organ system(s).

◈ **Detailed**—an extended examination of the affected body area(s) and other symptomatic or related organ system(s).

◈ **Comprehensive**—a general multisystem examination or complete examination of a single organ system.

For purposes of examination, the following **body areas** are recognized:

◈ Head, including face

◈ Neck

◈ Chest, including breasts and axillae

◈ Abdomen

◈ Genitalia, groin, buttocks

◈ Back, including spine

◈ Each extremity

For purposes of examination, the following **organ systems** are recognized:

◈ Constitutional (eg, vital signs, general appearance)

◈ Eyes

◈ Ears, nose, mouth, throat

◈ Cardiovascular

◈ Respiratory

◈ Gastrointestinal

◈ Genitourinary

◈ Musculoskeletal

◈ Skin

◈ Neurological

◈ Psychiatric

◈ Hematologic/lymphatic/immunologic

The extent of examinations performed and documented is dependent upon clinical judgment and the nature of the presenting problem(s). They range from limited examinations of single body areas to general multisystem or complete single organ system examinations.

•*DG:* *Specific abnormal and relevant negative findings of the examination of the affected or symptomatic body area(s) or organ system(s) should be documented. A notation of "abnormal" without elaboration is insufficient.*

•*DG:* *Abnormal or unexpected findings of the examination of the unaffected or asymptomatic body area(s) or organ system(s) should be described.*

•*DG:* *A brief statement or notation indicating "negative" or "normal" is sufficient to document normal findings related to unaffected area(s) or asymptomatic organ system(s).*

•*DG:* *The medical record for a general multisystem examination should include findings about eight or more of the 12 organ systems.*

C. Documentation of the Complexity of Medical Decision-making

The levels of E/M services recognize four types of medical decision-making (straightforward, low complexity, moderate complexity, and high complexity). Medical decision-making refers to the complexity of establishing a diagnosis and/or selecting a management option as measured by

◈ The number of possible diagnoses and/or the number of management options that must be considered

◈ The amount and/or complexity of medical records, diagnostic tests, and/or other information that must be obtained, reviewed, and analyzed

◈ The risk of significant complications, morbidity, and/or mortality, as well as co-morbidities, associated with the patient's presenting problem(s), the diagnostic procedure(s), and/or the possible management options.

The chart on page 96 shows the progression of the elements required for each level of medical decision-making. To qualify for a given type of decision-making, **two of the three elements in the table must be either met or exceeded.**

Each of the elements of medical decision-making is described below.

Number of Diagnoses or Management Options	Amount and/or Complexity of Data to Be Reviewed	Risk of Significant Complications, Morbidity, and/or Mortality	Type of Decision-Making
Minimal	Minimal or none	Minimal	Straightforward
Limited	Limited	Low	Low complexity
Multiple	Moderate	Moderate	Moderate complexity
Extensive	Extensive	High	High complexity

Number of Diagnoses or Management Options

The number of possible diagnoses and/or the number of management options that must be considered is based on the number and types of problems addressed during the encounter, the complexity of establishing a diagnosis, and the management decisions that are made by the physician.

Generally, decision-making with respect to a diagnosed problem is easier than that for an identified but undiagnosed problem. The number and type of diagnostic tests employed may be an indicator of the number of possible diagnoses. Problems that are improving or resolving are less complex than those that are worsening or failing to change as expected. The need to seek advice from others is another indicator of complexity of diagnostic or management problems.

•**DG:** *For each encounter, an assessment, clinical impression, or diagnosis should be documented. It may be explicitly stated or implied in documented decisions regarding management plans and/or further evaluation.*

    ✻ *For a presenting problem with an established diagnosis the record should reflect whether the problem is: (a) improved, well controlled, resolving, or resolved; or (b) inadequately controlled, worsening, or failing to change as expected.*

    ✻ *For a presenting problem without an established diagnosis, the assessment or clinical impression may be stated in the form of a differential diagnoses or as "possible," "probable," or "rule out" (R/O) diagnoses.*

•**DG:** *The initiation of, or changes in, treatment should be documented. Treatment includes a wide range of management options including patient instructions, nursing instructions, therapies, and medications.*

•**DG:** *If referrals are made, consultations requested, or advice sought, the record should indicate to whom or where the referral or consultation is made or from whom the advice is requested.*

Amount and/or Complexity of Data to Be Reviewed

The amount and/or complexity of data to be reviewed is based on the types of diagnostic testing ordered or reviewed. A decision to obtain and review old medical records and/or obtain history from sources other than the patient increases the amount and complexity of data to be reviewed.

Discussion of contradictory or unexpected test results with the physician who performed or interpreted the test is an indication of the complexity of data being reviewed. On occasion the physician who ordered a test may personally review the image, tracing, or specimen to supplement information from the physician who prepared the test report or interpretation; this is another indication of the complexity of data being reviewed.

•**DG:** *If a diagnostic service (test or procedure) is ordered, planned, scheduled, or performed at the time of the E/M encounter, the type of service (eg, lab or x-ray) should be documented.*

•**DG:** *The review of lab, radiology, and/or other diagnostic tests should be documented. An entry in a progress note such as "WBC elevated" or "chest x-ray unremarkable" is acceptable. Alternatively, the review may be documented by initialing and dating the report containing the test results.*

•**DG:** *A decision to obtain old records or to obtain additional history from the family, caretaker, or other source to supplement that obtained from the patient should be documented.*

•**DG:** *Relevant findings from the review of old records and/or the receipt of additional history from the family, caretaker, or other source should be documented. If there is no relevant information beyond that already obtained, that fact should be documented. A notation of "old records reviewed" or "additional history obtained from family" without elaboration is insufficient.*

•**DG:** *The results of discussion of laboratory, radiology, or other diagnostic tests with the physician who performed or interpreted the study should be documented.*

•**DG:** *The direct visualization and independent interpretation of an image, tracing, or specimen previously or subsequently interpreted by another physician should be documented.*

Risk of Significant Complications, Morbidity, and/or Mortality

The risk of significant complications, morbidity, and/or mortality is based on the risks associated with the presenting problem(s), the diagnostic procedure(s), and the possible management options.

•**DG:** *Co-morbidities/underlying diseases or other factors that increase the complexity of medical decision making by increasing the risk of complications, morbidity, and/or mortality should be documented.*

•**DG:** *If a surgical or invasive diagnostic procedure is ordered, planned, or scheduled at the time of the E/M encounter, the type of procedure (eg, laparoscopy) should be documented.*

•**DG:** *If a surgical or invasive diagnostic procedure is performed at the time of the E/M encounter, the specific procedure should be documented.*

•**DG:** *The referral for or decision to perform a surgical or invasive diagnostic procedure on an urgent basis should be documented or implied.*

The following table may be used to help determine whether the risk of significant complications, morbidity, and/or mortality is **minimal, low, moderate,** or **high.** Because the determination of risk is complex and not readily quantifiable, the table includes common clinical examples rather than absolute measures of risk. The assessment of risk of the presenting problem(s) is based on the risk related to the disease process anticipated between the present encounter and the next one. The assessment of risk of selecting diagnostic procedures and management options is based on the risk during and immediately following any procedures or treatment. The highest level of risk in any one category (presenting problem(s), diagnostic procedure(s), or management options) determines the overall risk.

D. Documentation of an Encounter Dominated by Counseling or Coordination of Care

In the case where counseling and/or coordination of care dominates (more than 50%) the physician/patient and/or family encounter (face-to-face time in the office or other outpatient setting or floor/unit time in the hospital or nursing facility), time is considered the key or controlling factor to qualify for a particular level of E/M services.

•**DG:** *If the physician elects to report the level of service based on counseling and/or coordination of care, the total length of time of the encounter (face-to-face or floor time, as appropriate) should be documented and the record should describe the counseling and/or activities to coordinate care.*

Table of Risk			
Level of Risk	**Presenting Problem(s)**	**Diagnostic Procedure(s) Ordered**	**Management Options Selected**
Minimal	⦿ One self-limited or minor problem, eg, cold, insect bite, tinea corporis	⦿ Laboratory tests requiring venipuncture ⦿ Chest x-rays ⦿ EKG/EEG ⦿ Urinalysis ⦿ Ultrasound, eg, echocardiography ⦿ KOH prep	⦿ Rest ⦿ Gargles ⦿ Elastic bandages ⦿ Superficial dressings

Table of Risk (*continued*)

Level of Risk	Presenting Problem(s)	Diagnostic Procedure(s) Ordered	Management Options Selected
Low	⚬ Two or more self-limited or minor problems ⚬ One stable chronic illness, eg, well-controlled hypertension or non–insulin-dependent diabetes, cataract, BPH ⚬ Acute uncomplicated illness or injury, eg, cystitis, allergic rhinitis, simple sprain	⚬ Physiologic tests not under stress, eg, pulmonary function tests ⚬ Non-cardiovascular imaging studies with contrast, eg, barium enema ⚬ Superficial needle biopsies ⚬ Clinical laboratory tests requiring arterial puncture ⚬ Skin biopsies	⚬ Over-the-counter drugs ⚬ Minor surgery with no identified risk factors ⚬ Physical therapy ⚬ Occupational therapy ⚬ IV fluids without additives
Moderate	⚬ One or more chronic illnesses with mild exacerbation, progression, or side effects of treatment ⚬ Two or more stable chronic illnesses ⚬ Undiagnosed new problem with uncertain prognosis, eg, lump in breast ⚬ Acute illness with systemic symptoms, eg, pyelonephritis, pneumonitis, colitis ⚬ Acute complicated injury, eg, head injury with brief loss of consciousness	⚬ Physiologic tests under stress, eg, cardiac stress test, fetal contraction stress test ⚬ Diagnostic endoscopies with no identified risk factors ⚬ Deep needle or incisional biopsy ⚬ Cardiovascular imaging studies with contrast and no identified risk factors, eg, arteriogram, cardiac catheterization ⚬ Obtain fluid from body cavity, eg, lumbar puncture, thoracentesis, culdocentesis	⚬ Minor surgery with identified risk factors ⚬ Elective major surgery (open, percutaneous, or endoscopic) with no identified risk factors ⚬ Prescription drug management ⚬ Therapeutic nuclear medicine ⚬ IV fluids with additives ⚬ Closed treatment of fracture or dislocation without manipulation
High	⚬ One or more chronic illnesses with severe exacerbation, progression, or side effects of treatment ⚬ Acute or chronic illnesses or injuries that pose a threat to life or bodily function, eg, multiple trauma, acute MI, pulmonary embolus, severe respiratory distress, progressive severe rheumatoid arthritis, psychiatric illness with potential threat to self or others, peritonitis, acute renal failure ⚬ An abrupt change in neurologic status, eg, seizure, TIA, weakness, or sensory loss	⚬ Cardiovascular imaging studies with contrast with identified risk factors ⚬ Cardiac electrophysiological tests ⚬ Diagnostic endoscopies with identified risk factors ⚬ Discography	⚬ Elective major surgery (open, percutaneous, or endoscopic) with identified risk factors ⚬ Emergency major surgery (open, percutaneous, or endoscopic) ⚬ Parenteral controlled substances ⚬ Drug therapy requiring intensive monitoring for toxicity ⚬ Decision not to resuscitate or to de-escalate care because of poor prognosis

1997 Documentation Guidelines for Evaluation and Management Services

I. Introduction

What Is Documentation and Why Is It Important?

Medical record documentation is required to record pertinent facts, findings, and observations about an individual's health history including past and present illnesses, examinations, tests, treatments, and outcomes. The medical record chronologically documents the care of the patient and is an important element contributing to high-quality care. The medical record facilitates

- The ability of the physician and other health care professionals to evaluate and plan the patient's immediate treatment and to monitor his/her health care over time
- Communication and continuity of care among physicians and other health care professionals involved in the patient's care
- Accurate and timely claims review and payment
- Appropriate utilization review and quality of care evaluations
- Collection of data that may be useful for research and education

An appropriately documented medical record can reduce many of the "hassles" associated with claims processing and may serve as a legal document to verify the care provided, if necessary.

What Do Payers Want and Why?

Because payers have a contractual obligation to enrollees, they may require reasonable documentation that services are consistent with the insurance coverage provided. They may request information to validate

- The site of service
- The medical necessity and appropriateness of the diagnostic and/or therapeutic services provided
- That services provided have been accurately reported

II. General Principles of Medical Record Documentation

The principles of documentation listed below are applicable to all types of medical and surgical services in all settings. For Evaluation and Management (E/M) services, the nature and amount of physician work and documentation varies by type of service, place of service, and the patient's status. The general principles listed below may be modified to account for these variable circumstances in providing E/M services.

1. The medical record should be complete and legible.
2. The documentation of each patient encounter should include
   - Reason for the encounter and relevant history, physical examination findings, and prior diagnostic test results
   - Assessment, clinical impression, or diagnosis
   - Plan for care
   - Date and legible identity of the observer
3. If not documented, the rationale for ordering diagnostic and other ancillary services should be easily inferred.
4. Past and present diagnoses should be accessible to the treating and/or consulting physician.
5. Appropriate health risk factors should be identified.
6. The patient's progress, response to and changes in treatment, and revision of diagnosis should be documented.
7. The *CPT* and *ICD-10-CM* codes reported on the health insurance claim form or billing statement should be supported by the documentation in the medical record.

III. Documentation of E/M Services

This publication provides definitions and documentation guidelines for the three key components of E/M services and for visits that consist predominantly of counseling or coordination of care. The three key components—history, examination, and medical decision making—appear in the descriptors for office and other outpatient services, hospital observation services, hospital inpatient services, consultations, emergency department services, nursing facility services, domiciliary care services, and home services. While some of the text of *CPT* has been repeated in this publication, the reader should refer to *CPT* for the complete descriptors for E/M services and instructions for selecting a level of service. Documentation guidelines are identified by the symbol •*DG.*

The descriptors for the levels of E/M services recognize seven components that are used in defining the levels of E/M services. These components are

* History
* Examination
* Medical decision making
* Counseling
* Coordination of care
* Nature of presenting problem
* Time

The first three of these components (ie, history, examination, and medical decision making) are the key components in selecting the level of E/M services. In the case of visits that consist *predominantly* of counseling or coordination of care, time is the key or controlling factor to qualify for a particular level of E/M service.

Because the level of E/M service is dependent on two or three key components, performance and documentation of one component (eg, examination) at the highest level does not necessarily mean that the encounter in its entirety qualifies for the highest level of E/M service.

These Documentation Guidelines for E/M services reflect the needs of the typical adult population. For certain groups of patients, the recorded information may vary slightly from that described here. Specifically, the medical records of infants, children, adolescents, and pregnant women may have additional or modified information recorded in each history and examination area.

As an example, newborn records may include under history of the present illness (HPI) the details of mother's pregnancy, and the infant's status at birth; social history will focus on family structure; family history will focus on congenital anomalies and hereditary disorders in the family. In addition, the content of a pediatric examination will vary with the age and development of the child. Although not specifically defined in these documentation guidelines, these patient group variations on history and examination are appropriate.

A. Documentation of History

The levels of E/M services are based on four types of history (problem focused, expanded problem focused, detailed, and comprehensive). Each type of history includes some or all of the following elements:

* Chief complaint (CC)
* History of present illness (HPI)
* Review of systems (ROS)
* Past, family, and/or social history (PFSH)

The extent of history of present illness; review of systems; and past, family, and/or social history that is obtained and documented is dependent upon clinical judgment and the nature of the presenting problem(s).

The chart on page 101 shows the progression of the elements required for each type of history. To qualify for a given type of history all three elements in the table must be met. (A chief complaint is indicated at all levels.)

History of Present Illness	Review of Systems	Past, Family, and/or Social History	Type of History
Brief	N/A	N/A	Problem focused
Brief	Problem pertinent	N/A	Expanded problem focused
Extended	Extended	Pertinent	Detailed
Extended	Complete	Complete	Comprehensive

•**DG:** *The CC, ROS, and PFSH may be listed as separate elements of history or they may be included in the description of the history of the present illness.*

•**DG:** *A ROS and/or a PFSH obtained during an earlier encounter does not need to be rerecorded if there is evidence that the physician reviewed and updated the previous information. This may occur when a physician updates his or her own record or in an institutional setting or group practice where many physicians use a common record. The review and update may be documented by*

⊛ *Describing any new ROS and/or PFSH information or noting there has been no change in the information*

⊛ *Noting the date and location of the earlier ROS and/or PFSH*

•**DG:** *The ROS and/or PFSH may be recorded by ancillary staff or on a form completed by the patient. To document that the physician reviewed the information, there must be a notation supplementing or confirming the information recorded by others.*

•**DG:** *If the physician is unable to obtain a history from the patient or other source, the record should describe the patient's condition or other circumstance that precludes obtaining a history.*

Definitions and specific documentation guidelines for each of the elements of history are listed below.

Chief Complaint (CC)

The CC is a concise statement describing the symptom, problem, condition, diagnosis, physician recommended return, or other factor that is the reason for the encounter, usually stated in the patient's words.

•**DG:** *The medical record should clearly reflect the chief complaint.*

History of Present Illness (HPI)

The HPI is a chronological description of the development of the patient's present illness from the first sign and/or symptom or from the previous encounter to the present. It includes the following elements:

⊛ Location
⊛ Quality
⊛ Severity
⊛ Duration
⊛ Timing
⊛ Context
⊛ Modifying factors
⊛ Associated signs and symptoms

Brief and *extended* HPIs are distinguished by the amount of detail needed to accurately characterize the clinical problem(s).

A *brief* HPI consists of one to three elements of the HPI.

•**DG:** *The medical record should describe one to three elements of the present illness (HPI).*

An *extended* HPI consists of at least four elements of the HPI or the status of at least three chronic or inactive conditions.

•**DG:** *The medical record should describe at least four elements of the present illness (HPI), or the status of at least three chronic or inactive conditions.*

Chapter 4: Evaluation and Management Documentation Guidelines/CMS 1997 Documentation Guidelines for Evaluation and Management Services

Review of Systems (ROS)

A ROS is an inventory of body systems obtained through a series of questions seeking to identify signs and/or symptoms that the patient may be experiencing or has experienced.

For purposes of ROS, the following systems are recognized:

- Constitutional symptoms (eg, fever, weight loss)
- Eyes
- Ears, nose, mouth, throat
- Cardiovascular
- Respiratory
- Gastrointestinal
- Genitourinary
- Musculoskeletal
- Integumentary (skin and/or breast)
- Neurological
- Psychiatric
- Endocrine
- Hematologic/lymphatic
- Allergic/immunologic

A *problem-pertinent* ROS inquires about the system directly related to the problem(s) identified in the HPI.

•**DG:** *The patient's positive responses and pertinent negatives for the system related to the problem should be documented.*

An *extended* ROS inquires about the system directly related to the problem(s) identified in the HPI and a limited number of additional systems.

•**DG:** *The patient's positive responses and pertinent negatives for two to nine systems should be documented.*

A *complete* ROS inquires about the system(s) directly related to the problem(s) identified in the HPI plus all additional body systems.

•**DG:** *At least 10 organ systems must be reviewed. Those systems with positive or pertinent negative responses must be individually documented. For the remaining systems, a notation indicating all other systems are negative is permissible. In the absence of such a notation, at least 10 systems must be individually documented.*

Past, Family, and/or Social History (PFSH)

The PFSH consists of a review of three areas

- Past history (the patient's past experiences with illnesses, operations, injuries, and treatments)
- Family history (a review of medical events in the patient's family, including diseases that may be hereditary or place the patient at risk)
- Social history (an age-appropriate review of past and current activities)

For certain categories of E/M services that include only an interval history, it is not necessary to record information about the PFSH. Those categories are subsequent hospital care, follow-up inpatient consultations, and subsequent nursing facility care.

A *pertinent* PFSH is a review of the history area(s) directly related to the problem(s) identified in the HPI.

•**DG:** *At least one specific item from any of the three history areas must be documented for a pertinent PFSH.*

A *complete* PFSH is of a review of two or all three of the PFSH history areas, depending on the category of the E/M service. A review of all three history areas is required for services that by their nature include a comprehensive assessment or reassessment of the patient. A review of two of the three history areas is sufficient for other services.

- **•DG:** *At least one specific item from two of the three history areas must be documented for a complete PFSH for the following categories of E/M services: office or other outpatient services, established patient; emergency department; domiciliary care, established patient; and home care, established patient.*
- **•DG:** *At least one specific item from each of the three history areas must be documented for a complete PFSH for the following categories of E/M services: office or other outpatient services, new patient; hospital observation services; hospital inpatient services, initial care; consultations; comprehensive nursing facility assessments; domiciliary care, new patient; and home care, new patient.*

B. Documentation of Examination

The levels of E/M services are based on four types of examination

- ◉ **Problem Focused**—a limited examination of the affected body area or organ system.
- ◉ **Expanded Problem Focused**—a limited examination of the affected body area or organ system and any other symptomatic or related body area(s) or organ system(s).
- ◉ **Detailed**—an extended examination of the affected body area(s) or organ system(s) and any other symptomatic or related body area(s) or organ system(s).
- ◉ **Comprehensive**—a general multisystem examination or complete examination of a single organ system and other symptomatic or related body area(s) or organ system(s).

These types of examinations have been defined for general multisystem and the following single organ systems:

- ◉ Cardiovascular
- ◉ Ears, nose, mouth, throat
- ◉ Eyes
- ◉ Genitourinary (female)
- ◉ Genitourinary (male)
- ◉ Hematologic/lymphatic/immunologic
- ◉ Musculoskeletal
- ◉ Neurological
- ◉ Psychiatric
- ◉ Respiratory
- ◉ Skin

A general multisystem examination or a single organ system examination may be performed by any physician regardless of specialty. The type (general multisystem or single organ system) and content of examination are selected by the examining physician and are based upon clinical judgment, the patient's history, and the nature of the presenting problem(s).

The content and documentation requirements for each type and level of examination are summarized below and described in detail in tables beginning on page 105. In the tables, organ systems and body areas recognized by *CPT* for purposes of describing examinations are shown in the left column. The content, or individual elements, of the examination pertaining to that body area or organ system are identified by bullets (•) in the right column.

Parenthetical examples, "(eg, ...)", have been used for clarification and to provide guidance regarding documentation. Documentation for each element must satisfy any numeric requirements (such as "Measurement of *any three of the following seven...*") included in the description of the element. Elements with multiple components but with no specific numeric requirement (such as "Examination of *liver* and *spleen*") require documentation of at least one component. It is possible for a given examination to be expanded beyond what is defined here. When that occurs, findings related to the additional systems and/or areas should be documented.

- **•DG:** *Specific abnormal and relevant negative findings of the examination of the affected or symptomatic body area(s) or organ system(s) should be documented. A notation of "abnormal" without elaboration is insufficient.*
- **•DG:** *Abnormal or unexpected findings of the examination of any asymptomatic body area(s) or organ system(s) should be described.*

•*DG:*   *A brief statement or notation indicating "negative" or "normal" is sufficient to document normal findings related to unaffected area(s) or asymptomatic organ system(s).*

General Multisystem Examinations

General multisystem examinations are described in detail beginning on page 105. To qualify for a given level of multisystem examination, the following content and documentation requirements should be met:

❋ **Problem-Focused Examination**—should include performance and documentation of one to five elements identified by a bullet (•) in one or more organ system(s) or body area(s).

❋ **Expanded Problem-Focused Examination**—should include performance and documentation of at least six elements identified by a bullet in one or more organ system(s) or body area(s).

❋ **Detailed Examination**—should include at least six organ systems or body areas. For each system/area selected, performance and documentation of at least two elements identified by a bullet is expected. Alternatively, a detailed examination may include performance and documentation of at least 12 elements identified by a bullet in two or more organ systems or body areas.

❋ **Comprehensive Examination**—should include at least nine organ systems or body areas. For each system/area selected, all elements of the examination identified by a bullet should be performed, unless specific directions limit the content of the examination. For each area/system, documentation of at least two elements identified by a bullet is expected.

Single Organ System Examinations

The single organ system examinations recognized by *CPT* are described in detail in the tables starting on page 108. Variations among these examinations in the organ systems and body areas identified in the left columns and in the elements of the examinations described in the right columns reflect differing emphases among specialties. To qualify for a given level of single organ system examination, the following content and documentation requirements should be met:

❋ **Problem-Focused Examination**—should include performance and documentation of one to five elements identified by a bullet, whether in a shaded or unshaded area.

❋ **Expanded Problem-Focused Examination**—should include performance and documentation of at least six elements identified by a bullet, whether in a shaded or unshaded area.

❋ **Detailed Examination**—examinations other than the eye and psychiatric examinations should include performance and documentation of at least 12 elements identified by a bullet, whether in a shaded or unshaded area.

❋ Eye and psychiatric examinations should include the performance and documentation of at least nine elements identified by a bullet, whether in a shaded or unshaded area.

❋ **Comprehensive Examination**—should include performance of all elements identified by a bullet, whether in a shaded or unshaded area. Documentation of every element in a shaded area and at least one element in each category in each unshaded area is expected.

General Multisystem Examination

System/Body Area	Elements of Examination
Constitutional	• Measurement of **any three of the following seven** vital signs: 1) sitting or standing blood pressure, 2) supine blood pressure, 3) pulse rate and regularity, 4) respiration, 5) temperature, 6) height, 7) weight (may be measured and recorded by ancillary staff) • General appearance of patient (eg, development, nutrition, body habitus, deformities, attention to grooming)
Eyes	• Inspection of conjunctivae and lids • Examination of pupils and irises (eg, reaction to light and accommodation, size and symmetry) • Ophthalmoscopic examination of optic discs (eg, size, C/D ratio, appearance) and posterior segments (eg, vessel changes, exudates, hemorrhages)
Ears, Nose, Mouth, and Throat	• External inspection of ears and nose (eg, overall appearance, scars, lesions, masses) • Otoscopic examination of external auditory canals and tympanic membranes • Assessment of hearing (eg, whispered voice, finger rub, tuning fork) • Inspection of nasal mucosa, septum, and turbinates • Inspection of lips, teeth, and gums • Examination of oropharynx: oral mucosa, salivary glands, hard and soft palates, tongue, tonsils, and posterior pharynx
Neck	• Examination of neck (eg, masses, overall appearance, symmetry, tracheal position, crepitus) • Examination of thyroid (eg, enlargement, tenderness, mass)
Respiratory	• Assessment of respiratory effort (eg, intercostal retractions, use of accessory muscles, diaphragmatic movement) • Percussion of chest (eg, dullness, flatness, hyperresonance) • Palpation of chest (eg, tactile fremitus) • Auscultation of lungs (eg, breath sounds, adventitious sounds, rubs)
Cardiovascular	• Palpation of heart (eg, location, size, thrills) • Auscultation of heart with notation of abnormal sounds and murmurs Examination of: • Carotid arteries (eg, pulse amplitude, bruits) • Abdominal aorta (eg, size, bruits) • Femoral arteries (eg, pulse amplitude, bruits) • Pedal pulses (eg, pulse amplitude) • Extremities for edema and/or varicosities
Chest (Breasts)	• Inspection of breasts (eg, symmetry, nipple discharge) • Palpation of breasts and axillae (eg, masses or lumps, tenderness)

Chapter 4: Evaluation and Management Documentation Guidelines/CMS 1997 Documentation Guidelines for Evaluation and Management Services

General Multisystem Examination (*continued*)

System/Body Area	Elements of Examination
Gastrointestinal (Abdomen)	• Examination of abdomen with notation of presence of masses or tenderness • Examination of liver and spleen • Examination for presence or absence of hernia • Examination (when indicated) of anus, perineum, and rectum, including sphincter tone, presence of hemorrhoids, rectal masses • Obtain stool sample for occult blood test when indicated

System/Body Area	Elements of Examination
Genitourinary	*Male* • Examination of the scrotal contents (eg, hydrocele, spermatocele, tenderness of cord, testicular mass) • Examination of the penis • Digital rectal examination of prostate gland (eg, size, symmetry, nodularity, tenderness) *Female* • Pelvic examination (with or without specimen collection for smears and cultures) including • Examination of external genitalia (eg, general appearance, hair distribution, lesions) and vagina (eg, general appearance, estrogen effect, discharge, lesions, pelvic support, cystocele, rectocele) • Examination of urethra (eg, masses, tenderness, scarring) • Examination of bladder (eg, fullness, masses, tenderness) • Cervix (eg, general appearance, lesions, discharge) • Uterus (eg, size, contour, position, mobility, tenderness, consistency, descent, or support) • Adnexa/parametria (eg, masses, tenderness, organomegaly, nodularity)
Lymphatic	Palpation of lymph nodes in **two or more** areas: • Neck • Axillae • Groin • Other
Musculoskeletal	• Examination of gait and station • Inspection and/or palpation of digits and nails (eg, clubbing, cyanosis, inflammatory conditions, petechiae, ischemia, infections, nodes) Examination of joints, bones, and muscles of **one or more of the following six areas:** 1) head and neck; 2) spine, ribs, and pelvis; 3) right upper extremity; 4) left upper extremity; 5) right lower extremity; and 6) left lower extremity. The examination of a given area includes: • Inspection and/or palpation with notation of presence of any misalignment, asymmetry, crepitation, defects, tenderness, masses, effusions • Assessment of range of motion with notation of any pain, crepitation, or contracture

General Multisystem Examination (*continued*)

System/Body Area	Elements of Examination
Musculoskeletal (*continued*)	• Assessment of stability with notation of any dislocation (luxation), subluxation, or laxity • Assessment of muscle strength and tone (eg, flaccid, cog wheel, spastic) with notation of any atrophy or abnormal movements
Skin	• Inspection of skin and subcutaneous tissue (eg, rashes, lesions, ulcers) • Palpation of skin and subcutaneous tissue (eg, induration, subcutaneous nodules, tightening)
Neurological	• Test cranial nerves with notation of any deficits • Examination of deep tendon reflexes with notation of pathological reflexes (eg, Babinski) • Examination of sensation (eg, by touch, pin, vibration, proprioception)
Psychiatric	• Description of patient's judgment and insight Brief assessment of mental status including: • Orientation to time, place, and person • Recent and remote memory • Mood and affect (eg, depression, anxiety, agitation)

Content and Documentation Requirements

Level of Exam	Perform and Document
Problem Focused	One to five elements identified by a bullet.
Expanded Problem Focused	At least six elements identified by a bullet.
Detailed	At least two elements identified by a bullet from each of six areas/systems OR at least 12 elements identified by a bullet in two or more areas/systems.
Comprehensive	Perform all elements identified by a bullet in at least nine organ systems or body areas and document at least two elements identified by a bullet from each of nine areas/systems.

Chapter 4: Evaluation and Management Documentation Guidelines/CMS 1997 Documentation Guidelines for Evaluation and Management Services

Cardiovascular Examination

System/Body Area	Elements of Examination
Constitutional	• Measurement of **any three of the following seven** vital signs: 1) sitting or standing blood pressure, 2) supine blood pressure, 3) pulse rate and regularity, 4) respiration, 5) temperature, 6) height, 7) weight (may be measured and recorded by ancillary staff) • General appearance of patient (eg, development, nutrition, body habitus, deformities, attention to grooming)
Head and Face	
Eyes	• Inspection of conjunctivae and lids (eg, xanthelasma)
Ears, Nose, Mouth, and Throat	• Inspection of teeth, gums, and palate • Inspection of oral mucosa with notation of presence of pallor or cyanosis
Neck	• Examination of jugular veins (eg, distension; a, v, or cannon a waves) • Examination of thyroid (eg, enlargement, tenderness, mass)
Respiratory	• Assessment of respiratory effort (eg, intercostal retractions, use of accessory muscles, diaphragmatic movement) • Auscultation of lungs (eg, breath sounds, adventitious sounds, rubs)
Cardiovascular	• Palpation of heart (eg, location, size, and forcefulness of the point of maximal impact; thrills; lifts; palpable S3 or S4) • Auscultation of heart including sounds, abnormal sounds, and murmurs • Measurement of blood pressure in two or more extremities when indicated (eg, aortic dissection, coarctation) Examination of • Carotid arteries (eg, waveform, pulse amplitude, bruits, apical-carotid delay) • Abdominal aorta (eg, size, bruits) • Femoral arteries (eg, pulse amplitude, bruits) • Pedal pulses (eg, pulse amplitude) • Extremities for peripheral edema and/or varicosities
Chest (Breasts)	
Gastrointestinal (Abdomen)	• Examination of abdomen with notation of presence of masses or tenderness • Examination of liver and spleen • Obtain stool sample for occult blood from patients who are being considered for thrombolytic or anti-coagulant therapy
Genitourinary (Abdomen)	
Lymphatic	

Cardiovascular Examination (*continued*)

System/Body Area	Elements of Examination
Musculoskeletal	• Examination of the back with notation of kyphosis or scoliosis • Examination of gait with notation of ability to undergo exercise testing and/or participation in exercise programs • Assessment of muscle strength and tone (eg, flaccid, cog wheel, spastic) with notation of any atrophy and abnormal movements
Extremities	• Inspection and palpation of digits and nails (eg, clubbing, cyanosis, inflammation, petechiae, ischemia, infections, Osler's nodes)
Skin	• Inspection and/or palpation of skin and subcutaneous tissue (eg, stasis dermatitis, ulcers, scars, xanthomas)
Neurological/ Psychiatric	Brief assessment of mental status including: • Orientation to time, place, and person • Mood and affect (eg, depression, anxiety, agitation)

Content and Documentation Requirements

Level of Exam	Perform and Document
Problem Focused	**One to five** elements identified by a bullet.
Expanded Problem Focused	**At least six** elements identified by a bullet.
Detailed	**At least 12** elements identified by a bullet.
Comprehensive	Perform **all** elements identified by a bullet; document every element in each shaded area and at least one element in each category in each unshaded area.

Chapter 4: Evaluation and Management Documentation Guidelines/CMS 1997 Documentation Guidelines for Evaluation and Management Services

Ear, Nose, and Throat Examination

System/Body Area	Elements of Examination
Constitutional	• Measurement of **any three of the following seven** vital signs: 1) sitting or standing blood pressure, 2) supine blood pressure, 3) pulse rate and regularity, 4) respiration, 5) temperature, 6) height, 7) weight (may be measured and recorded by ancillary staff) • General appearance of patient (eg, development, nutrition, body habitus, deformities, attention to grooming) • Assessment of ability to communicate (eg, use of sign language or other communication aids) and quality of voice
Head and Face	• Inspection of head and face (eg, overall appearance, scars, lesions, and masses) • Palpation and/or percussion of face with notation of presence or absence of sinus tenderness • Examination of salivary glands • Assessment of facial strength
Eyes	• Test ocular motility including primary gaze alignment
Ears, Nose, Mouth, and Throat	• Otoscopic examination of external auditory canals and tympanic membranes including pneumo-otoscopy with notation of mobility of membranes • Assessment of hearing with tuning forks and clinical speech reception thresholds (eg, whispered voice, finger rub) • External inspection of ears and nose (eg, overall appearance, scars, lesions, and masses) • Inspection of nasal mucosa, septum, and turbinates • Inspection of lips, teeth, and gums • Examination of oropharynx: oral mucosa, hard and soft palates, tongue, tonsils, and posterior pharynx (eg, asymmetry, lesions, hydration of mucosal surfaces) • Inspection of pharyngeal walls and pyriform sinuses (eg, pooling of saliva, asymmetry, lesions) • Examination by mirror of larynx including the condition of the epiglottis, false vocal cords, true vocal cords, and mobility of larynx (use of mirror not required in children) • Examination by mirror of nasopharynx including appearance of the mucosa, adenoids, posterior choanae, and eustachian tubes (use of mirror not required in children)
Neck	• Examination of neck (eg, masses, overall appearance, symmetry, tracheal position, crepitus) • Examination of thyroid (eg, enlargement, tenderness, mass)
Respiratory	• Inspection of chest including symmetry, expansion, and/or assessment of respiratory effort (eg, intercostal retractions, use of accessory muscles, diaphragmatic movement) • Auscultation of lungs (eg, breath sounds, adventitious sounds, rubs)

Ear, Nose, and Throat Examination (continued)

System/Body Area	Elements of Examination
Cardiovascular	• Auscultation of heart with notation of abnormal sounds and murmurs • Examination of peripheral vascular system by observation(eg, swelling, varicosities) and palpation (eg, pulses, temperature, edema, tenderness)
Chest (Breasts)	
Gastrointestinal (Abdomen)	
Genitourinary	
Lymphatic	• Palpation of lymph nodes in neck, axillae, groin, and/or other location
Musculoskeletal	
Extremities	
Skin	
Neurological/ Psychiatric	• Test cranial nerves with notation of any deficits Brief assessment of mental status including: • Orientation to time, place, and person • Mood and affect (eg, depression, anxiety, agitation)

Content and Documentation Requirements

Level of Exam	Perform and Document
Problem Focused	One to five elements identified by a bullet.
Expanded Problem Focused	At least six elements identified by a bullet.
Detailed	At least 12 elements identified by a bullet.
Comprehensive	Perform all elements identified by a bullet; document every element in each shaded area and at least one element in each category in each unshaded area.

Chapter 4: Evaluation and Management Documentation Guidelines/CMS 1997 Documentation Guidelines for Evaluation and Management Services

Eye Examination

System/Body Area	Elements of Examination
Constitutional	
Head and Face	
Eyes	• Test visual acuity (does not include determination of refractive error) • Gross visual field testing by confrontation • Test ocular motility including primary gaze alignment • Inspection of bulbar and palpebral conjunctivae • Examination of ocular adnexae including lids (eg, ptosis or lagophthalmos), lacrimal glands, lacrimal drainage, orbits, and preauricular lymph nodes • Examination of pupils and irises including shape, direct and consensual reaction (afferent pupil), size (eg, anisocoria), and morphology • Slit lamp examination of the corneas including epithelium, stroma, endothelium, and tear film • Slit lamp examination of the anterior chambers including depth, cells, and flare • Slit lamp examination of the lenses including clarity, anterior and posterior capsule, cortex, and nucleus • Measurement of intraocular pressures (except in children and patients with trauma or infectious disease) Ophthalmoscopic examination through dilated pupils (unless contraindicated) of: • Optic discs including size, C/D ratio, appearance (eg, atrophy, cupping, tumor elevation), and nerve fiber layer • Posterior segments including retina and vessels (eg, exudates and hemorrhages)
Ears, Nose, Mouth, and Throat	
Neck	
Respiratory	• Inspection of chest including symmetry, expansion, and/or assessment of respiratory effort (eg, intercostal retractions, use of accessory muscles, diaphragmatic movement) • Auscultation of lungs (eg, breath sounds, adventitious sounds, rubs)
Cardiovascular	
Chest (Breasts)	
Genitourinary	
Lymphatic	
Musculoskeletal	
Extremities	

Eye Examination (continued)

System/Body Area	Elements of Examination
Skin	
Neurological/ Psychiatric	Brief assessment of mental status including: • Orientation to time, place, and person • Mood and affect (eg, depression, anxiety, agitation)

Content and Documentation Requirements

Level of Exam	Perform and Document
Problem Focused	One to five elements identified by a bullet.
Expanded Problem Focused	At least six elements identified by a bullet.
Detailed	At least nine elements identified by a bullet.
Comprehensive	Perform all elements identified by a bullet; document every element in each shaded area and at least one element in each category in each unshaded area.

Genitourinary Examination

System/Body Area	Elements of Examination
Constitutional	• Measurement of any three of the following seven vital signs: 1) sitting or standing blood pressure, 2) supine blood pressure, 3) pulse rate and regularity, 4) respiration, 5) temperature, 6) height, 7) weight (may be measured and recorded by ancillary staff) • General appearance of patient (eg, development, nutrition, body habitus, deformities, attention to grooming)
Head and Face	
Eyes	
Ears, Nose, Mouth, and Throat	
Neck	• Examination of neck (eg, masses, overall appearance, symmetry, tracheal position, crepitus) • Examination of thyroid (eg, enlargement, tenderness, mass)
Respiratory	• Assessment of respiratory effort (eg, intercostal retractions, use of accessory muscles, diaphragmatic movement) • Auscultation of lungs (eg, breath sounds, adventitious sounds, rubs)
Cardiovascular	• Auscultation of heart with notation of abnormal sounds and murmurs • Examination of peripheral vascular system by observation (eg, swelling, varicosities) and palpation (eg, pulses, temperature, edema, tenderness)
Chest (Breasts)	[See Genitourinary (female)]
Gastrointestinal (Abdomen)	• Examination of abdomen with notation of presence of masses or tenderness • Examination for presence or absence of hernia • Examination of liver and spleen • Obtain stool sample for occult blood test when indicated
Genitourinary	**Male** • Inspection of anus and perineum Examination (with or without specimen collection for smears and cultures) of genitalia including: • Scrotum (eg, lesions, cysts, rashes) • Epididymides (eg, size, symmetry, masses) • Testes (eg, size, symmetry, masses) • Urethral meatus (eg, size, location, lesions, discharge) • Penis (eg, lesions, presence or absence of foreskin, fore-skin retractability, plaque, masses, scarring, deformities) Digital rectal examination including: • Prostate gland (eg, size, symmetry, nodularity, tenderness) • Seminal vesicles (eg, symmetry, tenderness, masses, enlargement) • Sphincter tone, presence of hemorrhoids, rectal masses

Genitourinary Examination (*continued*)

System/Body Area	Elements of Examination
Genitourinary (*continued*)	**Female** Includes **at least seven of the following 11 elements** identified by bullets: • Inspection and palpation of breasts (eg, masses or lumps, tenderness, symmetry, nipple discharge) • Digital rectal examination including sphincter tone, presence of hemorrhoids, rectal masses Pelvic examination (with or without specimen collection for smears and cultures) including: • External genitalia (eg, general appearance, hair distribution, lesions) • Urethral meatus (eg, size, location, lesions, prolapse) • Urethra (eg, masses, tenderness, scarring) • Bladder (eg, fullness, masses, tenderness) • Vagina (eg, general appearance, estrogen effect, discharge, lesions, pelvic support, cystocele, rectocele) • Cervix (eg, general appearance, lesions, discharge) • Uterus (eg, size, contour, position, mobility, tenderness, consistency, descent, or support) • Adnexa/parametria (eg, masses, tenderness, organomegaly, nodularity) • Anus and perineum
Lymphatic	• Palpation of lymph nodes in neck, axillae, groin, and/or other location
Musculoskeletal	
Extremities	
Skin	• Inspection and/or palpation of skin and subcutaneous tissue (eg, rashes, lesions, ulcers)
Neurological/Psychiatric	Brief assessment of mental status including: • Orientation (eg, time, place, and person) • Mood and affect (eg, depression, anxiety, agitation)

Content and Documentation Requirements

Level of Exam	Perform and Document
Problem Focused	One to five elements identified by a bullet.
Expanded Problem Focused	At least six elements identified by a bullet.
Detailed	At least 12 elements identified by a bullet.
Comprehensive	Perform **all** elements identified by a bullet; document every element in each shaded area and at least one element in each category in each unshaded area.

Chapter 4: Evaluation and Management Documentation Guidelines/CMS 1997 Documentation Guidelines for Evaluation and Management Services

Chapter 4: Evaluation and Management Documentation Guidelines/CMS 1997 Documentation Guidelines for Evaluation and Management Services

Hematologic/Lymphatic/Immunologic Examination

System/Body Area	Elements of Examination
Constitutional	• Measurement of any three of the following seven vital signs: 1) sitting or standing blood pressure, 2) supine blood pressure, 3) pulse rate and regularity, 4) respiration, 5) temperature, 6) height, 7) weight (may be measured and recorded by ancillary staff) • General appearance of patient (eg, development, nutrition, body habitus, deformities, attention to grooming)
Head and Face	• Palpation and/or percussion of face with notation of presence or absence of sinus tenderness
Eyes	• Inspection of conjunctivae and lids
Ears, Nose, Mouth, and Throat	• Otoscopic examination of external auditory canals and tympanic membranes • Inspection of nasal mucosa, septum, and turbinates • Inspection of teeth and gums • Examination of oropharynx (eg, oral mucosa, hard and soft palates, tongue, tonsils, posterior pharynx)
Neck	• Examination of neck (eg, masses, overall appearance, symmetry, tracheal position, crepitus) • Examination of thyroid (eg, enlargement, tenderness, mass)
Respiratory	• Assessment of respiratory effort (eg, intercostal retractions, use of accessory muscles, diaphragmatic movement) • Auscultation of lungs (eg, breath sounds, adventitious sounds, rubs)
Cardiovascular	• Auscultation of heart with notation of abnormal sounds and murmurs • Examination of peripheral vascular system by observation (eg, swelling, varicosities) and palpation (eg, pulses, temperature, edema, tenderness)
Chest (Breasts)	
Gastrointestinal (Abdomen)	• Examination of abdomen with notation of presence of masses or tenderness • Examination of liver and spleen
Genitourinary	
Lymphatic	• Palpation of lymph nodes in neck, axillae, groin, and/or other location
Musculoskeletal	
Extremities	• Inspection and palpation of digits and nails (eg, clubbing, cyanosis, inflammation, petechiae, ischemia, infections, nodes)

Hematologic/Lymphatic/Immunologic Examination (continued)

System/Body Area	Elements of Examination
Skin	• Inspection and/or palpation of skin and subcutaneous tissue (eg, rashes, lesions, ulcers, ecchymoses, bruises)
Neurological/Psychiatric	Brief assessment of mental status including: • Orientation to time, place, and person • Mood and affect (eg, depression, anxiety, agitation)

Content and Documentation Requirements

Level of Exam	Perform and Document
Problem Focused	One to five elements identified by a bullet.
Expanded Problem Focused	At least six elements identified by a bullet.
Detailed	At least 12 elements identified by a bullet.
Comprehensive	Perform all elements identified by a bullet; document every element in each shaded area and at least one element in each category in each unshaded area.

Musculoskeletal Examination

System/Body Area	Elements of Examination
Constitutional	• Measurement of **any three of the following seven** vital signs: 1) sitting or standing blood pressure, 2) supine blood pressure, 3) pulse rate and regularity, 4) respiration, 5) temperature, 6) height, 7) weight (may be measured and recorded by ancillary staff) • General appearance of patient (eg, development, nutrition, body habitus, deformities, attention to grooming)
Head and Face	
Eyes	
Ears, Nose, Mouth, and Throat	
Neck	
Respiratory	
Cardiovascular	• Examination of peripheral vascular system by observation (eg, swelling, varicosities) and palpation (eg, pulses, temperature, edema, tenderness)
Chest (Breasts)	
Gastrointestinal (Abdomen)	
Genitourinary	
Lymphatic	• Palpation of lymph nodes in neck, axillae, groin, and/or other location
Musculoskeletal	• Examination of gait and station Examination of joint(s), bone(s), and muscle(s)/tendon(s) of **four of the following six** areas: 1) head and neck; 2) spine, ribs, and pelvis; 3) right upper extremity; 4) left upper extremity; 5) right lower extremity; and 6) left lower extremity. The examination of a given area includes: • Inspection, percussion, and/or palpation with notation of any misalignment, asymmetry, crepitation, defects, tenderness, masses, or effusions • Assessment of range of motion with notation of any pain (eg, straight leg raising), crepitation, or contracture • Assessment of stability with notation of any dislocation (luxation), subluxation, or laxity • Assessment of muscle strength and tone (eg, flaccid, cog wheel, spastic) with notation of any atrophy or abnormal movements *Note:* For the comprehensive level of examination, all four of the elements identified by a bullet must be performed and documented for each of four anatomic areas. For the three lower levels of examination, each element is counted separately for each body area. For example, assessing range of motion in two extremities constitutes two elements.

Musculoskeletal Examination (*continued*)

System/Body Area	Elements of Examination
Extremities	[See Musculoskeletal and Skin]
Skin	• Inspection and/or palpation of skin and subcutaneous tissue (eg, scars, rashes, lesions, cafe-au-lait spots, ulcers) in **four of the following six areas: 1)** head and neck, 2) trunk, 3) right upper extremity, 4) left upper extremity, 5) right lower extremity, and 6) left lower extremity. *Note:* For the comprehensive level, the examination of all four anatomic areas must be performed and documented. For the three lower levels of examination, each body area is counted separately. For example, inspection and/or palpation of the skin and subcutaneous tissue of two extremities constitutes two elements.
Neurological/ Psychiatric	• Test coordination (eg, finger/nose, heel/knee/shin, rapid alternating movements in the upper and lower extremities, evaluation of fine motor coordination in young children) • Examination of deep tendon reflexes and/or nerve stretch test with notation of pathological reflexes (eg, Babinski) • Examination of sensation (eg, by touch, pin, vibration, proprioception) Brief assessment of mental status including: • Orientation to time, place, and person • Mood and affect (eg, depression, anxiety, agitation)

Content and Documentation Requirements

Level of Exam	Perform and Document
Problem Focused	One to five elements identified by a bullet.
Expanded Problem Focused	At least six elements identified by a bullet.
Detailed	At least 12 elements identified by a bullet.
Comprehensive	Perform **all** elements identified by a bullet; document every element in each shaded area and at least one element in each category in each unshaded area.

Chapter 4: Evaluation and Management Documentation Guidelines/CMS 1997 Documentation Guidelines for Evaluation and Management Services

Neurological Examination

System/Body Area	Elements of Examination
Constitutional	• Measurement of any three of the following seven vital signs: 1) sitting or standing blood pressure, 2) supine blood pressure, 3) pulse rate and regularity, 4) respiration, 5) temperature, 6) height, 7) weight (may be measured and recorded by ancillary staff) • General appearance of patient (eg, development, nutrition, body habitus, deformities, attention to grooming)
Head and Face	
Eyes	• Ophthalmoscopic examination of optic discs (eg, size, C/D ratio, appearance) and posterior segments (eg, vessel changes, exudates, hemorrhages)
Ears, Nose, Mouth, and Throat	
Neck	
Respiratory	
Cardiovascular	• Examination of carotid arteries (eg, pulse amplitude, bruits) • Auscultation of heart with notation of abnormal sounds and murmurs • Examination of peripheral vascular system by observation (eg, swelling, varicosities) and palpation (eg, pulses, temperature, edema, tenderness)
Chest (Breasts)	
Gastrointestinal (Abdomen)	
Genitourinary	
Lymphatic	
Musculoskeletal	• Examination of gait and station Assessment of motor function including: • Muscle strength in upper and lower extremities • Muscle tone in upper and lower extremities (eg, flaccid, cog wheel, spastic) with notation of any atrophy or abnormal movements (eg, fasciculation, tardive dyskinesia)
Extremities	[See Musculoskeletal]
Skin	

Neurological Examination (continued)

System/Body Area	Elements of Examination
Neurological	Evaluation of higher integrative functions including: • Orientation to time, place, and person • Recent and remote memory • Attention span and concentration • Language (eg, naming objects, repeating phrases, spontaneous speech) • Fund of knowledge (eg, awareness of current events, past history, vocabulary) Test the following cranial nerves: • 2nd cranial nerve (eg, visual acuity, visual fields, fundi) • 3rd, 4th, and 6th cranial nerves (eg, pupils, eye movements) • 5th cranial nerve (eg, facial sensation, corneal reflexes) • 7th cranial nerve (eg, facial symmetry, strength) • 8th cranial nerve (eg, hearing with tuning fork, whispered voice, and/or finger rub) • 9th cranial nerve (eg, spontaneous or reflex palate movement) • 11th cranial nerve (eg, shoulder shrug strength) • 12th cranial nerve (eg, tongue protrusion) • Examination of sensation (eg, by touch, pin, vibration, proprioception) • Examination of deep tendon reflexes in upper and lower extremities with notation of pathological reflexes (eg, Babinski) • Test coordination (eg, finger/nose, heel/knee/shin, rapid alternating movements in the upper and lower extremities, evaluation of fine motor coordination in young children)
Psychiatric	

Content and Documentation Requirements

Level of Exam	Perform and Document
Problem Focused	One to five elements identified by a bullet.
Expanded Problem Focused	At least six elements identified by a bullet.
Detailed	At least 12 elements identified by a bullet.
Comprehensive	Perform all elements identified by a bullet; document every element in each shaded area and at least one element in each category in each unshaded area.

Psychiatric Examination

System/Body Area	Elements of Examination
Constitutional	• Measurement of any three of the following seven vital signs: 1) sitting or standing blood pressure, 2) supine blood pressure, 3) pulse rate and regularity, 4) respiration, 5) temperature, 6) height, 7) weight (may be measured and recorded by ancillary staff) • General appearance of patient (eg, development, nutrition, body habitus, deformities, attention to grooming)
Head and Face	
Eyes	
Ears, Nose, Mouth, and Throat	
Neck	
Respiratory	
Cardiovascular	
Chest (Breasts)	
Gastrointestinal (Abdomen)	
Genitourinary	
Lymphatic	
Musculoskeletal	• Assessment of muscle strength and tone (eg, flaccid, cog wheel, spastic) with notation of any atrophy and abnormal movements • Examination of gait and station
Extremities	
Skin	
Neurological	

Psychiatric Examination (*continued*)

System/Body Area	Elements of Examination

Psychiatric	• Description of speech including: rate, volume, articulation, coherence, and spontaneity with notation of abnormalities (eg, perseveration, paucity of language)
	• Description of thought processes including: rate of thoughts (eg, logical vs. illogical, tangential), abstract reasoning, and computation
	• Description of associations (eg, loose, tangential, circumstantial, intact)
	• Description of abnormal or psychotic thoughts including hallucinations, delusions, preoccupation with violence, homicidal or suicidal ideation, and obsessions
	• Description of the patient's judgment (eg, concerning everyday activities and social situations) and insight (eg, concerning psychiatric condition)
	Complete mental status examination including:
	  • Orientation to time, place, and person
	  • Recent and remote memory
	  • Attention span and concentration
	  • Language (eg, naming objects, repeating phrases)
	  • Fund of knowledge (eg, awareness of current events, past history, vocabulary)
	  • Mood and affect (eg, depression, anxiety, agitation, hypomania, lability)

Content and Documentation Requirements

Level of Exam	Perform and Document
Problem Focused	One to five elements identified by a bullet.
Expanded Problem Focused	At least six elements identified by a bullet.
Detailed	At least nine elements identified by a bullet.
Comprehensive	Perform all elements identified by a bullet; document every element in each shaded area and at least one element in each category in each unshaded area.

Chapter 4: Evaluation and Management Documentation Guidelines/CMS 1997 Documentation Guidelines for Evaluation and Management Services

Respiratory Examination

System/Body Area	Elements of Examination
Constitutional	• Measurement of any three of the following seven vital signs: 1) sitting or standing blood pressure, 2) supine blood pressure, 3) pulse rate and regularity, 4) respiration, 5) temperature, 6) height, 7) weight (may be measured and recorded by ancillary staff) • General appearance of patient (eg, development, nutrition, body habitus, deformities, attention to grooming)
Head and Face	
Eyes	
Ears, Nose, Mouth, and Throat	• Inspection of nasal mucosa, septum, and turbinates • Inspection of teeth and gums • Examination of oropharynx (eg, oral mucosa, hard and soft palates, tongue, tonsils, and posterior pharynx)
Neck	• Examination of neck (eg, masses, overall appearance, symmetry, tracheal position, crepitus) • Examination of thyroid (eg, enlargement, tenderness, mass) • Examination of jugular veins (eg, distension; a, v, or cannon a waves)
Respiratory	• Inspection of chest with notation of symmetry and expansion • Assessment of respiratory effort (eg, intercostal retractions, use of accessory muscles, diaphragmatic movement) • Percussion of chest (eg, dullness, flatness, hyper-resonance) • Palpation of chest (eg, tactile fremitus) • Auscultation of lungs (eg, breath sounds, adventitious sounds, rubs)
Cardiovascular	• Auscultation of heart including sounds, abnormal sounds, and murmurs • Examination of peripheral vascular system by observation (eg, swelling, varicosities) and palpation (eg, pulses, temperature, edema, tenderness)
Chest (Breasts)	
Gastrointestinal (Abdomen)	• Examination of abdomen with notation of presence of masses or tenderness • Examination of liver and spleen
Genitourinary	
Lymphatic	• Palpation of lymph nodes in neck, axillae, groin, and/or other location
Musculoskeletal	• Assessment of muscle strength and tone (eg, flaccid, cog wheel, spastic) with notation of any atrophy and abnormal movements • Examination of gait and station

Respiratory Examination (continued)

System/Body Area	Elements of Examination
Extremities	• Inspection and palpation of digits and nails (eg, clubbing, cyanosis, inflammation, petechiae, ischemia, infections, nodes)
Skin	• Inspection and/or palpation of skin and subcutaneous tissue (eg, rashes, lesions, ulcers)
Neurological/ Psychiatric	Brief assessment of mental status including: • Orientation to time, place, and person • Mood and affect (eg, depression, anxiety, agitation)

Content and Documentation Requirements

Level of Exam	Perform and Document
Problem Focused	One to five elements identified by a bullet.
Expanded Problem Focused	At least six elements identified by a bullet.
Detailed	At least 12 elements identified by a bullet.
Comprehensive	Perform all elements identified by a bullet; document every element in each shaded area and at least one element in each category in each unshaded area.

Skin Examination

System/Body Area	Elements of Examination
Constitutional	• Measurement of **any three of the following seven** vital signs: 1) sitting or standing blood pressure, 2) supine blood pressure, 3) pulse rate and regularity, 4) respiration, 5) temperature, 6) height, 7) weight (may be measured and recorded by ancillary staff) • General appearance of patient (eg, development, nutrition, body habitus, deformities, attention to grooming)
Head and Face	
Eyes	• Inspection of conjunctivae and lids
Ears, Nose, Mouth, and Throat	• Inspection of lips, teeth, and gums • Examination of oropharynx (eg, oral mucosa, hard and soft palates, tongue, tonsils, posterior pharynx)
Neck	• Examination of thyroid (eg, enlargement, tenderness, mass)
Respiratory	
Cardiovascular	• Examination of peripheral vascular system by observation (eg, swelling, varicosities) and palpation (eg, pulses, temperature, edema, tenderness)
Chest (Breasts)	
Gastrointestinal (Abdomen)	• Examination of liver and spleen • Examination of anus for condyloma and other lesions
Genitourinary	
Lymphatic	• Palpation of lymph nodes in neck, axillae, groin, and/or other location
Musculoskeletal	
Extremities	• Inspection and palpation of digits and nails (eg, clubbing, cyanosis, inflammation, petechiae, ischemia, infections, nodes)

Chapter 4: Evaluation and Management Documentation Guidelines/CMS 1997 Documentation Guidelines for Evaluation and Management Services

Skin Examination (continued)

System/Body Area	Elements of Examination

Skin	• Palpation of scalp and inspection of hair of scalp, eyebrows, face, chest, pubic area (when indicated), and extremities
	Inspection and/or palpation of skin and subcutaneous tissue (eg, rashes, lesions, ulcers, susceptibility to and presence of photo damage) in **eight of the following 10 areas:**
	  • Head, including face
	  • Neck
	  • Chest, including breasts and axillae
	  • Abdomen
	  • Genitalia, groin, buttocks
	  • Back
	  • Right upper extremity
	  • Left upper extremity
	  • Right lower extremity
	  • Left lower extremity
	Note: For the comprehensive level, the examination of at least eight anatomic areas must be performed and documented. For the three lower levels of examination, each body area is counted separately. For example, inspection and/or palpation of the skin and subcutaneous tissue of the right upper extremity and the left upper extremity constitutes two elements.
	• Inspection of eccrine and apocrine glands of skin and subcutaneous tissue with identification and location of any hyperhidrosis, chromhidroses, or bromhidrosis

Neurological/ Psychiatric	Brief assessment of mental status including:
	  • Orientation to time, place, and person
	  • Mood and affect (eg, depression, anxiety, agitation)

Content and Documentation Requirements

Level of Exam	Perform and Document
Problem Focused	**One to five** elements identified by a bullet.
Expanded Problem Focused	**At least six** elements identified by a bullet.
Detailed	**At least 12** elements identified by a bullet.
Comprehensive	Perform **all** elements identified by a bullet; document every element in each shaded area and at least one element in each category in each unshaded area.

C. Documentation of the Complexity of Medical Decision-Making

The levels of E/M services recognize four types of medical decision-making (straightforward, low complexity, moderate complexity, and high complexity). Medical decision-making refers to the complexity of establishing a diagnosis and/or selecting a management option as measured by

* The number of possible diagnoses and/or the number of management options that must be considered
* The amount and/or complexity of medical records, diagnostic tests, and/or other information that must be obtained, reviewed, and analyzed
* The risk of significant complications, morbidity, and/or mortality, as well as co-morbidities associated with the patient's presenting problem(s), the diagnostic procedure(s), and/or the possible management options

The chart below shows the progression of the elements required for each level of medical decision-making. To qualify for a given type of decision-making, two of the three elements in the table must be either met or exceeded.

Number of Diagnoses or Management Options	Amount and/or Complexity of Data to Be Reviewed	Risk of Significant Complications, Morbidity, and/or Mortality	Type of Decision-making
Minimal	Minimal or none	Minimal	Straightforward
Limited	Limited	Low	Low complexity
Multiple	Moderate	Moderate	Moderate complexity
Extensive	Extensive	High	High complexity

Each of the elements of medical decision-making is described below.

Number of Diagnoses or Management Options

The number of possible diagnoses and/or the number of management options that must be considered is based on the number and types of problems addressed during the encounter, the complexity of establishing a diagnosis, and the management decisions that are made by the physician.

Generally, decision-making with respect to a diagnosed problem is easier than that for an identified but undiagnosed problem. The number and type of diagnostic tests employed may be an indicator of the number of possible diagnoses. Problems that are improving or resolving are less complex than those that are worsening or failing to change as expected. The need to seek advice from others is another indicator of complexity of diagnostic or management problems.

•**DG:** *For each encounter, an assessment, clinical impression, or diagnosis should be documented. It may be explicitly stated or implied in documented decisions regarding management plans and/or further evaluation.*

  * *For a presenting problem with an established diagnosis, the record should reflect whether the problem is: a) improved, well controlled, resolving, or resolved or b) inadequately controlled, worsening, or failing to change as expected.*

  * *For a presenting problem without an established diagnosis, the assessment or clinical impression may be stated in the form of differential diagnoses or as a "possible," "probable," or "rule out" (R/O) diagnosis.*

•**DG:** *The initiation of, or changes in, treatment should be documented. Treatment includes a wide range of management options including patient instructions, nursing instructions, therapies, and medications.*

•**DG:** *If referrals are made, consultations requested, or advice sought, the record should indicate to whom or where the referral or consultation is made or from whom the advice is requested.*

Amount and/or Complexity of Data to Be Reviewed

The amount and complexity of data to be reviewed is based on the types of diagnostic testing ordered or reviewed. A decision to obtain and review old medical records and/or obtain history from sources other than the patient increases the amount and complexity of data to be reviewed.

Discussion of contradictory or unexpected test results with the physician who performed or interpreted the test is an indication of the complexity of data being reviewed. On occasion the physician who ordered a test may personally review the image, tracing, or specimen to supplement information from the physician who prepared the test report or interpretation; this is another indication of the complexity of data being reviewed.

- •DG: If a diagnostic service (test or procedure) is ordered, planned, scheduled, or performed at the time of the E/M encounter, the type of service (eg, lab or x-ray) should be documented.
- •DG: The review of lab, radiology, and/or other diagnostic tests should be documented. A simple notation such as "WBC elevated" or "chest x-ray unremarkable" is acceptable. Alternatively, the review may be documented by initialing and dating the report containing the test results.
- •DG: A decision to obtain old records or to obtain additional history from the family, caretaker, or other source to supplement that obtained from the patient should be documented.
- •DG: Relevant findings from the review of old records and/or the receipt of additional history from the family, caretaker, or other source to supplement that obtained from the patient should be documented. If there is no relevant information beyond that already obtained, that fact should be documented. A notation of "old records reviewed" or "additional history obtained from family" without elaboration is insufficient.
- •DG: The results of discussion of laboratory, radiology, or other diagnostic tests with the physician who performed or interpreted the study should be documented.
- •DG: The direct visualization and independent interpretation of an image, tracing, or specimen previously or subsequently interpreted by another physician should be documented.

Risk of Significant Complications, Morbidity, and/or Mortality

The risk of significant complications, morbidity, and/or mortality is based on the risks associated with the presenting problem(s), the diagnostic procedure(s), and the possible management options.

- •DG: Co-morbidities/underlying diseases or other factors that increase the complexity of medical decision making by increasing the risk of complications, morbidity, and/ or mortality should be documented.
- •DG: If a surgical or invasive diagnostic procedure is ordered, planned, or scheduled at the time of the E/M encounter, the type of procedure (eg, laparoscopy) should be documented.
- •DG: If a surgical or invasive diagnostic procedure is performed at the time of the E/M encounter, the specific procedure should be documented.
- •DG: The referral for or decision to perform a surgical or invasive diagnostic procedure on an urgent basis should be documented or implied.

The following table may be used to help determine whether the risk of significant complications, morbidity, and/or mortality is minimal, low, moderate, or high. Because the determination of risk is complex and not readily quantifiable, the table includes common clinical examples rather than absolute measures of risk. The assessment of risk of the presenting problem(s) is based on the risk related to the disease process anticipated between the present encounter and the next one. The assessment of risk of selecting diagnostic procedures and management options is based on the risk during and immediately following any procedures or treatment. **The highest level of risk in any one category (presenting problem(s), diagnostic procedure(s), or management options) determines the overall risk.**

D. Documentation of an Encounter Dominated by Counseling or Coordination of Care

In the case where counseling and/or coordination of care dominates (more than 50%) the physician/patient and/or family encounter (face-to-face time in the office or other outpatient setting, floor/unit time in the hospital or nursing facility), time is considered the key or controlling factor to qualify for a particular level of E/M services.

- •DG: If the physician elects to report the level of service based on counseling and/or coordination of care, the total length of time of the encounter (face-to-face or floor time, as appropriate) should be documented and the record should describe the counseling and/or activities to coordinate care.

Chapter 4: Evaluation and Management Documentation Guidelines/CMS 1997 Documentation Guidelines for Evaluation and Management Services

Table of Risk

Level of Risk	Presenting Problem(s)	Diagnostic Procedure(s) Ordered	Management Options Selected
Minimal	• One self-limited or minor problem, eg, cold, insect bite, tinea corporis	• Laboratory tests requiring venipuncture • Chest x-rays • EKG/EEG • Urinalysis • Ultrasound, eg, echo-cardiography • KOH prep	• Rest • Gargles • Elastic bandages • Superficial dressings
Low	• Two or more self-limited or minor problems • One stable chronic illness, eg, well controlled hypertension, non-insulin-dependent diabetes, cataract, BPH • Acute uncomplicated illness or injury, eg, cystitis, allergic rhinitis, simple sprain	• Physiologic tests not under stress, eg, pulmonary function tests • Non-cardiovascular imaging studies with contrast, eg, barium enema • Superficial needle biopsies • Clinical laboratory tests requiring arterial puncture • Skin biopsies	• Over-the-counter drugs • Minor surgery with no identified risk factors • Physical therapy • Occupational therapy • IV fluids without additives
Moderate	• One or more chronic illnesses with mild exacerbation, progression, or side effects of treatment • Two or more stable chronic illnesses • Undiagnosed new problem with uncertain prognosis, eg, lump in breast • Acute illness with systemic symptoms, eg, pyelonephritis, pneumonitis, colitis • Acute complicated injury, eg, head injury with brief loss of consciousness	• Physiologic tests under stress, eg, cardiac stress test, fetal contraction stress test • Diagnostic endoscopies with no identified risk factors • Deep needle or incisional biopsy • Cardiovascular imaging studies with contrast and no identified risk factors, eg, arteriogram, cardiac catheterization • Obtain fluid from body cavity, eg, lumbar puncture, thoracentesis, culdocentesis	• Minor surgery with identified risk factors • Elective major surgery (open, percutaneous, or endoscopic) with no identified risk factors • Prescription drug management • Therapeutic nuclear medicine • IV fluids with additives • Closed treatment of fracture or dislocation without manipulation
High	• One or more chronic illnesses with severe exacerbation, progression, or side effects of treatment • Acute or chronic illnesses or injuries that pose a threat to life or bodily function, eg, multiple trauma, acute MI, pulmonary embolus, severe respiratory distress, progressive severe rheumatoid arthritis, psychiatric illness with potential threat to self or others, peritonitis, acute renal failure • An abrupt change in neurological status, eg, seizure, TIA, weakness, sensory loss	• Cardiovascular imaging studies with contrast with identified risk factor • Cardiac electrophysiological tests • Diagnostic endoscopies with identified risk factors • Discography	• Elective major surgery (open, percutaneous, or endoscopic) with identified risk factors • Emergency major surgery (open, percutaneous, or endoscopic) • Parenteral controlled substances • Drug therapy requiring intensive monitoring for toxicity • Decision not to resuscitate or to de-escalate are because of poor prognosis

Time-Based Coding

Contents

Most procedures and services in *Current Procedural Terminology* (*CPT*®) are described by specific components of physician work (eg, **94011**, measurement of spirometric forced expiratory flows in an infant or child through 2 years of age). However, time (especially intraservice time) is also used as a proxy for physician work. Many services are reported based solely on time of service or, as in the case of many evaluation and management (E/M) services, may be reported based on key components of work (history, examination, and medical decision-making [MDM]) *or* typical intraservice time when most of the time of service was spent in counseling and/or coordination of care.

Understanding the correct application of time in code selection is important to reporting the code that most accurately describes the service provided. *Current Procedural Terminology* provides general and category/code-specific instructions for reporting services based on time. An understanding of these instructions is key to selecting codes that most accurately capture the services provided. This chapter will review the general guidelines for reporting time and guidelines specific to time-based reporting of E/M services. Service-specific instructions and examples are also provided throughout this manual to help illustrate time-based coding.

The Value of Documenting Time

Failure to document time of service may be costly even when it is possible to report a service without documenting time.

Example

➤ **Discharge summary: Continued on intravenous (IV) antibiotics until this morning, breastfeeding well, no further fevers.** Vital signs and general appearance and examination of the heart, lungs, abdomen, and skin are performed. Blood and urine cultures remain negative after 48 hours. Intravenous antibiotics discontinued. Final diagnosis: fever, likely viral infection. Patient discharged home with instructions for home care and follow-up. A total of 35 minutes was spent on the floor reviewing the hospital course, expected follow-up, and signs and symptoms of possible sepsis or infection with mother.

The physician documents that 35 minutes was spent in discharge management services. A summary of the activities is documented to support the time of service.	***CPT*** **99239** (hospital discharge day management; more than 30 minutes)
Viral infection is not reported because diagnoses documented as uncertain (eg, likely) are not reported. Instead codes for signs and symptoms, such as fever, are reported.	***International Classification of Diseases, 10th Revision, Clinical Modification (ICD-10-CM)*** **F90.1** (fever)

Teaching Point: If time were not documented, lesser code **99238** (hospital discharge day management; 30 minutes or less) would be reported because time of greater than 30 minutes must be documented to support code **99239**. Code **99238** has 2.05 total relative value units (RVUs), while code **99239** is assigned 3.04 total RVUs. Persistent failure to document the time of discharge day management services may result in significant loss of otherwise earned revenue. For example, a payer contract allows $40 per RVU, so a practice is paid $82 ($40 × 2.05) for code **99238** and $121.60 ($40 × 3.04) for code **99239**. Therefore, $39.60 of potential revenue is lost due to lack of documentation; for 10 services, $396 of potential revenue is lost.

Likewise, failure to document time eliminates the possibility of reporting prolonged services and may negatively affect the level of service reported when multiple episodes of care occur on the same date (eg, multiple hospital care services). Routinely noting the time spent face-to-face (outpatient) or on a patient's unit or floor (observation and inpatient) and those instances when more than 50% of that time is spent in counseling and/or coordination of care allows for recognition of occasions where reporting based on time is most advantageous.

Chapter 5: Time-Based Coding

General Guidelines

Current Procedural Terminology® provides overall instructions for time-based reporting in the "Instructions for Use of the *CPT* Codebook" found in the Introduction of the coding manual. These instructions are followed for reporting time-based services when there are no section guidelines, prefatory instructions, parenthetical instructions, or specified time requirements in code descriptors.

- ❉ If your electronic health record (EHR) or other coding reference does not include the prefatory and parenthetical instructions provided in *CPT*, consider whether secondary code verification prior to billing is necessary. Alternatively, it may be possible to insert instructions in the form of notes or alerts in an EHR.

> ||||||||| **Coding Pearl** |||||||||
>
> Section and prefatory instructions, code descriptors, and parenthetical instructions override the general instruction for time-based reporting.

- ❉ Time is the physician or other reporting provider's face-to-face time with the patient, unless otherwise stated. Time spent by clinical staff is reported only when specified in *CPT* or allowed under incident-to policy established by a payer. (Learn more about incident-to service in Chapter 14, Allied Health and Clinical Staff Services.)
- ❉ A unit of time is met when the midpoint is *passed* (eg, an hour is attained when 31 minutes have passed), unless otherwise specified by *CPT* or payer policy. (Some payers may require that the typical time assigned to a service be met or exceeded rather than approximated as allowed by *CPT*.) The midpoint rule is not applied when *CPT* includes category or code-specific instructions to the contrary. Examples of when the midpoint rule does and does not apply are included throughout this chapter.
- ❉ It is important to note that a code that is reported "per day" (eg, **99468**, initial inpatient neonatal critical care, *per day*, for the E/M of a critically ill neonate, 28 days of age or younger) is not reported for all services in a 24-hour period but, rather, all services on a single date. Likewise, a code describing services "on the same date" (eg, **99463**, initial hospital or birthing center care, per day, for E/M of normal newborn infant admitted and discharged *on the same date*) is reported only for services on a single date of service.

General Guidelines for Documentation of Time

- ❉ Documentation of time spent providing services should be evident in the medical record for each service reported based on time (eg, start and stop times or total minutes of service).
- ❉ Documentation of time may be automated in an EHR, but physicians should be able to demonstrate that the EHR functionality captures the correct time for code selection as specified by *CPT*. For instance, only intraservice time is used to select codes for moderate sedation. Documentation should clearly reflect the start and stop times for this service.
- ❉ When multiple services are provided on the same date, the time spent in time-based services must be clearly distinguished from time spent providing other services.
- ❉ In addition to documentation of start and stop or total time of service, documentation should clearly support the service reported. For example, documentation of psychotherapy should include factors such as modalities and frequency, functional status, mental status examination, diagnosis, treatment plan, prognosis, and progress.
- ❉ All documentation must be signed or electronically authenticated with the name and credentials of the physician or other provider of care and date of service.

Time of Evaluation and Management Services

There are very few E/M service codes for which typical time is never a factor in reporting the service. Other criteria are used for the selection of the specific codes (eg, defined components, services reported per day).

E/M Services Not Reported Based on Typical Time	
E/M Codes	**Description**
99217	Observation care discharge
99281–99285	Emergency department encounters
99381–99397	Initial and periodic comprehensive preventive medicine E/M
99450–99456	Disability exam
99460–99463	Newborn services
99464–99465	Attendance at delivery/resuscitation
99468–99476	Neonatal/pediatric critical care
99477–99480	Intensive care

Certain E/M services are always reported based on time (see discussion later in this chapter).

However, many E/M services are described by key components of physician work or typical time. For these services, time may be the basis for code selection in lieu of key components (history, examination, MDM) when appropriate per *CPT®* instruction.

Reporting Time in Lieu of Key Components

Key guidelines for using time as the controlling factor in the selection of an E/M service that may otherwise be reported based on key components include

- ✸ Time shall be used as the key component in the selection of an E/M code if there is an assigned typical time and counseling and/or coordination of care accounts for *more than 50%* of the physician face-to-face time (for outpatient) or floor or unit time (for inpatient) with the patient and/or family.
- ✸ When reporting based on time spent counseling and/or coordinating care, codes are selected based on typical times assigned to the E/M code in the category appropriate to the service rendered (eg, office or other outpatient visit). See the tables in Chapter 7, Evaluation and Management Services in the Office, Outpatient, Home, or Nursing Facility Setting, for typical times in the outpatient setting and Chapter 10, Noncritical Hospital Evaluation and Management Services, for typical times in the inpatient or observation setting.
- ✸ The time spent in counseling and/or coordination of care may be with the patient, family, and/or those who may have assumed responsibility for the care of the patient (eg, foster parents, legal guardian, person acting in loco parentis).

Coding Conundrum: Child Is Not Present

It is common in pediatrics to have a parent come into the office to discuss a child's condition or problem without the child present. *Current Procedural Terminology* clarifies that counseling and/or coordination of care can be provided to those who have assumed responsibility for the care of the patient or decision-making even if they are not family members (eg, foster parents, legal guardians, persons acting in loco parentis). Therefore, counseling of those responsible for the care of the patient without the patient present is reported with the various levels of E/M service. It does not matter if the patient is a new or an established patient, although, typically, counseling and/or coordination of care with family members alone is performed for established patients. The pediatrician can report this E/M service using time as the key factor even if the child is not present. However, some payers require that the patient be present. Be aware of payer-specific requirements. These services are performed on behalf of the patient and reported under the patient's name, and not the parent's name.

Chapter 5: Time-Based Coding

- The term *counseling* is broadly defined by *CPT®* as most activities that are not procedures and includes discussions about a condition and/or its management. Per *CPT*, counseling includes
  - Diagnostic results, impressions, and/or recommended diagnostic studies
  - Prognosis
  - Risks and benefits of management (treatment) options
  - Instructions for management (treatment) and/or follow-up
  - Importance of compliance with chosen management (treatment) options
  - Risk factor reduction
  - Patient and family education
- Counseling about a condition emerging as part of the information gathering for the primary diagnosis may appropriately be included in total time of counseling (eg, discussing ways to increase caloric intake in a patient with anorectic effects of medication for attention-deficit/hyperactivity disorder [ADHD]).
- Time of an E/M service is categorized as face-to-face or unit or floor time.
  - Face-to-face time applies in non-facility settings for services such as office and other outpatient E/M visits and consultations. Only the time that a physician or other qualified health care professional (QHP) spends face-to-face with a patient and/or caregiver(s) is used for determining the level of service provided.
  - Unit or floor time is used in a facility setting (including outpatient observation) and includes the physician's or QHP's time directed to care of a single patient, including face-to-face time and time spent on the unit or floor managing and coordinating that patient's care (eg, reviewing charts, communicating with clinical staff). Time spent off the unit or floor (eg, in radiology viewing images) is not included in the unit or floor time used in code selection.

CPT Definition of Face-to-Face Time	
Consultation or Visit in Office/Outpatient, Home, Domiciliary	Inpatient Hospital, Observation Setting, Nursing Home, Hourly Critical Care
Direct physician to patient and/or family member/other with responsibility for care of the patient	Floor/unit time dedicated to the one patient Includes the time spent at the patient's bedside, counseling the family/patient, and on the floor documenting and coordinating care with the patient's care team members

- Although codes are valued to include typical preservice and post-service time, only the typical time (face-to-face or unit/floor) is used in code selection.

Example

➤ The typical time assigned to a level 3 established patient office or other outpatient E/M service (**99213**) is 15 minutes. Code **99213** is valued to include 3 minutes of preservice time (eg, time reviewing history obtained by clinical staff) and 5 minutes of post-service time (eg, time documenting the service provided, care coordination, and communication with patient/caregivers between current and next encounter). Because services are valued to include preservice and post-service time, code selection is affected only when the time of service significantly exceeds the typical time (eg, prolonged service is reported only for 30 minutes or more beyond the 15-minute typical time of code **99213**).

  - Time spent on a particular calendar day does not have to be continuous. A physician may spend face-to-face time with a patient before and after clinical staff administer treatments or monitor the patient, but only the physician's total face-to-face time with the patient is considered in selecting a level of service unless otherwise specified.
  - When service time is discontinuous, each episode of care should include documentation of time.

Example

➤ A physician provides critical care services to an 8-year-old inpatient for 25 minutes in the morning and, later on the same date, provides an additional 25 minutes of critical care services. The aggregated time of 50 minutes of critical care services (**99291**) is reported based on the time documented at each encounter on the same date.

⚬ Only physicians or QHPs with their own National Provider Identifier may report services using time as the key component: "Incident-to policy as developed by Medicare generally allows for reporting of services by QHPs working under direct physician supervision as if the services were personally performed by the physician. However, most Medicare contractors will not allow reporting of incident-to services based on time of counseling and/or coordination of care." Please refer to the Medicare Incident-to Requirements: Supervision of Nonphysician Health Care Professionals section in Chapter 14, Allied Health and Clinical Staff Services. Keep in mind that the incident-to requirements are Medicare policy; commercial payers may have their own policies.

⚬ When time is used as the controlling factor in the selection of an E/M code and the service is provided by a resident, the time reported is based on the face-to-face time (for outpatient) or floor or unit time (for inpatient) spent by the teaching physician with the patient or caregiver. Refer to the Guidelines for Reporting E/M Services Under Teaching Physician Guidelines section in Chapter 4, Evaluation and Management Documentation Guidelines.

⚬ When a range of codes includes sequential times (eg, office or other outpatient E/M services) and the time of service is between the times assigned to codes, report the code with the typical time closest to the actual time of service. If the actual time of service falls exactly between the typical times of 2 codes, report the code with the lower typical time (ie, the midpoint must be passed to report the greater service).

Examples

➤ An established patient office visit includes 20 minutes of physician face-to-face time. The actual time of 20 minutes falls exactly at the midpoint between code **99213** (typical time 15 minutes) and code **99214** (typical time 25 minutes), so the midpoint was not passed. The appropriate code for this encounter would be **99213**.

➤ A physician provides counseling to parents of a child who may be a stem cell donor to an ill sibling. Discussion includes addressing the parent's questions about risks to the healthy child as a donor and the typical course of care. The physician documents 20 minutes of face-to-face time spent with the parents. Code **99401** (preventive medicine counseling and/or risk factor reduction intervention[s] provided to an individual [separate procedure]; approximately 15 minutes) is reported.

Teaching Point: If the time of service had been 23 minutes or more, the midpoint between code **99401** and **99402** (preventive medicine counseling…; approximately 30 minutes) would be exceeded and code **99402** would be reported.

➤ A 12-year-old boy presents for management of medications prescribed for predominantly hyperactive ADHD. Medication was prescribed 3 weeks earlier.

History: No improvement was seen after starting medication, continues to disrupt class, fidgeting more, and unable to focus on work; no weight loss, occasional trouble sleeping, loss of appetite, and no diarrhea. No changes in his school or home environment.

Behavioral rating scales: Parent- and teacher-completed NICHQ Vanderbilt ADHD scales are reviewed. Neither rating scale by either observer showed changes from pretreatment behaviors.

Physical examination: 3 organ systems documented (constitutional, cardiovascular, gastrointestinal).

Chapter 5: Time-Based Coding

Assessment/plan: New medication is prescribed, old discontinued; follow up in 2 weeks. Twenty-five minutes is spent discussing side effects of the medication, behavior modifications, changes at school, and when psychiatric referral may be needed. Total time of face-to-face visit was 36 minutes.

The physician documents that 35 minutes was spent face-to-face with the child and guardian and 25 minutes of that was spent on counseling. A summary of the issues discussed is documented. Time (35 minutes face-to-face) is the key controlling factor.	***ICD-10-CM*** **F90.1** (ADHD, predominantly hyperactive) ***CPT*** **New Patient** **Established Patient** **99203 25** (30 minutes) **99215 25** (40 minutes) **96127** × 2 (brief behavioral and emotional assessment, with scoring and documentation, per instrument [2 scales reviewed])

Teaching Point: When the actual time is between 2 typical times, select the code with a typical time closest to the total physician time spent. Code **99214** has a typical time of 25 minutes. The actual time spent in this encounter (36 minutes) is closer to the 40 minutes assigned to code **99215**. Because more than 50% of the 36 minutes was spent in counseling and/or coordinating care, code **99215** may be reported. If the patient were new to the physician, code **99203** would be reported, as 36 minutes is closer to the 30-minute typical time of **99203** than the 45-minute typical time of **99204**. (Some health plans and state Medicaid programs may require that the typical time assigned to a code be met or exceeded.)

> **|||||||| Coding Pearl ||||||||**
> When reporting code 96127, one unit is reported for each standardized instrument completed and scored. When reporting more than 2 units of service, it may be necessary to report additional units of service on a separate claim line with modifier 59 due to National Correct Coding Initiative edits. See the Medically Unlikely Edits section in Chapter 3, Modifiers and Coding Edits, for more information.

- Time-based services are reported based only on time devoted to that particular service. When a separately reportable service is performed concurrently with a time-based service, the time associated with providing the concurrent service *is not* counted toward the time used in reporting the time-based service.
- When separately reportable services are rendered in the same encounter as time-based services, the time spent in the separately reportable service should be distinguishable from that of the time-based service (eg, start and stop times of procedural services are noted).

Examples

> During an encounter with an adolescent who dove into a lake, hit his head, and was unconscious when pulled from the water, a physician spends 10 minutes performing cardiopulmonary resuscitation (CPR) and then another 45 minutes providing critical care before the patient is transferred to another facility. Critical care service (**99291**) time is documented and distinctly identifiable in the patient record from the time spent performing the separately reportable CPR (**92950**), for which start and stop times were documented.

> A physician provides and documents 15 minutes of face-to-face E/M service, of which 10 minutes was spent in counseling an established patient and caregivers about changes to a care plan for managing obesity and mild hypertension in the adolescent patient (**99213 25**). The physician also performed and will separately report evacuation of a subungual hematoma (**11740**) at the same encounter. Time spent in provision of the evacuation procedure cannot be included in the time of the E/M service and is separately noted in the medical record.

Documentation of Time Spent in Counseling and/or Coordination of Care

According to the guidelines as specified in the American Medical Association publication *Principles of CPT®* *Coding*, when selecting a code based on time, the medical record documentation must reflect

1. The amount of time and extent of counseling and/or coordination of care services provided
2. Distinguishing of that time from time spent performing key components by reporting time separately
3. The total time spent face-to-face (for outpatient) or floor or unit (for inpatient)
4. A summary of the discussion items and/or the coordination of care efforts

If the entire face-to-face encounter is spent in counseling only, the total time spent and a summary of the discussion items must be clearly documented.

In distinguishing the time and extent of counseling and/or coordination of care services for a service that includes time spent performing key components, physicians may document the estimated number of minutes or the percentage of the documented total face-to-face time that was spent in counseling and/or coordination of care.

The summary of discussion items and/or coordination of care efforts should be sufficient in detail to support the selection of a code based on time (eg, include options discussed, patient/caregiver concerns addressed, and summary of patient and family education).

Examples for Documenting Time

Counseling in the office might be documented as follows:

◉ Spoke with Ms Jones about _____, and
  ❖ 40-minute visit with approximately 25 minutes spent discussing Ms Jones, or
  ❖ T = # minutes*; C = # minutes; counseled regarding Ms Jones, or
  ❖ Total face-to-face time was 40 minutes with >50% spent in counseling and/or coordination of care.

*If you choose to use the second method for documentation of time, be sure to include a description of T (total time) and C (counseling and/or coordination of care time) in your office policy. Otherwise, the documentation should state "total time" or "counseling time."

Hospital/observation care progress notes might be documented as follows:

◉ 25 minutes spent on floor with patient, nursing staff, and physical therapy regarding Ms Jones, or document time in and time out.

◉ Timed chart entry in the progress notes or orders may be enough to support floor time. Caseworkers, physical therapists, etc, may document the time spent communicating with the physician. These documented entries may support total floor time.

If you use a template for your progress notes, include space for reporting face-to-face time, counseling time, and a summary of discussion items. If you are using an EHR, make software changes to accommodate the documentation requirements. Do not just use the "office time" as shown in your EHR because that does not reflect face-to-face time.

A summary of the patient/caregiver concerns and questions, your responses and recommendations, and plan of care must be documented to support the medical necessity of the time spent counseling and/or coordinating care.

E/M Services That Are Always Time-Based

Certain E/M services are never reported based on key components but, rather, are time-based services. These codes are often not subject to the general instructions for reporting based on time, as prefatory language and code descriptors provide reporting instructions.

Examples

➤ A single code is reported for all hospital discharge day services based on time of 30 minutes or less (**99238**) or of more than 30 minutes (**99239**). See The Value of Documenting Time section earlier in this chapter for more information on these codes.

99238   Hospital discharge day management; 30 minutes or less
99239   more than 30 minutes

➤ The code descriptor for **99291** is critical care, E/M of the critically ill or critically injured patient; first 30 to 74 minutes. Per prefatory instruction, code **99291** is not reported for critical care of less than 30 minutes (ie, the midpoint rule does not apply). Code **99291** is reported only once per date by the reporting individual even if time spent providing critical care is not continuous and only for time of at least 30 minutes.

99291   Critical care, evaluation and management of the critically ill or critically injured patient; first 30-74 minutes

+99292   each additional 30 minutes (List separately in addition to code for primary service)

➤ Prolonged service(s) with direct patient contact (**99354–99357**) is reported for a service that extends significantly beyond the typical time of an E/M or psychotherapy service (**90837**). Codes are selected based on whether the service is provided in the hospital/observation setting or in an office or other outpatient setting and on the extent of time beyond the typical time of the related service. With time-based reporting, prefatory instructions state that an initial prolonged service (**99354, 99356**) is reported when a physician or QHP provides service for 30 or more minutes beyond the typical time of the related services. In addition, codes **99355** and **99357** may be reported for each additional 30 minutes beyond the first hour of prolonged service and for the final 15 to 30 minutes of prolonged service on a given date. Service of less than 15 minutes beyond the first hour or less than 15 minutes beyond the final 30 minutes is not reported separately.

+99354   Prolonged evaluation and management or psychotherapy service(s) (beyond the typical service time of the primary procedure) in the office or other outpatient setting requiring direct patient contact beyond the usual service; first hour

+99355   each additional 30 minutes

+99356   Prolonged service in the inpatient or observation setting, requiring unit/floor time beyond the usual service; first hour

+99357   each additional 30 minutes

When an E/M service is reported using time as the key or controlling factor (>50% of the total face-to-face time was spent in counseling and/or coordination of care), prolonged service can be reported only when the prolonged service exceeds 30 minutes beyond the highest level of E/M service (eg, **99205, 99223**). Please see other important instructions for reporting prolonged service(s) in Chapter 7, Evaluation and Management Services in the Office, Outpatient, Home, or Nursing Facility Setting, and Chapter 10, Noncritical Hospital Evaluation and Management Services.

➤ Preventive medicine counseling (**99401–99404**) is reported based on face-to-face time spent in counseling an individual patient. The midpoint rule for code selection applies.

➤ Behavior change interventions, such as smoking and tobacco cessation counseling (**99406, 99407**), include specific time ranges for each code (eg, greater than 3 minutes up to 10 minutes is reported with code **99406**). Smoking and tobacco cessation counseling of 3 minutes or less is not separately reported.

Time of Clinical Staff

In recent years, there has been greater recognition of the need for payment to support activities such as care coordination that require clinical staff time performing services under physician supervision rather than direct delivery of care by the physician. Services such as chronic care management, psychiatric collaborative care management, and prolonged clinical staff service are now described by specific *CPT®* codes reported based on the time spent by clinical staff. However, as with time-based services provided by physicians and QHPs, documentation to support services based on clinical staff time requires specific elements. These include

* Documentation of an authenticated order for the service by the ordering or supervising physician.
* Documentation of the time and care activity performed for each episode of service rendered by clinical staff during the reporting period, including authentication (written or electronic signature with credentials and date of service).
* Documentation and authentication of physician time spent in care activities that might otherwise be performed by clinical staff and were not otherwise reportable during the reporting period, when applicable.
* Evidence of the supervising physician's ongoing involvement in the patient's care, such as review and/or revision of the patient care plan.
* Only the time of clinical staff whose services are a practice expense to the reporting physician are included in the time of service (ie, services by clinical staff of a facility are not reportable by a physician who has no contractual or employment relationship with the staff).

When multiple clinical staff members meet about a patient, count the time only once.

Example

> A 6-year-old has spastic quadriplegia, gastrostomy, gastroesophageal reflux with recurrent bouts of aspiration pneumonia and reactive airways disease, chronic seizure disorder, failure to thrive, and severe neurodevelopment delay. He receives home occupational, physical, and speech therapy services. During the course of a calendar month, the care plan is substantially revised. Clinical staff and the physician document each individual care management activity performed and the time of each service in the EHR using non-billable pseudocodes (eg, CCMHH for chronic care management activities related to coordinating the patient's home health) that identify the type of activity and time of service in minutes. After the end of the calendar month, billing staff create a report of all patients to whom pseudocodes for chronic care management services were entered during the month. The total time of chronic care management services is 110 minutes for this patient.

Time of 110 minutes of care management activities along with substantial revision of the patient's care plan support reporting of complex chronic care management.	**CPT®** **99487** (complex chronic care management services, with the following required elements: • multiple (two or more) chronic conditions expected to last at least 12 months, or until the death of the patient, • chronic conditions place the patient at significant risk of death, acute exacerbation/decompensation, or functional decline, • establishment or substantial revision of a comprehensive care plan, • moderate or high complexity medical decision making; • 60 minutes of clinical staff time directed by a physician or other qualified health care professional, per calendar month) **+99489** (each additional 30 minutes of clinical staff time directed by a physician or other qualified health care professional, per calendar month [List separately in addition to **99487**.])
	ICD-10-CM Code for conditions addressed in the calendar month.

As team-based care becomes more predominant in pediatric practice, knowledge of which clinical staff activities are separately reportable and the requirements for reporting will have significant effect on the profitability of this care model. See Chapter 8, Managing Chronic and Complex Conditions, for detailed review of chronic care management and other services that are reported based on time of care by clinical staff.

Documentation and tracking of time for services that are reported on a periodic basis, such as per calendar month, require establishment of routine processes that prevent lost revenue due to failure to capture all billable services. The previous example illustrates one manual method of using pseudocodes that are set to never bill out on claims but provide a basis for tracking time-based services. Some practices use manual systems, such as spreadsheets, while others have adapted their EHR with flow sheets to capture each activity and the related time throughout a period of service and provide a report of time per patient within each period of service. Practice and system capabilities vary. Collaboration with system vendors, professional colleagues, and practice management consultants may be invaluable to successful delivery, documentation, and reporting of time-based services.

> **Coding Pearl** ||||||||
>
> See the prefatory language in *CPT®* when reporting sequential time-based services, such as critical care, prolonged service, and moderate (conscious) sedation, to find specific instructions and helpful tables illustrating code assignment by time of service.

Time-Based Reporting of Non-E/M Services

In addition to time-based reporting of E/M services, many other services are reported based on the time of service. See Chapter 15 for other information on reporting anesthesia or therapeutic and surgical procedures.

Examples

➤ Moderate (conscious) sedation services are reported based on 15-minute time increments of intraservice time beginning with administration of a sedating agent(s) and ending after the procedure is completed and the physician or QHP providing the sedation is no longer in personal continuous face-to-face contact with the patient.

➤ Intra-arterial and IV infusions are reported based on time and whether the infusion is the initial infusion service or a subsequent infusion service.

➤ Several types of psychological and neuropsychological testing are reported per hour based on whether a physician or QHP administers the tests and provides interpretation and report or tests are administered by a technician with interpretation and report by a physician or QHP.

➤ Care plan oversight services for ventilator management of a patient in a home or domiciliary setting are reported for 30 minutes or more per month.

Guidelines for Time-Based Procedural Services

Only include time spent in activities such as interpretation and report when the code descriptor indicates time spent in such activities is used in code selection.

Examples

➤ Code **96125** (standardized cognitive performance testing [eg, Ross Information Processing Assessment] per hour of a qualified health care professional's time, both face-to-face time administering tests to the patient and time interpreting these test results and preparing the report) specifically states that *the physician's time of interpreting tests and preparing the report is counted toward the time of service.*

➤ Code **94780** (car seat/bed testing for airway integrity, neonate, with continual nursing observation and continuous recording of pulse oximetry, heart rate and respiratory rate, with interpretation and report; 60 minutes) is reported based on the time spent (typically by clinical staff) monitoring the neonate during the testing period and not on time spent by the physician interpreting the outcome and preparing a report.

    Teaching Point: The physician's time interpreting the testing and preparing a report is not used in code selection, but the service was valued to include the typical post-service time that a physician spends in interpreting and preparing a report.

Time-based services may overlap 2 dates of service (ie, begin prior to midnight and continue on the next date). If the service is continuous, report as if provided on the initial date of service. However, once the initial service has ended, any new service provided on the second date is reported as an initial service.

Examples

➤ **A physician provides remote intraoperative neurophysiology monitoring from 8:00 pm on one date to 1:00 am on the next date.** The service is reported as performed on the date the service began with code **95941** (continuous intraoperative neurophysiology monitoring, from outside the operating room [remote or nearby] or for monitoring of more than one case while in the operating room, per hour) times 5 units.

➤ **A facility may report 2 initial IV push services (96374) when provided from 11:30 to 11:40 pm and again from 1:30 to 1:40 am, as the service was not continuous.** However, an IV push started at 11:55 pm and ending at 12:05 am is reported as one continuous service on the date the service started.

Key Takeaways for Reporting Time

Examples of time-based reporting are included throughout this manual to further the understanding of time-based reporting. The examples emphasize some key tips for reporting based on time.

- Time must be documented to support coding of time-based services. Failure to document time may lead to lost revenue.
- Time is met when the midpoint is passed unless otherwise specified in *CPT*® instruction or code descriptors.
- Time is that of the physician or other individual reporting the service unless otherwise specified (eg, code descriptor specifies clinical staff time).
- Documentation should include the context of time spent in counseling and/or coordination of care, when applicable.

Chapter 5: Time-Based Coding

||||||||

Preventive Services

||||||||

Contents

Preventive Care

Preventive care is the hallmark of pediatrics. The Patient Protection and Affordable Care Act (PPACA) recognized the importance of preventive care for children, a critical provision of which ensures that most health care plans cover, *without cost sharing,* the gold standard of pediatric preventive care—the American Academy of Pediatrics (AAP) *Bright Futures: Guidelines for Health Supervision of Infants, Children, and Adolescents,* 4th Edition.

Coverage of and appropriate payment for these pediatric preventive services should, at a minimum, reflect the total relative value units (RVUs) outlined for the current year under the Medicare Resource-Based Relative Value Scale (RBRVS) Physician Fee Schedule, inclusive of all separately reported codes for these services. Section 2713 of the PPACA includes the following 2 sets of services that must be provided to children without cost sharing:

1. The standard set of immunizations recommended by the Advisory Committee on Immunization Practices (ACIP) of the Centers for Disease Control and Prevention (CDC) with respect to the individual involved .
2. Evidence-informed preventive care and screenings provided for in the comprehensive guidelines supported by the Health Resources and Services Administration (HRSA), which include
   ❖ Bright Futures recommendations for preventive pediatric health care
   ❖ Recommendations of the Secretary's Advisory Committee on Heritable Disorders in Newborns and Children

The Bright Futures periodicity schedule, "Recommendations for Preventive Pediatric Health Care," is a great tool to identify recommended age-appropriate services; in addition, it can be used to identify those services that can and should be reported with their own *Current Procedural Terminology* (*CPT*®) or Healthcare Common Procedure Coding System code and it identifies appropriate diagnosis coding. This tool can be found at the end of this book as an insert or accessed online at www.aap.org/periodicityschedule.

Although all recommended preventive services are covered, physicians and practice managers should be aware of health plan policies that may affect payment.

⚙ Specific diagnosis codes may be required to support claims adjudication under preventive medicine benefits. Be sure to link the appropriate diagnosis to each service provided (eg, code **Z71.3**, dietary counseling, may be linked to risk-factor reduction counseling code **99401**).

⚙ Some payers bundle certain services when the services are provided on the same date. For instance, some plans will not allow separate payment for obesity counseling on the same date as a well-child examination but will cover obesity counseling when no other evaluation and management (E/M) service is provided on the same date. It is beneficial to monitor and maintain awareness of the payment policies of those plans most commonly billed by your practice. Most policies are available on payers' Web sites with notification of changes provided in payer communications, such as electronic newsletters.

Quality Initiatives and Preventive Care

Quality initiatives and measurement are becoming standard practice in health care. Many physicians have participated in quality measurement through programs such as the Centers for Medicare & Medicaid Services (CMS) Electronic Health Records Incentive Program and medical home recognition programs. In pediatrics, many quality measures are associated with preventive care (eg, provision of one meningococcal vaccine on or between the patient's 11th and 13th birthdays).

> |||||||| **Coding Pearl** ||||||||
>
> It is important to note that a request for medical records is less likely when you submit claims with procedure and diagnosis codes associated with pediatric quality measures.

Quality measurement is also required of health plans funded by government programs or offered through health exchanges created to support health insurance adoption under the PPACA. These health plans must collect and submit Quality Rating System measure data to the CMS. This entails collecting clinical quality measures, including a subset of the National Committee for Quality Assurance Healthcare Effectiveness Data and Information Set (HEDIS) measures and a Pharmacy Quality Alliance measure. (See Chapter 16, Common Testing and Therapeutic Services, for more information on HEDIS and quality reporting.) Physicians contracting with these plans may be asked to provide evidence that quality measures were met through claims data or medical records. It is important to note that a request for medical records is less likely when you submit claims with

Chapter 6: Preventive Services

procedure and diagnosis codes associated with pediatric quality measures. Examples of HEDIS measures related to preventive care include

- Percentage of members 12 to 21 years of age who had at least one comprehensive well-care visit with a primary care provider or obstetrician-gynecologist during the measurement year
- Percentage of members who were 3, 4, 5, or 6 years of age who received one or more well-child visits with a primary care provider during the measurement year
- Percentage of members who turned 15 months old during the measurement year and who had 6 or more well-child visits with a primary care provider during the first 15 months after birth
- Members 3 to 17 years of age who had an outpatient visit with a primary care provider and who had the following services in the current year:
  - ❖ Body mass index (BMI) percentile documentation
  - ❖ Counseling for nutrition
  - ❖ Counseling for physical activity

Certain preventive services, such as measuring height, weight, and BMI, are components of the preventive medicine service and require no additional procedure coding for payment purposes. However, associated diagnosis codes may be reported to support quality reporting initiatives. For instance, a group practice may decide to participate in a quality improvement program that requires calculation and reporting of BMI percentiles at all well-child visits for children aged 2 to 17 years. *International Classification of Diseases, 10th Revision, Clinical Modification (ICD-10-CM)* codes (**Table 6-1**) may be used in support of this effort.

Certain procedure codes also support quality measurement. For example, submission of claims containing codes for meningococcal (**90644**, **90734**); tetanus, diphtheria, and acellular pertussis (**90715**); and 3 doses of human papillomavirus (HPV) vaccine (**90649–90651**) provided to an adolescent before the patient's 13th birthday is indicative of meeting the measure for the immunization of adolescents. For a list of HEDIS measures and related codes, go to www.aap.org/cfp (access code AAPCFP23).

Table 6-1. Diagnosis Codes for Body Mass Index Percentile	
BMI	*ICD-10-CM*
BMI <5th percentile	**Z68.51**
BMI 5th–<85th percentile	**Z68.52**
BMI 85th–95th percentile	**Z68.53**
BMI ≥95th percentile	**Z68.54**

Abbreviations: BMI, body mass index; ICD-10-CM, International Classification of Diseases, 10th Revision, Clinical Modification.

Preventive Medicine E/M Services

Well-child or preventive medicine services are a type of E/M service and are reported with codes **99381–99397**. Most health plans provide a 100% benefit (no patient out-of-pocket cost) for the 31 recommended preventive medicine service encounters when provided by in-network providers. The selection of the pediatric-specific codes **99381–99395** is based simply on the age of the patient and whether the patient is new or established (**Table 6-2**) to the practice. In brief, an established patient has been seen by the physician or another physician of the same specialty and group practice within the last 3 years. Generally, other qualified health care professionals (QHPs) are considered to be working in the same specialty as the physicians with whom they work. Refer to Chapter 4, Evaluation and Management Documentation Guidelines, for more information about *new* versus *established* patients.

Table 6-2. New and Established Preventive Medicine Codes

Code Description	New Patient Code	Established Patient Code
Comprehensive preventive medicine evaluation and management; infant (age <1 year)	99381	99391
early childhood (age 1–4 years)	99382	99392
late childhood (age 5–11 years)	99383	99393
adolescent (age 12–17 years)	99384	99394
age 18–39 years	99385	99395

⁕ Most health plans will limit the benefits for preventive medicine E/M services covered in a year based on the patient's age.

  ❖ Six visits before the first birthday (recommended at 3–5 days and 1, 2, 4, 6, and 9 months)

  ❖ Three visits before the second birthday (recommended at 12, 15, and 18 months)

  ❖ Two visits before the third birthday (recommended at 24 and 30 months)

  ❖ Once per year beginning with the third birthday

⁕ Preventive medicine services include counseling, anticipatory guidance, and risk-factor reduction interventions. No average or typical times are assigned to these services, unlike the times found in many other E/M codes.

⁕ Immunizations, laboratory tests, and other special procedures or screening tests (eg, vision, hearing, developmental screening) that have their own specific *CPT®* codes are reported separately *in addition to* preventive medicine E/M services.

> ### ~ More From the AAP ~
> See "History in the Preventive Service" in the June 2015 *AAP Pediatric Coding Newsletter*™ at http://coding.aap.org (subscription required).

⁕ Most payers will require reporting modifier **25** with the preventive medicine service when immunizations or other services are also performed and reported.

⁕ A comprehensive history and physical examination must reflect an age- and gender-appropriate history and examination and are *not* synonymous with the "comprehensive" history and examination described in the E/M documentation guidelines from the CMS (see Chapter 4, Evaluation and Management Documentation Guidelines).

⁕ The comprehensive history performed as part of a preventive medicine visit does not require a chief complaint or history of present illness. It does require a comprehensive age-appropriate review of systems with an updated past, family, and social history (PFSH). The history should also include a comprehensive assessment or history of age-pertinent risk factors.

  ❖ Generally, the review of systems of a preventive medicine service is not a list of systems with pertinent positive and negative responses but, rather, a list of inquiries and patient responses for those areas of risk identified in preventive medicine guidelines as pertinent for patients of that age and gender. However, some payers may require review of all systems regardless of age and gender (eg, required by some Medicaid plans under Early and Preventive Screening, Diagnosis, and Treatment [EPSDT] benefits).

⁕ Routine management of contraception is considered part of the comprehensive preventive medicine E/M service when it is provided during the well-care health supervision visit.

⁕ A comprehensive physical examination is a multisystem examination that may include a routine pelvic and breast examination (when performed in the absence of specific symptoms of a separate problem) depending on the age of the patient and/or sexual history. If the pelvic examination is performed because of a gynecologic problem during a routine preventive medicine service, it may be appropriate to report a problem-oriented E/M service in addition to the preventive medicine service if this required additional physician work and required key components of the E/M code are met.

⁕ State Medicaid programs have requirements for performing, documenting, and reporting certain services in their EPSDT programs. Review your state Medicaid policies for the specific documentation and reporting requirements for services to patients in these programs.

Chapter 6: Preventive Services

- *ICD-10-CM* well-care diagnosis codes should be linked to the appropriate preventive medicine code (**99381–99395**). *ICD-10-CM* codes for well-child examinations include developmental, hearing, and vision screening.
  - ❖ **Z00.110** (health supervision for newborn <8 days)
  - ❖ **Z00.111** (health supervision for newborn 8–28 days old)
  - ❖ **Z00.121** (routine child health examination [29 days and older] with abnormal findings)
  - ❖ **Z00.129** (routine child health examination [29 days and older] without abnormal findings)
  - ❖ **Z00.00** (encounter for general adult medical examination without abnormal findings)
  - ❖ **Z00.01** (encounter for general adult medical examination with abnormal findings)
- For the purpose of assigning codes from this category, an *abnormal finding* is a newly discovered condition or a known or chronic condition that has increased in severity (eg, uncontrolled, acutely exacerbated). Assign additional codes for any abnormal findings.
- When an existing problem is addressed at the preventive medicine service but is not a newly discovered condition or a known or chronic condition that has increased in severity, report routine child health examination without abnormal findings and code also the condition addressed.
- Code **Z23** must be reported in addition to the routine health examination codes (eg, **Z00.129**) when immunizations are administered at the preventive medicine encounter. *ICD-10-CM* instructs to code **Z00** first, followed by code **Z23**.

Sports/Camp Physicals

Current Procedural Terminology® guidelines recommend that preventive medicine service codes (**99381–99397**) be reported when possible for physicals performed to determine eligibility for participation because they most accurately describe the services performed in that they are preventive and age appropriate in nature and physicians offer counseling on, for example, appropriate levels of exercise or injury prevention. However, the need for these services often arises after the child has had a yearly preventive medicine service, thereby rendering this service non-covered by some health plans, which allow only one preventive service per year. In this case, the parent may be billed if the payer contract allows because the service is non-covered.

> ### ~ More From the AAP ~
>
> For more information on reporting preparticipation physicals, see "Sports and Camp Physicals" in the June 2017 *AAP Pediatric Coding Newsletter*™ at http://coding.aap.org (subscription required).

Office visit codes (**99211–99215**) may be used if a problem is discovered during the service. Outpatient consultation codes (**99241–99245**) might be considered if the coach or school nurse requested the physician's opinion of a suspected problem (ie, exercise cough associated with reduced performance in cold weather). The medical record must include documentation of the written or verbal request and a copy of the written report with the physician's opinion or advice sent back to the coach or school nurse. *ICD-10-CM* code **Z02.5** is reported for an encounter for examination for participation in sports. If the school physical is incorporated into the annual well visit, use code **Z00.121** or **Z00.129**. Any problems or conditions that are addressed during the course of the visit would also be reported.

When reporting sports or camp physicals for patients with Medicare or Medicaid managed care plans, check the plan's policy on payment for these services and instructions for coding and billing. These physicals may be covered even when the child has already had an annual preventive medicine service under some Medicaid plans.

Immunizations

Vaccine services are reported using 2 families of *CPT* codes—one for the vaccine serum (the product) and one for the services associated with the administration of the vaccine.

Vaccines and Toxoids

Codes **90476–90748** are used to report the vaccine or toxoid product only. They do not include the administration of a vaccine.

* The exact vaccine product administered needs to be reported to meet the requirements of immunization registries, vaccine distribution programs, and reporting systems (eg, Vaccine Adverse Event Reporting System), as well as for payment.
* Codes may be specific to the product manufacturer and brand, schedule (number of doses or timing), chemical formulation, dosage, appropriate age guidelines, and/or route of administration.
* Codes for combination vaccines (eg, **90707**, measles, mumps, rubella and varicella [MMRV] virus vaccine) are available, as are separate codes for single-component vaccines (eg, **90716**, varicella virus vaccine).
* It is not appropriate to code each component of a combination vaccine separately using separate vaccine product codes when a combination vaccine is administered. However, if a combination vaccine is commercially available but a physician elects to administer the component vaccines due to nonavailability or other clinical reason, each vaccine product administered would be separately reported. See Appendix II, Vaccine Products: Commonly Administered Pediatric Vaccines, for a list of vaccine product codes.

> |||||||| **Coding Pearl** ||||||||
>
> The administration of immune globulins (including palivizumab [Synagis]) is not reported using the immunization administration codes. See codes **96365–96368, 96372, 96374**, and **96375**.

New Vaccines/Toxoids

The *CPT* Editorial Panel, in recognition of the public health interest in vaccine products, has chosen to publish new vaccine product codes prior to US Food and Drug Administration (FDA) approval. The American Medical Association (AMA) uses its *CPT* site (https://www.ama-assn.org/practice-management/cpt-category-i-vaccine-codes) to provide updates of *CPT* Editorial Panel actions on new vaccine products. Once approved by the *CPT* Editorial Panel, vaccine/toxoid product codes are typically made available for release on a semiannual basis (July 1 and January 1). As part of the electronic distribution, there is a 6-month implementation period from the initial release date (ie, codes released on January 1 are eligible for use on July 1; codes released on July 1 are eligible for use on January 1). These codes are indicated with a lightning bolt symbol (⚡) and will be tracked by the AMA to monitor FDA approval status. The lightning bolt symbol will be removed once the FDA status changes to "approved." Refer to the AMA Web site indicated earlier for the most up-to-date information on codes with this symbol. More rapid code release and implementation may occur when a government agency has identified the need for a vaccine as urgent to address an emergent health issue and the FDA has granted an expedited review process for the vaccine. In such cases, codes may be approved and released on an immediate (outside the normal code consideration schedule) or rapid basis (within the normal code consideration schedule but released shortly after approval with an implementation date within 3 months of release).

Before administering any new vaccine product or product with new recommendations, make certain the CDC, in the *Morbidity and Mortality Weekly Report,* or the AAP, in *Pediatrics,* has endorsed the use or recommendations of the vaccine. You may also want to verify with your carriers if the vaccine will be covered.

If a vaccine enters the market this year and is FDA approved, recommendations for use are published by the CDC or AAP, and no code exists for the specific vaccine, use code **90749** (unlisted vaccine/toxoid) and list the specific vaccine given.

Immunization Administration

Current Procedural Terminology® codes **90460** and **90461** *or* **90471–90474** are reported *in addition to* vaccine/toxoid code(s) **90476–90749**. If a significant, separately identifiable E/M service (eg, office or other outpatient services, preventive medicine services) is performed, the appropriate E/M service code appended with modifier **25** should be reported in addition to the vaccine and toxoid administration codes. If vaccines are given during the course of a preventive medicine service and another E/M service, both E/M services will need modifier **25** if required by the payer.

Codes 90460 and 90461

90460   Immunization administration through 18 years of age via any route of administration, with counseling by physician or other qualified health care professional; first or only component of each vaccine or toxoid administered

+90461   each additional vaccine or toxoid component administered
(List separately in addition to code for primary procedure.)

When reporting codes **90460** and **90461**

- Physicians or other QHPs must provide *face-to-face* counseling to the patient and/or family (patient aged ≤18 years) at the time of the encounter for the administration of a vaccine. (See the Codes **90471–90474** section later in this chapter for immunization administration [IA] without physician counseling or to patients older than 18 years.)

- *Current Procedural Terminology* defines a physician or other QHP as follows:

    A "physician or other qualified health care professional" is an individual who by education, training, licensure/regulation, facility credentialing (when applicable), and facility privileging (when applicable) performs a professional service within his/her scope of practice and independently reports that professional service. These professionals are distinct from "clinical staff." A clinical staff member is a person who works under the supervision of a physician or other qualified health care professional and who is allowed by law, regulation, and facility policy to perform or assist in the performance of a specified professional service, but who does not individually report that professional service. Other policies may also affect who may report specific services.

- Therefore, although nurses may be allowed by state scope of practice laws to explain risks and benefits of vaccines, their counseling does not fall under the description of code **90460** or **90461**, and codes **90471–90474** must be reported.

- When a private payer contract does not allow QHPs to report services under their own name and National Provider Identifier (NPI), check with the payer to determine eligibility of these professionals to report immunization counseling (**90460**, **90461**) and report under the name and number of the supervising physician.

- Documentation of immunization counseling should include a listing of all vaccine components with notation that counseling was provided for all listed components with authentication (electronic or written signature and date) by the physician or other QHP. Supply of the Vaccine Information Statement (VIS) without discussion of risks and benefits does not constitute counseling. Some payers require documentation of parent or caregiver questions or concerns that were addressed during counseling.

- Code **90460** is reported for the *first (or only) component of each vaccine administered* (whether single or combination) on a day of service and includes the related vaccine counseling.

- Code **90461** is only reported in conjunction with **90460** and is used to report the work of counseling for *each additional component(s) beyond the first* in a given combination vaccine. (See Vaccines for Children Program section later in this chapter for reporting administration of vaccines containing multiple components to this program.)

- Combination vaccines are those vaccines that contain multiple vaccine components. Refer to Appendix II, Vaccine Products: Commonly Administered Pediatric Vaccines, for the number of components in the most commonly reported pediatric vaccines.

❋ The IA codes include the physician or other QHP's work of discussing risks and benefits of the vaccines, providing parents with a copy of the appropriate CDC VIS for each vaccine given, the cost of clinical staff time to record each vaccine component administered in the medical record and statewide vaccine registry, giving the vaccine, observing and addressing reactions or side effects, and cost of supplies (eg, syringe, needle, bandages).

For each individual vaccine administered, report code **90460** because every vaccine will have, at minimum, one vaccine component. Depending on the specific vaccine, code **90461** is additionally reported for counseling on each additional component of each combination vaccine. No modifier is typically required for reporting multiple units of the immunization administration codes. Most payers advise reporting multiple units of the same service on a single line of the claim. However, individual payer guidance may vary.

Examples

➤ **A 15-year-old patient receives the 9-valent HPV (9vHPV) vaccine from his physician.** The ordering physician discusses risks of the vaccine and the disease for which it provides protection. The parent/guardian is given the CDC VIS. The parent/guardian consents; the nurse provides the VIS and prepares the vaccine. The patient receives the vaccine by a single injection, and the nurse charts the required information and accesses and enters vaccine data into the statewide immunization registry. The patient is discharged home after the nurse confirms that there are no serious immediate reactions.

ICD-10-CM	CPT®
Z23 (encounter for immunization)	**90651** (9vHPV) **90460**

Teaching Point: Because the physician personally performed the counseling, code **90460** is reported for this single-component vaccine. No other services are reported because the purpose of the visit was for administration of the vaccine only.

➤ **An 11-year-old girl (new patient) presents to a pediatrician for a preventive medicine service.** In addition to the preventive E/M service with no abnormal findings, the physician discusses risks of the HPV vaccine and the disease for which it provides protection. The parent/guardian is given the CDC VIS. The parent/guardian consents; the nurse prepares to administer the vaccine. However, the patient then refuses to receive the immunization, and counseling by the nurse does not change her decision. The physician returns to the examination room and provides additional counseling, but the patient becomes tearful and continues to refuse the vaccine. The patient's mother wishes to discuss with the child's father and return on a later date. A follow-up appointment is scheduled.

ICD-10-CM	CPT
Z00.129 **Z28.21** (immunization not carried out because of patient refusal)	**99383**

Teaching Point: Because the vaccine was not administered, no charge for the product or the administration would be reported. When the patient returns for follow-up, the codes reported will depend on the outcome of the encounter. If the vaccine is administered after additional physician counseling at the same encounter, code **90460** would be reported in addition to the appropriate vaccine product code. If the patient returns for administration by a nurse without additional counseling by a physician, code **90471** would be reported in lieu of **90460**. Additional counseling at the follow-up visit that does not result in immunization may be reported with a preventive medicine counseling code (**99401–99404**) based on the physician's face-to-face time with the patient.

Chapter 6: Preventive Services

➤ **You administer measles, mumps, rubella (MMR) vaccine and a varicella vaccine at the same encounter.**
Report code **90460** with 2 units (1 unit for the first component of each vaccine given) and code **90461** with 2 units for counseling related to additional components of the combination vaccine. Link the vaccine and administration *CPT®* codes to *ICD-10-CM* code **Z23** on health insurance claims.

➤ **A patient receives the diphtheria, tetanus toxoids, acellular pertussis; inactivated poliovirus; and *Haemophilus influenzae* type b (DTaP-IPV/Hib) vaccine as a combination vaccine and an influenza vaccine.**
Report **90460** for each vaccine administered (2 units) and **90461** with 4 units for counseling related to additional components of the combination vaccine (DTaP-IPV/Hib). The DTaP-IPV/Hib vaccine product is reported with code **90698**. *Note:* While not as common, some physicians provide single-component vaccines versus combinations. Therefore, for this example, **90460** would be reported with 4 units for the first components of the 4 vaccine products and **90461** with 2 units for the additional components of the DTaP vaccine. Link the vaccine and administration *CPT* codes to *ICD-10-CM* code **Z23** on health insurance claims.

➤ **A 4-month-old established patient receives the DTaP-IPV/Hib combination vaccine, rotavirus vaccine (RV5), and pneumococcal conjugate vaccine (PCV13) from her physician at the time of her preventive medicine visit.** The ordering physician discusses the risks of each vaccine component (eg, tetanus, pertussis) and the diseases for which each vaccine component provides protection. The parent/guardian is given the CDC VIS for all vaccine components and consents for each of the additional vaccine components. The nurse charts the required information and enters data into the statewide immunization registry for each vaccine component.

ICD-10-CM	CPT
Z00.129 (routine infant or child check without abnormal findings) **Z23** (encounter for immunization)	**99391 25** (preventive medicine visit; younger than 1 year) **90698** (DTaP-IPV/Hib) **90680** (RV5) **90670** (PCV13) **90460** × 3 units for counseling for first component of each of 3 vaccines **90461** × 4 units for counseling for additional components (eg, tetanus, pertussis, IPV, Hib)

Teaching Point: Code **90460** is reported for each vaccine administered and includes the work of counseling for the first component of each vaccine administered (diphtheria, rotavirus, and pneumococcus). Code **90461** is reported in conjunction with **90460** for each additional component that is part of the combination vaccine DTaP-IPV/Hib. Payers who have adopted the Medicare National Correct Coding Initiative (NCCI) edits will require that modifier **25** be appended to code **99391** to signify that it was significant and separately identifiable. (For more information on NCCI edits, see Chapter 3, Modifiers and Coding Edits.) *ICD-10-CM* code **Z00.129** is reported first, followed by code **Z23**.

➤ **A 12-year-old established patient is seen for his preventive medicine visit by the certified pediatric nurse practitioner (CPNP), who bills under her own NPI.** The patient complains of an increasingly severe itchy rash on his hands, arms, and legs for 3 days. A problem-focused history related to the complaint is performed. He is diagnosed and treated for a moderately severe case of poison ivy, requiring a prescription for a topical steroid. He has not yet received his tetanus, diphtheria, and acellular pertussis (Tdap), meningococcal (MenACWY, intramuscular), or human papillomavirus (9vHPV) vaccines. The CPNP counsels the parents on the risks and protection from each of the diseases. The CDC VISs are given to the parents and the nurse administers the vaccines.

ICD-10-CM	CPT®
Z00.121 (well-child check with abnormal findings) **L23.7** (allergic contact dermatitis due to plants, except food) **Z23**	**99394 25** (preventive medicine visit, established patient, age 12 through 17 years) **90715** (Tdap, 7 years or older, intramuscular) **90734** (MenACWY) **90651** (9vHPV) **90460** × 3 units **90461** × 2 units **99212 25** (office/outpatient E/M, established patient)

Teaching Point: Medical record documentation supports that a significant, separately identifiable E/M service was provided and is reported in addition to the preventive medicine service. Modifier **25** is appended to code **99212** to signify that it is significant and separately identifiable from the preventive medicine service. Modifier **25** is also appended to code **99394** to signify it is significant and separately identifiable from IA. Because the child is younger than 18 years and vaccine counseling was performed by the CPNP with her own NPI, codes **90460** and **90461** may be reported as appropriate.

Coding Conundrum: Vaccine Counseling on Day Different From Administration

Current Procedural Terminology states that codes **90460** and **90461** are reported when the physician or QHP provides face-to-face counseling of the patient and family during the administration of a vaccine. However, there are situations in which vaccine counseling is performed on a day different from the actual administration. For example, the physician or QHP might provide vaccine counseling during an encounter, but because the child is ill, the vaccines are deferred to a later date. Or the physician or QHP may counsel the patient and parent on all vaccines needed during the annual preventive medicine service visit, but the parent refuses multiple vaccines on the same day, and some of the vaccines are given over a series of encounters for vaccine administration only. How would a physician then report IA?

Because these circumstances split the actual administration from vaccine counseling, codes **90460** and **90461** cannot be reported. In these situations, IA is reported using codes **90471–90474** on the day the vaccines are administered.

Codes 90471–90474

90471 Immunization administration (includes percutaneous, intradermal, subcutaneous, or intramuscular injections); one vaccine (single or combination vaccine/toxoid)

+90472 each additional vaccine (single or combination vaccine/toxoid) (List separately in addition to code for primary procedure.) (Use code **90472** in conjunction with **90460, 90471**, or **90473**.)

90473 Immunization administration by intranasal or oral route; one vaccine (single or combination vaccine/toxoid)

+90474 each additional vaccine (single or combination vaccine/toxoid) (List separately in addition to code for primary procedure.) (Use code **90474** in conjunction with **90460, 90471**, or **90473**.)

Codes **90471–90474** will be reported when criteria for reporting the 2 pediatric IA codes (**90460** and **90461**) have not been met (ie, physician or QHP does not counsel patient/family or does not document that the counseling was personally performed, or when the patient is ≥19 years).

The Centers for Medicare & Medicaid Services (CMS) has assigned 0.72 RVUs to codes **90460, 90471**, and **90473** and 0.36 RVUs to codes **90461, 90472**, and **90474**. Appropriate reporting of codes **90460** and **90461** in lieu of codes **90471–90474** should result in higher payment based on reporting of multiple units of code **90461** for *each additional vaccine component* versus reporting of codes **90472** and **90474** for *each additional vaccine product*. Individual payers may or may not assign payment values based on the RVUs published by the CMS.

Chapter 6: Preventive Services

(Administration of vaccines provided through the Vaccines for Children [VFC] program is paid differently. See more about the Vaccines for Children Program later in this chapter.)

When reporting codes **90471–90474**

◉ Codes **90471–90474** are reported for each vaccine administered, whether single or combination vaccines.

◉ *Only one* "first" IA code (**90460**, **90471**, or **90473**) may be reported on a calendar day.

The "first" IA code can be reported from either family or either route of administration (eg, when a patient receives an immunization via injection and a second one via intranasal route, IA services can be reported with codes **90471** and **90474** or with codes **90473** and **90472**).

◉ The Medicare NCCI edits pair code **90460** with codes **90471** and **90473**, not allowing codes from both sets to be reported on the same day of service by the same physician or physician of the same group and specialty. If a physician personally performs counseling on one vaccine but not on another when given during the same encounter, IA will be reported using codes **90460** (and **90461** if appropriate) and either **90472** (IA, each additional vaccine via injection) or **90474** (each additional vaccine via intranasal or oral route).

For more information on vaccine administration, please see the following examples and Appendix II, Vaccine Products: Commonly Administered Pediatric Vaccines.

Examples

➤ **A 4-year-old patient is seen by a nurse per physician's order to follow up on impetigo and clearance to return to preschool.** The father also requests that his daughter receive influenza vaccination. The nurse performs an interval history and very brief examination and finds the impetigo has resolved. After assessing the patient and verifying she is in good health, the nurse confirms there are no contraindications to the immunization per CDC guidelines. Next, the nurse reviews the VIS with the father and the antipyretic dosage for weight and obtains the father's consent for the immunization. The nurse then administers the influenza vaccine and observes for immediate reactions.

ICD-10-CM	CPT®
Z09 (encounter for follow-up examination after completed treatment for conditions other than malignant neoplasm) **Z87.2** (personal history of diseases of the skin and subcutaneous tissue) **Z23** (encounter for immunization)	**99211 25** (E/M service) **90686** (influenza vaccine [IIV4], preservative free, 0.5 mL, intramuscular) **90471** (IA, first injection)

Teaching Point: If the payer follows NCCI edits, *CPT* code **99211** will never be paid for separately from vaccine administration (eg, **90473**), even with modifier **25**. See Coding Conundrum: Reporting E/M Services With IA later in this chapter for more information on reporting code **99211** with immunization administration.

➤ **A 5-year-old established patient presented 2 weeks ago for her 5-year check and vaccines.** At that appointment, her physician provided counseling for each recommended vaccine component and corresponding VISs. The patient's mother asked that the vaccines be split, so only the DTaP and IPV vaccines were given at that encounter. The patient returns today for an immunization-only visit to get the MMR and varicella (VAR) vaccines.

ICD-10-CM	CPT
Z23 (encounter for immunization)	**90707** (MMR, live) **90471** (IA, first injection) **90716** (VAR) **90472** (IA, subsequent injection)

Teaching Point: Despite that counseling for all vaccines occurred at the last encounter and all VISs were handed out, only administration occurred today. *Current Procedural Terminology*® codes **90460** and **90461** would be reported with the appropriate codes for DTaP and IPV vaccines that were administered during the previous encounter. However, services on this date did not include physician counseling. (See Coding Conundrum: Vaccine Counseling on Day Different From Administration earlier in this chapter.)

➤ **A 19-year-old established patient presents for college entrance examination.** In addition to providing a preventive medicine service, the physician counsels the patient on the need for meningococcal serogroup B (MenB-4C) immunization. The vaccine is administered and a medical history and physical form provided by the college are completed.

ICD-10-CM	CPT
Z02.0 (encounter for examination for admission to educational institution) **Z23** (encounter for immunization)	**99395 25** (preventive medicine service, established patient, 18–39 years old) **90620** (MenB-4C) **90471** (IA, first injection)

Teaching Point: Because the patient is older than 18 years, code **90460** cannot be reported even though the physician provided counseling for the vaccine provided. Code **Z00.00** (encounter for general adult medical examination without abnormal findings) is not reported because *ICD-10-CM* excludes reporting of code **Z00.00** in conjunction with codes in category **Z02**. Code **Z02.0** is appropriate as the reason the patient presented for the encounter.

See FAQ: Immunization Administration online at www.aap.org/cfp, access code AAPCFP23, for further discussion of coding for immunization administration.

Coding Conundrum: Reporting E/M Services With IA

Evaluation and management services most often reported with the vaccine product and IA include new and established patient preventive medicine visits (*CPT* codes **99381–99395**), problem-oriented visits (**99201–99215**), and preventive medicine counseling services (**99401–99404**).

The E/M service must be medically indicated, significant, and separately identifiable from the IA.

Payers may require modifier **25** (significant, separately identifiable E/M service by the same physician on the same day of the procedure or other service) to be appended to the E/M code to distinguish it from the administration of the vaccine.

If a patient is seen for the administration of a vaccine only, it is not appropriate to report an E/M visit if it is not medically necessary, significant, and separately identifiable.

Current Procedural Terminology code **99211** (established patient E/M, minimal level, not requiring physician presence) *should not* be reported when the patient encounter is for vaccination only because Medicare RBRVS relative values for IA codes include administrative and clinical services (ie, greeting the patient, routine vital signs, obtaining a vaccine history, presenting the VIS and responding to routine vaccine questions, preparation and administration of the vaccine, and documentation and observation of the patient following administration of the vaccine). However, if the service is medically necessary, significant, and separately identifiable, it may be reported with modifier **25** appended to the E/M code (**99211**). The medical record must clearly state the reason for the visit, brief history, physical examination, assessment and plan, and any other counseling or discussion items. The progress note must be signed with the physician's countersignature. For more information and clinical vignettes on the appropriate use of E/M services during IA, visit www.aap.org/cfp, access code AAPCFP23. Payers who do not follow the Medicare RBRVS may allow payment of code **99211** with IA. Know your payer guidelines, and if payment is allowed, make certain the guidelines are in writing and maintained in your office. Be aware that a co-payment will be required when the "nurse" visit is reported.

The same guidelines apply to physician visits (**99201–99215**).

Chapter 6: Preventive Services

National Drug Code

Many payers, specifically Medicare, Medicaid, and other government payers (eg, Tricare) and other private payers, require the use of the National Drug Code (NDC) when reporting vaccine product codes. The NDCs are universal product identifiers for medications, including vaccines. These codes are 10-digit, 3-segment numbers that identify the product, labeler, and trade package size. The Health Insurance Portability and Accountability Act of 1996 standards require an 11-digit code. If you are not currently reporting vaccines with NDCs, be sure to coordinate the requirements with your billing software company. For more information on NDCs, visit www.fda.gov/Drugs/InformationOnDrugs/ucm142438.htm or link through www.aap.org/cfp.

> ### ~ More From the AAP ~
>
> For more information on reporting NDCs, see "Reporting the National Drug Code: A Refresher" in the August 2014 *AAP Pediatric Coding Newsletter*™ at http://coding. aap.org (subscription required).

Vaccines for Children Program

The VFC program makes vaccines available to children up to 19 years of age who meet any of the following criteria: are enrolled in the Medicaid program, do not have health insurance, have no coverage of immunizations under their health plan, or are American Indians or Alaska Natives. Vaccines are provided at no cost to the participating physician or patient and payment is made only for administration of the vaccine.

If reporting the VFC vaccine with administration codes and not the product code, data for the vaccine products administered must be captured for registry and quality initiatives. This can be accomplished by entering the vaccine codes with a $0 charge (if your billing system allows) and appending modifier **SL** (state-supplied vaccine) to the vaccine code. However, follow individual payer rules for reporting.

According to the VFC Web site, providers are encouraged to use code **90460** for administration of a vaccine under the VFC program. If code **90461** is used for a vaccine with multiple antigens or components, it should be given a $0 value for a child covered under the VFC program. This applies to Medicaid-enrolled VFC-entitled children as well as non–Medicaid-enrolled VFC-entitled children (ie, uninsured, underinsured, and American Indian or Alaska Native children not enrolled in Medicaid). Please be aware that some state Medicaid programs do have reporting rules that differ from VFC. *Be sure to get this policy in writing from your state Medicaid program* and follow it to avoid denied payment. The AAP continues to advocate to the CMS to allow for recognition and payment for component-based vaccine counseling and administration (ie, code **90461**). Under the current statute, administration can only be paid "per vaccine" and not component.

Participants in the VFC program should be aware of program-specific guidance, including storage of VFC vaccine separate from privately purchased vaccines. For more information on the VFC program, visit www.cdc.gov/vaccines/programs/vfc/index.html.

Screening Tests and Procedures

Recommendations for age-appropriate screening services are outlined in the AAP "Recommendations for Preventive Pediatric Health Care" (www.aap.org/periodicityschedule) or in your state's EPSDT plan.

Hearing Screening

92551	Screening test, pure tone, air only
92552	Pure tone audiometry (threshold); air only (full assessment)
92558	Evoked otoacoustic emissions, screening (qualitative measurement of distortion product or transient evoked otoacoustic emissions), automated analysis
92583	Select picture audiometry
92567	Tympanometry (impedance testing)
92568	Acoustic reflex testing, threshold portion

Audiometric tests require the use of calibrated electronic equipment, recording of results, and a written report with interpretation. Services include testing of both ears. If the test is applied to one ear only, modifier **52** (reduced services) must be appended to the code.

- Code **92551** (screening test, pure tone, air only) is used when earphones are placed on the patient and the patient is asked to respond to tones of different pitches and intensities. This is a limited study.

- Code **92552** (full pure tone audiometric assessment) is used when earphones are placed on the patient and the patient is asked to respond to tones of different pitches and intensities. The threshold, which is the lowest intensity of the tone that the patient can hear 50% of the time, is recorded for a number of frequencies. Bone thresholds are obtained in a similar manner. The air and bone thresholds are compared to differentiate among conductive, sensorineural, or mixed hearing losses.

- Code **92558** (evoked otoacoustic emissions screening) is used when a probe tip is placed in the ear canal to screen for normal hearing function. The probe tip emits a repeated clicking sound (transient evoked emissions) or 2 tones at 2 frequencies (distortion product emissions). The sounds pass through the tympanic membrane, middle ear, and to the inner ear. In the inner ear, the sound is picked up by the hair cells in the cochlea, which in turn bounce the sound back in low-intensity sound waves (OAE). These OAEs are recorded and analyzed by computerized equipment and the results are automated.

- Code **92583** (select picture audiometry) is typically used for younger children. The patient is asked to identify different pictures with the instructions given at different sound intensity levels.

- Other commonly performed procedures include codes **92567** (tympanometry [impedance testing]) and **92568** (acoustic reflex testing, threshold portion). However, both codes may have limited coverage; check with payers.

- Automated audiometry testing is reported with Category III codes **0208T–0212T**. See Chapter 1, New and Revised *CPT*® Codes for 2018, for a listing of these codes.

> ||||||| **Coding Pearl** |||||||
>
> Report hearing tests conducted following a failed hearing screening with code **Z01.110** if results are normal. If findings are abnormal, report code **Z01.118** and a code to identify the abnormality.

Vision Screening

99173	Screening test of visual acuity, quantitative, bilateral
99174	Instrument-based ocular screening (eg, photoscreening, automated-refraction), bilateral; with remote analysis and report
99177	with on-site analysis
▲0333T	Visual evoked potential, screening of visual acuity, automated, with report
●0469T	Retinal polarization scan, ocular screening with on-site automated results, bilateral

- Screening test of visual acuity (**99173**) must use graduated visual stimuli that allow a quantitative estimate of visual acuity (eg, Snellen chart).
  - Medical record documentation must include a measurement of acuity for both eyes, not just a pass or fail score.
  - Code **99173** is only reported when vision screening is performed in association with a preventive medicine visit. It is not reported when it is performed as part of an evaluation for an eye problem or condition (eg, examination to rule out vision problems in a patient presenting with problems with schoolwork) because the assessment of visual acuity is considered an integral part of the eye examination.
- Instrument-based ocular screening (**99174**, **99177**) is used to report screening for a variety of conditions, including esotropia, exotropia, isometropia, cataracts, ptosis, hyperopia, myopia, and others, that affect or have the potential to affect vision. These tests are especially useful for screening infants, preschool patients, and those older patients whose ability to participate in traditional acuity screening is limited or very time intensive.
- Code **99177** specifies screening using an instrument that provides an on-site (ie, in-office) pass or fail result.

Chapter 6: Preventive Services

- Code 99174 specifies the use of a screening instrument that incorporates remote analysis and report.
- These screenings cannot be reported in conjunction with codes 92002–92700 (general ophthalmologic services), 99172 (visual function screening), or 99173 (screening test of visual acuity, quantitative) because ocular screening is inherent to these services. An AAP policy statement on instrument-based pediatric vision screening is available online at http://pediatrics.aappublications.org/content/130/5/983.full.
- Vision screening performed using an automated visual evoked potential system is reported with code 0333T. This code applies to automated screening using an instrument-based algorithm with a pass or fail result. Code 0333T was revised to indicate that a report of the result must be documented. Report code 95930 only for comprehensive visual evoked potential testing with physician interpretation and report.
- Retinal polarization scanning (0469T) is used to detect amblyopia due to strabismus and defocus. Similar to code 99177, results of each scan are generated on-site.

Developmental Screening

96110   Developmental screening with scoring and documentation, per standardized instrument

> **||||||| Coding Pearl |||||||**
>
> *ICD-10-CM* code **Z13.4**, encounter for screening for certain developmental disorders in childhood, is not reported for routine developmental testing of an infant or child at the time of a preventive service. An Excludes1 note directs to codes in subcategory **Z00.1⁻**.

Structured screening for developmental delay is a universal recommendation of the "Recommendations for Preventive Pediatric Health Care" at 18-month and 2-year visits for autism spectrum disorder (ASD)-specific screening (eg, Modified Checklist for Autism in Toddlers [M-CHAT]) and at 9-month, 18-month, and 2- or 2½-year visits for other developmental screening (eg, Ages & Stages Questionnaire [ASQ]). When reporting these screenings, code 96110 represents developmental screening with scoring and documentation per standardized instrument. (Note that screening results should be included in the patient medical record.)

Code 96110

- Is reported for standardized developmental screening instruments. It is not reported when the pediatrician conducts an informal survey or surveillance of development as part of a comprehensive preventive medicine service (which is considered part of the history and is not separately billed).
- May be reported for each standardized developmental screening instrument administered.
- Includes standardized screening tools, such as ASQ, Australian Scale for Asperger's Syndrome, M-CHAT, or Parents' Evaluation of Developmental Status (PEDS). Other tools are also used for developmental screening.

Example

➤ **A 20-month-old girl presents to her primary physician with a complaint of pulling at her ears and signs suggesting an upper respiratory infection. She missed her 18-month well-child checkup. A preventive visit is offered, but mother prefers to come back when she has scheduled more time off work. The mother is given the PEDS and M-CHAT (a standardized screening instrument for ASD in children 16–30 months of age) by the nursing assistant, who explains why the instruments are given and how they should be completed. After the child's mother completes both forms, the nursing assistant scores and attaches them to the child's medical chart. The physician evaluates the patient's upper respiratory symptoms and diagnoses allergic rhinitis. The physician also interprets and records the normal results of the PEDS and M-CHAT in the medical record and requests that the mother schedule a full preventive service for the child within the next month.**

Code 96110 is reported with 2 units of service (see Claim Form Example 1 for Multiple Units of Service), or 96110 and 96110 59 are reported (see Claim Form Example 2 for Multiple Units of Service), depending on payer requirements. *ICD-10-CM* code Z13.4 may be reported to indicate screening for developmental disability in children when the screening is not performed in conjunction with a well-child visit.

Claim Form Example 1 for Multiple Units of Service

21. Diagnosis or nature of illness or injury (Relate A–L to service line below 24E)					ICD Ind. 0						
A. **J30.9**		B. **Z13.4**		C.	D.						
24. A. Dates of service	B. Place of service	C. EMG	D. Procedures, services or supplies CPT/HCPCS	Modifier	E. Diagnosis Pointer	F. Charges	G. Days or units	H. EPSDT	I. ID Qual	J. Rendering Provider #
1/1/2018–1/1/2018	11		**99213**	**25**	A	$$$	1		NPI	123456789
1/1/2018–1/1/2018	11		**96110**		B	$$$	2		NPI	123456789

Abbreviations: CPT, Current Procedural Terminology; EMG, emergency; EPSDT, Early and Periodic Screening, Diagnosis, and Treatment; HCPCS, Healthcare Common Procedure Coding System; ICD, International Classification of Diseases; NPI, National Provider Identifier.

Claim Form Example 2 for Multiple Units of Service

21. Diagnosis or nature of illness or injury (Relate A–L to service line below 24E)					ICD Ind. 0						
A. **J30.9**	B. **Z13.4**		C.	D.							
24. A. Dates of service	B. Place of service	C. EMG	D. Procedures, services or supplies CPT/HCPCS	Modifier	E. Diagnosis Pointer	F. Charges	G. Days or units	H. EPSDT	I. ID Qual	J. Rendering Provider #
1/1/2018–1/1/2018	11		**99213**	**25**	A	$$$	1		NPI	123456789
1/1/2018–1/1/2018	11		**96110**		B	$$$	1		NPI	123456789
1/1/2018–1/1/2018	11		**96110**	**59**	B	$$$	1		NPI	123456789

Abbreviations: CPT, Current Procedural Terminology; EMG, emergency; EPSDT, Early and Periodic Screening, Diagnosis, and Treatment; HCPCS, Healthcare Common Procedure Coding System; ICD, International Classification of Diseases; NPI, National Provider Identifier.

Chapter 6: Preventive Services

Teaching Point: There is a Medically Unlikely Edit (MUE) on code **96110**. The MUE is 2; therefore, if the payer follows MUEs, you cannot report more than two **96110** codes per line on the claim form. (See Chapter 3, Modifiers and Coding Edits, for more details.) Proactive delivery and recommendations for preventive services support quality initiatives.

Emotional/Behavioral Assessment

96127   Brief emotional/behavioral assessment (eg, depression inventory, ADHD scale), with scoring and documentation, per standardized instrument

Code **96127**

* Is reported for standardized emotional/behavioral assessment instruments.
* Represents the practice expense of administering, scoring, and documenting each standardized instrument. No physician work value is included. Physician interpretation is included in a related E/M service.
* Is not reported in conjunction with **99401–99404**, **96101–96103**, or **96118–96120**.
* Can involve 2 or more separately reported completions of the same form (eg, attention-deficit/hyperactivity disorder [ADHD] rating scales by teacher and by parent). Note that MUEs limit reporting to 2 units per claim line. When reporting to payers adopting MUEs, additional units beyond the first 2 must be reported on a separate claim line with an NCCI modifier (eg, **59**, distinct procedural service). As always, documentation should support the appropriateness of the additional units of service.
* Can be reported for standardized depression instruments that are required under US Preventive Services Task Force (USPSTF) and Bright Futures recommendations (see AAP/Bright Futures "Recommendations for Preventive Pediatric Health Care" insert).

Examples of assessment and screening tools by code are available in Appendix I, Sample Assessment/Testing Tools, or online at www.aap.org/cfp, access code AAPCFP23.

Example

➤ **An 11-year-old boy is seen for an established patient well-child health supervision and sports physical encounter.** In addition to the preventive medicine service, the physician's staff administers and scores a recommended depression screening instrument. The physician reviews the score, documents that the screening result is negative for symptoms of depression, and completes the preventive medicine service. Clearance is given to participate in sports.

The preventive medicine service code (**99393**) would be reported in addition to code **96127**. The diagnosis code reported is **Z00.129** (encounter for routine child health examination without abnormal findings). Link **Z00.129** to the claim service line for code **96127**. Remember that *ICD-10-CM* guidelines state to link routine screening services to the well-child/adolescent code. A code for the sports physical (**Z02.5**) is not reported because *ICD-10-CM* excludes reporting of codes in category **Z02** in conjunction with codes in category **Z00**.

When screening results are positive and the physician performs further evaluation leading to a diagnosis of depression, code the preventive service with abnormal findings (**Z00.121**) followed by the appropriate code for the diagnosed depression (eg, **F32.0**, major depressive disorder, single episode, mild). When appropriate, a significant and separately identifiable E/M service to evaluate and manage depression may be reported by appending modifier **25** to an office or other outpatient E/M code (eg, **99213**). Documentation should clearly support the key components of the separate service or if billing based on time spent in counseling and/or coordination of care, the time and a summary of the service provided (eg, education on the condition, questions answered, patient and/or caregiver concerns, management options discussed, and plan of care).

Health Risk Assessment

96160   Administration of patient-focused health risk assessment (eg, health hazard appraisal) with scoring and documentation, per standardized instrument

96161   Administration of caregiver-focused health risk assessment (eg, depression inventory) for the benefit of the patient, with scoring and documentation, per standardized instrument

Code **96160** is reported for a patient-focused health risk assessment. This is differentiated from code **96161**, which is used to report a health risk assessment focused on a caregiver for the benefit of the patient.

* Code **96160** is reported for administration (with scoring and documentation) of a standardized patient-focused health risk assessment instrument (eg, health hazard appraisal). Code **96160** cannot be used in conjunction with codes **99408** and **99409**. Check individual payer guidance to determine if and for what purposes code **96160** is included as a covered and payable service under the payer's policies (eg, some Medicaid plans pay for adolescent health questionnaires, such as HEADSSS [*h*ome, *e*ducation (ie, school), *a*ctivities/employment, *d*rugs, *s*afety, *s*exuality, and *s*uicidality/depression], reported with **96160**).

* Code **96161** is reported for administration of a health risk assessment to a patient's caregiver. Examples are a postpartum depression inventory administered to the mother of a newborn and administration of a validated caregiver strain instrument to parents of a seriously injured or ill child.

* Report 1 unit of **96160** or **96161** for each standardized instrument administered.

Example

➤ **As part of a health supervision visit for a 2-month-old established patient, the physician directs clinical staff to administer a screening for postpartum depression.** Clinical staff explain the purpose of the instrument to the infant's mother. After the mother has completed the screening instrument, clinical staff score and document the result in the patient record. The physician completes the preventive medicine service. Included is anticipatory guidance advising the mother that her screening indicates no current signs of postpartum depression and of symptoms that should prompt a call to her physician.

ICD-10-CM	CPT®
Z00.129 (encounter for routine child health examination without abnormal findings)	99391 (preventive medicine visit) 96161 (administration of caregiver-focused health risk assessment [eg, depression inventory] for the benefit of the patient, with scoring and documentation, per standardized instrument)

Teaching Point: The screening for postpartum depression is caregiver-focused (sign/symptoms of depression in mother) but performed in this setting for the benefit of the infant. This service is reported as a service provided to the child with code **96161**. Check payer policy on adoption of code **96161** versus a requirement to report as a service to the mother (ie, to mother's health plan) with code **96127** (brief emotional/behavioral assessment [eg, depression inventory, ADHD scale], with scoring and documentation, per standardized instrument). Many Medicaid plans provide separate payment for maternal depression screening at well-child visits, but specific reporting instructions may apply.

Prevention of Dental Caries

Application of Fluoride Varnish

99188   Application of topical fluoride varnish by a physician or other qualified health care professional

❋ Topical fluoride application by primary care physicians is a recommended preventive service for children from birth through 5 years of age (Grade B rating by the USPSTF). This service may be covered when provided alone or in conjunction with other services. Coverage is usually limited to once every 6 months.

❋ ICD-10-CM code **Z29.3** is reported to identify encounter for prophylactic fluoride administration. When applicable, diagnosis of dental caries may be reported as a secondary diagnosis with codes in category **K02**. Encounter for prophylactic fluoride administration is reported separately from the encounter for routine child health examination (**Z00.121** or **Z00.129**) when both services are provided at the same encounter.

❋ Although code **99188** specifies application by a physician or QHP, payers may allow billing of services by trained clinical staff under direct physician supervision (incident to). Some Medicaid plans require training of clinical staff through specific programs. It is important to identify the requirements of individual payers prior to providing this service.

❋ *Code on Dental Procedures and Nomenclature* (*CDT®*) codes also exist for topical application of fluoride varnish and fluoride. In addition, *CDT* codes exist for nutrition counseling to prevent dental disease, oral hygiene instruction, and oral evaluations. However, acceptance of these codes by health plans may be limited.

> ||||||| **Coding Pearl** |||||||
>
> National Correct Coding Initiative edits bundle codes **96160, 96161** with codes **96110** and with immunization administration (**90460–90474**) services, but a modifier is allowed when each code represents a distinct service and is clinically appropriate. Append modifier **59** to the bundled code (second column of NCCI edits) when these services are reported on the same date to a payer that has adopted NCCI edits.

Counseling to Prevent Dental Caries

Some payers will provide coverage for oral evaluation and health risk assessment or other dental preventive services when provided on the same day as a preventive medicine visit; other payers will allow services only when they are provided at an encounter separate from a preventive medicine visit. Know payer requirements for reporting.

❋ Preventive counseling for oral health may be included as part of the preventive medicine service (**99381–99397**) or, if performed at a separate encounter, reported under the individual preventive medicine counseling service codes (**99401–99404**) or with an office or outpatient E/M service code (**99201–99215**). *ICD-10-CM* code **Z13.84** may be reported for an encounter for screening for dental disorders.

> ~ **More From the AAP** ~
>
> An oral health coding fact sheet is available online at https://www.aap.org/en-us/ Documents/coding_factsheet_ oral_health.pdf.

Chapter 6: Preventive Services

❖ For those carriers (particularly state Medicaid plans under EPSDT) that cover oral health care, some will require a modifier. These modifiers are payer specific and should only be used as directed by your state Medicaid agency or other private payer.

SC Medically necessary service or supply

EP Services provided as part of Medicaid EPSDT program

U5 Medicaid Level of Care 5, as defined by each state

> **~ More From the AAP ~**
>
> The Section on Oral Health also has state-specific information; see https://www.aap.org/en-us/about-the-aap/Committees-Councils-Sections/Oral-Health/Map/Pages/State-Information-and-Resources-Map.aspx.

Screening Laboratory Tests

❖ A test performed in the office laboratory should be billed using the appropriate laboratory code and, if performed, the appropriate blood collection code (**36400–36416**).

❖ Codes **36415** (collection of venous blood by venipuncture) and **36416** (collection of capillary blood specimen [eg, finger, heel, ear stick]) are used for any age child when the physician is not needed to perform the procedure.

❖ When a physician's skill is required to perform venipuncture (eg, access is too difficult for other staff to attain) on a child younger than 3 years, codes **36400–36406** are reported based on the anatomic site of the venipuncture. Report code **36400** when performed on a femoral or jugular vein, code **36405** when on the scalp vein, or code **36406** when another vein is accessed.

❖ When a physician's skill is required to perform venipuncture on a child 3 years or older, code **36410** (venipuncture, age 3 years and older, necessitating physician's skill, for diagnostic or therapeutic purposes [not to be used for routine venipuncture]) is reported.

❖ If the physician performs the venipuncture as a convenience or because staff is not trained in the procedure, code **36415** is reported because the physician's skill was not required.

❖ Although typically not required, some payers will require that modifier **25** be appended to the E/M code if a separate and significant E/M service is reported on the same day of service.

❖ Laboratories and physician offices performing waived tests may need to append modifier **QW** to the *CPT®* code for Clinical Laboratory Improvement Amendments (CLIA)-waived procedures. The use of modifier **QW** is payer specific. To review the list of CLIA-waived procedures, go to http://cms.hhs.gov/Regulations-and-Guidance/Legislation/CLIA/Categorization_of_Tests.html.

❖ *ICD-10-CM* allows separate reporting of special screening examinations (codes in categories **Z11** –**Z13**) in addition to the codes for routine child health examinations when these codes provide additional information. A screening code is not necessary if the screening is inherent to a routine examination. Payer guidelines for reporting screening examinations may vary. When specific *ICD-10-CM* codes are required to support payment for a screening service, be sure to link the appropriate *ICD-10-CM* code to the claim line for the screening service.

Screening for Anemia

85018 QW   Blood count; hemoglobin

Screening for anemia is reported with *ICD-10-CM* code **Z13.0** , encounter for screening for diseases of the blood and blood-forming organs and certain disorders involving the immune mechanism.

Lead Testing

83655 QW   Lead, quantitative analysis

❖ This test does not specify the specimen source or method of testing. Alternative tests sometimes (though now rarely) used for lead screening are **82135** (aminolevulinic acid, delta), **84202** (protoporphyrin, red blood cell count, quantitative), and **84203** (protoporphyrin, red blood cell count, screen).

❖ Some states provide lead testing at no cost to patients covered under the Medicaid EPSDT program. Check your state Medicaid requirements for reporting this service.

- Report *ICD-10-CM* code **Z13.88** (encounter for screening for disorder due to exposure to contaminants) when performing lead screening. Some payers require **Z77.011**, contact with and (suspected) exposure to lead, in lieu of **Z13.88**.

Tuberculosis Skin Test (Mantoux)

86580   Tuberculosis, intradermal (includes administration)

- The tuberculosis (TB) skin test (Mantoux) using intradermal administration of purified protein derivative (PPD) is the recommended diagnostic skin test for TB. (This is not the BCG TB vaccine.)
- Code **99211** is the appropriate code to report when the patient returns for the reading of a PPD test. In the case of a positive test result, when the physician sees the patient and forms a further diagnostic or treatment plan, the complexity may lead to a higher-level code (ie, **99212–99215**). The appropriate *ICD-10-CM* code is **Z11.1** (encounter for screening for respiratory TB).
- There is not a separate administration code reported when the TB test is performed.

Dyslipidemia Screening

80061 QW   Lipid panel (must include total serum cholesterol, lipoprotein by direct measurement high-density cholesterol [HDL], and triglycerides) *or*
82465 QW   Cholesterol, serum, total
83718 QW   Lipoprotein, direct measurement, high-density cholesterol (HDL cholesterol)
84478 QW   Triglycerides

The appropriate *ICD-10-CM* code for dyslipidemia screening is **Z13.220** (encounter for screening for lipoid disorders).

Screening for Sexually Transmitted Infection

86701 QW   Antibody; HIV-1
G0433 QW   Infectious agent antibody detection by enzyme-linked immunosorbent assay (ELISA) technique, HIV-1 and/or HIV-2, screening

- Screening laboratory tests for chlamydia, gonorrhea, and syphilis require more than waived testing laboratory certification. These include

     86631   Antibody; chlamydia
     86632   Antibody; chlamydia, IgM
     86703   Antibody; HIV-1 and HIV-2; single assay
     87081   Culture, presumptive, pathogenic organisms, screening only
     87110   Culture, chlamydia, any source
     87205   Smear, primary source with interpretation; Gram or Giemsa stain for bacteria, fungi, or cell types

- *ICD-10-CM* codes supporting screening laboratory tests are **Z11.8**, encounter for screening for other infectious and parasitic diseases (eg, chlamydia); **Z11.3**, encounter for screening for infections with a predominantly sexual mode of transmission (eg, syphilis and gonorrhea); and **Z11.4**, encounter for screening for HIV. Codes in category **Z72**, problems related to lifestyle, may also be required to support screening of a sexually active adolescent.

Preventive Care Provided Outside the Preventive Visit

Counseling and/or Risk-Factor Reduction

Codes **99401–99404**, **99411**, and **99412** are used to report risk-factor reduction services provided for the purpose of promoting health and preventing illness or injury in persons without a specific illness.

Table 6-3 lists the codes for counseling individuals and groups.

Chapter 6: Preventive Services

- Services will vary with age and address issues such as diet, exercise, sexual activity, dental health, injury prevention, safe travel, and family problems.
- Services are reported based on time.
- Counseling, anticipatory guidance, and risk-factor reduction interventions provided at the time of an initial or periodic comprehensive preventive medicine examination are components of the periodic service and not separately reported.
- Risk-factor reduction may be reported separately with other E/M services.
  - ❖ Evaluation and management services reported on the same day must be separate and distinct.
  - ❖ Time spent in the provision of risk-factor reduction may not be used as a basis for the selection of the other E/M code.
- When reporting a distinct E/M service, append modifier **25** to the code for the distinct E/M service.

> **|||||||| Coding Pearl ||||||||**
>
> Codes **99401–99404**, **99411**, and **99412** are time-based codes. Once the midpoint is passed, you may report the code with the closet time. To report code **99401**, the midpoint to pass is 8 minutes.

Table 6-3. Preventive Medicine Counseling and/or Risk-Factor Reduction

Code	Description
99401	Preventive medicine counseling and/or risk-factor reduction intervention(s) provided to an individual (separate procedure); approximately 15 minutes
99402	approximately 30 minutes
99403	approximately 45 minutes
99404	approximately 60 minutes
99411	Preventive medicine counseling and/or risk-factor reduction intervention(s) provided to individuals in a group setting; approximately 30 minutes
99412	approximately 60 minutes

However, preventive medicine service codes (**99381–99397**) include counseling, anticipatory guidance, and/or risk-factor reduction interventions that are provided at the time of the periodic comprehensive preventive medicine examination. *Current Procedural Terminology®* states to "refer to codes **99401**, **99402**, **99403**, **99404**, and **99411–99412** for reporting those counseling/anticipatory guidance/risk-factor reduction interventions that are provided at an encounter separate from the preventive medicine examination." Therefore, according to *CPT*, do not report **99401–99404**, **99411**, or **99412** in addition to **99381–99397**.

Examples

➤ **Parents of a 2-month-old patient come to their physician's office to discuss immunizations.** To date, they have refused to have their child immunized. Although the physician has discussed the need for vaccines during the child's previous visits, the parents indicate they have further questions. The physician spends 25 minutes counseling the parents about current recommendations, safety and efficacy of vaccines, and their importance in preventing disease.

ICD-10-CM	CPT
Z71.89 (other specified counseling) **Z28.3** (personal history of under-immunization status) **Z28.82** (vaccination not carried out because of caregiver refusal)	**99402** (risk-factor reduction counseling)

➤ A group of 4 overweight patients attend a 30-minute session in the physician's office to discuss diet and exercise. The physician conducts the counseling session.

ICD-10-CM	CPT
Z71.3 (dietary counseling and surveillance) Use additional code from category **Z68** to identify BMI. **Z71.82** (exercise counseling)	**99411** (risk-factor reduction counseling, group)

Teaching Point: Services are documented in each patient's medical record and are reported for each child. Services provided to a group of patients may not be reported as individual office E/M visits (**99201–99215**) because only face-to-face time spent counseling the individual patient may be reported based on time spent counseling and/or coordinating care when reporting office or other outpatient E/M visits. See **Table 6-1** for more information on BMI codes in category **Z68**. Counseling for exercise and physical activity is reported with code **Z71.82** (new in 2018).

Behavior Change Intervention

Behavior change interventions are for persons who have a behavior that is often considered an illness itself, such as tobacco use and addiction or substance abuse or misuse. Behavior change services may be reported when performed as part of the treatment of conditions related to or potentially exacerbated by the behavior or when performed to change the harmful behavior that has not yet resulted in illness.

Table 6-4 lists behavior change intervention codes.

> ||||||||| **Coding Pearl** |||||||||
>
> *ICD-10-CM* guidelines state that substance use codes should only be assigned when the use is associated with a mental or behavioral disorder and such a relationship is documented by the provider.

- ◉ Behavior change intervention codes **99406–99409** are reported when
  - ❖ Services are provided by a physician or QHP for patients who have a behavior that is often considered an illness (eg, tobacco use and addiction, substance abuse or misuse).
  - ❖ Services involve specific validated interventions, including assessing readiness for and barriers to change, advising change in behavior, providing specific suggested actions and motivational counseling, and arranging for services and follow-up care.
- ◉ Codes **99406–99409** include specific time requirements that must be met (eg, at least 15 minutes must be spent in counseling to support reporting of code **99408**).
- ◉ Medical record documentation supports the total time spent in the performance of the service, and a detail of the behavior change intervention is provided.
- ◉ Behavior change intervention services cannot be performed on a parent or guardian of a patient and reported under the patient's name.
- ◉ Behavior change interventions may be reported separately with preventive medicine or other E/M services.
  - ❖ Evaluation and management services reported on the same day must be separate and distinct.
  - ❖ Time spent in the provision of behavior change intervention may not be used as a basis for the selection of the other E/M code.
- ◉ When reporting a distinct E/M service, append modifier **25** to the code for the distinct E/M service (eg, **99213**).
- ◉ Code **99078** is reported when a physician counsels groups of patients with symptoms or an established illness. This service is reported for each participating child. (See the Physician Group Education Services section in Chapter 16, Common Testing and Therapeutic Services, for an example of how code **99078** is used.)

Table 6-4. Behavior Change Intervention

99406	Smoking and tobacco use cessation counseling visit; intermediate, >3 minutes up to 10 minutes
99407	intensive, >10 minutes
99408	Alcohol and/or substance (other than tobacco) abuse structured screening (eg, AUDIT, DAST), and brief intervention services; 15–30 minutes
99409	>30 minutes

Abbreviations: AUDIT, Alcohol Use Disorders Identification Test; DAST, Drug Abuse Screening Test.

Examples

➤ **During an office visit for a 14-year-old new patient for an unrelated problem, it is learned that he has been smoking for 2 years.** After counseling him about the dangers and potential health problems associated with smoking, he and his mother express interest in assistance to help him stop using tobacco. The physician spends 10 minutes discussing specific methods to overcome barriers, pharmacological options, behavioral techniques, and nicotine replacement. The patient is referred to a community support group and a follow-up visit is scheduled in 2 weeks to provide additional encouragement and counseling as needed. Diagnosis is tobacco use.

ICD-10-CM	CPT®
Use diagnosis code appropriate for problem addressed. **Z72.0** (tobacco use) **Z71.6** (tobacco abuse counseling)	**99201–99205 25** (based on service performed and documented) **99406**

Teaching Point: If only general advice and encouragement to stop smoking had been provided, it would be considered part of the new patient office visit. Counseling time must be documented.

➤ **During a preventive medicine service for a 14-year-old established patient, it is learned that he drinks beer at a friend's house.** The physician uses a structured screening tool to interview the patient about substance use. The result is positive and the physician spends a total of 20 minutes interviewing the patient about substance use history and counseling the patient about risks associated with alcohol and drug use, not driving or riding with someone under the influence, and seeking an agreement to avoid future use.

ICD-10-CM	CPT
Z00.129 (routine child health examination without abnormal findings) **Z71.89** (other specified counseling)	**99394 25** (preventive medicine visit) **99408**

Preventive Medicine Services Modifier

33   Preventive services

As a result of the PPACA, the *CPT* Editorial Panel created a modifier to communicate with payers that a preventive medicine service (defined by the PPACA provisions listed as follows) was performed on a patient enrolled in an individual and group non-grandfathered health care plan and, therefore, should not be subject to cost sharing.

⚬ The appropriate use of modifier **33** will reduce claim adjustments related to preventive services and corresponding payments to members.

- Modifier **33** should only be appended to codes represented in one or more of the following 4 categories:
  - ❖ Services rated A or B by the USPSTF
  - ❖ Immunizations for routine use in children, adolescents, and adults as recommended by ACIP of the CDC
  - ❖ Preventive care and screenings for children as recommended by Bright Futures (AAP) and newborn testing (American College of Medical Genetics and Genomics)
  - ❖ Preventive care and screenings provided for women supported by HRSA
- **DO *NOT* USE MODIFIER 33**
  - ❖ **When the *CPT* code(s) is identified as inherently preventive (eg, preventive medicine counseling)**
  - ❖ **When the service(s) is not indicated in the categories noted previously**
  - ❖ **With an insurance plan that continues to implement the cost-sharing policy on preventive medicine services (grandfathered health plan)**
- Check with your payers before fully implementing the use of modifier **33** to verify any variations in reporting requirements. Modifier **33** *is not used for benefit determination by some payers* and may be required by others only for services that may be either diagnostic/therapeutic or preventive.

Examples

➤ **A 9-month-old patient presents for her age-appropriate preventive medicine service.** The physician completes the age-appropriate history and physical examination and provides anticipatory guidance. While reviewing immunization history, the physician notes the patient is behind on her Hib vaccine because of a recent shortage from the manufacturer. The physician counsels the mother on the vaccine (ActHIB) and orders it. The physician also reviews the periodicity schedule and notes the patient is due for a developmental screening as part of the Bright Futures recommendations. The nurse administers the screening to the mother and scores it. The physician reviews the unremarkable results with the mother and the next routine visit is scheduled for 12 months.

ICD-10-CM	CPT®
Z00.129 Z23	99391 96110 33 (developmental screen) 90648 33 (Hib) 90460 33

Teaching Point: Append modifier **33** to those services that fall within the 4 listed categories previously discussed. In this case, the developmental screening falls under Bright Futures recommendations for a 9-month-old and the vaccine product and administration fall under routine immunizations recommended by ACIP. Note that the modifier does not have to be appended to code **99391** because that service is inherently preventive.

➤ **An 11-year-old is seen for an established patient office visit on Monday for a rash.** The physician provides an E/M service with a problem-focused history and physical examination and straightforward medical decision-making (MDM). The physician notes the patient is scheduled for a preventive medicine service one afternoon next week and has not been screened for dyslipidemia. The physician orders a fasting lipid panel to be performed prior to the preventive service. The patient returns the next morning and the in-office laboratory performs the lipid panel test. The results are reported to the physician.

ICD-10-CM	CPT
Monday: **R21** (rash)	Monday: **99212**
Tuesday: **Z13.220** (encounter for screening for lipoid disorders)	Tuesday: **80061 QW 33**

Teaching Point: Append modifier **33** to code **80061** to indicate the test was performed as a preventive service, even though it is ordered and performed on a date when no preventive medicine service was provided. Modifier **QW** is also appended when required by the payer to indicate the test is CLIA waived.

Chapter 6: Preventive Services

Other Preventive Medicine Services

99429   Unlisted preventive medicine service

Code **99429** may be reported if these options are not suitable. If the unlisted code is used, most payers will require a copy of the progress notes filed with the claim.

Reporting a Preventive Medicine Visit With a Problem-Oriented Visit

When a problem or abnormality is addressed *and requires significant additional work* (eg, symptomatic atopic dermatitis, exercise-induced asthma, migraine headache, poor academic performance in a patient with ADHD) to perform the required key components and is medically necessary, it may be reported using the office or other outpatient services codes (**99201–99215**) in addition to the preventive medicine services code.

> ||||||||| *Coding Pearl* |||||||||
>
> Although a separate E/M service is not reported when a minor problem or chronic condition requires less than significant additional work, the diagnosis code for the problem or chronic condition may be reported in addition to code **Z00.121** (routine child health examination with abnormal findings).

When reporting both E/M services

◉ The levels of history and examination performed and documented relative to the problem or abnormality may be limited by the work already included in the preventive medicine service (ie, elements that are included in the preventive service cannot be counted toward the level of service for the problem-oriented service). Because of this, typically, the level of E/M service reported will be one level lower than if the patient presented solely for the problem, unless coding is based on time.

   ❖ An age- and gender-appropriate examination is included in the preventive medicine service, but an extended examination of the affected body area(s) and other symptomatic or related organ system(s) would be separately considered in determining the level of E/M service provided to address the problem.

   ❖ Because *CPT®* states that the comprehensive history of a preventive medicine service includes a comprehensive or interval PFSH, the level of problem-oriented history on the same date may be limited to expanded problem focused unless you can show that elements of the PFSH were obtained only in relation to the problem being addressed.

   ❖ Payers may require MDM as 1 of the 2 key components met (ie, history and MDM or examination and MDM) to support an established patient visit.

◉ Documentation for each service should be maintained in the medical record. That documentation may be on a separate progress note (preferred) or, if included on the same progress note, must clearly reflect the additional work performed. If the problem-oriented visit is reported based on time, documentation must clearly reflect the total time spent in the face-to-face encounter addressing the issue(s) or problem(s), the total time spent in counseling and/or coordination of care, and a summary of the issues discussed.

◉ *ICD-10-CM* well-care diagnosis codes (see code list on page 150) should be linked to the appropriate preventive medicine service code (**99381–99395**) and the sick care diagnosis code linked to the problem-oriented service code (**99201–99215**).

◉ It is important to make parents aware of any additional charges that may occur at the preventive medicine encounter. This includes, but is not limited to, a significant, separately identifiable E/M service. The AAP has developed a template letter that can be used to outline what may not be covered under the no-cost-sharing preventive medicine services (www.aap.org/en-us/professional-resources/practice-transformation/getting-paid/Coding-at-the-AAP/Pages/Evaluation-and-Management.aspx).

In the following claim form example, a patient received an established patient preventive service (**99392**) and a problem-oriented E/M service (**99213**) to address recurrent bilateral otitis media on the same date. The claim form example shows diagnosis codes **Z00.121** and **H65.196** (recurrent bilateral otitis media) listed in fields 21 A and 21 B. The A and B are diagnosis pointers used in column 24E to link the appropriate diagnosis codes to the procedure codes included on each service line. Note that diagnosis code **H65.196** (diagnosis pointer B) is linked to the preventive and problem-oriented services in column 24E. Modifier **25** is appended to code **99213** (field 24D under "Modifier") to indicate the significant, separately identifiable E/M service was provided in addition to the preventive medicine service (**99392**).

Claim Form Example: Preventive and Problem-Oriented Services

21. Diagnosis or nature of illness or injury (Relate A–L to service line below 24E) A. **Z00.121** B. **H65.196** C. D.				ICD Ind. 0					
24. A. Dates of service B. Place of service	C. EMG	D. Procedures, services or supplies CPT/HCPCS	Modifier	E. Diagnosis Pointer	F. Charges	G. Days or units	H. EPSDT	I. ID Qual	J. Rendering Provider #
1/1/2018– 1/1/2018	11	**99392**		A, B	$$$	1		NPI	123456789
1/1/2018– 1/1/2018	11	**99213**	**25**	B	$$$	1		NPI	123456789

Abbreviations: CPT, Current Procedural Terminology; EMG, emergency; EPSDT, Early and Periodic Screening, Diagnosis, and Treatment; HCPCS, Healthcare Common Procedure Coding System; ICD, International Classification of Diseases; NPI, National Provider Identifier.

- The presence of a chronic condition(s) in and of itself does not change a preventive medicine visit to a problem-oriented visit, nor does it unilaterally support a separate problem-oriented E/M service (**99201–99215**) with the well visit, unless it is significant and has been separately addressed.
- An insignificant problem or condition (eg, minor diaper rash, stable chronic problem, renewal of prescription medications) that does not require additional work to perform the required key components cannot be reported as a separate E/M service.
- Modifier **25** (significant, separately identifiable E/M service by the same physician on the same day of the procedure or other service) should be appended to the problem-oriented service code (eg, **99212**). If vaccines are given at the same encounter, append modifier **25** to the problem-oriented E/M service code and the preventive medicine service code.

Coding Conundrum: Reporting 2 New Patient Codes on the Same Day

When a preventive medicine visit and problem-oriented E/M service are performed on the same day to a new patient, both codes may be reported with the appropriate new patient codes (eg, **99381** and **99203 25**).

Before reporting 2 new patient codes on the same patient on the same day of service, consider

- A new patient office or outpatient visit requires that all 3 key components (history, physical examination, and MDM) or typical time (if more than 50% of the total face-to-face encounter is spent in counseling and/or coordination of care) be met.
- If only 2 of the 3 required key components are met (eg, the physical examination was part of the comprehensive preventive medicine service), the code selection would have to be based on an established patient code (**99212–99215**).
- The physical examination can be counted as a key component only in situations in which the examination component of the problem-oriented visit would be considered as distinct or in addition to what is normally performed during the preventive medicine examination.

- Some patients will be required to provide a co-payment for the non–preventive medicine visit code under the terms of their plan benefit even when there is no co-payment required for the preventive medicine visit. Legally, this co-payment cannot routinely be written off. The AAP has developed a letter addressing this issue that can be found at www.aap.org/cfp (access code AAPCFP23).
- The AAP has developed forms that promote good documentation of preventive medicine services. Examples can be ordered from the AAP by calling 888/227-1770 or visiting http://shop.aap.org/Pediatric-Documentation-Forms-Economy-Package. Additionally, some state Medicaid programs have developed documentation templates for preventive services delivered in their EPSDT program.

Examples

➤ **A 13-year-old with complaint of earache is seen as a new patient.** The patient has not had his annual preventive medicine service. Parents agree to provision of the preventive medicine service at this encounter. Immunizations are up-to-date. Depression screening is performed and scored with a standardized instrument. In addition to the age- and gender-appropriate components of the preventive medicine service, the physician documents an expanded problem-focused history of illness; problem-focused examination of ear, nose, mouth, and throat; and diagnosis and plan for acute right otitis externa in an otherwise healthy and active boy with a BMI at the 55th percentile. Medical decision-making is straightforward.

Preventive medicine visit	*ICD-10-CM* **Z00.121** (well-child check with abnormal findings) **Z68.52** (BMI 5th to 85th percentile)
	CPT® **99384** **96127** (brief emotional/behavioral assessment)
Problem-oriented visit *MDM:* straightforward complexity *History:* Problem focused *Physical examination:* Problem focused	*ICD-10-CM* **H60.501** (unspecified acute noninfective otitis externa, right ear)
	CPT **99201 25**

Teaching Point: Provision of preventive services at this encounter reflects proactive delivery of recommended services and may support successful participation in quality initiatives. Documentation of the expanded problem-focused history, examination, assessment, and plan related to the earache should be readily identifiable in the patient record. Because all 3 key components are required for reporting a new patient visit, code **99201** (problem-focused history and examination with straightforward MDM) is supported. If documentation did not support code **99201**, an established patient office or other outpatient E/M code (**99212**) would be reported instead.

➤ **A mother of a new patient who presents for a well-child examination reports that her 6-year-old has been very disruptive at home and school since their move to the community.** The physician conducts a well-child examination with documentation of BMI at the 65th percentile. In addition to the preventive medicine service, a total of 20 minutes is specifically spent by the physician counseling the mother and child on the disruptive behavior. Diagnosis for the problem-oriented service is adjustment disorder with conduct disturbance.

Preventive medicine visit	*ICD-10-CM* **Z00.121** (well-child check with abnormal findings) **Z68.52** (BMI 5th to 85th percentile)
	CPT **99383**
Problem-oriented visit 20 minutes spent counseling	*ICD-10-CM* **F43.24** (adjustment disorder with disturbance of conduct)
	CPT **99202 25**

Teaching Point: The level of service for the problem-oriented E/M service was selected based on time spent counseling and/or coordinating care. Physician documentation must clearly support the time spent in providing the problem-oriented service versus time spent in anticipatory counseling as part of the preventive service. In support of quality measurement, code **Z68.52** is reported for the BMI percentile.

➤ A 12-month-old girl is seen for a new patient visit for painful urination. Mother states that the girl has been crying when voiding for 2 days and her urine "smells bad." Review of systems reveals that she had a fever of 100.0 °F (37.8°C) last night, is voiding more frequently, and is irritable. A history of present illness and comprehensive physical examination are performed. Urinalysis is consistent with a urinary tract infection (UTI). A urine culture is ordered. A full preventive medicine service is completed, including age-appropriate counseling and anticipatory guidance, and vaccines are deferred. She is placed on antibiotics for 10 days. Mother is advised to follow up in 2 weeks.

Preventive medicine visit	ICD-10-CM Z00.121 (well-child check with abnormal findings) Z28.01 (immunization not carried out because of acute illness of patient)
	CPT® 99382
Problem-oriented visit MDM: Moderate complexity History: Expanded problem focused Physical examination: Included in preventive medicine visit	ICD-10-CM N39.0 (UTI)
	CPT 99213 25

Teaching Point: Examination of external genitalia and back does not constitute examination beyond the comprehensive examination included in the preventive service. Because the physical examination was included as part of the preventive medicine visit, only 2 of the required 3 components needed to select the code for a new patient office or outpatient visit were provided and considered in the selection of the problem-oriented service. Therefore, the problem-oriented service is reported using the established patient visit code **99213**. By including code **Z28.01**, the practice indicates delay in immunization due to an acute illness and may use the diagnosis code as part of a recall system to follow up with patients who miss appointments for immunization.

➤ A 2-year-old boy with history of macrocephaly is seen for a preventive medicine visit. He is referred to an ophthalmologist because of strabismus noted by photoscreening with remote analysis. All other findings are normal, including BMI at the 75th percentile.

Preventive medicine visit Photoscreening	ICD-10-CM Z00.121 (well-child check with abnormal findings) H50.9 (strabismus, unspecified) Q75.3 (macrocephaly) Z68.52 (BMI 5th to 85th percentile)
	CPT New Patient Established Patient 99382 99392 99174 (instrument-based ocular screening, bilateral, with remote analysis and report)

Teaching Point: Because this scenario includes no additional workup of the strabismus, only the preventive medicine and photoscreening services are reported. The diagnosis code for strabismus discovered during the preventive medicine service is reported as an additional diagnosis to the code for the well-child check. If more work is needed or required a separate E/M service could be reported based on documentation.

Chapter 6: Preventive Services

Evaluation and Management Services in the Office, Outpatient, Home, or Nursing Facility Setting

Contents

Selecting the Appropriate Evaluation and Management (E/M) Codes

This chapter includes tables with descriptions of the required key components (ie, history, physical examination, medical decision-making [MDM], and, if appropriate, time) for all the evaluation and management (E/M) services that are reported in the office, outpatient, home, nursing facility and domiciliary, and rest home settings. Table 7-1 provides the key components and specific details on required elements within each level of history and physical examination (eg, problem focused, expanded) and MDM (eg, straightforward, moderate) of an E/M code. Refer to this table when using some of the other tables in this chapter. These tables can be downloaded at www.aap.org/cfp (access code AAPCFP23).

Chapter 7: Evaluation and Management Services in the Office, Outpatient, Home, or Nursing Facility Setting

Table 7-1. Evaluation and Management Key Components				
History (must meet or exceed HPI, ROS, and PFSH)	**Problem Focused** HPI: 1–3 elements ROS: 0 PFSH: 0	**Expanded** HPI: 1–3 elements ROS: 1 PFSH: 0	**Detailed** HPI: 4+ elements or status of 3 chronic or inactive conditions ROS: 2–9 PFSH: 1	**Comprehensive** HPI: 4+ elements or status of 3 chronic or inactive conditions ROS: 10+ PFSH: 2 (established patient) or 3 (new patient)
Physical Examination	**Problem Focused** 1995: 1 body area/organ system 1997: Performance and documentation of 1–5 elements identified by a bullet (●) in one or more areas or systems	**Expanded** 1995: Limited exam—affected body area/organ system and other related areas/systems 1997: Performance and documentation of at least 6 elements identified by a bullet (●) in one or more areas or systems	**Detailed** 1995: Extended exam—affected body area(s) and other symptomatic or related organ system(s) 1997: Performance and documentation of at least 2 elements identified by a bullet (●) in at least 6 areas or systems or at least 12 elements identified by a bullet (●) in at least 2 areas or systems	**Comprehensive** 1995: 8+ organ systems or complete exam of a single organ system 1997: Multisystem exam—9 systems or areas with performance of all elements identified by a bullet (●) in each area/system examined Documentation of at least 2 elements identified by a bullet (●) of each area(s) or system(s) Single organ system exam—Performance of all elements identified by a bullet (●) and documentation of every element in box with shaded border and at least one element in box with unshaded border
Medical Decision-making (must meet 2 of diagnoses/options, data, and risk)	**Straightforward** Presenting problem: Usually self-limited or minor severity # diagnoses/options: Minimal Data: Minimal Risk: Minimal	**Low Complexity** Presenting problem: Usually moderate severity # diagnoses/options: Limited Data: Limited Risk: Low	**Moderate Complexity** Presenting problem: Usually moderate to high severity # diagnoses/options: Multiple Data: Moderate Risk: Moderate	**High Complexity** Presenting problem: Usually moderate to high severity # diagnoses/options: Extensive Data: Extensive Risk: High

Abbreviations: HPI, history of present illness; PFSH, past, family, and social history; ROS, review of systems.

Note: All E/M code descriptors and their specific instructions reflect the exclusion of references to provider/professional type, whenever not essential, throughout the code set. The codes also reflect the inclusion of a qualified health care professional (QHP) when the word "physician" is included.

See Chapter 4, Evaluation and Management Documentation Guidelines, for a detailed description of the guidelines and components of E/M services with documentation requirements and tips.

Office and Other Outpatient Visits (99201–99205, 99211–99215)

Use **tables** 7-2 and 7-3 to guide you in the selection of the appropriate codes in the following clinical examples. Clinical vignettes are provided to illustrate correct coding applications and are not intended to offer advice on the practice of medicine.

Codes **99201–99205** and **99212–99215** are reported when services are provided in an outpatient setting (eg, physician office, outpatient hospital clinic, walk-in urgent care clinic, health department clinic).

- ❋ The place of service code (eg, **22**, on campus—outpatient hospital) is used to indicate whether office or other outpatient services are provided in a facility or non-facility setting. (See Chapter 19, The Business of Medicine: Working With Current and Emerging Payment Systems, for more information on place of service codes.)

> |||||||| **Coding Pearl** ||||||||
>
> When reporting office or other outpatient services, place of service codes may affect payment. Never report place of service **11** (office) for care in a hospital clinic or other facility.

- ❋ Codes are subcategorized into new patient and established patient visits.
- ❋ New patient E/M visits (**99201–99205**) require performance and documentation of all 3 key components unless billing based on time. See Chapter 4, Evaluation and Management Documentation Guidelines, for information on new versus established patient.
- ❋ Established patient visits (**99212–99215**) are reported based on the performance and documentation of 2 of the 3 key components unless billing based on time. Some payers require selection of the level of service based on the performed and documented MDM and either history or examination.
- ❋ Code **99211** is used to report E/M services that do not require a physician's presence but are usually performed incident to the physician. (See Chapter 14, Allied Health and Clinical Staff Services, for more information on incident-to services.) There are no required key components. Physicians and other QHPs should not report **99211** for face-to-face encounters with patients.
- ❋ Any service with its own code (eg, immunizations, laboratory procedures) should be reported in addition to E/M visit codes when performed as a separate service and documented. (Modifiers may be necessary; see Chapter 3, Modifiers and Coding Edits, for more information.)
- ❋ Time may be used as the key controlling factor in the selection of the code, when appropriate, in lieu of key components. (See Chapter 5, Time-Based Coding, for specific guidelines to follow when reporting an E/M service based on time.)

> ~ **More From the AAP** ~
>
> Read more about reporting E/M services based on time in the March 2016 *AAP Pediatric Coding Newsletter*™ at http://coding.aap.org (subscription required).

The examples included here and throughout the chapter are based on the 1995 E/M documentation guidelines. Medical decision-making is listed before history and physical examination because some payers require that the level of MDM be 1 of the 2 key components met to support the level of service for an established patient encounter. See the Examination in the E/M Guidelines: 1995 or 1997 box later in this chapter for an example based on the 1997 guidelines.

Table 7-2. Office Visit Codes: New Patient

Key Components (For a description of key components, see Table 7-1.)
3 of 3 key components must be performed to at least the degree specified for the code.

CPT® Code/Time[a]	Medical Decision-making	History	Examination
99201 10 min	Straightforward PP: Usually self-limited or minor severity	Problem focused	Problem focused
99202 20 min	Straightforward PP: Usually low to moderate severity	Expanded	Expanded
99203 30 min	Low complexity PP: Usually moderate severity	Detailed	Detailed
99204 45 min	Moderate complexity PP: Usually moderate to high severity	Comprehensive	Comprehensive
99205 60 min	High complexity PP: Usually moderate to high severity	Comprehensive	Comprehensive

Abbreviations: CPT, Current Procedural Terminology; PP, presenting problem.

[a] Typical time is an average and represents a range of times that may be higher or lower depending on clinical circumstances. The presenting problem is considered to be a contributory factor and does not need to be present to the degree specified.

Table 7-3. Office Visit Codes: Established Patient

Key Components (For a description of key components, see Table 7-1.)
2 of 3 key components must be performed to at least the degree specified for the code. Some payers may require medical decision-making as 1 of the 2 components performed and documented.

CPT® Code/Time[a]	Medical Decision-making	History	Examination
99211 5 min	Not required; may not require the presence of a physician PP: Usually minimal severity	Not required	Not required
99212 10 min	Straightforward PP: Usually self-limited or minor severity	Problem focused	Problem focused
99213 15 min	Low complexity PP: Usually moderate severity	Expanded	Expanded
99214 25 min	Moderate complexity PP: Usually moderate to high severity	Detailed	Detailed
99215 40 min	High complexity PP: Usually moderate to high severity	Comprehensive	Comprehensive

Abbreviations: CPT, Current Procedural Terminology; PP, presenting problem.

[a] Typical time is an average and represents a range of times that may be higher or lower depending on clinical circumstances. The presenting problem is considered to be a contributory factor and does not need to be present to the degree specified.

Examples

➤ A 2-year-old patient is seen with chief complaint of vomiting and diarrhea.

History: Vomiting and watery diarrhea since last evening; fussy. No fever.

Brief history of present illness (HPI), including

- ◉ Timing: last evening
- ◉ Quality: watery
- ◉ Associated signs/symptoms: fussy

Chapter 7: Evaluation and Management Services in the Office, Outpatient, Home, or Nursing Facility Setting

Review of 1 system
- Constitutional: no fever

Physical examination: 4 organ systems documented (a limited examination of the affected body area or organ system and other symptomatic or related organ system[s])
- Constitutional
- Cardiovascular
- Respiratory
- Gastrointestinal

Assessment/plan: Acute noninfectious gastroenteritis. Mother is told to give fluids and watch for dehydration. Call if no improvement or condition worsens.

MDM: Low (acute uncomplicated illness and low risk) *History:* Expanded (brief HPI and review of 1 system) *Physical examination:* Expanded (a limited examination of the affected body area or organ system and other symptomatic or related organ system[s])	***International Classification of Diseases, 10th Revision, Clinical Modification (ICD-10-CM)*** **K52.9** (noninfectious gastroenteritis and colitis, unspecified)
	Current Procedural Terminology (CPT®) **New Patient Established Patient** **99202 99213**

Teaching Point: The level of service for new patient visits must be supported by all 3 key components, while the level of service for the established patient encounter requires meeting 2 of 3 key components. Although low-complexity MDM would support a **99203** service, detailed history and examination are required to support this level of service. Although only 2 of 3 key components are required to support **99213**, all 3 were met.

Physicians participating in quality initiatives may elect to additionally report *CPT* Category II performance measure codes to indicate specific elements of care were provided (eg, **2030F**, hydration status documented, normally hydrated, and **4058F**, pediatric gastroenteritis education provided to caregiver). Category II codes are not used for direct fee-for-service payment. For more on Category II codes, see Chapter 17, Coding to Demonstrate Quality and Value.

➤ **The 2-year-old patient from the previous example is seen later the same day by another pediatrician in the same group practice due to continued vomiting and diarrhea and concerns of dehydration.** The physician reviews the documentation from the visit earlier that day and obtains an interval history, including documentation of multiple episodes of vomiting within minutes of fluid intake, lack of appetite, and continued loose, watery stools. Review of systems is updated to include 4 additional systems. Past medical history is reviewed, including previous urinary tract infections and up-to-date immunization status. Social and family history is negative for recent illness in family or known infectious contacts at child care. Examination includes constitutional; eyes, ears, nose, and throat; cardiovascular; respiratory; abdomen; and extremities. Urinalysis is performed and the result is negative. The physician directs a nurse to provide oral rehydration per a time-based rehydration plan and reassess the patient periodically until completed. On completion of the rehydration plan, the physician reevaluates the patient, who is now tolerating fluids and showing overall improvement. The patient is discharged to home from the office. Diagnoses are lethargy and dehydration due to noninfectious gastroenteritis.

Combined key components of the 2 encounters *MDM:* Moderate (established problem worsening with manifestations and moderate risk) *History:* Detailed (≥4 HPI and review of 5 systems; past, family, and social history [PFSH]) *Physical examination:* Detailed (expanded examination of the affected and related organ systems or body areas)	***ICD-10-CM*** **K52.9** (noninfectious gastroenteritis and colitis, unspecified) **E86.0** (dehydration) **R53.83** (other fatigue, lethargy)
	CPT® **New Patient** **Established Patient** **99203** **99214**

Teaching Point: The combined work of the 2 encounters is reported as a single E/M service (typically by the physician who provided the greater portion of the service). The level of service is based on the combined history, examination, and MDM of the physicians.

Time spent by clinical staff providing oral rehydration services may be separately reportable if the total accumulated clinical staff time for this service is greater than 45 minutes beyond the typical time of the related physician E/M service. See discussion of prolonged clinical staff service codes **99415** and **99416** in Chapter 14, Allied Health and Clinical Staff Services.

➤ **A 6-month-old is seen for a follow-up visit 2 weeks after a visit for an ear infection and cough.**

History: No fever or cough. Acting fine.

Physical examination: 3 organ systems documented (constitutional; ears, nose, mouth, and throat; respiratory).

Assessment: Resolved acute otitis media, right ear. Follow up as necessary.

MDM: Straightforward *History:* Problem focused *Physical examination:* Expanded problem focused	***ICD-10-CM*** **Z09** (encounter for follow-up examination after complete treatment for conditions other than malignant neoplasm) **Z86.69** (personal history of other diseases of the nervous system and sense organs)
	CPT **New Patient** **Established Patient** **99201** **99212**

Teaching Point: Otitis media should not be reported because it is resolved. If your payers require this, remind them that *ICD-10-CM* guidelines stipulate that resolved conditions are not reported in the outpatient setting or by providers. *ICD* guidelines are part of the Health Insurance Portability and Accountability Act of 1996 (HIPAA) standard code set and any violation of *ICD* guidelines is a direct HIPAA violation.

➤ **A 12-year-old boy presents for management of medications prescribed for predominantly hyperactive attention-deficit/hyperactivity disorder (ADHD). Medication was prescribed 3 weeks earlier.**

History: No improvement was seen after starting medication; continues to disrupt class, fidgeting more, and unable to focus on work; no weight loss; occasional trouble sleeping, loss of appetite, and no diarrhea. No changes in his school or home environment.

Behavioral rating scales: Parent NICHQ Vanderbilt ADHD scale is strongly positive for inattention and hyperactivity; teacher NICHQ Vanderbilt scale also strongly positive for inattention and hyperactivity. Neither rating scale by either observer showed changes from pretreatment behaviors.

Physical examination: 3 organ systems documented (constitutional [weight, height, and blood pressure documented], cardiovascular, gastrointestinal).

Assessment/plan: New medication is prescribed, old discontinued; follow up in 2 weeks. Twenty-five minutes is spent discussing side effects of the medication, behavior modifications, changes at school, and when psychiatric referral may be needed. Total visit time is 35 minutes.

The physician documents that 35 minutes was spent face-to-face with the child and guardian and 25 minutes of that was spent on counseling. A summary of the issues discussed is documented. Time (35 minutes face-to-face) is the key controlling factor.	**ICD-10-CM** **F90.1** (ADHD, predominantly hyperactive) **CPT®** **New Patient** **Established Patient** **99203 25** (30 minutes) **99215 25** (40 minutes) **96127** × 2 (brief behavioral and emotional assessment, with scoring and documentation, per instrument [2 scales reviewed])

Teaching Point: Because more than 50% of the physician's 35-minute face-to-face time was spent in counseling and/or coordinating care, code selection may be based on time rather than key components. Per *CPT* instruction, when the physician's total face-to-face time falls between the typical times of 2 codes, report the code with the closest typical time. (Some state Medicaid programs may require that the typical time assigned to a code be met or exceeded.) See Chapter 5, Time-Based Coding, for more information on reporting E/M services based on time.

Health plans may include follow-up care for children aged 6 to 12 years with ADHD in the collection of Healthcare Effectiveness Data and Information Set (HEDIS) measurement. Office visits linked to an *ICD-10-CM* code for ADHD would prompt payer identification of the visit provided within 30 days of when the first ADHD medication was dispensed (performance measure for ADHD). This measure also calls for 2 additional follow-up visits within the 31 to 300 days after start of medication for patients who remain on the medication for at least 210 days. When *ICD-10-CM* and *CPT* codes provide information necessary for measurement, time-consuming manual chart review might be avoided. For more on HEDIS, see Chapter 17, Coding to Demonstrate Quality and Value.

> |ı||ı|||| **Coding Pearl** |ı|||ı|||
>
> When reporting code **96127**, National Correct Coding Initiative edits may require reporting of 2 units of service per claim line. Modifier **59** is appended to the second claim line to indicate the additional units of service are for separately completed screening instruments.

➤ **A 5-year-old is seen by an office nurse in follow-up to a physician office visit 3 days earlier at which nonbullous impetigo was diagnosed and a topical antibiotic was prescribed. The area of infection shows improvement and the child's temperature is normal. Based on the physician's orders, the nurse advises the parents to continue the antibiotic until the skin is clear and completes a form provided by the child's school indicating the child has improved sufficiently to return to class.**

History: Here for follow-up of nonbullous impetigo per Dr Good's order. Started antibiotic ointment on Monday evening. Mother reports no fever and feels the sores are healing quickly. Needs form completed for return to school.

Physical assessment: Small area of sores remains. Temperature 36.8°C (98.2°F).

Plan: Discussed with Dr Good. Mother is told to continue antibiotic ointment until all sores are gone. Form completed. Call if no improvement or condition worsens.

Office or other outpatient visit for the E/M of an established patient that may not require the presence of a physician or other QHP. Usually, the presenting problem(s) is minimal. Typically, 5 minutes are spent performing or supervising these services.	**ICD-10-CM** **L01.01** (non-bullous impetigo) **CPT** **99211**

➤ A 5-year-old is seen by an office nurse in follow-up to a physician office visit 3 days earlier at which nonbullous impetigo was diagnosed and a topical antibiotic was prescribed. The area of infection shows improvement and the child's temperature is normal, but the nurse is not sure if improvement is sufficient for return to class. The physician provides a face-to-face E/M service and advises the parents to continue the antibiotic until the skin is clear and completes a form provided by the child's school indicating the child has improved sufficiently to return to class.

History: No complaints. No fever. Has followed instructions in using antibiotic ointment.

Physical examination: Small area of sores remains but otherwise healing well with no indication of complications.

Assessment/plan: Resolving impetigo. Instructed patient's mother to continue antibiotic ointment until all sores are gone. Return to school form completed. Call if no improvement or condition worsens.

MDM: Straightforward *History:* Problem focused *Physical examination:* Problem focused	**ICD-10-CM** **L01.01** (non-bullous impetigo)
	CPT® **99212**

➤ **A 13-year-old girl is seen with complaints of severe headaches.**

History: Throbbing headaches on left side of face and head a few times over the last few months, each lasting about 24 hours. Has nausea but no vomiting. Over-the-counter pain medication does not relieve the pain. No family history of migraines; doing well in school; no known allergies. No specific triggers noted. Headaches do not awaken from sleep and intensity does not seem to be increasing. Naproxen and acetaminophen have not been effective.

Review of systems: Last menstrual period 2 weeks ago; no gastrointestinal complaints other than nausea with headaches; appetite normal; no complaints of visual disturbance or eye problems; neurologic normal other than headaches; denies stress, worry, or fatigue and is negative for all other systems.

> ||||||||| **Coding Pearl** |||||||||
>
> Do not code diagnoses documented as "possible" or other similar terms indicating uncertainty. Rather, code the condition(s) to the highest degree of certainty for that encounter/visit, such as symptoms, signs, abnormal test results, or other reason for the visit.

(History level is comprehensive with chief complaint of severe headaches; extended HPI—location [left side of face and head], duration [about 24 hours], quality [throbbing], timing [over last few months], associated signs and symptoms [nausea, no vomiting], and modifying factors [unrelieved by over-the-counter medication]; complete review of systems—systems directly related to problems identified in HPI and all other body systems; and PFSH with one element each of past [no allergies], family [no history of migraines], and social history [doing well in school].)

Physical examination: Detailed examination of the neurologic system with additional 4 organ systems documented.

(The level of physical examination is detailed based on 1995 guidelines requiring an extended examination of the affected body area or organ system [neurologic] and other symptomatic or related organ system[s]. See the Examination in the E/M Guidelines: 1995 or 1997 box later in this chapter for examination requirements when using 1997 E/M guidelines.)

Assessment/plan: Headaches, possible migraine. Given headache diary to complete and counseled on triggers and treatment of migraines. Follow-up visit scheduled.

(The level of MDM is moderate, as the problem is an undiagnosed new problem and the risk is moderate [undiagnosed new problem].)

MDM: Moderate *History:* Comprehensive *Physical examination:* Detailed	***ICD-10-CM*** **R51** (headache) **R11.0** (nausea without vomiting)
	***CPT*®** **New Patient** **Established Patient** **99203** **99214**

Teaching Point: If the physician spent more than 50% of the face-to-face time of this visit counseling the patient and caregiver on questions and concerns (eg, possibility of tumor, indications for imaging studies), the service may be reported based on time spent counseling and/or coordinating care. Documentation should include sufficient detail about the nature of the counseling and/or coordination of care (eg, discussed mother's concerns about possible tumor and lack of indications for imaging or other diagnostic testing) and both the total face-to-face time of the visit and the portion spent in counseling and/or coordination of care (percentage or amount of time). For more, see Chapter 5, Time-Based Coding.

Telephone Services (99441–99443, 98966–98968)

99441	Telephone E/M service by a physician or other qualified health care professional who may report evaluation and management services provided to an established patient, parent, or guardian not originating from a related E/M service provided within the previous 7 days nor leading to an E/M service or procedure within the next 24 hours or soonest available appointment; 5–10 minutes of medical discussion
99442	11–20 minutes of medical discussion
99443	21–30 minutes of medical discussion
98966	Telephone assessment and management services provided by a qualified nonphysician health care professional to an established patient, parent, or guardian not originating from related assessment and management service provided within the previous 7 days nor leading to an assessment and management service or procedure within the next 24 hours or soonest available appointment; 5–10 minutes of medical discussion
98967	11–20 minutes of medical discussion
98968	21–30 minutes of medical discussion

Telephone services (**99441–99443**) are non–face-to-face E/M services provided to a patient using the telephone by a physician or other QHP who may report E/M services. Codes **98966–98968** are used to report telephone assessment and management services by qualified nonphysician health care professionals who may not report E/M services.

Guidelines for reporting of telephone assessment and management services are the same as those for physician and QHP telephone E/M service.

Examples

➤ **A 6-month-old was seen in the office 3 days ago for treatment of otitis media.** Mother calls to discuss problems with diarrhea. The discussion of antibiotic-associated diarrhea, probiotics, and symptoms that may require change in treatment lasts for 10 minutes.

Code **99441** cannot be reported because it is related to the E/M visit performed within the previous 7 days.

Examination in the E/M Guidelines: 1995 or 1997

The examination of a 13-year-old girl with complaints of severe headache in the example on page 183 indicated that a detailed examination was reported based on the 1995 examination guidelines (an extended examination of the affected body area or organ system [neurologic] and other symptomatic or related organ system[s]). The examples[a] below demonstrate elements of a detailed examination based on the 1997 documentation guidelines using the multisystem or single-organ (neurologic) examination. See Chapter 4, Evaluation and Management Documentation Guidelines, for more on the 1997 examination guidelines.

Multisystem examination: performance and documentation of at least 2 elements identified by a bullet (●) in at least 6 organ systems or body areas *or* performance and documentation of at least 12 elements identified by a bullet (●) in 2 or more organ systems or body areas

Constitutional
Temperature, pulse rate and regularity, blood pressure
General appearance

Eyes
Examination of pupils and irises (eg, reaction to light and accommodation, size and symmetry)
Ophthalmoscopic examination of optic discs (eg, size, cup to disc ratio, appearance) and posterior segments (eg, vessel changes, exudates, hemorrhages)

Ears, Nose, Mouth, Throat
Otoscopic examination of auditory canals and tympanic membranes
Inspection of nasal mucosa, septum, and turbinates

Neck
Examination of neck (eg, masses, overall appearance, symmetry, tracheal position, crepitus)

Cardiovascular
Auscultation of heart with notation of abnormal sounds and murmurs

Gastrointestinal
Examination of liver and spleen

Musculoskeletal
Assessment of muscle strength and tone (eg, flaccid, cog wheel, spastic) with notation of any atrophy or abnormal movements

Skin
Inspection of skin and subcutaneous tissue (eg, rashes, lesions, ulcers)

Neurologic
Test cranial nerves with notation of any deficits

Psychiatric
Brief assessment of mental status, including orientation to time, place, and person; recent and remote memory; mood and affect (eg, depression, anxiety, agitation)

Single organ system examination: performance and documentation of at least 12 elements identified by a bullet (●), whether in a box with a shaded or unshaded border (See guidelines for exceptions for eye and psychiatric examinations.)

Constitutional
Temperature, pulse rate and regularity, blood pressure
General appearance

Eyes
Ophthalmic examination of optic discs and posterior segments

Cardiovascular
Auscultation of heart with notation of abnormal sounds and murmurs

Musculoskeletal
Muscle strength in upper and lower extremities
Muscle tone in upper and lower extremities (eg, flaccid, cog wheel, spastic) with notation of any atrophy or abnormal movements (eg, fasciculation, tardive dyskinesia)

Neurologic
Orientation
Attention span
Concentration
Language
Third, fourth, and sixth cranial nerves (eg, pupils, eye movements)
Test coordination (eg, finger/nose, heel/knee/shin, rapid alternating movements in the upper and lower extremities, evaluation of fine motor coordination in young children)

[a] Example only; documentation elements may vary. The guidelines were developed for the adult population. Physicians and coders should recognize that different or additional information may be included in the pediatric population (eg, examination of head circumference in children).

Chapter 7: Evaluation and Management Services in the Office, Outpatient, Home, or Nursing Facility Setting

➤ **Mother calls because her 12-year-old has poison ivy after being in the woods 2 days ago.** Physician spends 10 minutes confirming poison ivy and prescribing a treatment plan.

ICD-10-CM	CPT®
L23.7 (allergic contact dermatitis due to plants, except food)	**99441** (physician telephone E/M, 5–10 minutes)

➤ **Father calls to discuss son's anxiety since his mother left for a tour of duty.** Physician spends 20 minutes discussing how the father can help with the child's anxiety.

ICD-10-CM	CPT
F43.22 (adjustment disorder with anxiety) **Z63.31** (absence of family member due to military deployment)	**99442** (physician telephone E/M, 11–20 minutes)

See Chapter 8, Managing Chronic and Complex Conditions, for more information on when telephone services may be separately reported.

Online Medical Services (99444, 98969)

99444   Online E/M service by a physician or other qualified health care professional who may report evaluation and management services provided to an established patient or guardian not originating from a related E/M service provided within the previous 7 days, using the Internet or similar electronic communications network

98969   Online assessment and management service provided by a qualified nonphysician health care professional to an established patient or guardian not originating from a related assessment and management service provided within the previous 7 days, using the Internet or similar electronic communications network

An online electronic medical evaluation (**99444**) is a non–face-to-face E/M service by a physician or other QHP who may report E/M services to a patient using Internet resources in response to a patient's online inquiry. This is in contrast with telemedicine services, which represent interactive audio and video telecommunications systems that permit real-time communication between the physician, at the distant site, and the patient, at the originating site. Code **98969** is used by a qualified allied health provider whose scope of practice does not include E/M services to report an online assessment and management service. The reporting guidelines for code **98969** are the same as those required for online services provided by the physician or QHP (**99444**).

> **~ More From the AAP ~**
>
> Online transmission of personal health information requires appropriate technical safeguards, such as encryption, authentication, and integrity controls. Learn more at https://www.aap.org/en-us/professional-resources/practice-support/practice-management/HIPAA/Pages/HIPAA-and-HITECH.aspx.

The Centers for Medicare & Medicaid Services has not assigned relative value units (RVUs) to online medical evaluation codes and considers them non-covered services. As a result, most third-party payers do not pay for them.

Before providing online medical services, understand local and state laws, ensure that communications will be HIPAA compliant, establish written guidelines and procedures, educate payers and negotiate for payment, and educate patients.

See Chapter 8, Managing Chronic and Complex Conditions, for more information on when online services may be separately reported.

Office or Other Outpatient Consultations (99241–99245)

Codes **99241–99245** are used to report consultations provided in the physician's office or in an outpatient or other ambulatory facility, including hospital observation services, home services, domiciliary, rest home, custodial care, or emergency department (ED). (See Chapter 10, Noncritical Hospital Evaluation and Management Services, to learn the reporting guidelines for inpatient consultations.)

The Medicare program no longer covers consultation codes **99241–99245** but has guidelines for reporting the services with office or outpatient E/M codes **99201–99215**. Check with your state Medicaid program and commercial payers to learn their coding policies.

Consultations are defined by *CPT®* as services provided by a physician at the request of another physician or "other appropriate source" to provide advice or opinion about the management or evaluation of a specific problem or to determine whether to accept responsibility for ongoing management of the patient's entire care or for the care of a specific condition/problem. The "other appropriate source" is not explicitly defined in *CPT.* It may mean any interested source (eg, schools, juvenile court, attorney, psychologist, dentist, physician extender, occupational therapist).

Guidelines for reporting consultations include

* A physician or other appropriate source must request the consultation for opinion and/or advice. Consultations may be requested of a child's primary care physician by other physicians or sources such as a school counselor or coach.
* Documentation must include
  * The request (written or verbal from the consultant; if verbal, still must be documented).
  * Name of the requesting physician or other appropriate source who requested the consultation.
  * Reason or need for the consultation (advice or opinion requested).
  * Opinion, recommendations, and services performed or ordered.
  * Written report back to the requesting physician or other appropriate source. A copy of the report must be maintained in the medical record. The report may be in letter form, a copy of the progress note, or a completed form (eg, preoperative form, consultation report). In a large group practice with shared medical records, it is acceptable to include the consultant's report as part of the documentation and a separate letter or report is not required.
  * The requesting physician or other appropriate source must also document the request (even if it is a verbal request) for consultation in his or her patient medical record.
* The consultant may initiate diagnostic or therapeutic services at the same or subsequent visit. Any identifiable procedures performed on or after the date of initial consultation (eg, endoscopy, cardiac catheterization, biopsy) should be reported separately.
* The management of the patient remains with the requesting or attending physician and is released in whole or in part only by the written notation of the requesting or attending physician in the medical record.
* Physicians in a group practice can provide consultations at the request of another member of the same practice if they are a different specialty or have an expertise in a specific medical area. For example, you may refer a patient to your partner who has expertise in the treatment of asthma and is an allergist.
* Consultations for preoperative clearance may be reported when the surgeon requests an opinion and/or advice and a written report is sent to the requesting physician. Be aware of Medicaid program and commercial payer guidelines—some do not allow preoperative clearance consultations.
* Follow-up visits that are initiated by the physician consultant are reported using codes for established patients appropriate to the place of service (office, home, domiciliary, rest home, custodial care).
* If an additional request for an opinion or advice on the same or a new problem is received from the attending physician and documented, the office consultation codes may be used again.
* Consultations mandated by a third party (eg, payer, regulatory authority) are reported with modifier **32**.

> ||||||| *Coding Pearl* |||||||
>
> Do not report a consultation code for an encounter requested by a patient or parent/guardian.

Chapter 7: Evaluation and Management Services in the Office, Outpatient, Home, or Nursing Facility Setting

Examples

Use **Table 7-4** to determine the appropriate consultation codes in the following examples:

➤ **A 3-month-old with a right indirect inguinal hernia is seen by the pediatric general surgeon for evaluation of the need for repair at the request of the primary care physician.** A comprehensive history and detailed physical examination are performed.

    Assessment/plan: Surgery is scheduled. Patient will have preoperative laboratory testing performed at primary care physician's office. A letter with these recommendations is sent to the primary care physician.

MDM: Moderate (new problem, laboratory tests ordered, high risk for surgery due to age) *History:* Comprehensive *Physical examination:* Detailed	**ICD-10-CM** **K40.90** (inguinal hernia, without mention of obstruction or gangrene, unilateral or unspecified)
	CPT® **99243** or, if payer does not recognize consultations, **New Patient** **Established Patient** **99203** **99214**

    Teaching Point: When a decision for surgery is made during an E/M service on the day before or day of a procedure, it may be necessary to append modifier **57**, decision for surgery, to indicate the service should not be included in the global period for the procedure. (See Chapter 3, Modifiers and Coding Edits, for more information on modifier **57** and the global period for procedures.)

➤ **A 5-year-old boy is referred from his family physician for opinion and recommendations for the treatment of sickle cell anemia.** A comprehensive history and physical examination are performed. Recent laboratory test results are reviewed and a recent chest radiograph is independently visualized. The child reports minimal pain and no ED visits in the last year. A written report is sent back to the referring family physician with recommendations of dosage and monitoring of hydroxyurea therapy.

MDM: Moderate (new problem with no additional workup, review of laboratory results and independent visualization of chest radiograph, high risk of prescription drug therapy requiring intensive monitoring for toxicity) *History:* Comprehensive *Physical examination:* Comprehensive	**ICD-10-CM** **D57.1** (sickle cell disease without crisis)
	CPT **99244** or, if payer does not recognize consultations, **New Patient** **Established Patient** **99204** **99215**

    Teaching Point: If a payer requires MDM as 1 of the 2 key components to support the level of service for an established patient office or other outpatient E/M encounter, moderate MDM would support code **99214** rather than **99215**. High MDM would require 2 of the following 3 conditions: new problem with additional workup planned; extended amount and/or complexity of medical records, diagnostic tests, and/or other information that must be obtained, reviewed, and analyzed; or high risk (eg, acute or chronic illness or injuries that may pose a threat to life or bodily function [eg, myocardial infarction, embolus]). Although high risk is supported by monitoring for drug toxicity (blood counts related to hydroxyurea therapy), the other 2 elements of MDM are not supportive of high MDM.

➤ **A 6-year-old is seen at the request of his surgeon for preoperative clearance prior to an adenoidectomy and tonsillectomy.** The child has had 6 episodes of streptococcal tonsillitis in the past 15 months, with one episode that resulted in a peritonsillar abscess that required surgical drainage. He has a history of seasonal allergies and intermittent asthma, takes montelukast and inhaled corticosteroids daily, and is allergic to penicillin. A comprehensive history and physical examination are performed and the results of the complete blood cell count and coagulation profile that was ordered by the surgeon are reviewed. The child is currently healthy and determined to be at standard anesthetic risk for the surgery. Medical record documentation includes the request for the consultation, findings, and a copy of the written report that is sent to the requesting physician. Diagnoses are preoperative examination, chronic tonsillitis with history of peritonsillar abscess, and mild intermittent asthma.

MDM: Low *History:* Comprehensive *Physical examination:* Comprehensive	**ICD-10-CM** **Z01.818** (preoperative examination, unspecified) **J35.01** (chronic tonsillitis) **Z87.09** (personal history of diseases of respiratory system) **J45.20** (mild intermittent asthma, uncomplicated)
	CPT® **99243** or, if payer does not recognize consultations, **New Patient** **Established Patient** **99203** **99214**

Teaching Point: In this scenario, if the patient did not have a history of a chronic (respiratory) problem or other preexisting risk factors, some payers may not allow the consultation. The comprehensive history and physical examination described in this example could be used to support reporting of code **99215** based on the *CPT* requirement of 2 of 3 key components. However, physicians should always consider medical necessity (eg, was the level of examination performed reasonable in relation to reason for encounter) and overall complexity of the service when selecting a level of service. Medical decision-making was low for the currently healthy patient with laboratory results reviewed and elective major surgery planned. Payers may require MDM as 1 of the 2 required components for established patient visits.

> ‖‖‖‖ **Coding Pearl** ‖‖‖‖
>
> For patients receiving preoperative evaluations only, sequence first a code from subcategory **Z01.81**, encounter for preprocedural examinations. Assign additional codes for the condition to describe the reason for the surgery and any findings related to the preoperative evaluation.

Table 7-4. New or Established Office/Outpatient Consultation Codes (99241–99245)

Key Components (For a description of key components, see Table 7-1.)
3 of 3 key components must be performed to at least the degree specified under the code.

CPT® Code/Timeª	Medical Decision-making	History	Examination
99241 15 min	Straightforward PP: Usually self-limited or minor	Problem focused	Problem focused
99242 30 min	Straightforward PP: Usually low to moderate severity	Expanded	Expanded
99243 40 min	Low complexity PP: Usually moderate severity	Detailed	Detailed
99244 60 min	Moderate complexity PP: Usually moderate to high severity	Comprehensive	Comprehensive
99245 80 min	High complexity PP: Usually moderate to high severity	Comprehensive	Comprehensive

Abbreviations: CPT, Current Procedural Terminology; *PP, presenting problem.*

ª *Typical time is an average and represents a range of times that may be higher or lower depending on clinical circumstances. The presenting problem is considered to be a contributory factor and does not need to be present to the degree specified.*

Chapter 7: Evaluation and Management Services in the Office, Outpatient, Home, or Nursing Facility Setting

Guidelines Used by Payers That Follow Medicare Consultation Guidelines

It is important that you check with your major payers to determine if they have adopted the Medicare policy or if they have established their own policy and guidelines for reporting consultations. You can access the American Academy of Pediatrics (AAP) position on Medicare consultation policy at www.aap.org/cfp (access code AAPCFP23) and the letter to major payers and their responses at www.aap.org/en-us/professional-resources/practice-support/financing-and-payment/Pages/Private-Payer-Advocacy-Letters-to-Carriers.aspx (AAP members only).

- See Chapter 10, Noncritical Hospital Evaluation and Management Services, for Medicare requirements for reporting consultations performed in the hospital setting.
- Consultations performed on patients in the office or outpatient setting are reported with the office or outpatient E/M codes **99201–99215**.
- If the patient is new to the consulting physician (ie, has not received any face-to-face professional services from the physician or another physician of the same specialty who belongs to the same group practice within the past 3 years), code **99201–99205** is reported based on the performance and documentation of the required key components or time, if appropriate.
- If the patient does not meet the requirements of a new patient, an established patient office or outpatient E/M code (**99211–99215**) is reported.
- If the service is provided in the ED, ED codes **99281–99285** are reported.
- The referring physician must document the request for consultation in his or her medical record, and the consulting physician must document the request and communicate the results back to the referring physician.

Coding Conundrum: Consultation or Transfer of Care?

Consultation codes (**99241–99245**, **99251–99255**) should not be reported by the physician who has agreed to accept transfer of care (ie, takes over the responsibility of management of the patient's entire care, or the care of a specific condition or problem, at the request of another physician) before an initial evaluation. Consultation codes are appropriate to report if the decision to accept transfer of care cannot be made until after the initial consultation evaluation, regardless of site of service. Any services that constitute transfer of care are reported with the appropriate new or established patient codes for office or other outpatient visits, domiciliary services, rest home services, or home services. The medical record should reflect the transfer of care to the service of the receiving physician.

Examples

Consultation	**Transfer of Care**
Primary Care Pediatrician to Specialist	**Pediatrician to Endocrinologist**
"Consultation requested for opinion regarding treatment of 8-year-old with joint pain, limited range of motion, malaise, and fatigue."	*"Please accept ongoing care of uncontrolled diabetes in this 4-year-old."*
	Subsequent to a consultation, the physician accepts the responsibility of ongoing management of the patient or care for the specific condition or problem.
Specialist to Pediatrician	
Written summary of findings and recommended treatment plan for treatment of juvenile arthritis sent.	
Consulting physician is unable to accept the responsibility of ongoing management for the specific condition or problem until he or she has performed an E/M service.	**Endocrinologist to Pediatrician**
	"Thank you for referring this patient to us for the management of her diabetes."
Pediatrician to Specialist	Transferring physician no longer provides care for the management of a patient or for those problems for which another physician has agreed to accept.
"Consultation requested for consideration of assuming management of juvenile arthritis on this 8-year-old patient."	
Specialist to Pediatrician	
Written summary of findings and agreement to assume ongoing care of the problem.	

Interprofessional Telephone/Internet Consultation (99446–99449)

99446   Interprofessional telephone/Internet assessment and management service provided by a consultative physician including a verbal and written report to the patient's treating/requesting physician/qualified health care professional; 5–10 minutes of medical consultative discussion and review

99447   11–20 minutes of medical consultative discussion and review

99448   21–30 minutes of medical consultative discussion and review

99449   31 minutes or more of medical consultative discussion and review

A consultation request by a patient's attending or primary physician or other QHP soliciting opinion and/or treatment advice by telephone or Internet from a physician with specialty expertise (consultant) is reported by the consultant with interprofessional consultation codes **99446–99449**. This consultation does not require face-to-face contact with the patient by the consultant and often takes place when a timely face-to-face service with the consultant is not feasible (eg, consultant is geographically distant). The patient may be in the inpatient or outpatient setting.

Guidelines for the consultant reporting interprofessional telephone/Internet consultations include

- Telephone/Internet consultations of less than 5 minutes are not reported. Most of the time reported as interprofessional consultation must have been spent in medical consultative discussion (verbal or Internet).

- A single interprofessional consultation code is reported for the cumulative time spent in discussion and information review regardless of the number of telephone or Internet contacts. The service is not reported more than once in a 7-day interval.

- Time spent in telephone or online consultation with the patient and/or family may be reported using codes **99441–99444** or **98966–98968**.

- When the purpose of communication is to arrange a transfer of care or face-to-face patient encounter, interprofessional consultation codes are not reported.

- Interprofessional consultation services are not reported if the consultant has provided a face-to-face service to the patient within the past 14 days or when the consultation results in scheduling of a face-to-face service within the next 14 days or at the consultant's next available appointment date.

- Time spent by the consultant reviewing pertinent medical records, studies, or other data is included in the telephone/Internet consultation and not separately reported.

- As with all consultations, the request for advice or opinion should be documented in the patient record. A verbal opinion report and a written opinion report from the consultant must also be documented. This may require creation of a new patient record by the consultant.

See Chapter 10, Noncritical Hospital Evaluation and Management Services, for examples for reporting interprofessional telephone/Internet consultations in the inpatient setting.

The requesting physician or QHP may report time spent in discussion with the consultant with an appropriate E/M service code according to site of service (when the patient is present for service) and/or prolonged service codes if the total time of discussion exceeds 30 minutes beyond the typical time of the associated E/M service. See Prolonged Services later in this chapter for more information.

Example

➤ **A 10-year-old boy with ADHD has become increasingly aggressive at home and school.** The child's pediatrician arranges a telephone consultation with a child and adolescent psychiatrist and forwards the child's history records prior to the telephone consultation. The pediatrician and psychiatrist spend a total of 16 minutes in discussion. The child and mother are present in the pediatrician's office and included in the discussion. A new care plan is developed for achieving better control of the child's predominantly hyperactive ADHD and agreed to by the mother. The total face-to-face time for the pediatrician is approximately 25 minutes.

Chapter 7: Evaluation and Management Services in the Office, Outpatient, Home, or Nursing Facility Setting

ICD-10-CM	CPT®	
Both physicians report **F90.1** (ADHD, predominantly hyperactive type)	The consultant reports **99447** (11–20 minutes of medical discussion and review)	The pediatrician reports **99214** (16 of 25 minutes [face-to-face] spent in counseling/coordination of care)

Teaching Point: In this vignette, the patient and mother are present and counseled on the revised care plan, allowing the pediatrician to report the encounter based on time spent counseling and/or coordinating care. If time had not been the controlling factor of the visit, the pediatrician would report the encounter based on key components of the E/M service rendered and, if applicable, prolonged service codes **99354** and **99355**.

If the child's pediatrician has established the capabilities to provide psychiatric collaborative care management (PCCM) or general behavioral health integration services, as described in Chapter 8, Managing Chronic and Complex Conditions, this encounter with the interprofessional assessment might be an initiating visit at which the pediatrician introduces the service to the patient and caregivers and orders PCCM.

Critical Care (99291, 99292)

Critical care services provided in the office or outpatient setting are reported with hourly critical care codes (**99291** and **99292**) regardless of the patient's age (**Table 7-5**). If the same patient requires outpatient and inpatient critical care services on the same day, the physician or a physician of the same group and specialty would report his or her services based on where the services were provided as well as the patient's age. See Chapter 12, Critical and Intensive Care, for reporting guidelines.

Table 7-5. Critical Care by Setting and Age		
Critical Care Provided in	**Age**	**Report**
Outpatient setting only	Any	**99291–99292** (minimum of 30 min) or **99205** or **99215** (<30 min)
Outpatient and inpatient setting	≤5 years	Initial inpatient neonatal or pediatric critical care (**99468, 99471, 99475**) only
Outpatient and inpatient setting	>6 years	**99291–99292** (minimum of 30 min) Combine inpatient and outpatient time. Report **99291** only once per day.

Note: This chart references the same physician or same physician group practice providing care only.

Example

➤ **A 3-year-old girl is seen with complaints of shortness of breath and wheezing.** She has a history of moderate persistent childhood asthma. The patient goes into respiratory failure with hypoxia and vital signs are deteriorating. The physician initiates critical care. An ambulance is called and the physician continues critical care services until the transport team accepts care of the patient. The total time for critical care services provided in the office was 35 minutes. The patient is admitted to the pediatric intensive care unit at the local university hospital under a pediatric intensivist. The pediatrician provides no more hands-on care for the patient that day and reports outpatient critical care services with a diagnosis of status asthmaticus.

ICD-10-CM	CPT
J96.01 (acute respiratory failure with hypoxia) **J45.42** (moderate persistent asthma with status asthmaticus)	**99291** (critical care, first 30–74 minutes)

Teaching Point: If the same physician or physician group of the same specialty provided outpatient and inpatient critical care services, due to the patient's age, only the per-day critical care code (**99475**) would be reported. Had the patient been 6 years or older, the time spent in outpatient critical care would be combined with time spent in the inpatient setting.

After-hours Services (99050–99060)

99050	Service(s) provided in office at times other than regularly scheduled office hours, or days when the office is normally closed (eg, holidays, Saturday, Sunday), in addition to basic service
99051	Service(s) provided in the office during regularly scheduled evening, weekend, or holiday office hours, in addition to basic service
99053	Services(s) provided between 10:00 pm and 8:00 am at 24-hour facility, in addition to basic service
99056	Service(s) typically provided in the office, provided out of the office at request of patient, in addition to basic service
99058	Service(s) provided on an emergency basis in the office, which disrupts other scheduled office services, in addition to basic service
99060	Service(s) provided on an emergency basis, out of the office, which disrupts other scheduled office services, in addition to basic service

Codes **99050–99060** are used to report services that are provided after hours or on an emergency basis and are an adjunct to the basic E/M service provided.

Third-party payers will have specific policies for coverage and payment. Some carriers pay practices for extended hours because they recognize the cost benefit they realize from decreased urgent care and ED visits. Communicate with individual payers to understand their definition or interpretation of the service and their coverage and payment policies. As part of this negotiation and education process, it is important to demonstrate the cost savings recognized by the payer for these adjunct services. If appropriate, more than one adjunct code may be reported on the same day of service (eg, **99058** and **99051**). However, most payers will pay only for the use of a single special services code per encounter and may manually review, question, or deny payment for a claim with stacked codes.

After-hours service codes are used by physicians or other QHPs (under their state scope of practice and when billing with their own National Provider Identifier [NPI]) to identify the services that are adjunct to the basic services rendered. These codes

* Describe the special circumstances under which a basic procedure is performed.
* Are only reported in addition to an associated basic service (eg, E/M, fracture care).
* Are reported without a modifier appended to the basic service because they only further describe the services provided.

99050	Service(s) provided in office at times other than regularly scheduled office hours, or days when the office is normally closed (eg, holidays, Saturday, Sunday), in addition to basic service

* Office hours must be posted. *Current Procedural Terminology*® does not define a holiday or posted office hours. While most commonly applied to evening, weekend, or holiday hours, code **99050** could be applied to services provided at the patient request on a weekday provided the office is typically closed on that day.
* Code **99050** is *not* reported when a physician or other QHP is behind schedule and sees patients after posted office hours.
* The service must be requested by the patient, and the physician or other QHP must agree to see the patient.
* Documentation must indicate the time and date of the encounter and the request to be seen outside of normal posted hours.

99051	Service(s) provided in the office during regularly scheduled evening, weekend, or holiday office hours, in addition to basic service

* Regularly scheduled office hours must be posted.
* Documentation must include the time and date of the encounter.
* Evenings and holidays are not defined by *CPT*, but holidays can generally refer to national and/or state holidays, and evenings are generally 6:00 pm and later. Check with payers.

Chapter 7: Evaluation and Management Services in the Office, Outpatient, Home, or Nursing Facility Setting

99053   Services(s) provided between 10:00 pm and 8:00 am at 24-hour facility, in addition to basic service

◉ Emergency department physicians who are scheduled during these hours will not typically report code **99053**, although they are not precluded by *CPT®*.

◉ Documentation must include the time and date of the encounter.

◉ Use the appropriate place of service code.

99056   Service(s) typically provided in the office, provided out of the office at request of patient, in addition to basic service

◉ It is not appropriate for an ED physician to report code **99056**.

◉ Documentation should include the patient's request to be seen outside of the office.

99058   Service(s) provided on an emergency basis in the office, which disrupts other scheduled office services, in addition to basic service

◉ Report when an office patient's condition, in the clinical judgment of the physician, warrants the physician interrupting care of another patient to deal with the emergency.

◉ Code **99058** may not be reported when patients are simply fit into the schedule or for walk-ins.

◉ Document that the patient was seen immediately and the reason for the emergent care.

99060   Service(s) provided on an emergency basis, out of the office, which disrupts other scheduled office services, in addition to basic service

◉ Documentation should indicate that the physician was called away during scheduled office hours to attend to a patient in another location (eg, ED).

Example

➤ **A child is seen for severe exacerbation of moderate persistent asthma on a Saturday at 9:00 am.** The child arrives and is immediately taken to an examination room by the triage nurse, and the physician disrupts his schedule to see the child urgently. The office is open on Saturday mornings from 8:00 am to 12:00 noon.

ICD-10-CM	CPT
J45.41 (moderate persistent asthma with acute exacerbation)	99201–99215 (new or established office E/M) 99058 (service provided on an emergency basis in office, disrupting other scheduled services) 99051 (service provided in office during regularly scheduled weekend hours)

    Teaching Point: If the Saturday hours were for walk-in visits only (ie, no scheduled appointments), code **99058** would not be reported.

Prolonged Services

Prolonged Service With Direct Patient Contact (99354, 99355)

+99354   Prolonged evaluation and management or psychotherapy service(s) (the service beyond the typical service time) in the office or other outpatient setting requiring direct patient contact; first hour

+99355   each additional 30 minutes

    Prolonged service codes **99354** and **99355** are used to report 30 minutes or more of a physician's or QHP's prolonged face-to-face E/M service provided on the same date as designated office or other E/M services that have a typical or designated time published in *CPT* or for prolonged service in conjunction with psychotherapy of 60 minutes or more (**90837**) (Table 7-6).

    Chapter 10, Noncritical Hospital Evaluation and Management Services, addresses reporting prolonged services performed in the observation and inpatient hospital setting.

These codes may *not* be reported with initial- or subsequent-day observation care services (**99218–99220** and **99224–99226**). The American Medical Association has clarified that although observation care services are performed in an "outpatient" setting, intraservice times for the observation care codes are defined as unit or floor time rather than face-to-face time as required in the office or outpatient setting.

Table 7-6. Prolonged Services Descriptors

Code	Description of Face-to-face Prolonged Services
+99354	Prolonged evaluation and management or psychotherapy service(s) (the service beyond the typical service time) in the office or other outpatient setting requiring direct patient contact; first hour (List separately in addition to code for office or other outpatient Evaluation and Management or psychotherapy service) (Use code **99354** in conjunction with codes **90837, 99201–99215, 99241–99245, 99324–99337, 99341–99350**.) (Do not report **99354** in conjunction with **99415** or **99416**)
+99355	each additional 30 minutes (List separately in addition to code for prolonged service.) (Use code **99355** in conjunction with **99354**.) (Do not report **99355** in conjunction with **99415** or **99416**)
Code	**Description of Prolonged Clinical Staff Services**
+99415	Prolonged clinical staff service (the service beyond the typical service time) during an evaluation and management service in the office or outpatient setting, direct patient contact with physician supervision; first hour (List separately in addition to code for outpatient Evaluation and Management service) (Use **99415** in conjunction with **99201–99205, 99211–99215**) (Do not report **99415** in conjunction with **99354** or **99355**)
+99416	each additional 30 minutes (List separately in addition to code for prolonged service) (Use **99416** in conjunction with **99415**) (Do not report **99416** in conjunction with **99354** or **99355**)
Code	**Description of Non–face-to-face Prolonged Services**
99358	Prolonged evaluation and management service before and/or after direct patient care; first hour
+99359	each additional 30 minutes (List separately in addition to code for prolonged service.) (Use code **99359** in conjunction with code **99358**.) (Do not report **99358, 99359** during the same month with **99487–99489**.) (Do not report **99358, 99359** when performed during the service time of codes **99495–99496**.)

Here are guidelines for reporting direct (face-to-face) physician or other QHP prolonged services when performed in the office or outpatient setting.

- Use codes **99354** and **99355** in conjunction with E/M codes **99201–99215, 99241–99245, 99324–99337**, and **99341–99350** or psychotherapy code **90837** (psychotherapy, 60 minutes with patient and/or family member).
- Only the time spent face-to-face between the physician or other QHP and the patient/family may be reported.
- Time does not have to be continuous but is reported for services provided in a calendar day.
- Reported with any level E/M service that is assigned a typical time.

> ||||||| *Coding Pearl* |||||||
>
> Codes **99354** and **99355** may not be reported with initial- or subsequent-day observation care services (**99218–99220** and **99224–99226**).

Chapter 7: Evaluation and Management Services in the Office, Outpatient, Home, or Nursing Facility Setting

- When an E/M service is reported using time as the key or controlling factor (>50% of the total face-to-face time was spent in counseling and/or coordination of care), prolonged service can be reported only when the prolonged service exceeds 30 minutes beyond the highest level of E/M service (eg, **99205**, **99245**).
- The total time of and medical necessity for the service must be documented.
- The first-hour prolonged service code (**99354**) is reported for the total duration of prolonged service of 30 (minimum) to 74 minutes' duration on a given day of service. Prolonged service of less than 30 minutes is included in the E/M service performed (eg, **99203**) and may not be reported separately (**Table 7-7**).
- Each additional 30 minutes beyond the first hour (**99355**) is reported. Code **99355** may be used to report the final 15 to 30 minutes of prolonged service on a given date.
- Less than 15 minutes beyond the first hour or less than 15 minutes beyond the final 30 minutes is not reported separately.
- Time spent providing separately reported services other than E/M (eg, inhalation therapy) is not counted toward the prolonged service time.
- Codes for prolonged service by a physician or QHP are never reported in conjunction with prolonged service provided by clinical staff (**99415**, **99416**).

Table 7-7. How to Code Prolonged Services (Office or Outpatient)

Total Duration of Prolonged Services, min (Time begins after typical time of related E/M service.)	Code(s)
<30	Not reported separately
30–74	**99354** or **99358** × 1 (First hour includes 30–74 min beyond the typical time of the related E/M service.)
75–104	**99354** or **99358** × 1 (first 74 min) AND **99355** or **99359** × 1 (75–104 min)
≥105 (≥1 h 45 min)	**99354** or **99358** × 1 (first 74 min) AND **99355** or **99359** × 2 (1 unit for 75–104 min and 1 for 105–134 min) or more for each additional 30 or final 15–30 min

Abbreviation: E/M, evaluation and management.

Examples

➤ **A 9-month-old previously healthy infant is seen in follow-up for failure to gain weight and increasing irritability with recurrent bouts of constipation.** A comprehensive history and detailed physical examination are performed. Medical decision-making is moderate. Because of a family history of gluten intolerance, the physician wants to refer the child to a pediatric gastroenterologist. The parents are resistant to the referral. A total of 35 minutes was spent providing the key components of the face-to-face E/M service and another 30 minutes was spent counseling the parents.

| Office/outpatient visit
Prolonged service of 30–74 minutes | *ICD-10-CM*
R62.51 (failure to thrive, child)
K59.00 (constipation, unspecified)
R45.4 (irritability and anger) |
| | *CPT*®
99214 (25 minutes typical time)
99354 (additional 40 minutes) |

Teaching Point: The total face-to-face time of this visit was 65 minutes. The 30 minutes spent counseling does not exceed 50% of the total face-to-face time, so this encounter is not reported based on time spent counseling and/or coordinating care (ie, code **99215** [typical time 40 minutes] is not reported). Code **99214**

is supported by the comprehensive history, detailed physical examination, and moderate MDM. Code **99354** is supported by the total time of the face-to-face service that extended 40 minutes beyond the typical time of 25 minutes assigned to code **99214**.

> **A 9-month-old previously healthy infant is seen in follow-up for failure to gain weight and increasing irritability with recurrent bouts of constipation.** A comprehensive history and detailed physical examination are performed. Medical decision-making is moderate. Because of a family history of gluten intolerance, the physician wants to refer the infant to a pediatric gastroenterologist. The parents are resistant to the referral. A total of 35 minutes was spent providing the face-to-face E/M service and another 40 minutes was spent counseling the parents.

Office/outpatient visit Prolonged service of 30–74 minutes	*ICD-10-CM* **R62.51** (failure to thrive, child) **K59.00** (constipation, unspecified) **R45.4** (irritability and anger)
	CPT® **99215** (40 minutes typical time) **99354** (additional 35 minutes)

 Teaching Point: The total face-to-face time spent by the physician was 75 minutes, with more than half spent in counseling and/or coordination of care. Code **99215** with a typical time of 40 minutes may be reported using time spent counseling as the key or controlling factor. The face-to-face time exceeds the typical time of 40 minutes and supports 1 unit of prolonged service with direct patient contact. When an E/M service is reported using time as the key or controlling factor (>50% of the total face-to-face time was spent in counseling and/or coordination of care), prolonged service can be reported only when the prolonged service exceeds 30 minutes beyond the highest level of E/M service (eg, **99205**, **99245**).

> **A 6-year-old established patient is seen for acute exacerbation of mild persistent asthma.** An expanded history and physical examination are performed and MDM is moderately complex. The patient receives 2 nebulizer treatments and is reexamined by the physician after each treatment. The physician spends a total of 20 minutes providing face-to-face care. The child returns later that afternoon and is examined and 2 additional nebulizer treatments are administered. The physician documents the initial care, each subsequent reevaluation following treatments, the subsequent care, the assessment, and the plan. A total of 60 minutes is spent in face-to-face E/M services (not including the time spent providing nebulizer treatments).

Office/outpatient visit Prolonged service of 30 minutes	*ICD-10-CM* **J45.31** (acute exacerbation of mild persistent asthma)
	CPT **99214** (25 minutes average time) **99354** (additional 35 minutes) **94640 76** × 4 (nebulizer treatments)

 Teaching Point: Time spent performing separately reported services, such as nebulizer treatments, is not counted toward the time of prolonged E/M service.

Current Procedural Terminology stipulates that modifier **76** (repeat procedure) be used to report multiple nebulizer treatments. At time of publication, Medicaid National Correct Coding Initiative policy does not allow for the reporting of multiple **94640** codes for the same encounter.

Prolonged Service Without Direct Patient Contact (99358, 99359)

99358   Prolonged evaluation and management service before and/or after direct patient care; first hour

+99359   each additional 30 minutes (Use in conjunction with code **99358**.)

Prolonged service without direct patient contact (ie, non–face-to-face) is reported when a physician provides prolonged service that does not involve face-to-face care. The prolonged service must relate to a service and patient where direct (face-to-face) patient care has occurred or will occur and to ongoing patient management. Only time spent by a physician or other QHP may be counted toward the time of prolonged service. Prolonged service of less than 30 minutes on a given date is not separately reported. Report code **99359** for 15 or more minutes beyond the first hour or the last full 30-minute period of prolonged service. See Chapter 8, Managing Chronic and Complex Conditions, for more information and another coding example.

Example

➤ **A child is seen in the physician's office with a long history of recurring ill-defined symptoms.** Tests are ordered. On a later date, when the physician receives the test results, she spends 30 minutes reviewing the results in light of the patient's signs and symptoms and researching options for further investigating the cause of the patient's symptoms. Code **99358** may be reported based on *CPT®* instruction.

Prolonged Clinical Staff Service (99415, 99416)

+99415   Prolonged clinical staff service (the service beyond the typical service time) during an evaluation and management service in the office or outpatient setting, direct patient contact with physician supervision; first hour

+99416   each additional 30 minutes

Codes **99415** and **99416** are used to report 45 minutes or more of clinical staff time spent face-to-face providing care to a patient under the supervision of a physician or other QHP who has provided an office or other outpatient E/M service at the same session. *Never report both* prolonged service by a physician or other QHP (**99354–99355**) and prolonged clinical staff services together. Codes **99415** and **99416** were assigned RVUs based only on clinical staff's intraservice time, as the preservice and post-service times were considered to be included in the value of the related E/M service. Relative value units assigned are 0.25 for **99415** and 0.13 for **99416**.

The following guidelines apply to reporting of prolonged clinical staff services:

❀ Prolonged clinical staff services are reported only in conjunction with E/M services in the office or other outpatient setting. Report **99415** and **99416** in addition to office or other outpatient E/M codes **99201–99215**.

❀ Supervision must be provided by a physician or other QHP during the provision of prolonged clinical staff services.

❀ Prolonged clinical staff services are reported only when the face-to-face time spent by clinical staff is 45 minutes or more beyond the typical time of the related E/M service on the same date. (See **tables 7-2** and **7-3** for typical times assigned to office and other outpatient services.)

❀ Do not report prolonged service of less than 45 minutes beyond the typical time of the related E/M service.

❀ The total time of and medical necessity for the service must be documented.

❀ Time spent providing separately reported services, such as intravenous medication administration or inhalation treatment, is not counted toward the time of prolonged service.

❀ It is not required that the clinical staff time be continuous, but each episode of face-to-face time should be documented.

❀ Report code **99416** for each additional 30 minutes of clinical staff time beyond the first hour and for the last 15 to 30 minutes of prolonged clinical staff service. Do not report **99416** for less than 15 minutes beyond the first hour or last 30-minute period.

Table 7-8 shows the time requirements for reporting codes **99415** and **99416**.

Table 7-8. How to Code Prolonged Clinical Staff Services

Total Duration of Prolonged Services, min	Code(s)
<45	Not reported separately
45–74	**99415** × 1 (First hour includes 45–74 min beyond the typical time of the related E/M service.)
75–104	**99415** × 1 (first 45–74 min) AND **99416** × 1 (from 75–104 min beyond typical time of related E/M service)
≥105 (≥1 h 45 min)	**99415** × 1 (first 45–74 min) AND **99416** × 2 (1 unit for 75–104 min and 1 unit for 105–134 min) or more for each additional 30 min or last period of 15–30 min

Abbreviation: E/M, evaluation and management.

Examples

➤ **A child is seen for diarrhea and concerns of dehydration.** The physician diagnoses moderate dehydration due to viral gastroenteritis. Oral rehydration is ordered. The physician completes his or her documentation and selects code **99214** for service to this established patient. The physician remains in the office suite while a nurse delivers and monitors a time-based oral rehydration plan using an electrolyte solution. The nurse's total direct care time is 2 hours. The first 25 minutes are included in the practice expense of the physician service. The additional 95 minutes following the physician's service are reported as prolonged clinical staff service.

E/M service by physician Prolonged clinical staff time	**ICD-10-CM** **A08.4** (viral intestinal infection, unspecified) **E86.0** (dehydration)
	CPT® **99214** (typical time of 25 minutes) **99415** × 1 (first hour) and **99416** × 1 (final 30-minute period)

Teaching Point: *CPT* instructs that prolonged clinical staff time begins 45 minutes after the typical time of the E/M service provided by the physician. In this scenario, the typical time of the physician service is 25 minutes, so prolonged clinical staff time is not reported until clinical staff have spent at least 70 minutes in face-to-face patient care. The final 5 minutes beyond the last 30-minute period reported with code **99416** is not separately reported, as only time of 15 to 30 minutes beyond the previous period is reported.

➤ **A new patient who has been vomiting for 2 days is seen in the physician's office.** After evaluation by a physician, she is given antipyretics and fluids and then monitored and reexamined by clinical staff for a total face-to-face clinical staff time of 90 minutes. At the end of the hour, the physician returns to the examination room and provides final instruction to the mother before releasing the child. The physician service includes a comprehensive history and examination with moderate MDM. Physician face-to-face time was 35 minutes, with 10 minutes spent in counseling and coordination of care.

E/M service by physician Prolonged clinical staff time	**ICD-10-CM** **K52.9** (gastroenteritis, unspecified)
	CPT® **99204** (typical time of 45 minutes) **99415** × 1 (first hour)

Teaching Point: Prolonged service by clinical staff under physician supervision is reported rather than the physician's prolonged service, as the physician's face-to-face time with the patient does not support reporting of prolonged service.

➤ **A physician provides treatment to an established patient with acute exacerbation of moderate persistent asthma.** Over the course of 2 hours, the patient is given fluids (oral) for mild dehydration and oxygen as needed, oral steroids, and 3 inhaled bronchodilators. Documentation supports a detailed history, detailed examination, and moderate MDM and total face-to-face time by the physician of 65 minutes. Clinical staff also document 60 minutes of direct patient care (eg, providing nebulizer treatments) following the physician's E/M service.

E/M service by physician Prolonged physician service	**ICD-10-CM** **J45.41** (acute exacerbation of moderate persistent asthma) **E86.0** (dehydration)
	CPT **99214** (typical time of 25 minutes) **99354** (additional 40 minutes) **94640 76** × 3 (nebulizer treatments)

Teaching Point: The physician's service described includes code **99214**, office or other outpatient encounter, and 1 unit of prolonged service with direct patient contact (**99354**). *Prolonged clinical staff service is not reported on the same date as prolonged service by a physician or QHP, and time spent providing separately reported services (eg, nebulizer treatment) is not included in prolonged service time.*

Home Care Services (99341–99350)

- ⊛ Home visits are reported with place of service code **12** (home location, other than hospital or other facility, where patient receives care in a private residence).
- ⊛ Do not report home visit codes for visits to patients in residential facilities or group homes. See codes for domiciliary, rest home, or custodial care services (**99324–99328** and **99334–99337**).
- ⊛ Code selection is based on the performance and documentation of the required key components or time if more than 50% of the time is spent in counseling and/or coordination of care, as seen in **tables 7-9** and **7-10**.
- ⊛ Travel time to and from a patient's home is assumed to be in the level of care, just as travel time to and from the hospital is included in hospital care codes and is not counted in the time spent. However, if escorting a patient to a medical facility becomes necessary, code **99082** (unusual travel) is available.
- ⊛ Services provided by a nonphysician provider who does not have his or her own NPI may not be billed unless the physician provides direct supervision. Refer to Chapter 14, Allied Health and Clinical Staff Services.
- ⊛ Any procedures performed by the physician may be separately reported.
- ⊛ Payers may have varied policies on coverage and reporting requirements for home visits and may not use Medicare incident-to guidelines. Check with them prior to reporting this service.

Table 7-9. Home Visits for New Patients

Key Components (For a description of key components, see Table 7-1.)
3 of 3 key components must be performed to at least the degree specified under the code.

CPT® Code/Timeª	Medical Decision-making	History	Examination
99341 20 min	Straightforward PP: Usually low severity	Problem focused	Problem focused
99342 30 min	Low complexity PP: Usually moderate severity	Expanded	Expanded
99343 45 min	Moderate complexity PP: Usually moderate to high severity	Detailed	Detailed
99344 60 min	Moderate complexity PP: Usually moderate to high severity	Comprehensive	Comprehensive
99345 75 min	High complexity PP: Usually patient is unstable or has developed a new problem requiring immediate physician attention.	Comprehensive	Comprehensive

Abbreviations: CPT, Current Procedural Terminology; *PP, presenting problem.*

ª *Typical time is an average and represents a range of times that may be higher or lower depending on clinical circumstances. The presenting problem is considered to be a contributory factor and does not need to be present to the degree specified.*

Table 7-10. Home Visits for Established Patients

Key Components (For a description of key components, see Table 7-1.)
2 of 3 key components must be performed to at least the degree specified under the code. Some payers may require medical decision-making as 1 of the 2 components performed and documented.

CPT® Code/Timeª	Medical Decision-making	History	Examination
99347 15 min	Straightforward PP: Usually self-limited or minor	Problem focused	Problem focused
99348 25 min	Low complexity PP: Usually low to moderate severity	Expanded	Expanded
99349 40 min	Moderate complexity PP: Usually moderate to high severity	Detailed	Detailed
99350 60 min	Moderate to high complexity PP: Usually moderate to high severity	Comprehensive	Comprehensive

Abbreviations: CPT, Current Procedural Terminology; *PP, presenting problem.*

ª *Typical time is an average and represents a range of times that may be higher or lower depending on clinical circumstances. The presenting problem is considered to be a contributory factor and does not need to be present to the degree specified.*

Domiciliary, Rest Home, or Custodial Care Services (99324–99337)

These services are provided in a facility that provides room and board and other personal assistance services (eg, assisted living facility) (**tables 7-11** and **7-12**).

- These codes are not reported for patients residing in a private residence (see codes **99341–99350**).
- Codes **99324–99328** and **99334–99337** are reported for services provided in facilities assigned the following place of service codes: **13** (assisted living) and **14** (group home), **33** (custodial care facility), and **55** (residential substance abuse facility).

✷ Prolonged services provided in a domiciliary, rest home, or custodial care are reported with codes **99354** and **99355**.

Table 7-11. Domiciliary, Rest Home, or Custodial Care Services: New Patient

Key Components (For a description of key components, see Table 7-1.)
3 of 3 key components must be performed to at least the degree specified under the code.

CPT® Code/Timeª	Medical Decision-making (meets 2 of 3 elements)	History (meets all 3 elements)	Examination
99324 20 min	Straightforward PP: Usually low severity	Problem focused	Problem focused
99325 30 min	Low complexity PP: Usually moderate severity	Expanded	Expanded
99326 45 min	Moderate complexity PP: Usually moderate to high severity	Detailed	Detailed
99327 60 min	Moderate complexity PP: Usually high severity	Comprehensive	Comprehensive
99328 75 min	High complexity PP: Usually patient is unstable or has developed a new problem requiring immediate physician attention.	Comprehensive	Comprehensive

Abbreviations: CPT, Current Procedural Terminology; PP, presenting problem.

ª Typical time is an average and represents a range of times that may be higher or lower depending on clinical circumstances. The presenting problem is considered to be a contributory factor and does not need to be present to the degree specified. Medical decision-making elements refer to number of diagnoses or management options, amount and/or complexity of data, and risk. History elements refer to history of present illness; past, family, and social history; and review of systems.

Table 7-12. Domiciliary, Rest Home, or Custodial Care Services: Established Patient

Key Components (For a description of key components, see Table 7-1.)
3 of 3 key components must be performed to at least the degree specified under the code. Some payers may require medical decision-making as 1 of the 2 components performed and documented.

CPT® Code/Timeª	Medical Decision-making (meets 2 of 3 elements)	History (meets all 3 elements)	Examination
99334 15 min	Straightforward PP: Usually self-limited to minor	Problem focused	Problem focused
99335 25 min	Low complexity PP: Usually low to moderate severity	Expanded	Expanded
99336 40 min	Moderate complexity PP: Usually moderate to high severity	Detailed	Detailed
99337 60 min	Moderate to high complexity PP: Usually moderate to high severity; patient may be unstable or develop new problem requiring immediate attention.	Comprehensive	Comprehensive

Abbreviations: CPT, Current Procedural Terminology; PP, presenting problem.

ª Typical time is an average and represents a range of times that may be higher or lower depending on clinical circumstances. The presenting problem is considered to be a contributory factor and does not need to be present to the degree specified.

Nursing Facility Care

Initial Nursing Facility Care (99304–99306)

- The level of service reported is dependent on performance and documentation of the 3 key components (history, physical examination, and MDM) or time if more than 50% of the floor or unit time is spent in counseling and/or care coordination (Table 7-13).
- Services are reported for a new or an established patient.
- When the patient is admitted to the nursing facility in the course of an encounter at another site of service (eg, hospital ED, physician's office), all E/M services provided by that physician in conjunction with that admission are considered part of the initial nursing facility care when performed on the same date as the admission or readmission.
- The nursing facility care level of service reported by the admitting physician should include services related to the admission he or she provided in the other sites of service on the same date.
- Hospital discharge or observation discharge services performed on the same date of nursing facility admission or readmission may be reported separately. When a patient is discharged from inpatient or observation status on the same date of nursing facility admission or readmission, hospital discharge services (**99238**, **99239**, or **99217**) should be reported in addition to the initial nursing facility care. (For a patient admitted and discharged from observation or inpatient status on the same date, see codes **99234–99236**.)
- For nursing facility care discharge, see codes **99315** and **99316**.
- Prolonged services provided in conjunction with a face-to-face nursing facility service are reported with codes **99356** and **99357**. For more information on these codes, see Chapter 10, Noncritical Hospital Evaluation and Management Services.

Table 7-13. Initial Nursing Facility Care: New or Established Patient

Key Components (For a description of key components, see Table 7-1.)
3 of 3 key components must be performed to at least the degree specified under the code.

CPT® Code/Time[a]	Medical Decision-making	History	Examination
99304 25 min	Straightforward or low PP: Usually low severity	Detailed	Detailed
99305 35 min	Moderate complexity PP: Usually moderate severity	Comprehensive	Comprehensive
99306 45 min	High complexity PP: Usually high severity	Comprehensive	Comprehensive

Abbreviations: CPT, Current Procedural Terminology; PP, presenting problem.

[a] Typical time is an average and represents a range of time that may be higher or lower depending on clinical circumstances. The presenting problem is considered to be a contributory factor and does not need to be present to the degree specified.

Subsequent Nursing Facility Care (99307–99310)

- Codes are used to report services provided to residents of nursing facilities who do not require a comprehensive assessment and/or who have not had a major, permanent change of status.
- Code selection is based on the performance and documentation of 2 of the 3 key components or time if more than 50% of the floor or unit time is spent in counseling and/or coordination of care (Table 7-14).
- All levels of service include reviewing the medical record and results of diagnostic studies, noting changes in the resident's status and response to management since the last visit, and reviewing and signing orders.

Table 7-14. Subsequent Nursing Facility Care

Key Components (For a description of key components, see Table 7-1.)
2 of 3 key components must be performed to at least the degree specified under the code. Some payers may require medical decision-making as 1 of the 2 components performed and documented.

CPT® Code/Timeᵃ	Medical Decision-making (meets 2 of 3 elements)	History (meets all 3 elements)	Examination
99307 10 min	Straightforward PP: Usually stable, recovering, or improving	Problem focused	Problem focused
99308 15 min	Low complexity PP: Usually responding inadequately to therapy or minor complication	Expanded	Expanded
99309 25 min	Moderate complexity PP: Usually patient develops significant complication or new problem.	Detailed	Detailed
99310 35 min	High complexity PP: Usually patient is unstable or has a new problem requiring immediate attention.	Comprehensive	Comprehensive

Abbreviations: CPT, Current Procedural Terminology; PP, presenting problem.

ᵃ Typical time is an average and represents a range of times that may be higher or lower depending on clinical circumstances. The presenting problem is considered to be a contributory factor and does not need to be present to the degree specified.

Nursing Facility Discharge Services (99315, 99316)

❉ The nursing facility discharge day management codes (Table 7-15) are used to report the total time spent by a physician for the final nursing facility discharge of a patient, even if the time spent by the physician on that date is not continuous.

❉ The codes include, as appropriate, final patient examination and discussion of the nursing facility stay. Instructions are given to all relevant caregivers for continuing care, preparation of discharge records, prescriptions, and referral forms.

❉ If the work of performing the discharge management is more than 30 minutes, the total time must be documented in the medical record.

Table 7-15. Nursing Facility Discharge Services

99315 99316	Nursing facility discharge day management; 30 minutes or less more than 30 minutes

Annual Nursing Facility Assessment (99318)

Code **99318** is used to report a comprehensive annual assessment that includes a detailed interval history, comprehensive physical examination, and minimum data set or resident assessment instrument evaluation. The patient's and family's goals for care and preferences for medical interventions are assessed, including, if applicable, reassessment of advance directives and updates of contact information for surrogate decision-makers. Table 7-16 describes the 3 key components for code **99318**.

	Table 7-16. Annual Nursing Facility Assessment		
Key Components (For a description of key components, see Table 7-1.) 3 of 3 key components must be performed to at least the degree specified under the code.			
CPT® Code/Timeᵃ	**Medical Decision-making**	**History**	**Examination**
99318 30 min	Low to moderate complexity PP: Usually stable, recovering, or improving	Detailed interval history	Comprehensive

Abbreviations: CPT, Current Procedural Terminology; *PP, presenting problem.*

ᵃ *Typical time is an average and represents a range of times that may be higher or lower depending on clinical circumstances. The presenting problem is considered to be a contributory factor and does not need to be present to the degree specified.*

E/M Services and Care of Children With Chronic Medical Conditions

As electronic communications and adoption of the principles of the medical home have increased, so has the need for codes that capture services beyond the traditional face-to-face visit. See Chapter 8, Managing Chronic and Complex Conditions, for information on reporting E/M services provided to patients with chronic and/or complex health conditions. Chapter 8 includes information on services such as

- Chronic care management (**99487**, **99489**, **99490**)
- Transitional care management services (**99495** and **99496**)
- Medical team conferences (**99366–99368**)
- Care plan oversight (**99339**, **99340**; **99374–99380**)

See also Chapter 13, Telemedicine, for information on telemedicine services and Chapter 14, Allied Health and Clinical Staff Services, for information on services provided by nonphysician health care providers (eg, psychologist, nutritionist).

Continuum Models for Otitis Media, Attention-Deficit/Hyperactivity Disorder, and Asthma

Chapter 7: Evaluation and Management Services in the Office, Outpatient, Home, or Nursing Facility Setting

Continuum Model for Otitis Media

CPT® Code Vignette	History	Physical Examination	Medical Decision-making
99211[a] Nursing evaluations Follow-up on serous fluid or hearing loss with tympanogram (Be sure to code tympanogram [92567] and/or audiogram [92551 series] in addition to 99211.)	1. Chief complaint 2. History of treatment		1. Completion of medication 2. No need for further therapy 3. No need for further follow-up
99212 Follow-up otitis media, uncomplicated with primary examination being limited to ears	**Problem focused** 1. Chief complaint 2. History of treatment 3. Difficulties with medication 4. Hearing status	**Problem focused** 1. Ears	**Straightforward** 1. Completion of medication 2. No need for further therapy 3. No need for further follow-up

99213
2-year-old presents with tugging at her right ear. Afebrile. Mild upper respiratory infection symptoms and mild otitis media.
	Problem focused
	1. Chief complaint
	2. Brief HPI plus pertinent ROS
	  a. Symptoms
	  b. Duration of illness
	  c. Home management, including over-the-counter medications, and response
	  d. Additional symptoms from ROS
		Expanded problem focused
		1. Ears
		2. Nose
		3. Throat
		4. Conjunctiva
		5. Overall appearance
			Low complexity
			1. Observation and nonprescription analgesics

99214
Infant presents for suspected third episode within 2–3 months.
Infant presents with fever and cough.
	Detailed
	1. Chief complaint
	2. Detailed HPI plus pertinent ROS and pertinent PFSH
	  a. Symptoms of illness
	  b. Fever, other signs
	  c. Any other medications
	  d. Allergies
	  e. Frequency of similar infection in past and response to treatment
	  f. Environmental factors (eg, tobacco exposure, child care)
	  g. Immunization status
	  h. Feeding history
		Detailed
		1. Overall appearance
		2. Hydration status
		3. Eyes
		4. Ears
		5. Nose
		6. Throat
		7. Lungs
		8. Skin
			Moderate complexity
			1. Treatment including antibiotics and supportive care.
			2. Consider/discuss tympanocentesis (69420 or 69421).
			3. Hearing evaluation planned.
			4. Discuss possible referral to an allergist or otolaryngologist for tympanostomy.
			5. Discuss contributing environmental factors and supportive treatment.

Continuum Model for Otitis Media (continued)

CPT® Code Vignette	History	Physical Examination	Medical Decision-making

99215
3-month-old presents with high fever, vomiting, irritability.
	Detailed
	1. Chief complaint
	2. Detailed HPI plus pertinent ROS and pertinent PFSH
	  a. Symptoms of illness
	  b. Fever, other signs
	  c. Any other medications
	  d. Allergies
	  e. Frequency of similar infection in past and response to treatment
	  f. Environmental factors (eg, tobacco exposure, child care)
	  g. Immunization status
	  h. Feeding history
		Detailed
		1. Overall appearance
		2. Hydration status
		3. Eyes
		4. Ears
		5. Nose
		6. Throat
		7. Lungs
		8. Skin
			High complexity
			1. Laboratory tests: Consider a complete blood cell count with differential, blood culture, blood urea nitrogen, creatinine, electrolytes, urinalysis with culture, chest radiograph, and possible lumbar puncture based on history and clinical findings.
			2. Antibiotic therapy: Consider parenteral antibiotics.
			3. Consider hospitalization based on history, physical findings, and laboratory studies.
			4. Determine need for follow-up (eg, reassess later in same day by phone or follow-up visit as well as later follow-up).
			5. Attempt oral rehydration in office.

99214 or 99215 **NOTE:** Depending on the variables (ie, time), this example could be reported as **99214** or **99215.** Extended evaluation of child with chronic or recurrent otitis media **NOTE:** Time is the key factor when counseling and/or coordination of care are more than 50% of the face-to-face time with the patient. For **99214**, the total visit time would be 25 minutes; for **99215**, the total time is 40 minutes. You must document time spent on counseling and/or coordination of care and list the areas discussed.	**Detailed** History with extended HPI as in **99214**, but complete ROS and PFSH	**Detailed** or **comprehensive** General or single organ system (ears, nose, mouth, and throat)	**Moderate** or **high complexity** Tests: audiometry and/or tympanometry Extensive discussion of treatment options, including, but not limited to, 1. Continued episodic treatment with antibiotics 2. Myringotomy and tube placement 3. Adenoidectomy 4. Allergy evaluation 5. Steroid therapy with weighing of risk to benefit ratio of various therapies

Abbreviations: CPT, Current Procedural Terminology; HPI, history of present illness; PFSH, past, family, and social history; ROS, review of systems.

a There are no required key components for code **99211**; however, the nurse must document his or her history, physical examination, and assessment to support medical necessity.

Chapter 7: Evaluation and Management Services in the Office, Outpatient, Home, or Nursing Facility Setting

Chapter 7: Evaluation and Management Services in the Office, Outpatient, Home, or Nursing Facility Setting

Continuum Model for Attention-Deficit/Hyperactivity Disorder

CPT® Code Vignette	History	Physical Examination	Medical Decision-making
99211[a] Nurse visit to follow up growth or blood pressure prior to renewing prescription for psychoactive drugs	1. Chief complaint 2. Brief HPI, existing medications, and desired/undesired effects	1. Weight, blood pressure 2. Overall appearance	1. Refill existing prescription.
99212 Follow-up visit to recheck prior weight loss in patient with established ADHD otherwise stable on stimulant medication	**Problem focused** 1. Chief complaint 2. Brief HPI, existing medications, and desired/undesired effects	**Problem focused** 1. Weight, blood pressure 2. Overall appearance	**Straightforward** 1. Refill existing prescription.
99213 (Typical time: 15 min) 3- to 6-month follow-up of child with ADHD who is presently doing well using medication and without other problems OR May be reported based on time if more than 50% of the face-to-face encounter is spent in counseling and/or coordination of care	**Expanded problem focused** 1. Reason for the visit 2. Review of medications 3. Effect of medication on appetite, mood, sleep 4. Quality of schoolwork (eg, review report cards) 5. Absence of tics 6. Problem-pertinent ROS	**Expanded problem focused** 1. General multisystem examination or single organ system examination with special reference to neurologic examination	**Low complexity** 1. Review rating scale results and feedback materials from teacher. 2. Discuss 6-month treatment plan with adjustment of medication. 3. Plan for further monitoring.

99214 (Typical time: 25 min)
Follow-up evaluation of an established patient with ADHD with failure to improve on medication and/or weight loss
 	
OR
 	
May be reported based on time if more than 50% of the face-to-face encounter is spent in counseling and/or coordination of care
	Detailed
	All data implicit in **99213** expanded plus pertinent review of PFSH and extended ROS, including gastrointestinal and psychiatric
		Detailed
		1. General multisystem examination or detailed single organ system examination of neurologic system
			Moderate complexity
			1. Review rating scale results and feedback materials from teacher.
			2. Discussion of possible interventions, including, but not limited to
			  a. Educational intervention
			  b. Alteration in medications
			  c. Obtaining drug levels
			  d. Psychiatric intervention
			  e. Behavioral modification program

Continuum Model for Attention-Deficit/Hyperactivity Disorder (continued)

CPT® Code Vignette	History	Physical Examination	Medical Decision-making
99215 (Typical time: 40 min) Initial evaluation of an established patient experiencing difficulty in classroom, home, or social situation and suspected of having ADHD This could be billed as a consultation if the established patient is referred by school for opinion or advice (not transfer of care) and the criteria for reporting a consultation are met. May be reported based on time if more than 50% of the face-to-face encounter is spent in counseling and/or coordination of care	**Comprehensive** 1. Chief complaint 2. History of the problem, extended 3. Complete PFSH 4. Complete ROS	**Comprehensive** 1. General multisystem examination with special attention to neurologic examination and mental health status	**High complexity** Review of Vanderbilt scales, school record, any other formal evaluations completed to date; discussion of differential diagnoses; possible interventions including, but not limited to 1. Educational interventions 2. Initiation of medications 3. Obtaining drug levels or ruling out substance abuse, if appropriate 4. Laboratory tests as indicated (eg, complete blood cell count and iron studies, serum lead levels) 5. Psychological and/or psychiatric interventions 6. Behavioral modification program 7. Consideration of neurology consultation 8. Coordination of care services with school, family, and other providers

Abbreviations: ADHD, attention-deficit/hyperactivity disorder; CPT, Current Procedural Terminology; HPI, history of present illness; PFSH, past, family, and social history; ROS, review of systems.

[a] There are no required key components for code **99211**; however, the nurse must document his or her history, physical examination, and assessment to support medical necessity.

Chapter 7: Evaluation and Management Services in the Office, Outpatient, Home, or Nursing Facility Setting

Chapter 7: Evaluation and Management Services in the Office, Outpatient, Home, or Nursing Facility Setting

Continuum Model for Asthma

CPT® Code Vignette	History	Physical Examination	Medical Decision-making
99211 [a] Nurse reviews medication list and use and obtains a peak expiratory flow rate for a well 10-year-old established patient. Nurse reviews disease management protocol with mother and child, including acute exacerbations.			

99212
Follow-up visit for an 8-year-old with stable asthma who is in good health
	Problem focused
	1. Chief complaint
	2. Brief HPI
	  a. Cough
	  b. Wheeze
	  c. Labored breathing
		Problem focused
		1. Limited to respiratory system
			Straightforward
			1. Review of home peak flow data.
			2. Continue current medications.
			3. Routine follow-up.

99213
Follow-up visit for a 7-year-old with stable chronic asthma who is using a metered-dose steroid inhaler with β-agonist as needed
	Expanded problem focused
	1. Chief complaint
	2. Brief HPI
	  a. Cough, including nocturnal symptoms
	  b. Wheeze
	  c. Respiratory distress
	  d. Exercise tolerance
	  e. Frequency of rescue medication use
	  f. Peak flow monitoring at home
	  g. Associated illnesses and problem-pertinent ROS
		Expanded problem focused
		1. Examination of respiratory system, including lungs, nose, throat, and other pertinent organ systems
			Low complexity
			1. Review of home peak flow data
			2. Evaluation of medications
			3. Alteration of medications
			4. Criteria for urgent follow-up care
			5. Plans for routine follow-up care
			6. Spirometry performed

Continuum Model for Asthma (*continued*)

CPT® Code Vignette	History	Physical Examination	Medical Decision-making
99214 An 8-year-old with known unstable asthma is examined because of an acute exacerbation of the disease; already receiving inhaled albuterol and inhaled steroids by metered-dose inhaler.	**Detailed** 1. Chief complaint 2. Extended HPI 3. Pertinent PFSH	**Detailed** 1. General appearance 2. Ears, nose, throat 3. Neck, lymph 4. Lymph 5. Respiratory 6. Cardiovascular	**Moderate** As in **99213**, plus 1. Treatment with a nebulized β-agonist in office and at home 2. Use of oral steroids 3. Discussion of effects of medications 4. Limitations on physical activity 5. Pre- and post-bronchodilator spirometry done
99215 A 1-year-old known to have recurrent wheezing following respiratory syncytial virus bronchiolitis has had increasingly frequent attacks during the past 2 months. New infiltrates are revealed by chest radiograph. Laboratory evaluation since last visit documented a positive sweat test result. A diagnosis of cystic fibrosis is made.	**Comprehensive** 1. Chief complaint 2. Extended HPI 3. Complete ROS 4. Complete PFSH	**Comprehensive** As in **99214**, plus 1. Eyes 2. Skin 3. Gastrointestinal	**High complexity** 1. Review laboratory data and radiology results. 2. Consult with pulmonologist by telephone. 3. Initiate therapy with review of adverse effects and their duration. 4. Plan for alternatives if deterioration occurs. 5. Discuss implications of positive sweat test result with parent(s).

Abbreviations: CPT, Current Procedural Terminology; HPI, history of present illness; PFSH, past, family, and social history; ROS, review of systems.

ᵃThere are no required key components for code *99211*; however, the nurse must document his or her history, physical examination, and assessment to support medical necessity.

CHAPTER 8

Managing Chronic and Complex Conditions

Contents

Children with chronic and complex health care needs are patients who require greater levels and amounts of multidisciplinary medical, psychosocial, rehabilitation, and habilitation services than their same-aged peers. The child with special health care needs will require extra services, such as prolonged services, home care visits, and care management, with an increased frequency of evaluation and management (E/M) visits. Patient-centered medical home recognition programs and related quality initiatives have focused on care of children with chronic and episodic health conditions and complex care through planning and coordination, management between face-to-face encounters, and use of electronic technology for population management, increased access to care, and quality measurement. However, physician practices have faced challenges in receiving adequate funding for the infrastructure necessary to effectively coordinate and manage care for patients with multiple and complex conditions. In response, codes have been developed with the aim of capturing the components of care that go beyond those included in preservice, intraservice, and post-service values of the traditional face-to-face visit. Services such as chronic care management (CCM) and transitional care management (TCM) have been defined and valued and are separately reportable services in addition to other face-to-face services. New in 2018 are codes for reporting psychiatric collaborative care management (PCCM) services performed under the supervision of a physician or qualified health care professional (QHP) by a behavioral health care manager and in consultation with a psychiatric consultant.

Codes and payment policy for many of these services continue to evolve. Awareness of the codes for these services and the related coding instructions may offer additional opportunities for providing and/or coordinating comprehensive care for all children. Reporting these services and the diagnosis codes representing the patient's chronic and complex conditions can play an important role in demonstrating the higher quality, lower cost care that is a key element of emerging payment methodologies. (See Chapter 19, The Business of Medicine: Working With Current and Emerging Payment Systems, for information on emerging payment methodologies, such as value-based purchasing.) Payers that have adopted value-based or enhanced payment initiatives, such as per-member, per-month payment models, may consider certain care management services bundled into the services for which the enhanced payment is made. However, practices may choose to assign codes for use in internal calculations of the cost to provide enhanced care in comparison to any enhanced payments.

To take advantage of opportunities for providing and reporting services related to management of chronic conditions and complex health care needs, physicians must identify the services that their practice capabilities will support. For instance, provision of TCM services requires timely identification of patients who are discharged from an inpatient or observation stay such that contact may be made with the patient within 2 business days of facility discharge. Payers may also require specific electronic capabilities (eg, having a system that meets specifications required by the Medicaid electronic health record [EHR] incentive programs and/or Merit-based Incentive Payment System [MIPS]).

Identification of patients who may qualify for care management services must be accomplished through a standardized methodology. This may involve developing checklists or processes for identifying characteristics of patients with complex health care needs (eg, patients with chronic or episodic conditions that are expected to last at least 12 months and increase the risk of morbidity and mortality, acute exacerbation or decompensation, or functional decline may require CCM services). Examples of such characteristics (*examples only; not a practice guideline*) include

- Number of chronic conditions
- Number of visits for nonroutine care in the past year
- Number of days the child did not attend school due to health condition
- Emergency department (ED) visits or hospitalizations in the past 6 months
- Number of current medications or medications prescribed or revised in the last 6 months
- Number of physicians and other providers (eg, home health care provider, nutritionist)
- Lack of resources (eg, housing, health plan coverage, access to care in community)
- Assistance required for activities of daily living
- Other psychosocial considerations (eg, language barriers, multiple family members with complex care needs)

Electronic systems may be used to identify patients whose records include specific diagnoses and/or services that may indicate the need for care management. However, standardized procedures for identifying the need for services and documenting orders for and delivery of services are necessary to support billing and payment.

For more information on preparing your practice to provide care to patients with complex health care needs, see the American Academy of Pediatrics (AAP) policy statement, "Patient- and Family-Centered Care Coordination: A Framework for Integrating Care for Children and Youth Across Multiple Systems" (http://pediatrics.aappublications.org/content/early/2014/04/22/peds.2014-0318). This policy statement, coauthored by the AAP Council on Children With Disabilities and the Medical Home Implementation Project Advisory Committee, specifically outlines the essential partnerships that are critical to this framework. To further augment and facilitate application of the recommendations within this policy statement, the freely accessible Boston Children's Hospital Care Coordination Curriculum (www.childrenshospital.org/care-coordination-curriculum) provides content that can be adapted to the needs of any entity (eg, a single practice, a network of practices, parent and family organizations, a statewide organization). By design, most of the content is universally relevant, but the curriculum is optimally used when it is adapted and customized to reflect local needs, assets, and cultures.

Physicians may also choose to incorporate other health care professional services (eg, medical nutrition therapy, psychotherapy) into their medical practice to meet the needs of patients with complex health care needs. See Chapter 14, Allied Health and Clinical Staff Services, for information on reporting services by nonphysician providers (NPPs).

Provider Terminology

Of particular importance to correct reporting of services that include clinical staff and other NPPs is identifying the providers included when terms such as "physician or other qualified health care professional" or "qualified, nonphysician health care professional" are used in *Current Procedural Terminology* (*CPT®*) and/or payer instruction.

CPT Provider Definitions

Current Procedural Terminology provides definitions of *providers* as follows:
- **Physician or other qualified health care professional:** an individual who is qualified by education, training, licensure/regulation (when applicable), and facility privileging (when applicable) who performs a professional service within his or her scope of practice and independently reports that professional service
- **Clinical staff member:** a person who works under the supervision of a physician or other qualified health care professional and who is allowed by law, regulation, and facility policy to perform or assist in the performance of a specific professional service but does not individually report that professional service

   Throughout the *CPT* code set, the use of terms such as "physician," "qualified health care professional," or "individual" is not intended to indicate that other entities may not report the service. In selected instances, specific instructions may define a service as limited to professionals or to other entities (eg, hospital, home health agency).

Clinical staff member is used in *CPT* mostly in the context of staff who provide components of physician or QHP services, such as TCM and CCM, and services that are always billed by a supervising physician or QHP under incident-to guidelines (eg, nurse visit, medication administration).

The *CPT* definition of *physician or other QHP* creates a broad category of providers (eg, advanced practice providers, therapists, social workers). The definition of physician and other QHP is used in relation to services such as E/M services (**99201–99499**) and immunization administration with physician counseling (**90460, 90461**) and to codes *not reported* by physicians, such as genetic counseling (**96040**).

However, this definition may be confusing, as payer policies commonly differentiate QHPs such as advanced practice providers, who may perform and prescribe services much like a physician, from those who provide specialized services under the supervision and order of a physician or advanced practice provider. Payers may offer direct reporting by certain QHPs (eg, advanced practice provider, psychologist) while requiring others to report services in the name of the supervising physician or advanced practice QHP. To aid in differentiating how services are typically reported by these subcategories of QHPs, the following definitions will apply in discussions and examples in this chapter:

- **Physician**: signifies an individual licensed under state law to practice medicine or osteopathy (Medicare also includes individuals licensed to provide dental, podiatric, optometric, and chiropractic services in the definition of physician.)
- **Qualified health care professional**: signifies advanced practice providers, such as advanced practice nurses and physician assistants, whose scope of practice includes E/M services beyond minimal services incident to a physician (ie, **99211**) and who can individually report their professional services within their scope of practice
- **Clinical staff member** (as defined by *CPT*® in differentiating from a physician or QHP): a health care team member (eg, registered nurse, licensed practical nurse, medical assistant) who works under the supervision of a physician or other QHP and who is allowed by law, regulation, and facility policy to perform or assist in the performance of a specific professional service but does not individually report that professional service
- **Allied health professional** (AHP): represents a broad category of health care professionals (eg, social worker, nutritionist) who typically would not independently prescribe and manage, whose professional services are typically performed under the order and supervision of a physician or QHP, and whose scope of practice does not include E/M services beyond **99211**

Note that *CPT* does not include any requirements for licensure but, rather, advises physicians to follow state regulations and the related scopes of practice defined by regulations (eg, regulations defining services that require a nursing license).

Coding for Management of Complex Medical Conditions

Coordination and delivery of complex care may include use of technology such as access to the medical home through telephone and online medical evaluations and subspecialty care through telemedicine or interprofessional consultation. In addition, medical team conferences may be performed on occasion to coordinate or manage care and services or to present findings and recommendations that are used to develop or revise a plan of care that includes coordination across multiple disciplines. Several different types of non–face-to-face E/M services may be performed within the same calendar month, so practices must be cognizant of *CPT* coding guidelines.

Many inclusion and exclusion rules are applied to the services included in this chapter. These rules often bundle certain niche services (eg, management of end-stage renal disease [ESRD]) in addition to prohibiting separate reporting of services that may be considered components of care management during a period when more comprehensive care management is reported. Tables are provided to summarize the patient population, work, and potentially bundled services for each type of service.

Care Management Services

Chronic care management services are management and support services that are provided by physicians or QHPs or by clinical staff under the direction of a physician or other QHP to individuals with 2 or more chronic conditions who reside at home or in a domiciliary, rest home, or assisted living facility. The care management provider provides or oversees the management and/or coordination of services, as needed, for all the patient's medical conditions, psychosocial needs, and activities of daily living. A comprehensive care plan for all the patient's health problems is created, monitored, and revised as needed. Chronic care management codes **99487–99489** and **99490** represent 2 levels of care management. Codes **99487** and **99489** require additional elements of service and greater clinical staff time than code **99490**. The appropriate CCM code is reported once per calendar month by only one physician or other QHP who has assumed this management role for the patient's care. Face-to-face E/M services may be separately reported by the same physician or QHP during the same calendar month. See Appendix III for an example of a worksheet for tracking CCM services; it is also available online at www.aap.org/cfp (access code AAPCFP23).

Chapter 8: Managing Chronic and Complex Conditions

Guidelines Applicable to All Chronic Care Management (CCM) Services

⊛ Services include all face-to-face and non–face-to-face clinical staff time spent in CCM activities on days other than a date when the physician or other QHP reporting care management services also provides a separately reportable E/M service (eg, office visit). Time spent on the date of an E/M service (eg, time of prolonged clinical staff service [**99415,99416**]) may not be included to meet requirements for reporting CCM.

⊛ Includes care plan oversight services (**99339,99340,99374–99380**), prolonged services without direct patient contact (**99358,99359**), home international normalized ratio (INR) monitoring (**93792,93793**), medical team conferences (**99366–99368**), education and training (**98960–98962,99071,99078**), telephone services (**98966–98968,99441–99443**), online medical evaluation (**98969,99444**), preparation of special reports (**99080**), analysis of data (**99090,99091**), TCM services (**99495,99496**), and medication therapy management services (**99605–99607**).

⊛ Cannot be reported with ESRD services (**90951–90970**) during the same month.

⊛ Cannot be reported if performed within the postoperative portion of the global period of a surgery or procedure reported by the same physician or other physician of the same specialty and same group practice.

⊛ Cannot be reported for any post-discharge CCM services for any days within 30 days of discharge, if reporting **99495** or **99496** (TCM services).

⊛ When care management resumes after a discharge in a new month, start a new period or report TCM services (**99495,99496**), as appropriate.

⊛ If discharge occurs in the same month, continue the reporting period or report TCM services.

Guidelines Specific to CCM Based on Clinical Staff Time

Codes **99487,99489**, and **99490** are reported only once per calendar month.

⊛ These are reported in any calendar month when the clinical staff time requirements are met. Only time spent by clinical staff employed directly by or under contract with the reporting professional's practice is included. If multiple clinical staff members meet about one patient, count the time for only one staff member.

⊛ If the physician personally performs the clinical staff activities, his or her time may be counted toward the required clinical staff time to meet the elements of the code.

⊛ Time spent by clinical staff on the date of a visit to initiate CCM services *or any other E/M service* (including services reported with code **99211**) is not counted toward the time of CCM services.

Chronic Care Management (99490)

99490   CCM services, at least 20 minutes of clinical staff time directed by a physician or other qualified health care professional, per calendar month, with the following required elements:
   ⊛ multiple (two or more) chronic conditions expected to last at least 12 months, or until the death of the patient,
   ⊛ chronic conditions place the patient at significant risk of death, acute exacerbation/ decompensation, or functional decline,
   ⊛ comprehensive care plan established, implemented, revised, or monitored

Chronic care management code **99490** was developed to align with Centers for Medicare & Medicaid Services (CMS) benefit specifications for Medicare coverage of CCM. The CMS has outlined specific coverage criteria that may be adopted by Medicaid and private health plans, including 2 points of consideration for physicians who wish to provide CCM services.

1. Practices providing CCM services must have certain capabilities, including use of an EHR. Health plans may adopt the CMS requirement for use of an EHR that meets certification requirements of the Medicaid EHR incentive programs and/or MIPS in place on December 31 of the prior year.

2. Chronic care management activities are provided by clinical staff under the supervision of the physician or QHP reporting CCM services. Check with payers for the level of supervision required. The CMS has allowed an exception to the requirement for direct supervision (ie, physician presence in the office suite when staff perform activities) for CCM services provided to Medicare patients. This exception allows staff to perform CCM activities under the physician's or QHP's general supervision (ie, supervising provider is available as needed by phone) as long as all other incident-to requirements are met. See Chapter 14, Allied Health and Clinical Staff Services, for information on incident-to requirements.

To report code **99490**, physicians must meet the required practice capabilities, document the patient's care plan, and supervise clinical staff activities of CCM. At least 20 minutes of clinical staff time spent in CCM activities must be documented. Time spent in activities personally performed by a physician may be counted toward CCM when provided on a date when no face-to-face service was provided.

Chronic Care Management Required Practice Capabilities

- Use an electronic health record system that allows care providers timely access to clinical information.
- Use a medical record form and format that are standardized within the practice.
- Identify patients who require care management using a standardized methodology.
- Adopt an internal care management process to provide care management services in a timely manner following identification of need for these services.
- Provide access to care providers or clinical staff 24 hours a day, 7 days a week, including providing patients and caregivers with a means to make contact with health care professionals in the practice to address urgent needs, regardless of the time of day or day of the week.
- Provide continuity of care through scheduling of the patient's successive routine appointments with a designated member of the care team.
- Provide timely access and management for necessary follow-up when the patient is discharged from the emergency department or hospital.
- Engage and educate patients and caregivers.
- Coordinate care among all service providers, as appropriate for each patient.

Chronic Care Management Clinical Staff Activities

- Face-to-face and non–face-to-face time spent communicating with and engaging the patient and/or family, caregivers, other professionals, community services, and agencies
- Developing, revising, documenting, communicating, and implementing a comprehensive care plan
- Collecting health outcomes data and registry documentation
- Teaching patient and/or family/caregiver patient self-management, independent living, and activities of daily living
- Identifying community and health resources
- Facilitating access to care and other services needed by the patient and/or family
- Management of care transitions not reported as part of transitional care management (**99495, 99496**)
- Ongoing review of patient status, including review of laboratory and other studies not reported as part of an E/M service
- Assessment and support for adherence to the care plan

Table 8-1 provides an overview of the patient population, work, and services not separately reportable with CCM services.

CPT copyright 2017 American Medical Association. All rights reserved.

Chapter 8: Managing Chronic and Complex Conditions

Table 8-1. Chronic Care Management Services

Service	Services Not Separately Reported in Same Calendar Month
99490 Chronic care management services **Patient Population** Patients have multiple (2 or more) chronic or episodic conditions expected to last at least 12 months, or until the death of the patient, that place the patient at significant risk of death, acute exacerbation/decompensation, or functional decline. **Work Required** ◉ Comprehensive care plan established, implemented, revised, or monitored ◉ At least 20 minutes of clinical staff activity directed by a physician or other qualified health care professional, per calendar month	**90951–90970** End-stage renal disease performed in an outpatient setting **98960–98962** Education and training for patient self-management by AHP **98966–98968** Telephone A/M service provided by AHP **98969** Online A/M service provided by AHP **99071** Educational supplies **99078** Physician or other QHP educational services to a group **99080** Special reports such as insurance forms **99090** Analysis of clinical data stored in computers **99091** Collection and interpretation of physiologic data **99339–99340** Care plan oversight in home, domiciliary, or rest home **99358–99359** Prolonged E/M service before and/or after direct patient care **93792, 93793** Home INR management **99366–99368** Medical team conferences **99374–99375** Supervision of patient under care of home health agency in home, domiciliary, or equivalent environment **99377–99378** Supervision of hospice patient **99379–99380** Supervision of a nursing facility patient **99441–99443** Telephone E/M service by a physician or other QHP **99444** Online E/M service by a physician or other QHP **99487–99489** Care management services **99495–99496** Transitional care management services **99605–99607** Medication therapy management by a pharmacist

Abbreviations: AHP, allied health professional; A/M, assessment and management; E/M, evaluation and management; INR, international normalized ratio; QHP, qualified health care professional.

Example

➤ A 12-year-old has severe atopic disease and moderate persistent asthma, which has led to multiple ED visits, hospital admissions, lost school days, and behavioral adjustment reactions. Clinical staff spend 30 minutes in the calendar month providing education and care plan monitoring and facilitating access to community services.

Code **99490** is reported. *International Classification of Diseases, 10th Revision, Clinical Modification* (*ICD-10-CM*) codes reported are **J45.4-** (moderate persistent asthma [see *ICD-10-CM* reference for required fifth character]), **Z91.09** (other allergy status, other than to drugs and biological substances) or appropriate code for more specific atopic condition, **R43.2-** (adjustment disorders [fifth character required; see *ICD-10-CM* reference for specified disorder]), and codes for other acute or episodic conditions that affected CCM activities.

Complex Chronic Care Management (99487, 99489)

99487   Complex chronic care management (CCM) services, with the following required elements:
- multiple (two or more) chronic conditions expected to last at least 12 months, or until the death of the patient,
- chronic conditions place the patient at significant risk of death, acute exacerbation/decompensation, or functional decline,
- establishment or substantial revision of a comprehensive care plan,
- moderate or high complexity medical decision-making;

> **~ More From the AAP ~**
>
> For more examples and information on reporting complex chronic care management, see articles in the April 2017 *AAP Pediatric Coding Newsletter*™ at http://coding.aap.org (subscription required).

> 60 minutes of clinical staff time directed by a physician or other qualified health care professional, per calendar month

+99489   each additional 30 minutes of clinical staff time directed by a physician or other qualified health care professional, per calendar month (List separately in addition to **99487**.)

Complex CCM services (**99487** and **99489**) require additional physician work and clinical staff time. Medical decision-making (MDM) for the reporting period must be of moderate or high complexity. Code **99487** is reported when at least 60 minutes of clinical staff time is spent in care management activities. Code **99489** is reported in addition to **99487** when at least 90 minutes are spent in complex CCM and for each additional full 30 minutes of clinical staff time spent in care management activities during the calendar month. Do not report **99489** for care management services of less than 30 minutes beyond the first 60 minutes or last full 30 minutes of complex CCM services during a calendar month.

The reporting physician or other QHP must develop or substantially revise the plan of care for all health problems. (See the *CPT®* manual for a description of a typical care plan.) Complex CCM is not reported when the care plan is unchanged or requires minimal change (eg, medication change, adjustment of a treatment modality).

In contrast, substantial revision of the care plan is not required for CCM (**99490**). Code **99490** may be reported for 20 minutes or more of clinical staff time spent in CCM activities in a calendar month even if no substantial revision is made to the care plan.

The significant difference in work and practice expense required for delivery of complex CCM services is reflected in the total non-facility relative value units (RVUs) assigned to codes **99487** (2.61), **99489** (1.31), and **99490** (1.19). For more information on how RVUs affect payment, see Chapter 18, Preventing Fraud and Abuse: Compliance, Audits, and Paybacks.

Table 8-2 provides an overview of the patient population, work, and services not separately reported with complex CCM services.

Table 8-2. Complex Chronic Care Management Services

Service	Services Not Separately Reported in Same Calendar Month
99487, +99489 Complex chronic care management services **Patient Population** Patients have multiple (2 or more) chronic or episodic conditions expected to last at least 12 months, or until the death of the patient, that place the patient at significant risk of death, acute exacerbation/decompensation, or functional decline. **Work Required** • Establishment or substantial revision of a comprehensive care plan • Moderate- or high-complexity medical decision-making • At least 60 minutes of clinical staff activity directed by a physician or other qualified health care professional, per calendar month	**90951–90970** End-stage renal disease performed in an outpatient setting **98960–98962** Education and training for patient self-management by AHP **98966–98968** Telephone A/M service provided by AHP **98969** Online A/M service provided by AHP **99071** Educational supplies **99078** Physician or other QHP educational services to a group **99080** Special reports such as insurance forms **99090** Analysis of clinical data stored in computers **99091** Collection and interpretation of physiologic data **99339–99340** Care plan oversight in home, domiciliary, or rest home **99358–99359** Prolonged E/M service before and/or after direct patient care **93792, 93793** Home INR management **99366–99368** Medical team conferences **99374–99375** Supervision of patient under care of home health agency in home, domiciliary, or equivalent environment **99377–99378** Supervision of hospice patient **99379–99380** Supervision of a nursing facility patient **99441–99443** Telephone E/M service by a physician or other QHP **99444** Online E/M service by a physician or other QHP **99490** Chronic care management services **99495–99496** Transitional care management services **99605–99607** Medication therapy management by a pharmacist

Abbreviations: AHP, allied health professional; A/M, assessment and management; E/M, evaluation and management; INR, international normalized ratio; QHP, qualified health care professional.

Example

➤ **A 6-year-old has spastic quadriplegia, gastrostomy, gastroesophageal reflux with recurrent bouts of aspiration pneumonia and mild persistent asthma, myoclonic epilepsy, failure to thrive, and expressive language disorder.** He receives home occupational, physical, and speech therapy services. During the course of a calendar month, the care plan is substantially revised to address changes in nutritional requirements, side effects of treatment, and need for additional home health services to address activities of daily living that the primary caregivers can no longer handle on their own. Significant time is spent assisting with development of an individual education plan for the patient. A referral and prior authorization for neurology consultation is necessary due to changes to the patient's preferred provider network. Clinical staff confirm that the patient's medical records are received by the consulting neurologist prior to the child's appointment and assist with arranging transportation services to the appointment. Clinical staff time of CCM services is 110 minutes.

Codes **99487** and **99489** (1 unit) are reported. *ICD-10-CM* codes reported are **G80.0** (spastic quadriplegic cerebral palsy), **K21.9** (gastroesophageal reflux disease without esophagitis), **G40.409** (other generalized epilepsy and epileptic syndromes, not intractable, without status epilepticus), **R62.51** (failure to thrive [child]), and **F80.1** (expressive language disorder). If applicable during the reporting period, report **J69.0** (pneumonitis due to inhalation of food and vomit), **J45.3-** (mild persistent asthma [see *ICD-10-CM* reference for required fifth character]), and codes for other acute or episodic conditions that affected CCM activities.

Transitional Care Management Services

99495 Transitional care management services with the following required elements:
- Communication (direct contact, telephone, electronic) with the patient and/or caregiver within 2 business days of discharge
- Medical decision-making of at least moderate complexity during the service period
- Face-to-face visit, within 14 calendar days of discharge

99496 Transitional care management services with the following required elements:
- Communication (direct contact, telephone, electronic) with the patient and/or caregiver within 2 business days of discharge
- Medical decision-making of high complexity during the service period
- Face-to-face visit, within 7 calendar days of discharge

Transitional care management includes services provided to a new or an established patient whose medical and/or psychosocial problems require moderate- or high-complexity MDM during the transition from an inpatient hospital setting, observation care setting, or skilled nursing facility to the patient's home, domiciliary, rest home, or assisted living facility.

- The reporting physician or other QHP oversees the management and/or coordination of services.
- Only one physician or other QHP may report these services and only once per patient within 30 days of discharge.
- The TCM services begin on the date of discharge and continue for the next 29 days.
- One face-to-face visit is included in addition to non–face-to-face services performed by the physician or other QHP and/or licensed clinical staff under the direction of the physician or other QHP.
- Non–face-to-face services provided by the physician or other QHP may include obtaining and reviewing the discharge information; reviewing, ordering, or following up on pending diagnostic tests and treatments; communication or interaction with or education provided to family, caregivers, or other QHPs; scheduling assistance for necessary follow-up services; and arranging referrals and community resources as necessary.
- Clinical staff time (under the direction of the physician or other QHP) may include
  - ❖ Face-to-face and non–face-to-face time spent communicating with the patient and/or family, caregivers, other professionals, and agencies
  - ❖ Revising, documenting, and implementing the care plan
  - ❖ Collecting health outcomes data and registry documentation

Chapter 8: Managing Chronic and Complex Conditions

- ❖ Teaching patient and/or family/caregiver patient self-management
- ❖ Assessment and support for adherence to treatment plan and medication management
- ❖ Facilitating access to care and other services needed by the patient and/or family, including identification of community and health resources

Codes **99495** and **99496**

- ◉ Require a face-to-face visit, initial patient contact, and medication reconciliation within specified time frames.
- ◉ *Medication reconciliation* refers to the process of avoiding such inadvertent inconsistencies across transitions in care by reviewing the patient's complete medication regimen at the time of admission, transfer, and discharge and comparing it with the regimen being considered for the new setting of care.
- ◉ Medication management must occur *no later than* the date of the face-to-face visit.
- ◉ Code selection is based on the level of MDM and the date of the first face-to-face visit, as shown in **Table 8-3**. Note that all 3 components (communication within 2 business days, type of MDM, and timing of face-to-face visit) must be met to report TCM services, although only the MDM and time of the face-to-face visit differentiate code selection.

Table 8-3. Levels of Transitional Care Management

Type of Medical Decision-making	Face-to-face Visit Within 7 Days	Face-to-face Visit Within 8 to 14 Days
Moderate complexity	99495	99495
High complexity	99496	99495

- ◉ The first face-to-face visit is included in the TCM service and is not reported separately.
- ◉ Additional E/M services on dates subsequent to that of the first face-to-face visit may be reported.
- ◉ Another TCM service may not be reported by the same provider (or provider of the same group) for any subsequent discharge(s) within the 30 days.
- ◉ Hospital or observation discharge services (**99238**, **99239**, or **99217**) can be reported by the same physician reporting TCM services. Discharge services do not qualify as the required face-to-face visit for TCM.
- ◉ The TCM services cannot be reported when provided during a postoperative portion of the global period of a service reported by the same physician or other physician of the same specialty and same group practice.
- ◉ Services include care plan oversight services (**99339**, **99340**, **99374–99380**), prolonged services without direct patient contact (**99358**, **99359**), home INR monitoring (**93792**, **93793**), medical team conferences (**99366–99368**), education and training (**98960–98962**, **99071**, **99078**), telephone services (**98966–98968**, **99441–99443**), ESRD services (**90951–90970**), online medical evaluation services (**98969**, **99444**), preparation of special reports (**99080**), analysis of data (**99090**, **99091**), CCM services (**99487–99490**), or medication therapy management services (**99605–99607**). These services may not be separately reported by the same physician or physicians of the same group practice during a period of TCM.
- ◉ Medical decision-making is defined by the E/M service guidelines. Medical decision-making over the service period reported is used to define the MDM of TCM. Documentation includes the timing of the initial post-discharge communication with the patient or caregivers, date of the face-to-face visit, and complexity of MDM.
- ◉ Only one individual may report these services and only once per patient within 30 days of discharge. Another TCM service may not be reported by the same individual or group for any subsequent discharge(s) within the 30 days.
- ◉ Follow payer guidelines for reporting. The CMS allows reporting of TCM services once the included face-to-face visit has been completed (ie, prior to the end of the service period). Other payers may not allow billing until the complete service period has elapsed.

Table 8-4 provides an overview of the patient population, work, and services not separately reported with TCM services.

Table 8-4. Transitional Care Management Services

Service	Services Not Separately Reported in Same Calendar Month
99495, 99496 Transitional care management services **Patient Population** ◉ Patients are new or established and have medical and/or psychosocial problems that require moderate- or high-complexity medical decision-making. ◉ Patients are transitioning from care in an inpatient hospital setting, partial hospital, observation status in a hospital, or skilled nursing facility/nursing facility to the patient's community setting. **Work Required** ◉ Communication (direct contact, telephone, electronic) with the patient and/or caregiver within 2 business days of discharge. ◉ Medication reconciliation and management (ie, updating and reviewing medications and dosages) must occur no later than the date of the face-to-face visit. ◉ Face-to-face visit within 7 or 14 calendar days of discharge. ◉ Medical decision-making of moderate or high complexity during the service period.	**90951–90970** End-stage renal disease performed in an outpatient setting **98960–98962** Education and training for patient self-management by AHP **98966–98968** Telephone A/M service provided by AHP **98969** Online A/M service provided by AHP **99071** Educational supplies **99078** Physician or QHP educational services to a group **99080** Special reports such as insurance forms **99090** Analysis of clinical data stored in computers **99091** Collection and interpretation of physiologic data **99339–99340** Care plan oversight in home, domiciliary, or rest home **99358–99359** Prolonged E/M service before and/or after direct patient care **93792, 93793** Home INR management **99366–99368** Medical team conferences **99374–99375** Supervision of patient under care of home health agency in home, domiciliary, or equivalent environment **99377–99378** Supervision of hospice patient **99379–99380** Supervision of a nursing facility patient **99441–99443** Telephone E/M service by a physician or other QHP **99444** Online E/M service by a physician or other QHP **99487–99490** Care management services **99605–99607** Medication therapy management by a pharmacist

Abbreviations: AHP, allied health professional; A/M, assessment and management; E/M, evaluation and management; INR, international normalized ratio; QHP, qualified health care professional.

Examples

➤ A child with cystic fibrosis is discharged from the hospital after an admission for recurrent *Pseudomonas aeruginosa* infection. Two days after discharge, the physician speaks with the mother. Clinical staff assesses adherence with the treatment plan and educates the parents on management of the child. The child is seen by the physician in follow-up 10 days after discharge. Medical decision-making is highly complex.

Code **99495** is reported. This service did not meet the requirements for code **99496** because the face-to-face visit did not occur within 7 days of discharge. Diagnosis codes may include **E84.0** (cystic fibrosis with pulmonary manifestations), **B96.5** (*Pseudomonas* as the cause of diseases classified elsewhere) and, if pneumonia persists, **J15.1** (pneumonia due to *Pseudomonas*).

➤ A 6-month-old born at 25 weeks' gestation with a diagnosis of bronchopulmonary dysplasia resulting in chronic lung disease requiring home oxygen, diuretics, bronchodilators, and high-caloric formula is discharged from the hospital after an admission for respiratory failure. The physician speaks with the mother the day after discharge. Clinical staff assesses adherence with the treatment plan and educates the parents on management of the child. The child is seen by the physician in follow-up in 5 days. Medical decision-making is highly complex.

Code **99496** is reported. Diagnosis is **P27.1** (bronchopulmonary dysplasia originating in the perinatal period) and **P07.24** (extreme immaturity of newborn, gestational age 25 completed weeks).

Medical Team Conferences

99366 Medical team conference with interdisciplinary team of health care professionals, face-to-face with patient and/or family, 30 minutes or more; participation by nonphysician qualified health care professional

99367 Medical team conference with interdisciplinary team of health care professionals, patient and/or family not present, 30 minutes or more; participation by physician

99368 Medical team conference with interdisciplinary team of health care professionals, patient and/or family not present, 30 minutes or more; participation by nonphysician qualified health care professional

Medical team conference codes are used to report participation by a minimum of 3 physicians and/or QHPs or NPPs of different specialties in conferences to coordinate or manage care and services for established patients with chronic or multiple health conditions (eg, child who is ventilator dependent with developmental delays, seizures, and gastrostomy tube for nutrition).

◈ Codes differentiate provider (physician vs other QHP or AHP) and between face-to-face and non–face-to-face (patient and/or family is not present) patient team conference services.

◈ *Current Procedural Terminology*® code descriptors for medical team conferences do not differentiate between NPPs who do not independently report E/M services and QHPs who may do so when state licensing and scope of practice allow. However, *CPT* instructs that physicians or other QHPs who may report E/M services should report their time spent in a team conference with the patient and/or family present using E/M codes (and time as the key controlling factor for code selection when counseling and/or coordination of care dominates the service).

◈ If licensed QHPs (including clinical nurse specialists and clinical nurse practitioners) participated in a conference without direct physician supervision, they may report the service (**99367**) if it is within the state's scope of practice and they use their own National Provider Identifier. State Medicaid and commercial payers may follow these Medicare requirements or have their own specific rules.

◈ Medical team conferences may not be reported if the facility or organization is contractually obligated to provide the service, they are informal meetings or simple conversations between physicians and other QHPs and NPPs, or less than 30 minutes of conference time is spent in the team conferences.

◈ Code **99367** is the only code that may be reported by a physician, and it can only be reported when the patient and/or family is not present at the team conference.

◈ When the physician participates in a medical team conference with the patient and/or family present, the appropriate-level E/M code (eg, **99212–99215** if an outpatient setting) will be reported based on the place of service and total face-to-face time spent in counseling and/or coordination of care.

◈ Medical team conferences may be reported separately from other E/M services provided on the same day of service with modifier **25** appended to the appropriate-level E/M code, with the exception of neonatal and pediatric critical care (**99468–99476**) and intensive care (**99477–99480**). However, the time reported for these conferences may not be used in the determination of time for care plan oversight (**99339**, **99340**; **99374–99380**), CCM services (**99487–99490**), TCM services (**99495** and **99496**), prolonged services (**99354–99359**), psychotherapy (**90832–90853**), or any E/M service.

Medical team conferences require

◈ Face-to-face participation by a minimum of 3 physicians and/or QHPs or NPPs from different subspecialties or disciplines (eg, speech-language pathologists, dietitians, social workers), with or without the presence of the patient, family member(s), community agencies, surrogate decision-maker(s) (eg, legal guardian), and/or caregiver(s).

◈ Active involvement in the development, revision, coordination, and implementation of health care services needed by the patient by each participant.

CPT copyright 2017 American Medical Association. All rights reserved.

- Face-to-face evaluations and/or treatments by the participant that are separate from any team conference within the previous 60 days.
- Only one individual from the same specialty may report codes **99366–99368** for the same encounter. However, physicians of different specialties may each report their participation in a team conference.
- Medical record documentation supporting the participation of the physician or other QHP, the time spent from the beginning of the review of an individual patient until the conclusion of the review, and the contributed information and subsequent treatment recommendations.

Table 8-5 provides an overview of the patient population, work, and services not separately reported with medical team conference services.

Table 8-5. Medical Team Conference Services	
Service	**Services Not Separately Reported in Same Calendar Month**
99366–99368 Medical team conference with interdisciplinary team of health care professionals (Physicians report other evaluation and management codes when patient or caregivers attend conference.) **Patient Population** Established patients with chronic and multiple health conditions or with congenital anomalies (eg, cleft lip and palate, craniofacial abnormalities) **Work Required** - At least 30 minutes of face-to-face services from different specialties or disciplines - Performed face-to-face evaluations or treatments of the patient, independent of any team conference, within the previous 60 days - Presentation of findings and recommendations - Formulation of a care plan and subsequent review/proofing of the plan	**99487–99490** Care management services **99495–99496** Transitional care management services

Examples

➤ **A 14-year-old girl with spinal muscular atrophy is wheelchair bound and receives her education at home.** Over the past 6 months, her respiratory compromise has progressed and she has required 2 inpatient admissions for pneumonia. She is on oxygen at night. She receives physical and occupational therapy services at home and twice-weekly visits from a respiratory therapist. She sees a pediatric pulmonologist every 4 months and a pediatric physiatrist every 6 months. You have started discussions with her parents about how aggressive the family wishes to be if she were to require assisted ventilation. The pediatrician, pulmonologist, physiatrist, occupational and physical therapists, respiratory therapist, home care coordinator, home educator, and social worker attend the conference to discuss the child's current medical status, prognosis for the short and long term, and the child's and family's wishes as her condition deteriorates. The conference lasts 60 minutes.

Each participating physician (if they are different specialties and/or from different practices [ie, separate tax identification numbers])	*ICD-10-CM* **G12.1** (other inherited spinal muscular atrophy) *CPT* **99367**
Each nonphysician AHP (eg, respiratory therapist, occupational therapist)	*CPT®* **99368**

> A patient with mixed cerebral palsy requires coordination with multiple health care professionals (eg, physical and occupational therapists, neurologist, pediatrician). Each participant in the conference has completed his or her evaluation of the patient within 60 days prior to the conference, and a team conference of 40 minutes is held to assess the current plan of care and therapy. The patient's family is present at this conference.

Because the patient's family is present, the participating physicians must report an appropriate E/M service rather than team conference services. The appropriate E/M code for the site of service (eg, **99215**) and typical time would be reported by each participating physician if they are different specialties and/or from different practices (ie, separate tax identification numbers). Code **99368** would be reported by the physical and occupational therapists. *ICD-10-CM* code **G80.8** (other cerebral palsy) is reported. Additional codes would be reported for any diagnoses addressed that are not integral to mixed cerebral palsy.

Care Plan Oversight Services

99339   Individual physician supervision of a patient (patient not present) in home, domiciliary, or rest home (eg, assisted living facility) requiring complex and multidisciplinary care modalities involving regular physician development and/or revision of care plans, review of subsequent reports of patient status, review of related laboratory and other studies, communication (including telephone calls) for purposes of assessment or care decisions with health care professional(s), family member(s), surrogate decision-maker(s) (eg, legal guardian), and/or key caregiver(s) involved in patient's care, integration of new information into the medical treatment plan, and/or adjustment of medical therapy, within a calendar month; 15-29 minutes

+99340   ≥30 minutes (Report in addition to **99339**)

99374   Supervision of a patient under care of home health agency (patient not present) in home, domiciliary or equivalent environment (eg, Alzheimer's facility) requiring complex and multidisciplinary care modalities involving regular development and/or revision of care plans by that individual, review of subsequent reports of patient status, review of related laboratory and other studies, communication (including telephone calls) for purposes of assessment or care decisions with health care professional(s), family member(s), surrogate decision-maker(s) (eg, legal guardian) and/or key caregiver(s) involved in patient's care, integration of new information into the medical treatment plan and/or adjustment of medical therapy, within a calendar month; 15-29 minutes

+99375   ≥30 minutes (Report in addition to **99374**)

99377   Supervision of a hospice patient (patient not present) requiring complex and multidisciplinary care modalities involving regular development and/or revision of care plans by that individual, review of subsequent reports of patient status, review of related laboratory and other studies, communication (including telephone calls) for purposes of assessment or care decisions with health care professional(s), family member(s), surrogate decision-maker(s) (eg, legal guardian) and/or key caregiver(s) involved in patient's care, integration of new information into the medical treatment plan and/or adjustment of medical therapy, within a calendar month; 15-29 minutes

+99378   ≥30 minutes (Report in addition to **99377**)

99379   Supervision of a nursing facility patient (patient not present) requiring complex and multidisciplinary care modalities involving regular development and/or revision of care plans by that individual, review of subsequent reports of patient status, review of related laboratory and other studies, communication (including telephone calls) for purposes of assessment or care decisions with health care professional(s), family member(s), surrogate decision-maker(s) (eg, legal guardian) and/or key caregiver(s) involved in patient's care, integration of new information into the medical treatment plan and/or adjustment of medical therapy, within a calendar month; 15-29 minutes

+99380   ≥30 minutes (Report in addition to **99379**)

Care plan oversight is recurrent physician or QHP supervision of a complex patient or a patient who requires multidisciplinary care and ongoing physician or QHP involvement. Chronic care management or TCM services would not be reported in conjunction with care plan oversight services. (When reporting criteria are met for

Chapter 8: Managing Chronic and Complex Conditions

CCM or TCM services and payer policy allows payment, it may be beneficial to report these services in lieu of care plan oversight.) Care plan oversight services are not face-to-face and reflect the complexity and time required to supervise the care of the patient. The codes are reported separately from E/M office visits.

Care plan oversight services

- ☀ Are reported only by the individual (physician/QHP) who has the predominant supervisory role in the care of the patient or is the sole provider of the services. A face-to-face service with the patient must have been provided by the physician prior to assuming care plan oversight.
- ☀ Include
  - ❖ Regular development and/or revision of care plans
  - ❖ Review of subsequent reports of the patient's status
  - ❖ Review of related laboratory or other diagnostic studies
  - ❖ Communication (including telephone calls) for purposes of assessment or care decisions with health care professionals, family members, surrogate decision-makers (eg, legal guardians), and/or key care-givers involved in the patient's care
  - ❖ Integration of new information into the medical treatment plan or adjustment of medical therapy
  - ❖ Team conferences
  - ❖ Prolonged E/M service before and/or after direct patient care when the same time is attributed to care plan oversight

- ☀ Require recurrent supervision of therapy. Provision of very low-intensity or infrequent supervision services is considered part of the pre- and post-encounter work for home, office/outpatient, hospital, and nursing facility or domiciliary visit codes. For example, a child is discharged from the hospital and requires weekly laboratory tests for 2 weeks. The test results are called to the physician's office and the physician relays the findings to the mother. These low-intensity services would be included in the post-service work of the hospital services.

> **||ılıllı Coding Pearl ılıllılı||**
>
> Unlike nonphysician chronic care management and transitional care management services, time included in care plan oversight is only that of the physician or other qualified health care professional and not that of clinical staff.

- ☀ Are reported once per month based on the amount of time spent by the physician during that calendar month.
- ☀ Cumulative time begins with the first day of the month and ends with the last day of the month.
- ☀ Are reported based on the patient's location or status (eg, home, hospice) and the total time spent by the physician within a calendar month. Less than 15 minutes' cumulative time within a calendar month cannot be reported.
- ☀ Are reported separately from other office or outpatient, hospital, home, nursing facility, or domiciliary E/M services.
- ☀ Do not require specific practice capabilities as are defined for CCM services.

Time spent on the following activities *may not* be considered care plan oversight:

- ☀ Travel time to or from the facility or place of domicile
- ☀ Services furnished by clinical staff (ancillary or incident-to staff)
- ☀ Very low-intensity or infrequent supervision services included in the pre- and post-encounter work for an E/M service
- ☀ Interpretation of laboratory or other diagnostic studies associated with a face-to-face E/M service
- ☀ Informal consultations with health professionals not involved in the patient's care
- ☀ Routine postoperative care provided during the global surgery period of a procedure
- ☀ Time spent on telephone calls or online medical evaluation or in medical team conferences if they are separately reported with codes **99441–99443**, **99444**, or **99367**

Table 8-6 provides a comparison of care plan oversight services, including patient population, work included, and services not separately reported for each.

Table 8-6. Care Plan Oversight Services

Service	Services Not Separately Reported in Same Calendar Month[a]
99339–99340[a] Care plan oversight in home, domiciliary, or rest home (eg, assisted living facility) **Patient Population** Patients require complex and multidisciplinary care modalities involving regular physician development and/or revision of care plans. **Work Included** ⚙ At least 15 minutes by physician in regular development and/or revision of care plans ⚙ Review of subsequent reports of the patient's status ⚙ Review of related laboratory or other diagnostic studies ⚙ Communication for purposes of assessment or care decisions ⚙ Integration of new information into the medical treatment plan or adjustment of medical therapy	**99358–99359** Prolonged E/M service before and/or after direct patient care (when time is included in care plan oversight) **99441–99443** Telephone E/M service by a physician or other QHP (when time is included in care plan oversight) **99444** Online E/M service by a physician or other QHP (when time is included in care plan oversight) **99487–99490** Care management services **99495–99496** Transitional care management services
99374–99375[a] Supervision of patient under care of home health agency in home, domiciliary, or equivalent environment **Patient Population** ⚙ Patients are under the care of a home health agency. ⚙ Patients require complex and multidisciplinary care modalities involving regular physician development and/or revision of care plans. **Work Included** Same as **99339–99340**	**98966–98968** Telephone A/M service provided by AHP (when time is included in care plan oversight) **98969** Online A/M service provided by AHP (when time is included in care plan oversight) **99358–99359** Prolonged E/M service before and/or after direct patient care (when time is included in care plan oversight) **99441–99443** Telephone E/M service by a physician or other QHP (when time is included in care plan oversight) **99444** Online E/M service by a physician or other QHP (when time is included in care plan oversight) **99487–99490** Care management services **99495–99496** Transitional care management services
99377–99378[a] Supervision of hospice patient **Patient Population** ⚙ Patients are under the care of a hospice agency. ⚙ Patients require complex and multidisciplinary care modalities involving regular physician development and/or revision of care plans. **Work Included** Same as **99339–99340**	**98966–98968** Telephone A/M service provided by AHP (when time is included in care plan oversight) **98969** Online A/M service provided by AHP (when time is included in care plan oversight) **99441–99443** Telephone E/M service by a physician or other QHP (when time is included in care plan oversight) **99444** Online E/M service by a physician or other QHP (when time is included in care plan oversight) **99487–99490** Care management services **99495–99496** Transitional care management services

Chapter 8: Managing Chronic and Complex Conditions

Table 8-6. Care Plan Oversight Services (*continued*)	
Service	**Services Not Separately Reported in Same Calendar Month**[a]
99379–99380[a] Supervision of a nursing facility patient **Patient Population** ◉ Patients reside in nursing facility. ◉ Patients require complex and multidisciplinary care modalities involving regular physician development and/or revision of care plans. **Work Included** Same as **99339–99340**	**98966–98968** Telephone A/M service provided by AHP (when time is included in care plan oversight) **98969** Online A/M service provided by AHP (when time is included in care plan oversight) **99358–99359** Prolonged E/M service before and/or after direct patient care (when time is included in care plan oversight) **99441–99443** Telephone E/M service by a physician or other QHP (when time is included in care plan oversight) **99444** Online E/M service by a physician or other QHP (when time is included in care plan oversight) **99487–99490** Care management services **99495–99496** Transitional care management services

Abbreviations: AHP, allied health professional; A/M, assessment and management; E/M, evaluation and management; QHP, qualified health care professional.

[a] Telephone and online assessments and prolonged physician service before and/or after direct patient care may be separately reported when the time of each service is distinct and nonoverlapping with time spent in care plan oversight.

Medicare requires the use of Level II Healthcare Common Procedure Coding System codes for care plan oversight services provided to patients under the care of a home health agency (**G0181**) or hospice (**G0182**). To report these G codes, Medicare requires a minimum of 30 minutes of physician supervision per calendar month. Because some state Medicaid programs may follow suit, check with your payer to learn its requirements for reporting these services.

A care plan oversight log serves as medical record documentation and as an encounter form for reporting purposes. An example is found in Appendix IV and online at www.aap.org/cfp (access code AAPCFP23). A completed care plan oversight log follows. The service elements represented by the letter in the second column are defined on the complete form in Appendix IV.

Home Care Plan Oversight Log[a]						
Total time for care plan oversight activities performed in August = 37 minutes (code **99340**)						
Date of Service	**Special Services Provided A–F**	**Contact Name and Agency**	**Start Time**	**End Time**	**Total Minutes**	**Monthly Subtotal**
August 4	C, D	Consultation with pediatric endocrinologist	12:00 pm	12:06 pm	6	6
August 4	D, A	Phone call to mother, change in medication	12:15 pm	12:21 pm	6	12
August 15	C	Review of individual education plan (IEP)	5:15 pm	5:25 pm	10	22
August 16	D	Phone calls to mother and teacher re: changes in IEP	5:30 pm	5:45 pm	15	37

[a] See worksheet in Appendix IV and online at www.aap.org/cfp; use access code AAPCFP23.

Advance Care Planning

99497   Advance care planning including the explanation and discussion of advance directives such as standard forms (with completion of such forms, when performed), by the physician or other qualified health care professional; first 30 minutes, face-to-face with the patient, family member(s) and/or surrogate

+99498   each additional 30 minutes (List separately in addition to code for primary procedure)

Codes **99497** and **99498** include

- Face-to-face service by a physician or QHP to a patient, family member, or surrogate spent in counseling and discussion of advance directives
- Completion of forms, when applicable (eg, Health Care Proxy, Durable Power of Attorney for Health Care, Living Will, and Medical Orders for Life-Sustaining Treatment)

Active management of problems is not included in advance care planning. Other E/M services provided on the same date as advance care planning may be separately reported with the exceptions of hourly critical care services (**99291**, **99292**), inpatient neonatal and pediatric critical care (**99468–99469**, **99471–99476**), and initial and continuing intensive care services (**99477–99480**). Do not report codes **99497** and **99498** in conjunction with codes **99291**, **99292**, **99468**, **99469**, **99471–99476**, or **99477–99480**.

Do not report code **99497** for less than 16 minutes of physician face-to-face time.

Advance care planning services may be considered bundled to enhanced payment methodologies and not separately paid. However, *CPT®* requires reporting of the code that is specific to the service provided regardless of payment policy. Advance care planning services should not be reported as another service (eg, office visit) in an effort to avoid denial as a bundled service.

Relative value units for a non-facility site of service assigned are 2.31 for **99497** and 2.02 for **99498** (based on 2017 Medicare Physician Fee Schedule), making the allowed amounts $82.91 and $72.50, respectively, when paid at the Medicare conversion factor of $35.89 per RVU.

Example

> **Expectant parents who have learned that their baby has a life-limiting anomaly at a recent visit with a neonatologist return for advance care planning.** The neonatologist spends 50 minutes face-to-face with the parents and assesses their understanding of the diagnosis, confirms the desire to carry the baby to term, and communicates expectations at and following delivery. A plan of care is developed and documented and an appointment with the supportive care team at the hospital is scheduled to provide additional counseling to the family and connection to other supportive services.

The neonatologist may report codes **99497** and **99498** for the 50 minutes of face-to-face time spent providing the advance care planning. Because the *CPT* prefatory language and code descriptors for advance care planning do not include other instruction on the time required for reporting, these services may be reported based on general *CPT* instruction to report when the midpoint is passed (eg, one unit of **99498** may be reported for services of 46–75 minutes). Exceptions may apply for payers with policy requiring that the time be met or exceeded.

Teaching Point: In this vignette, the service was aimed at advance planning of what care the parents wish to be provided to their baby following delivery. This is best described by advanced care planning codes **99497** and **99498**. *CPT* instructs that codes reported should accurately describe the service rendered and physicians should not report a code that merely approximates the service provided, so it would be inappropriate to report another service that may have higher RVUs and payment values. However, when a payer does not recognize these codes or the main reason for an encounter is other than advance care planning, consultation codes **99241–99245** or **99251–99255** or other E/M service codes (eg, **99212–99215**) may be appropriately reported (see Chapter 7, Evaluation and Management Services in the Office, Outpatient, Home, or Nursing Facility Setting, and Chapter 10, Noncritical Hospital Evaluation and Management Services, for discussion of reporting to payers that do not accept consultation codes).

Psychiatric Collaborative Care Management (PCCM) Services

Psychiatric collaborative care management services are provided to patients who have a new or existing psychiatric disorder that requires a behavioral health assessment; care plan implementation, revision, or monitoring; and provision of brief interventions. Psychiatric collaborative care management services involve the efforts of a team of 3 health care professionals: a treating physician or QHP, a behavioral health care manager, and a psychiatric consultant. The treating physician or QHP reports codes **99492–99494** when all requirements

Chapter 8: Managing Chronic and Complex Conditions

for reporting are met. Evaluation and management and other services may be reported separately by the same physician or QHP during the same calendar month.

●99492 Initial psychiatric collaborative care management, first 70 minutes in the first calendar month of behavioral health care manager activities, in consultation with a psychiatric consultant, and directed by the treating physician or other qualified health care professional, with the following required elements:

* outreach to and engagement in treatment of a patient directed by the treating physician or other qualified health care professional;
* initial assessment of the patient, including administration of validated rating scales, with the development of an individualized treatment plan;
* review by the psychiatric consultant with modifications of the plan if recommended;
* entering patient in a registry and tracking patient follow-up and progress using the registry, with appropriate documentation, and participation in weekly caseload consultation with the psychiatric consultant; and
* provision of brief interventions using evidence-based techniques such as behavioral activation, motivational interviewing, and other focused treatment strategies.

●99493 Subsequent psychiatric collaborative care management, first 60 minutes in a subsequent month of behavioral health care manager activities, in consultation with a psychiatric consultant, and directed by the treating physician or other qualified health care professional, with the following required elements:

* tracking patient follow-up and progress using the registry, with appropriate documentation;
* participation in weekly caseload consultation with the psychiatric consultant;
* ongoing collaboration with and coordination of the patient's mental health care with the treating physician or other qualified health care professional and any other treating mental health providers;
* additional review of progress and recommendations for changes in treatment, as indicated, including medications, based on recommendations provided by the psychiatric consultant;
* provision of brief interventions using evidence-based techniques such as behavioral activation, motivational interviewing, and other focused treatment strategies;
* monitoring of patient outcomes using validated rating scales; and
* relapse prevention planning with patients as they achieve remission of symptoms and/or other treatment goals and are prepared for discharge from active treatment.

●+99494 Initial or subsequent psychiatric collaborative care management, each additional 30 minutes in a calendar month of behavioral health care manager activities, in consultation with a psychiatric consultant, and directed by the treating physician or other qualified health care professional (List separately in addition to code for primary procedure)

(Use **99494** in conjunction with **99492**, **99493**)

Each team member's role is defined in *CPT®* as follows:

Treating Physician or QHP

The treating physician or QHP directs the behavioral health care manager and continues to oversee the patient's care, including prescribing medications, providing treatments for medical conditions, and making referrals to specialty care when needed. The treating physician or QHP engages the services of the psychiatric consultant who does not directly bill for PCCM services (ie, the treating physician's or QHP's practice contracts with the psychiatric consultant for this component of the PCCM service).

The treating physician or QHP acts in a supervisory role to the behavioral health care manager (may be a direct employee or contractual employee but should represent a practice expense similar to other clinical staff and AHPs). If the treating physician or QHP personally performs behavioral health care management (BHCM) activities and those activities are not used to meet criteria for a separately reported service, his or her time may be counted toward the required time for PCCM. As the reporting/billing provider for PCCM services, the treating physician or QHP is ultimately responsible for delivery, documentation, and billing of PCCM services in compliance with *CPT* and payer policies.

Behavioral Health Care Manager

The behavioral health care manager is an AHP or clinical staff member with either master's or doctoral-level education or specialized training in behavioral health who provides BHCM services under the treating physician's or QHP's supervision and in consultation with a psychiatric consultant. The behavioral health care manager provides the following services, as needed:

- Assessment of needs, including the administration of validated rating scales
- Development of a care plan
- Provision of brief interventions, face-to-face and non–face-to-face
- Ongoing collaboration with the treating physician or QHP
- Consultation with the psychiatric consultant at least weekly (typically non–face-to-face)
- Maintenance of a registry

The behavioral health care manager whose scope of practices includes services such as psychiatric evaluation (**90791**, **90792**), psychotherapy (**90832–90838**), psychotherapy for crisis (**90839**, **90840**), family psychotherapy (**90846**, **90847**), multiple family group psychotherapy (**90849**), group psychotherapy (**90853**), smoking and tobacco use cessation counseling (**99406**, **90407**), and alcohol and/or substance abuse structured screening and brief intervention services (**99408**, **99409**), may report these services separately when performed. However, the time of separately reported services is not included in the time of PCCM.

Psychiatric Consultant

The psychiatric consultant is a medical professional trained in psychiatry or behavioral health and qualified to prescribe a full range of medications. The psychiatric consultant typically does not see the patient or prescribe medications, except in rare circumstances. The psychiatric consultant advises and makes recommendations to the treating physician or QHP (typically via consultation with the behavioral health manager). The psychiatric consultant's services include recommending as needed

- Psychiatric and other medical differential diagnoses
- Treatment strategies for appropriate therapies
- Medication management
- Medical management of complications associated with treatment of psychiatric disorders
- Referral for specialty services

The psychiatric consultant may directly provide and separately report E/M or psychiatric services, such as psychiatric evaluation (**90791**, **90792**), to a patient within a calendar month when the same patient receives PCCM services. Activities for services reported separately are not included in the services reported with codes **99492–99494**.

PCCM Reporting Requirements

Reporting requirements for PCCM services include

- Psychiatric collaborative care management services are time-based services that are subject to the *CPT®* midpoint rule for reporting time. Time of service is met when the midpoint is passed. Documentation must support provision of PCCM services for
  - ❖ 36 minutes or more to report a 70-minute service (**99492**)
  - ❖ 31 minutes or more to report a 60-minute service (**99493**)
  - ❖ 16 minutes or more beyond the last full service period to report an additional 30 minutes of service (**99494**)
- Time spent by the behavioral health manager coordinating care with the ED may be included in time attributed to PCCM services. However, time spent while the patient is an inpatient or in observation status at a hospital may not be included in time of PCCM services.
- Psychiatric collaborative care management services are provided for an episode of care defined as beginning when the treating physician or QHP directs the patient to the behavioral health care manager and ending when any of the following scenarios is true:
  - ❖ The attainment of targeted treatment goals, which typically results in the discontinuation of care management services and continuation of usual follow-up with the treating physician or other QHP

❖ Failure to attain targeted treatment goals, culminating in referral to a psychiatric care provider for ongoing treatment

❖ Lack of continued engagement with no PCCM services provided over a consecutive 6-month calendar period (break in episode)

◉ A new episode of care starts after a break in episode of 6 calendar months or more.

◉ Medical necessity of PCCM services may be supported by documentation of a newly diagnosed condition, a patient's need for help engaging in treatment, or a patient who has not responded to standard care delivered in a nonpsychiatric setting or who requires further assessment and engagement prior to consideration of referral to a psychiatric care setting. (These are typical patient scenarios. Other reasons for services may support medical necessity.) Where health plans implement specific coverage criteria and/or prior authorization for PCCM services, documentation of the patient's behavioral health conditions, psychosocial needs, and other factors influencing patient care may help support the necessity of services.

◉ Unlike CCM services, PCCM services do not require establishment of a care plan for all the patient's health care needs. Psychiatric collaborative care management services are directed to behavioral health needs. Patients may or may not have comorbid conditions that affect treatment and management.

◉ Provision of PCCM services may support quality initiatives, such as use of an electronic clinical data system to track care and administration of a validated rating scale (eg, Patient Health Questionnaire-9) during a 4-month period for patients diagnosed with major depression or dysthymia.

General Behavioral Health Integration Care Management

●**99484**   Care management services for behavioral health conditions, at least 20 minutes of clinical staff time, directed by a physician or other qualified health care professional, per calendar month, with the following required elements:

◉ Initial assessment or follow-up monitoring, including the use of applicable validated rating scales;

◉ Behavioral health care planning in relation to behavioral/psychiatric health problems, including revision for patients who are not progressing or whose status changes;

◉ Facilitating and coordinating treatment such as psychotherapy, pharmacotherapy, counseling and/or psychiatric consultation; and

◉ Continuity of care with a designated member of the care team

Code **99484** was created to allow for reporting provision of behavioral health integration care management (or BHCM) services by other than the PCCM model. The services are performed by clinical staff for a patient with a behavioral health (including substance use) condition that requires care management services (face-to-face or non–face-to-face) of 20 or more minutes in a calendar month. The service must be initiated and supervised by a physician or QHP who may report E/M services (ie, is not reported by NPPs whose scope of practice does not include E/M services under state regulations or when not allowed by payer policy). A documented treatment plan is required as well as all activities specified in the code descriptor.

Behavioral health care integration clinical staff are not required to have qualifications that would permit them to separately report services (eg, psychotherapy), but, if qualified and they perform such services, they may report such services separately, as long as the time of the service is not used in reporting **99492**.

This code may or may not be included as a benefit under Medicaid or private health plans. Be sure to verify coverage of all PCCM and integrated behavioral health services prior to providing services.

◉ A treatment plan is required as well as the specified elements of the service description. The assessment and treatment plan is not required to be comprehensive and the office or practice is not required to have all the functions of CCM (**99487**, **99489**, **99490**).

◉ If the treating physician or other QHP personally performs BHCM activities and those activities are not used to meet criteria for a separately reported code, his or her time may be counted toward the required BHCM time to meet the elements of **99484**.

- Do not use **99484** in conjunction with **99492**, **99493**, or **99494** in the same calendar month.
- The same physician or QHP may report BHCM (**99484**) on the same date or during the same calendar month as other E/M services, including, but not limited to, CCM (**99487**, **99489**, **99490**) and TCM (**99495**, **99496**) or psychiatric services (**90785–90899**). However, activities and time attributed to support reporting of one code may not also be attributed to the time and activities described by another code reported for the same period.
- Time spent in BHCM activities while the patient is admitted to the hospital as an inpatient or in observation is not included in the time supporting code **99484**.
- Time spent coordinating care with the ED may be attributed to the time of **99484**.

Prolonged Services Without Direct Patient Contact

99358 Prolonged evaluation and management service before and/or after direct patient care; first hour
+99359 each additional 30 minutes (Use in conjunction with code **99358**.)

Guidelines for reporting non-direct prolonged services include

- Reported when a physician or QHP provides prolonged service that does not involve face-to-face care; does not include time spent by clinical staff.
- Service must be related to another physician or other QHP service. The primary service may be an E/M service (with or without an assigned average time), a procedure, or other non–face-to-face service codes that have a published maximum time (eg, telephone services). However, it must relate to a service or patient where direct (face-to-face) patient care has occurred or will occur and to ongoing patient management.
- May be reported on a different date than the related primary service.
- Cannot be reported for time spent in medical team conferences, online medical evaluations, care plan oversight services, CCM services, TCM services, or other non–face-to-face services that have more specific codes and no upper time limit assigned.
- The first-hour prolonged service code (**99358**) is reported for the total duration of prolonged service of 30 to 74 minutes' duration on a given day of service, and code **99359** is used to report each additional 30 minutes beyond the first hour, regardless of the place of service. Code **99359** may also be used to report the final 15 to 30 minutes of prolonged service on a given date.
- Less than 30 minutes' total duration on a given date cannot be reported.
- Less than 15 minutes beyond the first hour or beyond the final 30 minutes is not reported separately.

See Chapter 7, Evaluation and Management Services in the Office, Outpatient, Home, or Nursing Facility Setting, and Chapter 10, Noncritical Hospital Evaluation and Management Services, for discussion of face-to-face prolonged services in the outpatient and inpatient settings.

> ||||||| **Coding Pearl** |||||||
> Codes **99358** and **99359** must be related to an E/M service, procedure, or other non–face-to-face service with a published maximum time.

Example

➤ A physician requested and received medical records from the former physician of a 6-year-old who was born with hypoplastic left heart syndrome. The patient has undergone staged palliative reconstruction, including eventual Fontan procedure with extracardiac conduit. The child has residual supraventricular tachycardic arrhythmia. On a day separate from any face-to-face service, the physician spends 35 minutes reviewing and summarizing the medical records and documents his time in the medical record.

> ||||||| **Coding Pearl** |||||||
> Codes for congenital malformation or deformity may be used throughout the life of the patient. If a congenital malformation or deformity has been *completely repaired,* a personal history code should be used to identify the history of the (corrected) malformation or deformity.

Prolonged physician services without direct patient contact (30–74 minutes)	*ICD-10-CM* **Q23.4** (hypoplastic left heart syndrome) **I49.1** (supraventricular tachycardia) **Z95.818** (presence of other cardiac implants and grafts)
	CPT® **99358**

Interprofessional Telephone/Internet Consultations

99446   Interprofessional telephone/Internet assessment and management service provided by a consultative physician including a verbal and written report to the patient's treating/requesting physician/qualified health care professional; 5–10 minutes of medical consultative discussion and review

99447   11–20 minutes of medical consultative discussion and review

99448   21–30 minutes of medical consultative discussion and review

99449   31 minutes or more of medical consultative discussion and review

A consultation request by a patient's attending or primary physician or other QHP soliciting opinion and/or treatment advice by telephone or Internet from a physician with specialty expertise (consultant) is reported by the consultant with interprofessional consultation codes **99446–99449**. This consultation does not require face-to-face contact with the patient by the consultant and often takes place when a timely face-to-face service with the consultant is not feasible (eg, consultant is geographically distant). The patient may be in the inpatient or outpatient setting.

Guidelines for the consultant reporting interprofessional telephone/Internet consultations include

◉ Telephone/Internet consultations of less than 5 minutes are not reported. Most of the time reported as interprofessional consultation must have been spent in medical consultative discussion (verbal or Internet).

◉ A single interprofessional consultation code is reported for the cumulative time spent in discussion and information review regardless of the number of telephone or Internet contacts. The service is not reported more than once in a 7-day interval.

◉ Time spent in telephone or online consultation with the patient and/or family may be reported using codes **99441–99444** or **98966–98968**.

◉ When the purpose of communication is to arrange a transfer of care or face-to-face patient encounter, interprofessional consultation codes are not reported.

◉ Interprofessional consultation services are not reported if the consultant has provided a face-to-face service to the patient within the past 14 days or when the consultation results in scheduling of a face-to-face service within the next 14 days or at the consultant's next available appointment date.

◉ Time spent by the consultant reviewing pertinent medical records, studies, or other data is included in the telephone/Internet consultation and not separately reported.

◉ As with all consultations, the request for advice or opinion should be documented in the patient record. A verbal opinion report and a written opinion report from the consultant must also be documented. For a new patient with no record, one will have to be created to document this service.

The requesting physician or QHP may report time spent in discussion with the consultant with prolonged service codes if the total time of discussion exceeds 30 minutes beyond the typical time of the associated E/M service. The prefatory language for interprofessional telephone/Internet consultations states that prolonged service codes **99354** and **99355** may be reported when the patient is present (on-site) and accessible to the requesting physician in the office or other outpatient setting during the time of service. Prolonged services without the patient present are reported with codes **99358** and **99359**. For more information on prolonged services, see Chapter 7, Evaluation and Management Services in the Office, Outpatient, Home, or Nursing Facility Setting, for prolonged services in an outpatient setting and Chapter 10, Noncritical Hospital Evaluation and Management Services, for prolonged services in an inpatient setting.

Example

➤ **A 10-year-old boy with attention-deficit/hyperactivity disorder (ADHD) has become increasingly aggressive at home and school.** The child's pediatrician arranges a telephone consultation with a child and adolescent psychiatrist and forwards the child's history records prior to the telephone consultation. The pediatrician and psychiatrist spend a total of 16 minutes in discussion. On a second date, the child and mother are present in the pediatrician's office and included in the discussion. A new care plan is developed for achieving better control of the child's predominantly hyperactive ADHD and is agreed to by the mother. The total face-to-face time for the pediatrician is approximately 20 minutes.

ICD-10-CM	CPT®	
Both physicians report **F90.1** (ADHD, predominantly hyperactive type)	The consultant reports **99447** (11–20 minutes of medical discussion and review) for the service on the first date	The pediatrician reports **99214** (16 of 25 minutes [face-to-face] spent in counseling/coordination of care) for services on the second date

Teaching Point: In this vignette, the patient and mother are not present for the interprofessional consultation. If the time of the interprofessional consultation had been 30 minutes or more, the primary care physician may have reported prolonged service before and/or after direct patient care **99358** and **99359**. Prolonged service before and/or after direct patient care requires that a related face-to-face encounter take place in proximity to the non–face-to-face prolonged service.

|||||||| **Coding Pearl** ||||||||

See codes in the General Behavioral Health Integration Care Management section for a potential ongoing management option for the patient in this example.

Telephone Services

99441   Telephone E/M service by a physician or other qualified health care professional who may report evaluation and management services provided to an established patient, parent, or guardian not originating from a related E/M service provided within the previous 7 days nor leading to an E/M service or procedure within the next 24 hours or soonest available appointment; 5–10 minutes of medical discussion

99442   11–20 minutes of medical discussion

99443   21–30 minutes of medical discussion

98966   Telephone assessment and management services provided by a qualified nonphysician health care professional to an established patient, parent, or guardian not originating from a related assessment and management service provided within the previous 7 days nor leading to an assessment and management service or procedure within the next 24 hours or soonest available appointment; 5–10 minutes of medical discussion

98967   11–20 minutes of medical discussion

98968   21–30 minutes of medical discussion

Telephone services (**99441–99443**) are non–face-to-face E/M services provided to a patient using the telephone by a physician or other QHP, who may report E/M services. Codes **98966–98968** are used to report telephone assessment and management services by health care professionals who may not report E/M services. Guidelines for reporting of telephone assessment and management services are the same as those for physician and QHP telephone E/M services.

Chapter 8: Managing Chronic and Complex Conditions

Codes 99441–99443 *may* be reported when	Codes 99441–99443 are *not* reported when
The call was initiated by an established patient or guardian of an established patient.	The call results in a face-to-face encounter within 24 hours.
They include physician management of a new problem that does not result in an office visit within 24 hours from the telephone call or at the next available urgent visit appointment.	There was a face-to-face encounter related to the problem in the previous 7 days from the telephone call.
They include physician management of an existing problem for which the patient was not seen in a face-to-face encounter in the previous 7 days from the telephone call (physician requested or unsolicited patient follow-up) or within the postoperative period of a performed and reported procedure.	The call occurs within the postoperative period of a reported procedure.
The physician documentation of telephone calls includes the date of the call, name and telephone number of the patient, name of person and relationship of the caller, type of service provided (eg, provide consultation or medical management, initiate or adjust therapy, report results), and the time spent in the encounter.	The call occurs within 7 days of a previously reported telephone management service.
	Care plan oversight (99339, 99340, or 99374–99380), care management (99487–99490), or transitional care management (99495 and 99496) services are reported and the calls are included as part of these services.
	Non–face-to-face communication is between the physician and other health care professionals. If applicable, the services may be reported using non–face-to-face prolonged physician service codes 99358 and 99359 or as part of care plan oversight or care management services (99339 and 99340; 99374–99380; 99487–99490; 99495 and 99496).
	Performed by a provider who may not report E/M services. (See codes 98966–98968 for services by qualified providers who may not report E/M services.)

Online Medical Services

99444   Online E/M service by a physician or other qualified health care professional who may report evaluation and management services provided to an established patient or guardian not originating from a related E/M service provided within the previous 7 days, using the Internet or similar electronic communications network

98969   Online assessment and management service provided by a qualified nonphysician health care professional to an established patient or guardian not originating from a related assessment and management service provided within the previous 7 days, using the Internet or similar electronic communications network

~ More From the AAP ~

Personal health information should not be transmitted online without appropriate technical safeguards, such as encryption, authentication, and integrity controls. Learn more at https://www.aap.org/en-us/professional-resources/practice-transformation/managing-practice/Pages/HIPAA-Privacy-and-Security-Compliance-Manuals.aspx.

An online electronic medical evaluation (**99444**) is a non–face-to-face E/M service by a physician or other QHP who may report E/M services to a patient using Internet resources in response to a patient's online inquiry. This is in contrast with telemedicine services, which represent interactive audio and video telecommunications systems that permit real-time communication between the physician, at the distant site, and the patient, at the originating site. Code **98969** is used by a qualified AHP to report an online assessment and management service. The reporting guidelines for code **98969** are the same as those required for online services provided by the physician or QHP.

The CMS has not assigned RVUs to online medical evaluation codes and considers them non-covered services. As a result, most third-party payers do not pay for them.

Before providing online medical services, understand local and state laws, ensure communications will be Health Insurance Portability and Accountability Act of 1996 compliant, establish written guidelines and procedures, educate payers and negotiate for payment, and educate patients.

Online services *may* be reported	Online services are *not* reported
When Internet resources are used by a physician to an established patient (including parent or guardian) in response to a patient's or guardian's online inquiry	When the online medical evaluation refers to an E/M service previously performed and reported by the physician within the previous 7 days (physician requested or unsolicited patient follow-up) or within the postoperative period of the previously completed procedure; the service(s) is considered inherent to the previous E/M service or procedure.
When the service involves the physician's personal timely response to the patient's inquiry and there is permanent documentation (electronic or hard copy) of the encounter	When it had been reported in the previous 7 days
Only once for the same episode of care during a 7-day period, although multiple physicians could report their exchange with the same patient	When care plan oversight service codes (**99339** and **99340**; **99374–99380**) or care management service codes (**99487–99490**, **99495**, and **99496**) are reported and include the online service
Only one time per episode of care and encompasses the sum of communication (eg, related telephone calls, prescription provision, laboratory orders) pertaining to the online patient encounter	When the patient is new or for established patients with an emergent medical issue (eg, seizure, severe exacerbation) or condition that requires a face-to-face encounter to appropriately treat the condition (eg, atypical or complex rash)

After-hours and Special Services

Codes **99050–99060** are used to report services that are provided after hours or on an emergency basis and are an adjunct to the basic E/M service provided. Refer to Chapter 7, Evaluation and Management Services in the Office, Outpatient, Home, or Nursing Facility Setting, for more details on after-hours and special services codes.

Reporting a Combination of Non–face-to-face Services

When CCM or TCM services do not apply or a payer does not provide benefits for these services, it may be necessary to report a combination of codes for non–face-to-face services provided to a child with special health care needs. These may include care plan oversight, online or telephone E/M services, prolonged services, and team conference services.

Be sure to review payer guidance on reporting of these services, as National Correct Coding Initiative edits or other payment policy may require appending modifiers to indicate distinct periods were spent in the provision of each service. For instance, prolonged E/M service is bundled to care plan oversight, but a modifier may be appended to indicate distinct services within the same reporting period. Guidance for reporting and coverage may vary.

Chapter 8: Managing Chronic and Complex Conditions

Example

➤ On January 3, several days prior to performing a preventive medicine visit on a 4-year-old new patient with cerebral palsy, the physician reviews medical records that were brought in by the mother. It takes the physician 30 minutes at noon and another 20 minutes after regular office hours to complete the review. The total time spent is documented.

On January 5, the child is seen by the pediatrician in the morning and a preventive medicine visit is performed and documented. During the visit, the mother relates that the child has had wheezing for 1 day and increased gastroesophageal reflux. A detailed history is performed for the wheezing and reflux. Medications are prescribed and reflux precautions are reviewed in detail.

Later that day, the physician spends 40 minutes developing a care plan and an emergency information form to summarize the medical condition(s), medications, and special health care needs that will be used to inform other health care professionals of the child's special health conditions and needs. The nurse (under direction of the physician) spends 35 minutes scheduling appointments with a neurologist, physical therapist, and social worker.

The next day, an additional 12 minutes is spent by the physician on the telephone with the patient's mother to discuss the care plan and coordination of care. All services and the time spent are documented on the care plan oversight log. On January 16, the child's mother calls the physician because she is concerned that the child will have problems adjusting to his new school. The physician spends a total of 15 minutes on the telephone with the mother to discuss how she should handle the issue. The physician documents the time spent on the telephone call, the history, and issues discussed.

On January 24, the pediatrician attends a medical team conference with the child's neurologist, physical therapist, occupational therapist, and social worker to discuss the current plan of care and therapy and make appropriate revisions. The patient and family are not present at this conference. The conference lasts 35 minutes. Each participant documents the total time spent in conference and a summary of the treatment recommendations and plans.

Pediatrician reports		
	ICD-10-CM	**CPT**
January 3	**G80.9** (infantile cerebral palsy, unspecified)	**99358** (prolonged E/M service before and/or after direct patient care; first hour)
January 5	**Z00.129** (routine child health check with abnormal findings) **K21.9** (gastroesophageal reflux without esophagitis) **R06.2** (wheezing) **G80.9** (infantile cerebral palsy, unspecified)	**99382** (preventive medicine visit, 1–4 years of age, new patient) **99214 25** (detailed history, moderate-level MDM)
January 16	**Z71.89** (other specified counseling)	**99442** (telephone E/M service; 11–20 minutes of medical discussion) Alternatively, the time spent on the telephone call could be included in the care plan oversight time.
January 24	**G80.9**	**99367** (medical team conference)
January 31	**G80.9**	**99340** (care plan oversight, patient at home, ≥30 minutes) Total physician time spent over the course of the calendar month was 52 minutes (does not include time spent providing other reported services).

CHAPTER 9

Pre-birth Counseling and Care of the Newborn

Contents

Perinatal Care

This chapter focuses on coding for care of the typical newborn and those with conditions not requiring intensive monitoring or critical care. See Chapter 12, Critical and Intensive Care, for intensive or critical care services provided to a neonate.

The American Academy of Pediatrics (AAP) Section on Neonatal-Perinatal Medicine, in conjunction with state chapters and councils of the AAP, has developed strategies that have been successful in addressing payment concerns for neonatal care. Contact your state chapter, its pediatric council, your section district AAP Executive Committee representative, a neonatal trainer, or the AAP Committee on Coding and Nomenclature for assistance in addressing any payment inequities for neonatal services in your state.

Definitions of the Perinatal and Neonatal Periods

For coding purposes, the *perinatal period* commences at 32 completed weeks of gestation through the 28th day following birth (World Health Organization definition). Based on this definition, the *neonatal period* begins at birth and continues through the completed 28th day after birth, ending on the 29th calendar day after birth. The day of birth is considered day 0 (zero). Therefore, the day after birth is considered day 1. This definition is important to diagnosis code selection for conditions that originate in the perinatal period. (This is also important for selection of codes for neonatal critical care and initial intensive care. See Chapter 12, Critical and Intensive Care, for more information on codes for these services.)

Prenatal Counseling and Consultation Codes

Preventive Medicine, Individual Counseling Codes

99401	Preventive medicine counseling and/or risk factor reduction intervention(s) provided to an individual (separate procedure); approximately 15 minutes
99402	approximately 30 minutes
99403	approximately 45 minutes
99404	approximately 60 minutes

Current Procedural Terminology (*CPT®*) codes **99401–99404** may be reported if a parent or family is seen by the physician to discuss a risk-reduction intervention (ie, seeking advice to avoid a future problem or complication). If a family is referred by its obstetrician for an existing problem, the outpatient consultation should be reported using office-based consultation codes (**99241–99245**) or other appropriate evaluation and management (E/M) codes as directed by payer policy. (See Chapter 7, Evaluation and Management Services in the Office, Outpatient, Home, or Nursing Facility Setting, and Chapter 10, Noncritical Hospital Evaluation and Management Services.)

International Classification of Diseases, 10th Revision, Clinical Modification (*ICD-10-CM*) code **Z76.81** (expectant parent[s] pre-birth pediatrician visit) would be reported for pre-birth counseling visits in addition to other relevant *ICD-10-CM* codes as applicable. Family history codes may also be relevant for reporting the reason for pre-birth and/or preconception counseling (eg, **Z82.79**, family history of other congenital malformations, deformations, and chromosomal abnormalities).

>
> **|||||||| Coding Pearl ||||||||**
>
> *ICD-10-CM* codes for fetal conditions affecting management of the mother (categories **O35–O36**) are reported only when the fetal condition is actually responsible for modifying the management of the mother (ie, requiring diagnostic studies, additional observation, special care, or termination of pregnancy). That a fetal condition exists does not justify assigning a code to the mother's record.

Report codes **99401–99404**

⊛ Based on a physician or other qualified health care professional's face-to-face time spent providing counseling.

⊛ For a new or an established patient.

Chapter 9: Pre-birth Counseling and Care of the Newborn

❖ When the medical record includes documentation of the total counseling time and a summary of the issues discussed. Time is met when the midpoint is passed (eg, 8 minutes of service required to report a 15-minute service). Table 9-1 contains examples and time ranges for each code.

When counseling and risk-reduction interventions are provided to a mother or her fetus prior to delivery, report them under the mother's insurance. Verification of the payer's benefit policy for these services is recommended prior to service; if non-covered, an advance beneficiary notice should be signed by the patient. An advance beneficiary notice or waiver is a written notice to the patient of noncoverage or potential out-of-pocket costs provided prior to delivery of a service. Verify payer requirements and applicable state regulations prior to using waivers in your practice. A copy of the signed notice should be kept on file with the practice's billing records. An encounter for a meet and greet is not considered a medically necessary service and will most likely not be covered.

Table 9-1. Preventive Medicine Counseling and/or Risk-Factor Reduction Intervention(s) Provided to an Individual (Separate Procedure)

Code	Timeª	Documentation Examples
99401	15 min (8–22 min)	20 minutes spent with parents reviewing the risks of recurrent congenital heart disease; assured low risk of recurrence in next pregnancy
99402	30 min (23–37 min)	25 minutes spent in discussion with parents considering in vitro fertilization; discussed potential risks of multiple gestations and preterm delivery, types of problems, and hospital stay associated with preterm delivery; parents understand risks.
99403	45 min (38–52 min)	50 minutes spent with parents who request counseling on the fetal/maternal risks due to mother having insulin-dependent diabetes; reviewed maternal risks for infection, poor glucose control, and operative delivery; reviewed risks of fetal anomaly risk, macrosomia, and preterm delivery; postnatal risk for hypoglycemia, respiratory problems reviewed
99404	60 min (≥53 min)	60 minutes spent with parent(s) and maternal grandparents reviewing the hospital records and autopsy results of a previous child who died shortly after birth from congenital skeletal dysplasia and pulmonary hypoplasia; reviewed genetics, risk factors for recurrence, and screening studies that would be used to identify risk or recurrence

ª Unless Current Procedural Terminology® instructs otherwise for a code or code range, time is met when the midpoint is passed. Payers following Medicare policy may require that time be met or exceeded.

Consultations

A consultation is reported when a physician or other appropriate source requests an opinion and/or advice from another physician or appropriate source. The consulting physician renders advice, records it, and returns a report to the requesting physician or appropriate source. Chapter 7, Evaluation and Management Services in the Office, Outpatient, Home, or Nursing Facility Setting, and Chapter 10, Noncritical Hospital Evaluation and Management Services, detail the specific reporting, documentation, and coding requirements for the selection of consultation codes or other E/M service codes when consultation codes are not recognized. This request must be in writing or given verbally by the requestor.

See Table 7-4 for the key components and typical times of consultation codes used in reporting outpatient consultation codes (eg, office or observation) and Table 10-4 for inpatient consultation codes.

|||||||| **Coding Pearl** ||||||||

Consultations are not reported when they are requested by a patient or family member; office codes are used. See Chapter 7, Evaluation and Management Services in the Office, Outpatient, Home, or Nursing Facility Setting.

Examples

➤ **At the request of the obstetrician, you counsel a family that was just informed that its fetus has an enlarged bladder and dilated ureter.** You meet with the family in your office and spend 28 minutes counseling the family about the condition. The time spent in counseling and a summary of the issues discussed are documented in your medical record. Your consultation report is sent to the requesting physician and a copy is maintained in your medical record.

Time (30 minutes face-to-face) is the key controlling factor.	*ICD-10-CM* **Z76.81** (expectant parent pre-birth visit)
	CPT® **99242** (average 30 minutes) or, if payer does not recognize consultations, **New Patient** **Established Patient** **99203** (average 30 minutes) **99214** (average 25 minutes)

Teaching Point: If the findings of enlarged bladder and dilated ureter will modify management of the mother's pregnancy (eg, site of delivery, repeat ultrasounds), a code for fetal conditions affecting management of the mother's pregnancy (eg, **O35.8XX0**, maternal care for other [suspected] fetal abnormality and damage, single or unspecified fetus) would also be reported. Remember that you need a written or verbal request (which should be documented) to support consultation services. This service is reported under the mother's insurance.

➤ **At the request of a primary care physician, a neonatologist evaluates a 35-weeks' gestation neonate with recurrent hypoglycemia.** A detailed history is obtained from the mother, documenting hyperglycemia during pregnancy, but she was not overtly diabetic. Family history is negative for previous neonates with hypoglycemia or other metabolic diseases. Review of labor and delivery records is unremarkable. After birth, the newborn had 3 documented preprandial blood glucose concentrations less than 40 mg/dL and responded well to oral feeding. On physical examination, the neonate's earlobes showed no abnormal creases, the liver size was normal, and a complete neurologic examination was normal. Gestational age assessment by physical examination and growth parameters was consistent with 35 weeks' gestation. The neonatologist recommends more frequent feeding and rechecking blood glucose before feeds until 4 consecutive preprandial glucose concentrations are greater than 60 mg/dL. The neonatologist spends 10 minutes explaining the findings and reassuring the baby's parents. The neonatologist writes a detailed chart note and discusses her recommendations with the pediatrician by phone.

Medical decision-making (MDM): Low complexity *History:* Detailed *Physical examination:* Detailed	*ICD-10-CM* **P70.4** (hypoglycemia, newborn)
	CPT **99253** or, if payer does not recognize consultations, **99221** (initial hospital care)

Attendance at Delivery and Newborn Resuscitation

99464   Attendance at delivery (when requested by the delivering physician or other qualified health care professional) and initial stabilization of newborn

99465   Delivery/birthing room resuscitation, provision of positive pressure ventilation and/or chest compressions in the presence of acute inadequate ventilation and/or cardiac output

Chapter 9: Pre-birth Counseling and Care of the Newborn

Code **99464** is not reported when hospital-mandated attendance is the only underlying basis for providing the service. When physician on-call services are mandated by the hospital (eg, attending specific types of deliveries, such as all repeat cesarean deliveries) and are not physician requested, report code **99026** (hospital-mandated on-call service; in hospital, each hour) or **99027** (hospital-mandated on-call service; out of hospital, each hour). See Chapter 10, Noncritical Hospital Evaluation and Management Services, for guidelines for use of codes **99026** and **99027**.

Attendance at delivery (**99464**)

❋ Service is only reported when requested by the delivering physician and indicated for a newborn who may require immediate intervention (ie, stabilization, resuscitation, or evaluation for potential problems).

❋ Medical record documentation must include the request for attendance at the delivery and substantiate the medical necessity of the services performed. If there is no documentation by the delivering physician for attendance at delivery, the verbal request and the reason for the request should be documented in the attendance note.

❋ Includes initial drying, stimulation, suctioning, blow-by oxygen, or continuous positive airway pressure (CPAP) or high-flow air/oxygen without positive-pressure ventilation (PPV); a cursory visual inspection of the neonate; assignment of Apgar scores; and discussion of the care of the newborn with the delivering physician and parents. A quick look into the delivery room or examination after stabilization is not sufficient to report **99464**.

❋ Any medically necessary procedures to complete the resuscitation that are provided in the delivery room may be reported separately (eg, direct laryngoscopy without intubation).

❋ May be reported in addition to initial normal newborn (**99460**), initial sick newborn (**99221–99223**), initial intensive care of the neonate (**99477**), or critical care (**99468**; **99291–99292**) codes.

When qualifying resuscitative efforts are provided, code **99465** (delivery/birthing room resuscitation) is reported instead. Codes **99464** and **99465** cannot be reported on the same day of service.

Attendance at delivery with neonatal resuscitation (**99465**)

❋ Includes bag-and-mask or bag-to-endotracheal tube ventilation (PPV) and/or cardiac compressions.

❋ May be reported when positive-pressure breaths are administered by the T-piece resuscitator to a neonate exhibiting inadequate ventilation and/or cardiac output in lieu of a manual bag-mask resuscitator (documentation should support ventilatory or cardiac dysfunction and the necessity and provision of PPV). Do not report when T-piece resuscitator is used to provide CPAP only. See Chapter 12, Critical and Intensive Care, for further information.

❋ Other life support procedures that are performed as a necessary part of the resuscitation may be reported separately, such as **31500**, intubation, endotracheal, emergency procedure; **31515**, laryngoscopy, direct, for aspiration; **36510**, catheterization of umbilical vein for diagnosis or therapy, newborn; and **94610**, surfactant administration.

❋ May be reported in addition to any initial care service, including initial critical care (**99468**; **99291–99292**) or initial neonatal intensive care (**99477**).

> ### ~ More From the AAP ~
>
> Read more about code **99465** and CPAP/T-piece ventilation in the May 2015 *AAP Pediatric Coding Newsletter*™ at http://coding.aap.org (subscription required).

Examples

➤ **A physician attends a repeat cesarean delivery.** The services are provided because they are mandated by hospital policy. The delivering physician did not request the services.

Code **99026** (hospital-mandated on-call service; in hospital, each hour) is reported. This may be used for tracking purposes or in financial arrangements with the hospital.

➤ A physician is called at the request of an obstetrician to stand by during a delivery and spends 30 minutes waiting for the delivery before she attends the delivery of a typical newborn and admits him to her service.

    Codes **99464** (attendance at delivery) and **99460** (initial hospital or birthing center care, per day, for the E/M of normal newborn infant) are reported. Standby services are not reported in addition to attendance at delivery but may be reported with the newborn resuscitation services (**99465**) per *CPT®* guidelines.

➤ A physician provides brief resuscitation services, including PPV, to a neonate with mild primary apnea who recovered quickly and is later released to the newborn nursery for close monitoring over the next 4 hours. The neonate shows no further signs of distress.

    Codes **99465** and **99460** (initial newborn care) are reported. (Neonatal resuscitation is likely followed by initial neonatal intensive or critical care more often than normal newborn care.)

➤ A neonatologist is asked to be present at delivery by the delivering physician. The neonatologist documents a comprehensive examination of the neonate, in addition to the maternal and fetal history, and provides all the elements required for reporting of attendance at delivery. The neonate is typical and admitted to the newborn nursery under the orders of her general pediatrician.

    Code **99464** is the only code reported by the neonatologist. Although a history and examination were performed, this does not equate to initial hospital care of the newborn, which is reported by the attending physician who provides a comprehensive history and examination, ordering of screening tests and prophylactic interventions, and counseling the family on topics such as newborn feeding, sleep, and safety.

Coding Conundrum: When a Physician Arrives After Delivery, What Service Can Be Reported?

There are no specific time requirements for reporting attendance at delivery. Remember, this service requires a request for attendance at delivery by the delivering physician and includes physician work to perform the initial drying, stimulation, suctioning, blow-by oxygen, or CPAP without PPV; a cursory visual inspection of the neonate; assignment of Apgar scores; and discussion of the care of the newborn with the delivering physician and parents. When a physician arrives in the delivery room after the delivery and some or all this work has been performed, should attendance at delivery be reported? Physicians might want to consider

- When the newborn continues to require intervention or stabilization in the delivery room, code **99464** (attendance at delivery) may be reported if the physician work and medical necessity are related to the delivery, not a component of a sick, intensive, or critical admission, and the nature of the intervention is documented in the medical record.
- When the work provided in the delivery room is related more to the initial hospital care (neonate is examined and the physician sends him to the well-baby nursery), only the initial normal newborn code (**99460**) is reported.

For example, attendance at delivery was requested by the delivering physician and the physician arrives after the delivery.

→ The 1-minute Apgar score has been assigned and the neonate has been dried, stimulated, and suctioned by the nurses and is ready to be sent to the newborn nursery by the time the physician appears in the delivery room. The delivering physician acknowledges that assistance is no longer needed. The physician will report initial normal newborn care (**99460**) after completing his or her initial examination of the newborn. However, if the physician is not the attending pediatrician, no service can be reported.

→ In the previous example, the delivering physician continues to want assistance. The physician assigns the 5-minute Apgar score, performs a cursory examination, and discusses the care of the newborn with the delivering physician and parents. Code **99464** can be reported because most of the basic elements of the attendance at delivery were performed and documented in the medical record.

A stillborn neonate for whom resuscitation services are provided will be billed to the mother's insurer.
A stillborn neonate examined after birth at the request of the obstetrician should be reported on the mother's insurance as a consultation, with a report sent to the obstetrician.

Chapter 9: Pre-birth Counseling and Care of the Newborn

Normal Newborn Care

99460	Initial hospital or birthing center care, per day, for evaluation and management of normal newborn infant
99461	Initial care, per day, for evaluation and management of normal newborn infant seen in other than hospital or birthing center
99462	Subsequent hospital care, per day, for evaluation and management of normal newborn
99463	Initial hospital or birthing center care, per day, for evaluation and management of normal newborn infant admitted and discharged on the same date
99238	Hospital discharge day management; 30 minutes or less
99239	more than 30 minutes

Codes **99460**, **99462–99463**, **99238**, and **99239** are used to report E/M services provided to the healthy newborn in a hospital setting (including birthing room deliveries). They are reported when the neonate is cared for in the mother's room (rooming-in), a labor and delivery room, a postpartum floor, or a traditional newborn nursery and when a normal neonate is cared for after the mother is discharged (eg, awaiting adoption). Normal newborn codes are also used to report services to neonates who are being observed for onset of jaundice, low glucose, or other conditions or problems but are presently asymptomatic. A normal newborn is defined as a newborn who

- Transitions to life in the usual manner
- Requires delivery room intervention but is normal after transition
- May require some testing or monitoring (eg, bilirubin, complete blood cell count, culture)
- Will not require significant intervention
- Is being observed for illness but is not sick
- Is late preterm but requires no special care
- Is in house with sick mother/twin

Guidelines for reporting include

- The neonate is considered admitted at the time of arrival to the nursery.
- Code **99460** (history and examination of the normal newborn, initial service) is reported only once on the first day that the physician provides a face-to-face service in the facility. This date may not necessarily correlate with the date the patient is born or the hospital admission date.
- Code **99462** (subsequent hospital care, normal newborn) is reported once per calendar date on the date(s) subsequent to the initial normal newborn care service but *not* on the discharge date. This code is not reported for follow-up encounters in the office on the second or third day after birth with a newborn who is discharged early. See "Coding Conundrum: 3- to 5-Day-Old Post-discharge Encounter" later in this chapter for discussion of reporting initial office visits following the birth admission.
- Any additional procedures (eg, lumbar puncture, arterial puncture, circumcision, bladder tap) should be reported in addition to normal newborn care codes. Modifier **25** (significant, separately identifiable E/M service) should be appended to the E/M code when a procedure is performed on the same day of service.
- Discharge management services performed on a day subsequent to initial newborn care are reported with code **99238** (hospital discharge day management; 30 minutes or less) or **99239** (hospital discharge day management; more than 30 minutes), when discharging a normal newborn. Include time spent in final examination of the patient, discussion of the hospital stay, instructions for continuing care, and preparation of discharge records, prescriptions, and referral forms. Time must be documented when reporting **99239**.
- Code **99463** (history and examination of the normal newborn, including discharge) should be reported when an initial history and physical examination and the discharge management are performed on the same calendar date for a normal newborn.

> ||||||| **Coding Pearl** ||||||
>
> Normal newborn codes can be reported for care provided to neonates who are acting normally but recovering from fetal stress or a low Apgar score or who are being observed for a potential problem but are asymptomatic.

✳ Code **99461** (normal newborn care in other than hospital and birthing room) is reported when newborn care is provided in a setting other than the hospital or birthing room (eg, home, freestanding birthing center, physician office). The service includes a prenatal history, family and social history, the initial physical examination, and conference with the parent(s).

Do not report **99461** for the initial office encounter of a newborn when the baby was seen in the hospital setting by any provider.

ICD-10-CM codes from category **Z38** are used to report live-born neonates according to type of birth and are the first-listed codes for care by the attending or admitting physician during the entire birth admission. Category **Z38** codes for single live-born infant are shown in **Table 9-2**.

Table 9-2. *ICD-10-CM* Codes for Single Live-born Neonates

Z38.00	Single liveborn infant, delivered vaginally
Z38.01	Single liveborn infant, delivered by cesarean
Z38.1	Single liveborn infant, born outside hospital
Z38.2	Single liveborn infant, unspecified as to place of birth

Abbreviation: ICD-10-CM, International Classification of Diseases, 10th Revision, Clinical Modification.

See the *ICD-10-CM* manual for **Z38** codes for multiple birth neonates.

Report *ICD-10-CM* code **Z76.2** (encounter for health supervision and care of other healthy infant and child) when a healthy newborn continues to receive daily visits pending discharge of the mother, adoption, or other reasons. Code **Z76.2** is useful for indicating the reason for an extended stay of a healthy newborn.

Examples

➤ **The physician is not present at a repeat cesarean delivery of a healthy term male neonate.** The nursery calls the office and relates that the newborn has been admitted and seems fine. The physician's standing admission orders are followed and the physician examines the newborn the following morning. The physician reviews the record, examines the neonate, and speaks with the mother. The newborn and his mother remain in the hospital 2 additional days, when both are then discharged home. Discharge management takes 25 minutes.

Diagnosis code for all days	**ICD-10-CM** **Z38.01** (single liveborn by cesarean section)
Day 1 of hospital stay Day 2 Day 3 Day 4	**CPT®** No charge (no face-to-face services provided) **99460** (initial normal newborn care) **99462** (subsequent normal newborn care) **99238** (hospital discharge day management; 30 minutes or less)

➤ **A baby is born vaginally in the hospital on March 3 at 4:00 pm.** The pediatrician first sees the baby on March 4 and determines, after initial hospital assessment, that the newborn is ready for discharge. A history and examination of the newborn, discussion of the hospital stay with the parents, instructions for continuing care, family counseling, and preparation of the final discharge records are performed.

ICD-10-CM	**CPT**
Z38.00 (single liveborn without cesarean section)	**99463** (initial normal newborn care and discharge on the same date)

➤ **A subsequent hospital visit is performed in the well-baby nursery on a 2-day-old who is being observed due to risk of jaundice; however, no interventions are noted and baby is doing well.**

Code **99462** (subsequent normal newborn care) is reported.

➤ **A physician provides initial newborn care in her office to a neonate who was born at home earlier that day.**

Code **99461** (normal newborn care in other than hospital and birthing room) is reported. See Chapter 18, Preventing Fraud and Abuse: Compliance, Audits, and Paybacks, for appropriate place of service codes (eg, **11**, office; **12**, home) for these services.

➤ **A neonate fails a routine hearing examination.** During a subsequent newborn care visit, the attending physician spends 15 minutes discussing the results with the parents and refers to an audiologist for testing to confirm or rule out hearing abnormality.

ICD-10-CM	CPT®
Z38.00 (single liveborn without cesarean section) **R94.120** (abnormal auditory function study)	**99462** (subsequent normal newborn care)

Teaching Point: Only code **Z38.00** would be reported when the result of an auditory screening is normal. The audiologist performing the screening would report code **Z13.5**, encounter for screening for eye and ear disorders.

Diagnosis Codes for Perinatal Conditions

There are some important guidelines for reporting conditions that originate in the perinatal period. In *ICD-10-CM*, these conditions are classified to Chapter 16 and codes **P00–P96**. Codes in this chapter are used only on the neonate's record and not that of the mother. Other important guidelines include

⊚ Perinatal condition codes are assigned for any condition that is clinically significant.
⊚ In addition to clinical indications for reporting codes from other chapters, perinatal conditions are considered clinically significant if the condition has implications for future health care needs. Other clinical indications that apply to all conditions are those requiring
  ❖ Clinical evaluation
  ❖ Therapeutic treatment
  ❖ Diagnostic procedures
  ❖ Extended hospital stay
  ❖ Increased nursing care and/or monitoring
⊚ Should a condition originate in the perinatal period and continue throughout the life of the patient, the perinatal code should continue to be used regardless of the patient's age.
⊚ If a newborn has a condition that could be due to the birth process or community acquired and documentation does not indicate which it is, the condition is reported as due to the birth process. Community-acquired conditions are reported with codes other than those in Chapter 16.
⊚ Codes in categories **P00–P04**, newborn affected by maternal factors and by complications of pregnancy, labor, and delivery, may be reported when the conditions are suspected but not yet been ruled out. However, if a neonate is suspected of having an abnormal condition that, after examination and observation, is ruled out, assign codes for signs and symptoms or, in the absence of signs or symptoms, assign a code from category **Z05** (encounter for observation and evaluation of newborn for suspected diseases and conditions ruled out).

> The ordering of codes for neonates at the birth hospital are as follows:
> 1. Birth outcome (**Z38-**, reported only by the attending/admitting physician)
> 2. Codes from the perinatal chapter (**P00–P96**)
> 3. Codes from the congenital anomalies chapter (**Q00–Q99**)
> 4. All other chapters

Examples

➤ **The pediatrician admits a 3,500-g term neonate born vaginally to a mother who developed a low-grade fever during labor.** The neonate is hypothermic. A comprehensive history, including review of the maternal, prenatal, labor, and delivery history; history of present illness; and social and family history, is performed. A comprehensive examination is performed. Complete blood cell count and blood cultures are obtained and antibiotics are started. Infection is later ruled out. Medical decision-making is moderate due to a new problem with additional workup and prescribed antibiotic therapy.

MDM: Moderate complexity *History:* Comprehensive *Physical examination:* Comprehensive	**ICD-10-CM** **Z38.00** (single liveborn without cesarean section) **P80.8** (other hypothermia of newborn) **Z05.1** (observation and evaluation of newborn for suspected infectious condition ruled out)
	CPT® **99222**

Teaching Point: If test results are positive, use a diagnosis code appropriate to the findings.

➤ **A neonate was born to a mother who tested positive for group B β-hemolytic streptococcal infection and received 2 doses of prophylactic intravenous administration of penicillin during labor.** The newborn appeared typical in the delivery room and was admitted to the newborn nursery. A comprehensive maternal history and physical examination with review of intrapartum laboratory values were performed. The newborn is monitored for 48 hours with no indication of illness.

ICD-10-CM	CPT
Day 1 **Z38.00** (single liveborn without cesarean section) **P00.89** (newborn affected by other maternal conditions)	Day 1 **99460**
Day 2 **Z38.00** (single liveborn without cesarean section) **Z05.1** (observation and evaluation of newborn for suspected infectious condition ruled out)	Day 2 **99462**

Teaching Point: Note that on day 1, the patient was suspected of being affected by a localized maternal infection (**P00.89**), but by day 2, the condition was ruled out (**Z05.1**). Initial and subsequent normal newborn care codes are reported rather than initial and subsequent hospital care because the neonate, while at risk for infection in this case, was not treated but observed and did not develop infection.

- Codes in category **P05** are reported for the newborn affected by fetal growth restriction or slow intrauterine growth.
  - ❖ Codes in subcategory **P05.0** are used to report the neonate is light for dates but not small. (See definitions in the *ICD-10-CM Codes for Small and/or Light for Gestational Age* box later in this chapter.)
  - ❖ Codes in subcategory **P05.1** are used to report the neonate is small or small and light for dates.
- Code **P05.2** is provided for reporting fetal (intrauterine) malnutrition affecting a newborn who is not light or small for gestational age.

> Codes in subcategory **P07.0-** and **P07.1-** are not reported in conjunction with codes in category **P05,** disorders of the newborn due to slow fetal growth and fetal malnutrition. However, subcategory **P07.2-** and **P07.3-** may be reported in addition to category **P05.**

Chapter 9: Pre-birth Counseling and Care of the Newborn

ICD-10-CM Codes for Small and/or Light for Gestational Age

ICD-10-CM codes for small and/or light for gestational age are aligned to the World Health Organization definitions of these conditions. In the United States, many clinicians use the term *small for gestational age* for all newborns below the 10th (or fifth) percentile for gestational age and then subcategorize as *symmetric* when weight, length, and head circumference are all below the 10th percentile and *asymmetric* when only the weight is below the 10th percentile. Asymmetric fetal growth would fall in the light for gestational age group, whereas symmetric fetal growth would fall in the small for gestational age group. *Note that head circumference percentile is not a factor in choosing the correct code.*

The World Health Organization provides definitions to support diagnostic selection for these conditions.

Light for gestational age: Usually referred to as weight below but length above 10th percentile for gestational age.

Small for gestational age: Usually referred to as weight and length below 10th percentile for gestational age.

ICD-10-CM includes codes **P05.09** (newborn light for gestational age, 2500 grams and over) and **P05.19** (newborn small for gestational age, other) to allow for identification of all infants with fetal growth and malnutrition, fetal growth retardation, and preterm birth.

- Codes from category **P07**, disorders of newborn related to short gestation and low birth weight, are reported based on the recorded birth weight and estimated gestational age to indicate these conditions as the cause of morbidity or additional care of the newborn.
  - When both are documented, weight is sequenced before age.
  - These codes may be reported for a child or an adult who was preterm or had a low birth weight as a newborn and this is affecting the patient's current health status.

Hospital Care of the Ill Neonate

Initial Hospital Care

Codes **99221–99223** are used to report the initial hospital care of a sick neonate who does not require intensive observation and monitoring or critical care services. Refer to Chapter 10, Noncritical Hospital Evaluation and Management Services, and **Table 10-2** for the specific coding and documentation requirements for reporting initial hospital care.

Example

➤ **The pediatrician sees a newborn boy admitted to the well-baby nursery.** He was born to a mother with blood type O+ who has a history of 2 previous newborns with jaundice secondary to ABO incompatibility. Umbilical cord blood sent for blood typing and direct antibody (Coombs) test shows the baby is A+ DAT+. At 8 hours of age, the neonate appears jaundiced. A bilirubin and complete blood cell count with a reticulocyte count are ordered, results are evaluated, the newborn's risks for kernicterus are discussed with the family, and phototherapy is started. The pediatrician performs a comprehensive history and physical examination. Medical decision-making is of moderate complexity for this new problem with moderate risk.

MDM: Moderate *History:* Comprehensive *Physical examination:* Comprehensive	**ICD-10-CM** **Z38.00** (single liveborn without cesarean section) **P55.1** (hemolytic disease due to ABO isoimmunization)
	CPT® 99222

Teaching Point: When reporting initial hospital care, all 3 key components (history, physical examination, MDM), or average total floor/unit time if more than 50% of time spent is in counseling and/or coordination of care, must be met. The level of service is based on all hospital care services on the same date by the same physician or physicians of the same group practice and same specialty. If the minimum key components are not sufficiently met (eg, an expanded history is performed), the initial care must be reported using subsequent hospital care codes (**99231–99233**). See Chapter 10, Noncritical Hospital Evaluation and Management Services.

Subsequent Hospital Care and Discharge Management

Subsequent hospital care codes (**99231–99233**) are reported for each day of service subsequent to initial care for the newborn who continues to be sick (ie, not a typical neonate but not in critical condition and not requiring intensive observation and interventions). Code **99238** or **99239** (hospital day discharge management) is reported on the day the newborn is discharged (when on a separate day from the initial hospital care).

* When a neonate is not treated but only observed for the potential development of illness, normal newborn codes would be reported.
* If the neonate is sick but improves and requires no more care than a normal newborn, the subsequent normal newborn care code (**99462**) should be reported.

It is useful to consider the typical patient when reporting subsequent hospital care. These are

* **99231:** Usually, the patient is stable, recovering, or improving.
* **99232:** Usually, the patient is responding inadequately to therapy or has developed a minor complication.
* **99233:** Usually, the patient is unstable or has developed a significant complication or a significant new problem.

Refer to Chapter 10, Noncritical Hospital Evaluation and Management Services, and **Table 10-3** for detailed coding and documentation requirements for codes **99231–99233**. Chapter 10 also includes more information on discharge day management codes **99238** and **99239**.

Examples

➤ The physician performs an expanded problem-focused history and physical examination on a subsequent day on a term neonate born via cesarean delivery who has resolving mild tachypnea. The newborn requires intermittent low-flow oxygen by nasal cannula but is alternately nipple and gavage feeding. The physician then speaks with the mother. Medical decision-making is low based on resolving mild tachypnea, no data reviewed, and moderate risk.

MDM: Low complexity *History:* Expanded problem focused *Physical examination:* Expanded problem focused	**ICD-10-CM** **Z38.01** (single liveborn by cesarean section) **P22.1** (transitory tachypnea of newborn)
	CPT® **99232**

Teaching Point: Two of 3 key components are required to support the level of subsequent hospital care provided. If the payer requires MDM as 1 of the 2 key components met for subsequent hospital care, this service would be reported with code **99231** because MDM was low.

➤ The physician performs a follow-up visit for a neonate who was on intravenous antibiotics until this morning and is breastfeeding well, with no further fevers. Vital signs and general appearance and examination of the heart, lungs, abdomen, and skin are performed. Blood and urine cultures remain negative after 48 hours. Intravenous antibiotics are discontinued. Patient is discharged home with instructions for home care and follow-up. Thirty-five minutes was spent on the floor reviewing the hospital course, expected follow-up, and signs and symptoms of possible sepsis or infection with the mother.

| Time (35 minutes unit/floor time dedicated to the patient) is the key controlling factor. | *CPT*®
99239 (more than 30 minutes) |

Teaching Point: If time spent in discharge day management is not documented, code **99238** must be reported.

Car Seat Testing

Codes **94780** and **94781** (car seat testing) are reported for monitoring to determine if a neonate may be safely transported in a car seat or must be transported in a car bed. These services are most commonly provided to neonates who required critical care during their initial hospital stay. However, these codes may be reported in addition to the subsequent hospital or discharge day management codes when performed and documented. Note that you cannot report these codes in addition to critical or intensive care services. Time spent in car sear testing would not be counted as time spent in discharge day management. See Chapter 12, Critical and Intensive Care, for more information on car seat testing.

Prolonged Services (99354–99359)

❋ If direct (face-to-face) prolonged services (**99354–99357**) are required on the same day as a consultation (**99241–99245**, **99251–99255**), an initial hospital service (**99221–99223**), or a subsequent hospital service (**99231–99233**), they may be reported in addition to the basic E/M service (an add-on code).

❋ Direct prolonged services are not reported with normal newborn codes, intensive care codes, or neonatal/pediatric critical care codes because these services do not include an assigned typical time by *CPT*.

The specific coding guidelines for reporting face-to-face (**99354–99357**) and non–face-to-face (**99358** and **99359**) prolonged service codes are detailed in Chapter 7, Evaluation and Management Services in the Office, Outpatient, Home, or Nursing Facility Setting, and Chapter 10, Noncritical Hospital Evaluation and Management Services. See **tables 7-6** and **10-5** for the list of prolonged service codes. Prolonged clinical staff services (**99415** and **99416**) are not reported for inpatient care.

Examples

➤ **The physician performs an expanded problem-focused history and physical examination on a term neonate born via cesarean delivery who is experiencing mild tachypnea on a subsequent day.** The physician obtains and reviews a chest radiograph and complete blood cell count and requests that an oxygen saturation (Spo_2) monitor be placed on the neonate for 5 minutes. The chest radiograph and complete blood cell count are normal and the Spo_2 is persistently greater than 95%. The physician spends 65 minutes of total time on the floor with the patient, speaking with the mother and reviewing the chart.

| *MDM:* Low complexity
History: Expanded problem focused
Physical examination: Expanded problem focused | *CPT*
99232 (average time is 25 minutes)
99356 (direct prolonged services, first 30–74 minutes) |

Teaching Point: In addition to code **99232**, code **99356** will be reported based on total documented time spent on the floor or unit dedicated to the one patient. Time is not the controlling factor in selection of the subsequent hospital care code because there is no documentation of time spent counseling and coordinating care.

> **An infant is transferred from a Level III neonatal intensive care unit, following a 30-day hospital stay, to a community Level II unit to complete her recovery before home discharge.** A large volume of records accompanies the infant. A comprehensive history and physical examination are performed on admission; MDM is moderately complex. The provider spends another 1 hour and 20 minutes reviewing the extensive transfer records while off the unit.

MDM: Moderate complexity	***CPT*®**
History: Comprehensive	**99222**
Physical examination: Comprehensive	**99358** (prolonged non–face-to-face services, first hour)
	99359 (each additional 30 minutes)

Teaching Point: This service included 80 minutes of prolonged services. Code **99358** represents the first 60 minutes. Code **99359** is reported for the final 15 to 30 minutes of prolonged services; in this example, the final 20 minutes. If fewer than 75 minutes of prolonged services were provided, code **99359** would not be reported because this code is reported for time that goes at least 15 minutes beyond the first hour or final 30 minutes.

Coding for the Newborn Who Transitions to a Higher Level of Care

During a hospital stay, a newborn or readmitted neonate may require different levels of care. A normal newborn may end up becoming sick, intensively ill, or critical during the same hospital stay. Neonates who were initially sick may also improve to require lower levels of care (eg, normal neonatal care).

It is important to remember

* Normal newborn care (**99460** or **99462**) may be reported in addition to hospital care (**99221–99223**), initial intensive care (**99477**), or initial critical care (**99468**) or time-based critical care (**99291–99292**) on the same day when a patient qualifies for normal newborn care earlier in the day and, at a subsequent encounter on the same day, becomes ill and requires an additional encounter at a higher service level.

* Once an initial-day care code for a higher service level has been reported, an initial code for a lower service level within the same hospital stay will not be reported. If a patient has required intensive care (**99477**) but no longer qualifies for intensive care and is transferred to the care of a primary care pediatrician, the receiving physician will report sick visit codes. The receiving physician will not report initial hospital care (**99221–99223**) for the first encounter; rather, the physician will report subsequent hospital care (**99231–99233**) based on the level of service provided.

* An initial-day critical or intensive care code (eg, **99468**, **99477**) is reported only once per hospital stay. If the patient recovers and is later stepped up again to that higher level of care, only the subsequent-level codes (**99469**, **99478–99480**) are reported. See Chapter 12, Critical and Intensive Care, for more information on reporting care on dates when the level of care changes or the patient is transferred.

Circumcision

54150   Circumcision, using clamp or other device with regional dorsal penile or ring block

* If the circumcision using a clamp or other device is performed without dorsal penile or ring block, append modifier **52** (reduced services) to **54150**.

* Medicare has a global period of 0 (zero) assigned to code **54150**. When performing a circumcision and a separately identifiable E/M service on the same day (eg, **99462**, subsequent normal newborn care; **99238**, discharge services <30 minutes), append modifier **25** to the E/M code. Link the appropriate *ICD-10-CM* code (eg, **Z38.00**) to the E/M service and link *ICD-10-CM* code **Z41.2** (encounter for routine and ritual male circumcision) to the circumcision code.

54160   Circumcision, surgical excision other than clamp, device, or dorsal slit; neonate (28 days of age or less)

54161   older than 28 days

Unlike code **54150**, Medicare has a global period of 10 days assigned to codes **54160** and **54161**. A physician who performs a procedure with a 10-day global period must append modifier **24** (unrelated E/M service by the same physician or other qualified health care professional during a postoperative period) to the E/M code for subsequent newborn or hospital care or discharge management (eg, **99238 24**) provided in the 10-day period following the procedure for general care of the newborn unrelated to the procedure.

When circumcisions are performed in the office

⊛ If a payer does not base payment on a global surgical package, a supply code for the surgical tray can be reported with code **99070**. The description of the supply (circumcision tray) would need to be included on the claim form.

⊛ Anesthetic creams (eutectic mixture of local anesthetics) are included in the circumcision code itself and should not be reported unless a third-party payer pays separately for topical anesthetic agents. In that case, they would be reported with code **99070**.

Post-discharge Newborn Care

99391   Periodic comprehensive preventive medicine reevaluation and management of an individual including an age and gender appropriate history, examination, counseling/anticipatory guidance/risk factor reduction interventions, and the ordering of laboratory/diagnostic procedures, established patient; infant (age younger than 1 year)

See Chapter 7, Evaluation and Management Services in the Office, Outpatient, Home, or Nursing Facility Setting, for office and other outpatient E/M codes (**99211–99215**) and requirements for reporting E/M services to address problems or abnormal findings in the newborn.

Physicians often see a newborn in the office for a well-child visit (preventive medicine service) within 3 to 5 days after birth. In keeping with the *CPT®* guidelines on new and established patients, a physician, or physician of the same group practice and same specialty and subspecialty of the physician who provided care during the birth admission, has established a professional relationship with the newborn (ie, provided a professional service within the past 3 years). All office and other outpatient services, including preventive medicine services, provided to the newborn would be reported with *established* patient codes (**99211–99215** and **99391–99395**). This guideline also applies to nurse practitioners and physician assistants who work in the same group practice as a physician who has provided professional services to the newborn, as these professionals are considered to be working in the same specialty and subspecialty as the physician. Code **99381** is limited to reporting an initial preventive medicine service to a patient younger than 1 year who meets the definition of a new patient.

ICD-10-CM codes for newborn health examinations are

Z00.110   Health examination for newborn under 8 days old
Z00.111   Health examination for newborn 8–28 days old

Codes for any abnormal findings (eg, underfeeding of newborn, jaundice) should be reported in addition to the code for newborn health examination.

The appropriate level of office or other outpatient E/M service (**99212–99215**) may be reported in addition to a preventive medicine service when a significant and separately identifiable service is necessary to address a problem or abnormal finding. Modifier **25** is appended to codes **99212–99215** to indicate the separately reportable service.

> ||||||| *Coding Pearl* |||||||
>
> Per *CPT*, when advanced practice nurses and physician assistants are working with physicians, they are considered as working in the exact same specialty and exact same subspecialties as the physician.

Newborn Metabolic Screening

S3620   Newborn metabolic screening panel, includes test kit, postage, and the laboratory tests specified by the state for inclusion in this panel (eg, galactose; hemoglobin, electrophoresis; hydroxyprogesterone, 17-D; phenylalanine (phenylketonuria [PKU]); and thyroxine, total)

Early preventive services may include state-mandated metabolic screening panels and recommended second screenings. Healthcare Common Procedure Coding System code **S3620** reports use of a test kit specific to state requirements.

Coding Conundrum: 3- to 5-Day-Old Post-discharge Encounter

The AAP "Recommendations for Preventive Pediatric Health Care," or periodicity schedule, is the gold standard of care for preventive services. The Patient Protection and Affordable Care Act has adopted the recommendations under its required benefits for all non-grandfathered plans. On the schedule is the 3- to 5-day post-discharge visit. Therefore, this service should be included in the number of preventive medicine services a patient is allowed in the first year after birth. However, the AAP is often asked how to code for this encounter because, many times, this visit addresses follow-up of a problem or a new problem. The AAP recommends coding for the services provided and documented. If the visit is strictly a problem-oriented encounter because of a new or existing problem, report an office or outpatient encounter code (eg, **99213**). If, however, the focus of the encounter is growth, feeding, anticipatory guidance, and preventive counseling, report a preventive medicine service (ie, **99381** or **99391**). For more information on the recommendations, visit www.aap.org/periodicityschedule.

Collection of venous (**36415**) or capillary (**36416**) blood may be separately reported. States may have program-specific guidelines for reporting initial, secondary, and repeat screenings.

Review of metabolic screening panel results received after the patient is discharged from the hospital would typically not be separately reported from the first well-child visit. However, abnormal results that require additional workup may result in a reportable office E/M service (eg, **99212–99215**).

ICD-10-CM code **Z00.110** or **Z00.111** may be reported with **Z13.228**, encounter for screening for other metabolic disorders (includes inborn errors), or **Z13.0**, encounter for screening for diseases of the blood and blood-forming organs and certain disorders involving the immune mechanism (**Table 9-3**). However, a payer may require reporting of individual codes supporting each included screening.

Table 9-3. *ICD-10-CM* Codes for Newborn Metabolic Screening

Code	Description
Z00.110	Health supervision, newborn, <8 days old
Z00.111	Health supervision, newborn, 8–28 days old
Z13.29	Encounter for screening for other suspected endocrine disorder (except diabetes)
Z13.228	Encounter for screening for other metabolic disorders (eg, galactosemia, cystic fibrosis, phenylketonuria)
Z13.0	Encounter for screening for diseases of the blood and blood-forming organs and certain disorders involving the immune mechanism (eg, sickle cell trait)

Abbreviation: ICD-10-CM, International Classification of Diseases, 10th Revision, Clinical Modification.

Additional Screenings

In addition to newborn metabolic screening, it is important that practices ensure that all newborns have also been screened for hearing loss, cardiac congenital anomalies, and bilirubin per the most recent "Recommendations for Preventive Pediatric Health Care." If performed in the hospital setting there is no need to repeat unless required. If not performed, these services should be performed in the office or referred out. For example, if the bilirubin test is performed in the physician's office, report **82247** (bilirubin, total) or **88720** (bilirubin, total, transcutaneous) with *ICD-10-CM* code **Z13.228** (encounter for screening for other metabolic disorder).

Lactation Counseling

Breastfeeding support, supplies, and counseling are preventive services when not provided in response to maternal or newborn or infant problems. These may be covered without out-of-pocket costs to the patient under coverage through a non-grandfathered health plan. (See Chapter 6, Preventive Services, for more information.) Coverage may vary by health plan, with some considering breastfeeding support and counseling bundled to the well-woman preventive service, while others allow separate benefits under the mother's, and not the baby's, plan.

When medically necessary, a standard medical benefit may apply along with deductible, coinsurance, or co-payment costs to the patient. The service may be provided to address a feeding problem of the newborn or infant or a lactation disorder of the mother. Services to address a mother's condition should be documented in a separate chart from that of her newborn or infant and reported to her health plan. Verification of benefits prior to service is recommended.

ICD-10-CM code **Z39.1** is reported for encounter for care and examination of lactating mother. When addressing lactation disorders, such as cracked nipple, suppressed lactation, or agalactia, see codes in category **O92**. It is important to verify benefits and bill for services to the mother separately from services to address a condition of the newborn. Feeding difficulty in the newborn is reported with codes in category **P92** (Table 9-4). Remember that codes that define or describe maternal conditions cannot be reported for the baby.

Table 9-4. *ICD-10-CM* Codes for Newborn Feeding Problems

Excludes1[a]: Feeding problems in child over 28 days old (R63.3)

Code	Description
P92.0	Vomiting of newborn **Excludes1:** Vomiting of child over 28 days old (R11.-)
P92.01	Bilious vomiting of newborn **Excludes1:** Bilious vomiting in child over 28 days old (R11.14)
P92.09	Other vomiting of newborn **Excludes1:** Regurgitation of food in newborn (P92.1)
P92.1	Regurgitation and rumination of newborn
P92.2	Slow feeding of newborn
P92.3	Underfeeding of newborn
P92.4	Overfeeding of newborn
P92.5	Neonatal difficulty in feeding at breast
P92.6	Failure to thrive in newborn **Excludes1:** Failure to thrive in child over 28 days old (R62.51)
P92.8	Other feeding problems of newborn
P92.9	Feeding problem of newborn, unspecified

Abbreviation: ICD-10-CM, International Classification of Diseases, 10th Revision, Clinical Modification.

[a] *Excludes1 is a convention of ICD-10-CM indicating that 2 codes are not reported for the same encounter.*

NOTE: *If the feeding problem begins when younger than 28 days and continues past the 28th day after birth, use the appropriate P code to account for the feeding problem that began in the perinatal period regardless of the patient's current age.*

Examples

➤ **A 1-month-old presents for a scheduled health supervision visit.** The infant appears to be thriving without problems. Mother indicates that she is supplementing breastfeeding with formula because she felt the baby was not satisfied with breastfeeding alone. The physician spends about 5 minutes discussing the mother's concerns and benefits of exclusive breastfeeding and recommends a lactation consultation.

Code **99391** (established patient preventive medicine visit, age younger than one year) is reported. The brief counseling is not a significant, separately reported service.

➤ **A 6-day-old is seen by a nurse following the physician's instruction to perform a weight check in follow-up to the newborn's well-baby visit 3 days earlier.** The nurse consults the physician because the newborn's weight is only slightly higher than the previous encounter. An interim history indicates a fussy newborn who feeds every 1 to 2 hours. The physician spends 30 minutes face-to-face with the patient and parents examining the newborn, observing a feeding, counseling the parents, and arranging a referral for a lactation consultation. Counseling and coordination time is documented as 18 of 30 minutes. Diagnosis is feeding problem of newborn.

Code **99214** is reported, based on time spent counseling and coordinating care, with *ICD-10-CM* code **P92.9**, unspecified feeding problems of newborn. See Chapter 5, Time-Based Coding, for more information on reporting E/M services based on time.

➤ **A newborn is seen in the office for a 5-day well-baby visit.** The mother expresses anxiety about breast-feeding her baby and wishes to receive lactation support and counseling services. The pediatrician completes the well-baby examination, confirming the newborn appears healthy and thriving. Mother and baby are also referred to a lactation class offered by the practice's registered nurse, a certified lactation counselor. Mother and baby return for a class 2 days later.

Code **99391** is reported by the physician for the 5-day well-baby visit along with *ICD-10-CM* code **Z00.110** for health examination for newborn younger than 8 days. The lactation class is reported according to payer specifications that may require specific certification in lactation counseling and credentialing of the counselor as a nonphysician provider. Payer policies vary and should be confirmed prior to providing these services. Healthcare Common Procedure Coding System code **S9443** may be accepted by some payers for this service to the mother. *ICD-10-CM* code **Z39.1** is reported for an encounter for care and examination of a lactating mother. Be sure to submit this claim under the mother's name.

Chapter 9: Pre-birth Counseling and Care of the Newborn

Noncritical Hospital Evaluation and Management Services

Contents

Evaluation and management (E/M) codes for noncritical hospital care services require adherence to the 1995 or 1997 Centers for Medicare & Medicaid Services (CMS) *Documentation Guidelines for Evaluation and Management Services.* (See Chapter 4, Evaluation and Management Documentation Guidelines, for specific documentation requirements.) This chapter includes tables with descriptions of the required key components (ie, history, physical examination, medical decision-making [MDM], and time) for all the E/M services that are reported in the observation and inpatient hospital setting.

Here are basic guidelines for reporting noncritical observation and inpatient hospital E/M services. There are no distinctions between new and established patients.

- Codes are reported based on the cumulative services (performance of the required key components and/or time when appropriate) provided by an individual physician or physicians or other qualified health care professionals (QHPs) of the same specialty within a group with the same tax identification number during a calendar day.
- Time in the observation and inpatient setting is defined as floor or unit time (dedicated to the one patient) and includes time spent
  - ❖ At the patient's bedside
  - ❖ Counseling family or patient (or those who may have assumed responsibility for the care of the patient, eg, foster parents, legal guardians, persons acting in loco parentis)
  - ❖ On the floor documenting care, performing the history and examination, and reviewing diagnostic tests
  - ❖ Coordinating care with care team members
- When time is used as the controlling factor in the selection of the code, the time spent and the notation that more than half the time was spent in counseling and/or coordination of care *must be documented* in the medical record. See reporting guidelines for using time as the controlling key component in Chapter 5, Time-Based Coding.
- Services may be performed and reported by any physician of any specialty (eg, hospitalist, primary care physician, specialist).
- Any procedure or other service with a *Current Procedural Terminology* (*CPT*®) code may be reported separately when performed by the reporting provider or group and documented.

Table 10-1 provides the key components and specific detail of required elements within each level of history and physical examination (eg, problem focused, expanded) and MDM (eg, straightforward, moderate) of an E/M code. Services may be reported using either the 1995 or 1997 documentation guidelines. The nature of the presenting problem (ie, reason for the encounter) is included as a contributory factor for levels of MDM but is not 1 of the 3 required elements.

Observation Care

- Hospital observation services are provided to patients who require monitoring for possible inpatient admission. For example, a patient with dehydration who requires hydration and is not quite sick enough to be at an inpatient level of care in the hospital would be admitted to observation.
- Hospitals do not need to designate a separate area for these patients; rather, designation of observation versus inpatient status is dependent on the physician's order and patient's diagnosis(es) and severity of illness.
- Initial observation care is reported by the admitting physician or QHP using codes **99218–99220**. Subsequent-day observation care is reported with codes **99224–99226** and observation care discharge management with code **99217**.
- Physicians of specialties other than the supervising physician (ie, attending physician) who provide care in the observation setting report outpatient consultation (**99241–99245**) or subsequent observation care codes. (See the Coding Conundrum: 2 Physicians Providing Initial Observation or Inpatient Hospital Day Services box later in this chapter for Medicare and *CPT* guidance.)
- Admission (ie, initial care) and discharge services (observation or inpatient status) provided on the same day are reported with codes **99234–99236**.

Chapter 10: Noncritical Hospital Evaluation and Management Services

Table 10-1. Evaluation and Management Key Components[a]

	Problem focused	Expanded	Detailed	Comprehensive
History (must meet or exceed HPI, ROS, and PFSH)	HPI: 1–3 elements ROS: 0 PFSH: 0	HPI: 1–3 elements ROS: 1 PFSH: 0	HPI: 4+ elements or status of 3 chronic or inactive conditions ROS: 2–9 PFSH: 1	HPI: 4+ elements or status of 3 chronic or inactive conditions ROS: 10+ PFSH: 3
Examination	**Problem focused** 1995: 1 body area/organ system 1997: Performance and documentation of 1–5 elements identified by a bullet (●) in one or more areas or systems	**Expanded** 1995: Limited exam—affected body area/organ system and other related areas/systems 1997: Performance and documentation of at least 6 elements identified by a bullet (●) in one or more areas or systems	**Detailed** 1995: Extended exam—affected body area(s) and other symptomatic or related organ system(s) 1997: Performance and documentation of at least 2 elements identified by a bullet (●) in at least 6 areas or systems or at least 12 elements identified by a bullet (●) in at least 2 areas or systems	**Comprehensive** 1995: 8+ organ systems or complete exam of a single organ system 1997: <u>Multisystem exam</u>—9 systems or areas with performance of all elements identified by a bullet (●) in each area/system examined and documentation of at least 2 elements identified by a bullet (●) of each area(s) or system(s) <u>Single organ system exam</u>—Performance of all elements identified by a bullet (●) and documentation of every element in box with shaded border and at least one element in box with unshaded border
MDM (must meet 2 of 3—diagnoses/options, data, and risk)	**Straightforward** # diagnoses/options: Minimal Data: Minimal Risk: Minimal Presenting problem: Usually self-limited or minor severity	**Low complexity** # diagnoses/options: Limited Data: Limited Risk: Low Presenting problem: Usually moderate severity	**Moderate complexity** # diagnoses/options: Multiple Data: Moderate Risk: Moderate Presenting problem: Usually moderate to high severity	**High complexity** # diagnoses/options: Extensive Data: Extensive Risk: High Presenting problem: Usually moderate to high severity

Abbreviations: HPI, history of present illness; MDM, medical decision-making; PFSH, past, family, and social history; ROS, review of systems.

[a] See Chapter 4, Evaluation and Management Documentation Guidelines, for a detailed description of the guidelines and components of evaluation and management services with documentation requirements and tips.

❋ When the patient's status changes from observation to inpatient status or the reverse (eg, physician is asked by utilization review staff to change status from inpatient to observation), the physician should write an order to reflect the change and report only the code that reflects care consistent with the patient's final status on that date.

❋ Typical times have not been established for code **99217**, so time spent in discharge management is not a factor in the selection of this code.

Coding Conundrum: 2 Physicians Providing Initial Observation or Inpatient Hospital Day Services

When Payers Follow Medicare Rules

Initial observation services: The admitting physician will report the initial observation care codes (**99218–99220**). Other physicians (ie, physicians belonging to a different group practice or of a different specialty) providing initial services to a patient in observation will report a new or established office or outpatient E/M code (**99201–99215**) based on the performance and documentation of the required key components.

Initial inpatient hospital services: Initial inpatient hospital care codes (**99221–99223**) may be reported by every physician who performs initial hospital care. The admitting physician will append modifier **AI** (principal physician of record) to codes **99221–99223**.

When Payers Do Not Follow Medicare Rules

Initial observation services: The admitting physician will report the initial observation care codes (**99218–99220**). The office or outpatient consultation codes (**99241–99245**) may be reported by other physicians if the service was requested by a physician or other appropriate source, opinion and/or advice was rendered by the consulting physician, and a written report was generated from the consulting physician to the referring physician. When the criteria for reporting a consultation are not met, the subsequent observation E/M codes (**99224–99226**) would be reported based on the level of care provided and documented.

Initial inpatient hospital services: The admitting physician will report the initial hospital care codes (**99221–99223**). Inpatient consultation codes (**99251–99255**) may be reported by other physicians if the requirements for reporting the services are met (ie, requested, opinion/advice rendered, written report to requesting source). Otherwise, subsequent hospital care E/M codes (**99231–99233**) are reported.

Initial Observation Care

99218–99220   Initial observation care, per day, for the evaluation and management of a patient

See the full code descriptors in **Table 10-2**. The examples included here and throughout the chapter are coded based on the 1995 E/M documentation guidelines.

Initial observation care codes are reported

❋ On the first day that the admitting physician provides face-to-face services to the patient in the observation setting

❋ Using the code that reflects the overall care provided to the patient on that calendar date (See the Unique Considerations for Hospital Services box later in this chapter for more details about coding for initial observation care initiated elsewhere [eg, office, emergency department (ED)].)

> ||||||||| **Coding Pearl** |||||||||
>
> Medicare limits reporting of observation services for less than 8 hours on the same calendar date. Only initial observation care (**99218–99220**) is reported. Codes including discharge management (**99217 or 99234–99236**) shall not be reported. Medicaid or private payers may or may not limit reporting.

When "observation status" is initiated in the course of an encounter in another site of service (eg, ED, physician's office), all E/M services performed by the same physician (or physicians of the same specialty in the same group practice) are considered part of the initial observation care when performed on the same calendar date.

Important guidelines to remember include

❋ If the patient is admitted for observation and subsequently is formally admitted to the hospital on the same day, only the initial inpatient hospital code (**99221–99223**) is reported.

Table 10-2. Initial Observation Care (99218–99220), Inpatient Hospital Care (99221–99223), and Observation or Inpatient Care Admission and Discharge Same Day (99234–99236)

Key Components (For a description of key components, see Table 10-1.)
3 of 3 key components must be performed to at least the degree specified for the codes in each row.

CPT® Code/Timeª	Medical Decision-making	History	Examination
99218 (I) 30 min 99221 (S) 30 min 99234 (A&D) 40 min	Straightforward to low PP: Usually low severity	Detailed	Detailed
99219 (I) 50 min 99222 (S) 50 min 99235 (A&D) 50 min	Moderate complexity PP: Usually responding inadequately to therapy or minor complication	Comprehensive	Comprehensive
99220 (I) 70 min 99223 (S) 70 min 99236 (A&D) 55 min	High complexity PP: Usually patient is unstable or develops significant complication or new problem.	Comprehensive	Comprehensive

Abbreviations: A&D, admission and discharge on same day; CPT, Current Procedural Terminology; I, initial day; PP, presenting problem; S, subsequent day.

ª Typical time is an average and represents a range of times that may be higher or lower depending on clinical circumstances. The presenting problem is considered to be a contributory factor and does not need to be present to the degree specified.

* Physicians from other groups providing services on the same date will report other appropriate outpatient E/M services based on the services provided and payer requirements. Chapter 7, Evaluation and Management Services in the Office, Outpatient, Home, or Nursing Facility Setting, addresses the guidelines for selection of codes **99241–99245** and **99201–99215**.

* Place of service code **22** (on campus—outpatient hospital) is reported with observation service codes. (See Chapter 19, The Business of Medicine: Working With Current and Emerging Payment Systems, for more information on place of service codes.)

* Selection of the code is dependent on the performance and documentation of all 3 key components. Time may be used as the key controlling factor in the selection of the code if more than 50% of the total face-to-face encounter and/or floor/unit time is spent in counseling and/or coordination of care.

* Observation care codes are not reported for initial care of hospital-born neonates.

Use **Table 10-2** to help you in the selection of the appropriate codes in the following clinical examples:

Examples

➤ **A 3-year-old girl is admitted to observation for vomiting and diarrhea with dehydration.** *History:* Parents report vomiting and diarrhea for 2 days and the patient is not keeping liquids down. She has had a fever to 102.0°F (38.9°C) and is sluggish with decreased urine output. She has no respiratory symptoms or rashes and remainder of a complete system review is negative. She attends child care. Past and family histories are noncontributory. Immunizations including rotavirus are up-to-date.

Physical examination: Detailed-level examination includes vital signs, general appearance, extended examination of abdomen (notations of no masses or tenderness, no enlargement of liver or spleen,

> Report code **A08.4**, viral intestinal infection, unspecified, as the infectious agent had not been identified at the end of this encounter.

and no hernia), and examination of related organ systems (ears, nose, mouth and throat, lymphatic, cardiovascular, respiratory, and skin).

Assessment/plan: Moderate dehydration secondary to acute viral gastroenteritis. Will rehydrate with intravenous (IV) fluids and monitor electrolytes, urine output, and weight. Stool is to be tested for rotavirus. Appropriate infection precautions are taken.

MDM: Moderate complexity *History:* Comprehensive *Physical examination:* Detailed	***International Classification of Diseases, 10th Revision, Clinical Modification (ICD-10-CM)*** **A08.4** (viral intestinal infection, unspecified) **E86.0** (dehydration)
	CPT® **99218** (requires at least detailed history and examination and straightforward or low MDM)

Teaching Point: Remember, all 3 key components must be met for the level of initial observation care reported. The level of history is comprehensive with extended history of present illness (duration: 2 days; severity: not keeping liquids down; associated signs and symptoms: fever and sluggish; context: immunizations up-to-date), complete review of systems, and complete past, family, and social history (social: attends child care; past and family: noncontributory). (*Note:* Some payers may not accept "noncontributory" as sufficient for documentation of past and family histories without further documentation. This would reduce the level of history to detailed but would not affect the level of service in this example.) The examination is detailed. Medical decision-making is moderate based on a new problem with additional workup and risk associated with an undiagnosed new problem. The detailed examination limits reporting of this service to code **99218**, even though the history and MDM meet or exceed requirements for code **99219**.

➤ **A 3-year-old girl is admitted to observation for vomiting and diarrhea with dehydration.** *History:* Parents report that she has vomited about 10 times over the last 24 hours with frequent watery, non-bloody stools. She has become sluggish and has a decreased urinary output. She is unable to keep any liquids down. She had a fever to 102.0°F (38.9°C) last night and was given acetaminophen but vomited it back up. Past history includes no food intolerances and no surgeries. Family history includes a maternal aunt who is lactose intolerant. Social history includes child care attendance and no tobacco use in the home.

Physical examination: Comprehensive-level examination includes vital signs, general appearance, and examination of the mucous membranes, neck, lymph nodes, ears, eyes, heart, lungs, gastrointestinal system, and skin.

Assessment/plan: Moderate dehydration secondary to acute viral gastroenteritis. Will rehydrate with IV fluids and monitor electrolytes, urine, and weight. Stool is to be tested for rotavirus. Appropriate infection precautions are taken.

MDM: Moderate complexity *History:* Comprehensive *Physical examination:* Comprehensive	***ICD-10-CM*** **A08.4** **E86.0**
	CPT **99219** (requires at least comprehensive history and examination and moderate MDM)

Teaching Point: The examination in this example includes 8 organ systems (constitutional; eyes; ears, nose, mouth, and throat; lymphatic; cardiovascular; respiratory; gastrointestinal; and skin) to support a comprehensive examination.

Chapter 10: Noncritical Hospital Evaluation and Management Services

➤ **An established patient presents to her physician's office on Monday.** During the evaluation of the patient, the physician decides to admit to observation care for further treatment and monitoring for acute pyelonephritis and dehydration. The physician does not see the patient in the observation setting until the next morning (Tuesday) but phones in orders and keeps in touch with the nursing staff. On Tuesday, the physician performs an initial observation care service (detailed history and examination, moderate-complexity MDM) on the patient and determines the patient is not improving enough to be discharged.

Monday's visit	*ICD-10-CM* **E86.0** **N10** (acute pyelonephritis)
	CPT® **99212–99215** (office E/M, established patient)
Tuesday's visit	*CPT* **99218** (initial observation care) Same diagnosis codes as Monday's visit

Teaching Point: Initial observation care and initial inpatient care (**99218–99220, 99221–99223**) require a face-to-face service with the patient by the reporting physician in the facility. Entry of the history, physical examination, and orders directly into a facility electronic health record by online connection without a face-to-face visit in the facility does not support reporting. Also, an outpatient office building connected physically to the hospital does not count as seen in facility.

➤ **Same patient; however, the physician sees the patient in the hospital on Monday.** The combined E/M service in the office and hospital results in a comprehensive history and physical examination with moderately complex MDM.

Monday's services	*CPT* **99219** (initial observation care)

Subsequent Observation Care

99224–99226   Subsequent observation care, per day, for the evaluation and management of a patient
* Codes include all E/M services by a physician or physician group provided on a given day.
* Level of service reported will be dependent on the total services provided and documented.
* Codes require that 2 of the 3 key components be performed and documented. Some payers may require MDM as 1 of the 2 key components performed and documented.
* Time may be used as the key controlling factor in the selection of the code if more than 50% of the total face-to-face encounter (ie, floor/unit time) is spent in counseling and/or coordination of care.
* The history component required for subsequent observation visits is considered interval history (ie, new history obtained since the last physician assessment, including history of present illness and problem-pertinent system review). A past, family, and social history is not required.
* Because the individual documentation for each encounter should contain all information necessary to determine the level of service provided, it is important to document the chief complaint and other factors of the patient presentation that affect management at each encounter.

When reporting subsequent observation services, the status of the patient is often an indicator of the medically necessary level of service. *Current Procedural Terminology* indicates the patient status for each level of subsequent observation care.

99224: Usually, the patient is stable, recovering, or improving.

99225: Usually, the patient is responding inadequately to therapy or has developed a minor complication.

99226: Usually, the patient is unstable or has developed a significant complication or a significant new problem.

Use **Table 10-3** to help you select the appropriate codes in the clinical example.

Table 10-3. Subsequent Observation and Inpatient Hospital Care				

Key Components (For a description of key components, see Table 10-1.)
2 of 3 key components must be performed to at least the degree specified for the codes in each row.

CPT® Code/Time[a]	Medical Decision-making[b]	History[c]	Examination
99224 15 min 99231 15 min	Straightforward to low PP: Usually stable, recovering, or improving	Problem focused	Problem focused
99225 25 min 99232 25 min	Moderate complexity PP: Usually responding inadequately to therapy or minor complication	Expanded	Expanded
99226 35 min 99233 35 min	High complexity PP: Usually patient is unstable or develops significant complication or new problem.	Detailed	Detailed

Abbreviations: CPT, Current Procedural Terminology; PP, presenting problem.

[a] Typical time is an average and represents a range of times that may be higher or lower depending on clinical circumstances. When counseling and/or coordination of care dominates the encounter, time shall be the controlling factor.

[b] The presenting problem is considered to be a contributory factor and does not need to be present to the degree specified.

[c] Past, family, and social histories are not required for interval history.

Example

➤ **7:00 am: A 3-year-old girl is seen for subsequent observation care for vomiting and diarrhea with dehydration.** She is experiencing occasional diarrhea and vomiting but is now tolerating sips of liquids. The patient has a low-grade fever without abdominal discomfort. Vital signs are stable and examination of skin, heart, lungs, and abdomen is normal. Diagnostic test results are negative. The plan is to continue IV fluids until vomiting and diarrhea decrease and patient is eating soft foods.

MDM: Straightforward or low complexity *History:* Expanded problem focused *Physical examination:* Expanded problem focused	***ICD-10-CM*** **E86.0** (dehydration) **R19.7** (diarrhea) **R11.10** (vomiting)
	CPT **99225**

Teaching Point: The patient in this example is improving. Medical decision-making is straightforward or low depending on whether tests reviewed were from one or more sections of *CPT* (laboratory, radiology, or medicine). A payer may require MDM as one of the 2 key components to support subsequent observation care, which would reduce the level of service to **99224**.

Observation Care Discharge Day Management

99217   Observation care discharge day management

Code **99217** is to be used to report all services provided to a patient on discharge from "observation status" (ie, final examination of the patient, discussion of the hospital stay, counseling, instructions for continuing care, and preparation of discharge records) if the discharge is on a day other than the initial date of observation status.

❖ Performance of the key components is not required.

❖ Observation care discharge services are not assigned a typical time.

Example

➤ **Same patient as previous example (ie, patient with dehydration).** Patient is fully alert and interactive. She experienced no vomiting overnight; diarrhea has decreased. The patient has a low-grade fever with no abdominal pain. She is tolerating fluids and had cereal this morning. Parents are now comfortable with discharge home.

Physical examination: vital signs and examination of skin, heart, lungs, and abdomen. *Assessment/plan:* resolving gastroenteritis, most likely viral. Instructions for home care and follow-up are given.

ICD-10-CM	CPT®
K52.9 (acute gastroenteritis)	**99217** (observation care discharge day management)

Observation or Inpatient Hospital Care Services (Including Admission and Discharge Services)

99234–99236 Observation or inpatient hospital care, for the evaluation and management of a patient including admission and discharge on the same date

When a patient is admitted and discharged from observation or inpatient services on the *same date of service,* report codes **99234–99236**.

❁ Selection of the code is based on the performance and documentation of all 3 key components and includes the combined services provided by the same physician or physician of the same specialty within a group during a calendar day.

❁ Time may be used as the key controlling factor in the selection of the code if more than 50% of the total face-to-face encounter (eg, floor/unit time) is spent in counseling and/or coordination of care.

❁ Except where payer guidance specifies otherwise, reporting of initial observation or inpatient care is based on the date of the face-to-face assessment, and not the date of admission or designation of a status by a facility on physician order.

Use **Table 10-2** to review the required components used to select level of service in the following examples:

Examples

➤ **6:00 am: A 3-year-old girl is admitted to observation for vomiting and diarrhea with dehydration.** Encounter includes comprehensive history and examination and MDM of moderate complexity. Physician returns to the hospital at 7:00 pm.

7:00 pm: Patient has occasional diarrhea without vomiting and is now tolerating sips of liquids. She has a low-grade fever without abdominal discomfort. Vital signs are stable and examination of skin, heart, lungs, and abdomen is normal. Diagnostic test results are negative. Diagnosis is resolving viral gastroenteritis. Parents are comfortable with taking child home. Discharge instructions are given.

Face-to-face services performed include initial care and discharge management. A code from the **99234–99236** series would be reported because observation admission and discharge services were provided on the same date.

| MDM: Moderate complexity
History: Comprehensive
Physical examination: Comprehensive | ICD-10-CM
A08.4 (viral gastroenteritis) |
| | CPT
99235 |

Teaching Point: Physicians participating in quality initiatives may elect to additionally report *CPT* Category II performance measure codes to indicate specific elements of care were provided (eg, **4058F**, pediatric gastroenteritis education provided to caregiver). Category II codes are not used for direct fee-for-service payment. For more on Category II codes, see Chapter 17, Coding to Demonstrate Quality and Value.

➤ **On Monday evening, a physician admits a 4-year-old patient by phone to observation care for acute viral laryngotracheitis (croup).** On Tuesday morning, the physician performs a face-to-face service in the observation setting. The physician performs a comprehensive history and physical examination with low-complexity MDM. Later that day, the physician determines the patient has improved enough to be discharged and performs the discharge service.

Monday's service	**CPT®** There is no *CPT* code to report for this service.
Tuesday's visit *MDM:* Low complexity *History:* Comprehensive *Physical examination:* Comprehensive	**ICD-10-CM** **J05.0** (croup)
	CPT **99234** (observation care, same-day admission and discharge)

Teaching Point: If reporting to a payer that has adopted Medicare policy on same-date admission and discharge services, the physician must document that the patient was in observation or inpatient status for a minimum of 8 hours and no more than 24 hours. Therefore, it is important that the physician document the length of time spent in observation or inpatient status when admission and discharge occur on the same date of service. See the Reporting to Payers Using Medicare Policy section later in this chapter for more information on Medicare requirements.

➤ **An established patient is seen in the physician's office with acute viral laryngotracheitis (croup) and admitted for observation at 6:00 pm on Tuesday.** The attending physician telephones the observation admission orders and does not see the child again until the next morning (Wednesday). On Wednesday, the physician completes a history and physical examination and discharges the child.

Tuesday's visit	**ICD-10-CM** **J05.0** (croup)
	CPT **99211–99215** (office E/M, established patient)
Wednesday's visit	**CPT** **99234–99236** (observation care, same-day admission and discharge) Same diagnosis code as was reported for Tuesday's visit

➤ **A 4-year-old patient with croup is admitted from the ED at 6:00 am on Monday.** A physician from a different group than the ED physician sees the child that morning and performs the initial history and physical examination. Another physician from the attending physician's group practice returns to the hospital at 5:00 pm and, after evaluation of the child, discharges the patient home. The combined service is a comprehensive history and physical examination with moderate-level MDM.

MDM: Moderate complexity *History:* Comprehensive *Physical examination:* Comprehensive	**ICD-10-CM** **J05.0** (croup)
	CPT **99235** (observation care, same-day admission and discharge)

➤ **A 14-year-old patient is seen in the ED at 8:00 am on Monday after falling while riding his skateboard to school.** Witnesses reported brief loss of consciousness and the emergency medical technician reported disorientation at the time of transport. The ED physician consults the patient's pediatrician, who orders observation care to rule out clinically significant brain injury. The pediatrician visits the patient and provides initial observation care, including a comprehensive history and physical examination with moderate-level MDM, finding the patient has a moderately severe headache and mild nausea. Later the same day, the patient experiences seizures and repeated vomiting. After reexamining the patient, the pediatrician orders admission, computerized tomography, and a neurologic consultation. The pediatrician's combined services include a comprehensive history and examination and high-complexity MDM. Assessment is closed head injury with concussion.

If payer or state mandates require reporting of all external cause of injury information, document and report the cause, intent (when applicable), place of occurrence, activity, and patient status (eg, employee, volunteer, at leisure) at the time of the event. Place of occurrence, activity, and status are reported only for the initial encounter for care of an injury.	
MDM: High complexity *History:* Comprehensive *Physical examination:* Comprehensive	***ICD-10-CM*** **S06.0X1A** (initial encounter for concussion with loss of consciousness of 30 minutes or less) **V00.131A** (initial encounter for fall from skateboard)
	***CPT*®** **99223** (initial hospital care)

Teaching Point: Observation care is not separately reported when initial hospital care is provided on the same date by the same physician or physicians of the same group and specialty.

Reporting to Payers Using Medicare Policy

Medicaid and private payers may adopt a Medicare policy that limits reporting of codes **99234–99236** to services provided to a patient who was admitted to observation or inpatient status for at least 8 hours and not more than 24 hours. Under this policy, when a patient is admitted to observation or inpatient care for less than 8 hours on the same calendar date, only the initial observation (**99218–99220**) or inpatient care (**99221–99223**) shall be reported by the physician. A separate code for discharge services is not reported.

Medicare also requires that there must be a medical observation record for the patient that contains dated and timed physician's orders for the observation services the patient is to receive, nursing notes, and progress notes prepared by the physician indicating physical presence and personal performance of services. This record must be in addition to any record prepared as a result of an ED or outpatient clinic encounter.

> **~ More From the AAP ~**
>
> For more information on reporting observation care services, see "Observation Care Services: *CPT* or Medicare" in the August 2014 *AAP Pediatric Coding Newsletter*™ at http://coding. aap.org (subscription required).

Inpatient Hospital Care

Initial Inpatient Hospital Care

99221–99223   Initial hospital care, per day, for the evaluation and management of a patient
* Initial inpatient hospital service codes are used to report initial face-to-face services provided to a hospital inpatient.
* Initial inpatient encounters by more than one physician must be reported based on payer guidelines. (See the Coding Conundrum: 2 Physicians Providing Initial Observation or Inpatient Hospital Day Services box earlier in this chapter.)

Chapter 10: Noncritical Hospital Evaluation and Management Services

- Selection of the code is based on performance and documentation of the 3 key components or time, if more than 50% of the encounter is spent in counseling and/or coordination of care (see **Table 10-2**).
- If the level of history and physical examination performed and documented is expanded or problem focused, initial inpatient hospital care must be reported using subsequent hospital visit codes **99231–99233** because the required key components for code **99221** (ie, at least a detailed history and detailed examination) have not been met.
- The code is reported on the first day that a face-to-face (physician-patient) service is provided.
- The date of initial hospital care that the physician reports does not need to correlate with the facility's date of admission.
- Report only an initial hospital care code when a patient is admitted to inpatient status from observation status. Use **Table 10-2** to review the required components used to select level of service in the following examples:

Examples

➤ **An 8-week-old is seen in the ED and admitted by physician A.** Over the past 2 days, the mother reported that the infant seemed warm to the touch, fed much less than normal, and had been harder to arouse. The mother had noticed only 2 wet diapers and one stool in the past 24 hours.

Review of systems: Fever, no history of heart murmur, no apnea or cyanosis, no wheeze or respiratory distress. *Past, family, and social history:* Full-term male, no reported problems with pregnancy or delivery, delivered by repeat cesarean. No maternal complications with delivery; rupture of membranes at the time of cesarean delivery, no fever prior to cesarean delivery; no prior ED visits or hospitalizations since birth hospitalization, no sick contacts at home, and lives with parents and 2 older female siblings. Two-month well-child vaccinations were received last week. *Physical examination:* Comprehensive examination includes vital signs and general appearance with examination of head, mucous membranes, clavicles, heart, lungs, abdomen, hips, genitalia, and skin. *Assessment:* Laboratory evaluation: complete blood cell count with white blood cells 12,000, no left shift on differential; urinalysis normal or negative with pH 7.0, specific gravity 1.020; fever, concern for sepsis or serious bacterial infection, doubt pyelonephritis given normal urinalysis, less likely meningitis given normal examination and not ill appearing, doubt bronchiolitis given lack of viral symptoms.

Plan: Admit for IV antibiotics, pending culture results. Continue breastfeeding ad lib. Discussed differential diagnoses, working diagnosis, current diagnostic and treatment plans, and anticipated hospital course with parents.

MDM: Moderate complexity History: Detailed Physical examination: Comprehensive	**ICD-10-CM** **R50.9** (fever, unspecified)
	CPT® **99221**

➤ **Later that same calendar day, physician B from the same group practice sees the infant.** She performs a more comprehensive history, examines the infant, and spends 20 minutes talking with the parents.

MDM: Moderate complexity History: Comprehensive Physical examination: Comprehensive	**ICD-10-CM** **R50.9**
	CPT **99222**

Teaching Point: The total E/M services provided on this date now meet the guidelines for a comprehensive history. Physician B may now report the service with code **99222**. Physician A would submit no bill for his work that day.

If physician A performed a comprehensive history and physical examination with moderate-complexity MDM at the initial hospital visit and documents that he spent 25 minutes on the floor with the patient and family, the service would be reported with code **99222**. However, later that same calendar day, physician

B (same specialty and from the same practice) sees the patient. She documents that 35 of her 40 minutes on the floor were spent counseling the parents and coordinating the patient's care. The code for all the care provided on that calendar day would now be reported using code **99223** based on the documented floor/unit time (total of 65 minutes between the 2 physicians, with 35 minutes spent in counseling/coordination of care). Physician A would submit no bill and physician B would submit the bill for the calendar day's service. Coding based on time is further discussed in Chapter 5, Time-Based Coding.

Subsequent Hospital Care

99231–99233   Subsequent hospital care, per day, for the evaluation and management of a patient

* Codes include all E/M services by a physician or physician group provided on a given subsequent day.
* The level of service reported will be dependent on the total services provided and documented.
* Selection of the code is based on performance and documentation of 2 of the 3 key components or time if more than 50% of the encounter is spent in counseling and/or coordination of care (see **Table 10-3**).
* The history component required for subsequent hospital visits is considered interval history (ie, new history information obtained since the last physician assessment, including chief complaint, history of present illness, and problem-pertinent system review).

> |||||||| **Coding Pearl** ||||||||
>
> Past, family, and social history is not required as part of an interval history.

Use **Table 10-3** to help you in the selection of the appropriate codes in the following examples:

Examples

➤ **No reported problems overnight; breastfeeding well, continues to have low-grade fever (100.7°F [38.2°C] maximum) overnight, no reported apnea or cyanosis, no respiratory distress.**
   Physical examination: Expanded-level examination, including vital signs and general appearance, heart, lungs, and skin.
   Laboratory: No growth in blood or urine cultures at less than 24 hours.
   Assessment/plan: Continued fever; concern for sepsis, suspect viral etiology given negative workup so far for common serious bacterial infections, such as pyelonephritis and bacteremia. Continue IV antibiotics until culture results are negative for 48 hours; continue breastfeeding ad lib. Spoke with mom and reviewed overnight events, morning laboratory results, current plan, and possible discharge home tomorrow.

MDM: Straightforward complexity *History:* Expanded interval history *Physical examination:* Expanded	***ICD-10-CM*** **R50.9** (fever)
	***CPT*®** **99232**

   Teaching Point: Time cannot be used as the controlling factor in selection of the code because the documentation does not indicate the total floor/unit time or time spent in counseling and/or coordination of care.
   In this example, the risk is moderate with an undiagnosed problem requiring IV antibiotics. However, the diagnosis and management options are limited to an established problem that is stable. The amount and complexity of data reviewed was limited to laboratory results. With 2 of 3 elements required to support the level of MDM, it is straightforward. A payer may require MDM as 1 of 2 key components supporting subsequent hospital care. This example would be limited to code **99231** if MDM were a required component.

➤ **Same progress note as in previous vignette but with additional documentation.**
   Spoke with mom for 30 minutes and reviewed overnight events, morning laboratory results, and current plan; anticipate discharge home tomorrow. Total visit time: 40 minutes.
   Time would be used as the controlling factor in selection of the code because a total of 40 minutes was spent on the unit/floor with the patient and more than 50% of the time was spent in counseling. The appropriate code would be **99233**.

Hospital Discharge Day Management

99238   Hospital discharge day management; 30 minutes or less
99239   more than 30 minutes

> |||||||| **Coding Pearl** ||||||||
>
> If the total time spent in performing discharge management is not documented in the medical record, report code **99238** instead of **99239**.

Codes **99238** (≤30 minutes) and **99239** (>30 minutes) are reported by the attending physician providing discharge services on a day subsequent to the date that the admission service was provided.

- A face-to-face physician-patient encounter in the hospital is required.
- Reporting is based on the total time (time does not have to be continuous) spent performing all final discharge services, including, as appropriate, examination of the patient, discussion of the hospital stay, patient and/or family counseling, instructions for continuing care to all relevant caregivers, and preparation of referral forms, prescriptions, and records.
- May be used to report discharge services provided to patients who die during their hospital stay.
- Services are reported on the day the physician sees the patient and performs discharge services, even if the patient leaves the hospital on a different day.
- Only the attending physician or physician providing services on behalf of the attending physician (eg, covering physician, physician of same group and same specialty) may report discharge management services. If another physician is providing concurrent care, his or her services would be reported using subsequent hospital visit codes (**99231–99233**).

> |||||||| **Coding Pearl** ||||||||
>
> Only unit or floor time spent on the date of the discharge management is reported with codes **99238** and **99239**. Do not include time spent documenting discharge on a date after the service was rendered.

- Time spent in discharge services must be documented in the medical record to report code **99239**. If the total time spent performing the discharge management is not documented in the medical record, report code **99238** instead of **99239**. Only time spent on the day of discharge may be counted.
- Time spent on the day of discharge performing separately reported services (eg, car seat testing) is not included in the discharge day management time.

Example

➤ **Continued on IV antibiotics until this morning, breastfeeding well, no further fevers.** Vital signs and general appearance and examination of the heart, lungs, abdomen, and skin are performed. Blood and urine culture results remain negative after 48 hours. Intravenous antibiotics are discontinued. Patient is discharged home with instructions for home care and follow-up. The physician spent 35 minutes on the floor reviewing the hospital course, expected follow-up, and signs and symptoms of possible sepsis or infection with mother.

This visit would be reported with code **99239** because 35 minutes was spent in the provision of discharge management services and the time was documented in the medical record.

Discharge Versus Subsequent Hospital Services

Codes **99238** and **99239** are underused and often reported incorrectly. Subsequent hospital visit codes should not be reported on the day of discharge alone or in addition to the discharge code. Code **99239** is one of the most underreported *CPT*® codes, even though it often more accurately reflects the service performed! Physicians often spend more than 30 minutes in discharge management, especially when the patient is seen several times that day. Time spent in charting *on the day of discharge* is counted in the total unit/floor time.

Note: The 2018 relative value units (RVUs) were not available at time of publication.

CPT Code	2017 Medicare RVUs
99231	1.11
99232	2.04
99233	2.95
99238	2.05
99239	3.04

Teaching Point: The RVUs for discharge service codes reflect the additional services provided on the day of discharge.

Unique Considerations for Hospital Services

Admission to the hospital after a visit in the office and hospital rounds by more than one physician can create unusual circumstances. Proper coding in these situations will be contingent on whether the attending physician and colleagues provide coverage, bill under the same group name and tax identification number, or bill independently using individual tax identification numbers.

Office Visit and Initial Hospital Care on Same Day of Service

The primary care physician examines the patient in the office and a colleague admits the patient to the hospital later the same day for the same problem. If using independent billing numbers, each physician would submit a separate bill (ie, the primary care physician would bill for the office visit; the colleague would bill for the observation or inpatient hospital admission). If using the same billing number, services should be combined into one initial hospital care code encompassing the combined work of the 2 encounters. If the 2 encounters are not related and have different diagnoses, there is a legitimate reason to submit a claim for 2 distinct E/M services on the same day, even by the same provider, but be prepared to justify payment. Alternatively, bundle the 2 encounters, including all appropriate *ICD-10-CM* codes. If 2 distinct E/M services are reported on the same day of service by the same provider, append modifier **25** to the second service.

Two Hospital Visits on Same Day of Service

The primary care physician admits the patient to the hospital in the morning and a colleague is called to see the patient in the evening. If using independent National Provider Identifiers, separate bills are submitted. If using the same National Provider Identifier number, the services are combined.

When office or outpatient E/M and hospital admissions occur on the same calendar day, coding will depend on whether the admitting physician and/or physician of the same group and specialty provides face-to-face care in the hospital setting.

Office Visit Without Face-to-face Encounter in Hospital

The primary care physician examines an established patient in the office and determines the patient needs admission. The admission history and physical examination are performed, and a treatment plan and orders are sent to the hospital. The physician remains in communication with the hospital nurses that night as the child improves and sees the child the next morning on rounds—he is stable but not ready for discharge. The office visit on day 1 would be reported with code **99212–99215** (office/outpatient E/M service, established patient) based on the performance and documentation of the required key components. The second day's work is reported using initial hospital care or observation care codes (**99221–99223** or **99218–99220**) based on the level of work (ie, history, physical examination, and MDM or time) performed on the hospital floor on that day of service. If the work performed on the second day did not meet the required key components, the service would be reported using subsequent-day codes (**99224–99226, 99231–99233**).

Office Visit and Inpatient Encounter on Same Day of Service

The physician (or physician of the same group) provides face-to-face services in the hospital later that same day. The level of initial hospital care service will then be based on the combination of the E/M services provided during that calendar day.

Coordinating billing is important. The office billing manager should have all hospital charges for each patient by the end of the next business day to coordinate billing and avoid delays in claims submissions.

Teaching Physician Encounter on Day After Admission

If a resident provides the only face-to-face encounter on the date a patient is admitted to inpatient or observation status and the attending physician provides an initial face-to-face encounter on the next day, the physician reports the encounter based on the extent of work performed. If documentation clearly supports the work of an initial encounter (**99221–99223** or **99218–99220**), this service may be reported because these services are reported for the initial encounter without regard to the date of admission. However, if the encounter involves a more limited interval assessment, subsequent encounter services (**99231–99233** or **99224–99226**) or same-day admission and discharge services (**99234–99236**) are likely more appropriate.

Consultations

Current Procedural Terminology® defines *consultations* as services provided by a physician at the request of another physician or "other appropriate source" to provide advice or opinion about the management or evaluation of a specific problem. Medicare does not recognize consultation codes but pays for the services using codes for other E/M services. Detailed information on the *CPT* and CMS Medicare guidelines for reporting consultations for office and outpatient consultations appears in Chapter 7, Evaluation and Management Services in the Office, Outpatient, Home, or Nursing Facility Setting. Please review those guidelines carefully as general guidelines that apply for all consultations.

Consultation codes should not be reported by the physician who has agreed to accept transfer of care before an initial evaluation. Consultation codes are appropriate to report if the decision to accept transfer of care cannot be made until after the initial consultation evaluation, regardless of site of service. See Chapter 7 for the definition of *transfer of care* versus consultation.

Guidelines Used by Payers That Do Not Follow Medicare Consultation Guidelines

Consultations for Patients in Observation

99241–99245   Office consultation for a new or established patient (includes consultations in other outpatient settings)

* Level of care is determined by performing and documenting the required 3 key components (history, physical examination, and MDM) or time (**Table 10-4**) as described for other E/M services that are assigned a typical time. Follow-up visits that are initiated by the physician consultant are reported using codes for subsequent observation care services (**99224–99226**).

* If an additional request for an opinion or advice on the same or a new problem is received from the attending physician and documented in the medical record, office or outpatient consultation codes, unlike inpatient consultation codes, may be used again.

* When reporting prolonged physician care with consultations that are performed in the observation care setting, report the office or other outpatient setting prolonged services code (**99354, 99355**) in addition to the appropriate outpatient consultation code (**99241–99245**) or appropriate other outpatient service code (**99201–99205, 99212–99215**). See Chapter 7, Evaluation and Management Services in the Office, Outpatient, Home, or Nursing Facility Setting, for more information.

Use **Table 10-4** to help you in the selection of the appropriate codes in the following example:

||||||| *Coding Pearl* |||||||

Consultation codes are not reported when a transfer of care occurs before the patient is seen.

Example

➤ **A 14-year-old is admitted to observation for closed head trauma and possible concussion after a fall from his skateboard with brief loss of consciousness.** The attending physician consults a pediatric neurologist for her opinion and advice. The neurologist performs a detailed history and physical examination, reviews computed tomography images, and orders additional diagnostic studies. Documentation of the written report is included in the shared medical record. Assessment is concussion with brief loss of consciousness. The neurologist reports the service with

MDM: Moderate History: Detailed Physical examination: Detailed	*ICD-10-CM* **S06.0X1A** (initial encounter for concussion with loss of consciousness of 30 minutes or less) **V00.131A** (initial encounter for fall from skateboard)
	CPT **99243** or, if payer does not recognize consultations, **New Patient** **Established Patient** **99203** (office/outpatient E/M) **99214** (office/outpatient E/M)

Table 10-4. Observation (99241–99245) and Inpatient (99251–99255) Consultation Codes

Key Components (For a description of key components, see Table 10-1.)
3 of 3 key components must be performed to at least the degree specified under the code.

CPT® Code/Time[a]	Medical Decision-making	History	Examination
99241 15 min 99251 20 min	Straightforward	Problem focused	Problem focused
99242 30 min 99252 40 min	Straightforward	Expanded	Expanded
99243 40 min 99253 55 min	Low complexity	Detailed	Detailed
99244 60 min 99254 80 min	Moderate complexity	Comprehensive	Comprehensive
99245 80 min 99255 110 min	High complexity	Comprehensive	Comprehensive

Abbreviation: CPT, Current Procedural Terminology.

[a] Typical time is an average and represents a range of times that may be higher or lower depending on clinical circumstances. The presenting problem is considered to be a contributory factor and does not need to be present to the degree specified.

Inpatient Consultations

99251–99255   Inpatient consultation for a new or established patient

❋ Codes **99251–99255** are to be used only once by the reporting physician for an individual hospital patient for a particular admission. There are no specific guidelines for the length of stay.

❋ Follow-up visits provided in the hospital by the same physician must be reported using subsequent care codes (**99231–99233**). Examples of a follow-up visit might be to complete the initial consultation when test results become available or in response to a change in the patient's status.

❋ If a consultation is requested by the attending physician for the same patient on a completely different problem during the same hospital stay, subsequent hospital care codes (**99231–99233**) must be reported. The subsequent role of a consultant in the ongoing care of the patient must be made clear in the medical record by the attending physician. If the attending physician turns over the care of the patient to the consultant, the consultant, now the new attending physician, should use subsequent hospital care codes (**99231–99233**) to indicate the level of service provided.

❋ The attending physician and consultant may continue to provide care to the patient. Each would code for subsequent hospital care as long as the problems they manage are different. (The attending and consulting physicians should use different *diagnosis* codes to indicate they are managing different problems. However, sometimes, the diagnosis will be the same.)

❋ If a patient is readmitted for the same or different problem (a new hospital stay), an initial inpatient consultation code may be reported if it meets the definition and requirements for reporting a consultation.

> A diagnosis of congenital volvulus would be reported with *ICD-10-CM* code **Q43.8**, other specified congenital malformation of the intestine.

Chapter 10: Noncritical Hospital Evaluation and Management Services

※ When an inpatient consultation is performed on a date a patient is admitted to the hospital, all E/M services provided by the consultant (including any outpatient encounters) related to the admission are reported with the inpatient consultation service code. If a patient is admitted after an outpatient consultation (eg, office, ED) and the patient is not seen on the unit on the date of admission, only the outpatient consultation code is reported.

Use **Table 10-4** to help you in the selection of the appropriate codes in the following examples:

Examples

➤ **A 3-month-old patient is seen by the pediatrician in the ED and is subsequently admitted for bilious vomiting, dehydration, and possible bowel obstruction.** A gastroenterologist is consulted and, following workup, diagnoses volvulus due to congenital malrotation of intestine. He documents his written report in the medical record, speaks to the parents, and agrees to follow the patient. The gastroenterologist reports his consultation service with

MDM: High complexity *History:* Comprehensive *Physical examination:* Comprehensive	**ICD-10-CM** **K56.2** (volvulus) **Q43.3** (congenital malformations of intestinal fixation)
	CPT® **99255** or, if payer does not recognize consultations, **99223** (initial hospital visit)

Teaching Point: Follow-up visits by the gastroenterologist are reported using the appropriate-level subsequent inpatient hospital codes (**99231–99233**).

➤ **A neonatologist is asked by an obstetrician to consult with a mother in preterm labor with triplets at 23 weeks' gestation.** She is being treated with steroids and magnesium sulfate. The neonatologist reviews the maternal prenatal and hospital record, interviews the mother, and meets with both parents to discuss fetal and neonatal risks and likely hospital course and complications if delivered in the next few days. The neonatologist spends a total of 65 minutes of floor/unit time devoted to this patient's consultation, which is dominated by discussing morbidity and mortality risks and resuscitation and possible treatment.

Inpatient floor/unit time (65 minutes) is the key controlling factor.	**ICD-10-CM** **O60.02** (preterm labor without delivery, second trimester) **O30.102** (triplet pregnancy, unspecified number of placenta and unspecified number of amniotic sacs, second trimester)
	CPT **99253** (typical time 55 minutes) or, if payer does not recognize consultations, **99223** (average 70 minutes)

Teaching Point: Pediatric hospital care may, at times, begin prior to birth with services provided to the mother during the peripartum period. Although it is atypical for pediatric claims to be submitted for services to adult patients, these services rendered to the mother are an exception. Services provided prior to delivery are reported as services to the mother (ie, to the mother's health insurance plan).

Guidelines Used by Payers That Follow Medicare Consultation Guidelines

Medicare guidelines require that consultations provided to patients in observation status will be reported with office or outpatient E/M codes **99201–99215**. If the patient is new to the physician (ie, has not received any face-to-face professional services from the physician or another physician of the same specialty who belongs to the same group practice within the past 3 years), codes **99201–99205** are reported based on the performance and documentation of the required key components. If the patient does not meet the requirements of a new patient, an established patient office or outpatient E/M code is reported.

Consultations provided to inpatient hospital patients are reported using initial inpatient hospital care codes (**99221–99223**). The admitting physician must report the initial hospital care services with modifier **AI** (principal physician of record) appended to the appropriate code to distinguish the services from the consulting physician. Subsequent face-to-face services, including new consultations within the same admission, are reported with subsequent hospital care codes **99231–99233**.

Check with your commercial payers to learn if they follow Medicare consultation guidelines or have otherwise adopted consultation guidelines that differ from *CPT®*.

Concurrent Care

Concurrent care is defined by *CPT* as the provision of similar services to the same patient by more than one physician on the same day. Concurrent care may be provided by physicians from different practices or physicians of the same practice but different specialties. When concurrent care is provided, the diagnosis code(s) reported by each physician should reflect the medical necessity for the provision of services by more than one physician on the same *date* of service. Although it is easier to justify concurrent care when each treating physician reports different diagnoses, if the *diagnosis* code is reported for the same condition, it does not prevent billing for the services.

> **~ More From the AAP ~**
>
> For more information on concurrent care, see "Concurrent Care: A Refresher" in the May 2014 *AAP Pediatric Coding Newsletter*™ at http://coding.aap.org (subscription required).

Example

➤ The attending physician wants the consultant to provide ongoing management of one problem (eg, heart failure) while the attending physician provides ongoing management for other active problems (eg, pneumonia, inadequate weight gain).

  Both physicians would report subsequent hospital care codes and link the *CPT* codes to the appropriate *diagnosis* codes.

Interprofessional Telephone/Internet Consultation

99446	Interprofessional telephone/Internet assessment and management service provided by a consultative physician including a verbal and written report to the patient's treating/requesting physician/qualified health care professional; 5–10 minutes of medical consultative discussion and review
99447	11–20 minutes of medical consultative discussion and review
99448	21–30 minutes of medical consultative discussion and review
99449	31 minutes or more of medical consultative discussion and review

A consultation request by a patient's attending or primary physician or other QHP soliciting opinion and/or treatment advice by telephone or Internet from a physician with specialty expertise (consultant) is reported by the consultant with interprofessional consultation codes **99446–99449**. This consultation does not require face-to-face contact with the patient by the consultant and often takes place when a timely face-to-face service with the consultant is not feasible (eg, consultant is geographically distant). The patient may be in the inpatient or outpatient setting. For information on reporting a face-to-face consultation provided via an interactive audiovisual telemedicine system, see Chapter 13, Telemedicine.

Guidelines for the consultant reporting interprofessional telephone/Internet consultations include

⁂ Telephone/Internet consultations of less than 5 minutes are not reported. Most of the time reported as interprofessional consultation must have been spent in medical consultative discussion (verbal or Internet).

⁂ A single interprofessional consultation code is reported for the cumulative time spent in discussion and information review regardless of the number of telephone or Internet contacts. The service is not reported more than once in a 7-day interval.

⁂ Time spent in telephone or online consultation with the patient and/or family may be reported using codes **99441–99444** or **98966–98968**.

⁂ When the purpose of communication is to arrange a transfer of care or face-to-face patient encounter, interprofessional consultation codes are not reported.

⁂ Interprofessional consultation services are not reported if the consultant has provided a face-to-face service to the patient within the past 14 days or when the consultation results in scheduling of a face-to-face service within the next 14 days or at the consultant's next available appointment date.

⁂ Time spent by the consultant reviewing pertinent medical records, studies, or other data is included in the telephone/Internet consultation and not separately reported.

⁂ As with all consultations, the request for advice or opinion should be documented in the patient record. A verbal opinion report and a written opinion report from the consultant must also be documented. This may require creation of a new patient record by the consultant.

See Chapter 7, Evaluation and Management Services in the Office, Outpatient, Home, or Nursing Facility Setting, for examples of interprofessional telephone/Internet consultations in the outpatient setting.

The requesting physician or QHP may report time spent in discussion with the consultant with an appropriate E/M service code according to site of service (when the patient is present for service) and/or prolonged service codes if the total time of discussion exceeds 30 minutes beyond the typical time of the associated E/M service. The prefatory language for interprofessional telephone/Internet consultations states that prolonged service codes **99354** and **99355** may be reported when the patient is present (on-site) and accessible to the requesting physician in the office or other outpatient setting during the time of service. Prolonged services without the patient present are reported with codes **99358** and **99359**. (See Chapter 7 for prolonged services in an outpatient setting.)

Examples

➤ **A physician at a rural hospital admits a child with acute lymphoblastic leukemia who developed a *Streptococcus pneumoniae* infection.** The physician communicates with the child's hematologist, who is located several hours away, via a secure health information exchange for advice about treatment. The hematologist spends a total of 25 minutes reviewing hospital records and communicating with the attending physician.

ICD-10-CM	CPT®	
Both physicians report **A49.1** (streptococcal infection, unspecified site) **C91.00** (acute lymphoblastic leukemia not having achieved remission)	The consultant reports **99448** (21–30 minutes of medical consultative discussion and review)	The pediatrician reports **99221–99223** (appropriate level of initial hospital care)
The categories for leukemia have codes indicating whether the leukemia has achieved remission. Coders are instructed to ask the physician for status if documentation is unclear.		

Teaching Point: The attending physician will report the appropriate level of hospital care (eg, **99223**); if the unit or floor time spent caring for this patient exceeds the typical time of the hospital care service by at least 30 minutes, the attending physician will also report inpatient prolonged services (**99356** and **99357**). Interprofessional consultation services would not be reported if the consultant has provided a face-to-face service to the patient within the past 14 days or if the consultation results in scheduling of a face-to-face service within the next 14 days or at the consultant's next available appointment date.

Chapter 10: Noncritical Hospital Evaluation and Management Services

► **A 2-day-old hospitalized newborn develops poor feeding and tachypnea and is diagnosed with group B streptococcal septicemia.** The patient's primary care physician telephones an infectious disease specialist located several hours away for treatment advice. The physicians spend 8 minutes discussing the child's condition and treatment options. The infectious disease specialist reports this service with

ICD-10-CM	CPT®
P36.0 (sepsis of newborn due to streptococcus, group B)	**99446** (interprofessional consultation, 5–10 minutes)

Teaching Point: The attending physician will include this work in the per diem charge for intensive or critical care services based on the type of care rendered.

Prolonged Evaluation and Management Services Provided in the Inpatient Setting

According to *CPT*, the prolonged services inpatient add-on codes **99356** and **99357** may be reported in addition to observation codes (**99218–99220, 99224–99226, 99234–99236**) because, although observation care services are performed in an "outpatient" setting, the intraservice times for the codes are defined as unit or floor time rather than face-to-face time as required in the office or outpatient setting. Prolonged service codes (**tables 10-5 and 10-6**) are reported when a physician provides services that are beyond the usual service duration described in an E/M code or other codes with a published maximum time. The codes for prolonged service are subdivided into the following categories: service with direct (ie, face-to-face) patient contact and service without direct patient contact.

Table 10-5. Prolonged Services in the Hospital Setting

Code	Description of Prolonged Services
+99356	Prolonged service in the inpatient or observation setting, requiring unit/floor time beyond the usual service; first hour (30–74 min) (List separately in addition to the code for inpatient evaluation and management service.) (Use code 99356 in conjunction with codes 90837, 99218–99220, 99221–99223, 99224–99226, 99231–99233, 99234–99236, 99251–99255, 99304–99310.)
+99357	each additional 30 minutes (List separately in addition to the code for prolonged physician service.) (Use code 99357 in conjunction with code 99356.)
99358	Prolonged evaluation and management service before and/or after direct patient care; first hour
+99359	each additional 30 minutes (Use code 99359 in conjunction with code 99358.)

Table 10-6. Coding Direct Prolonged Services for Inpatient and Observation Care

Total Duration of Prolonged Services, min	Code(s)
<30	Not reported separately
30–74	99356 × 1
75–104	99356 × 1 and 99357 × 1
≥105 (≥1 h 45 min)	99356 × 1 and 99357 × 2 or more for each additional 30 min

Refer to Chapter 7, Evaluation and Management Services in the Office, Outpatient, Home, or Nursing Facility Setting, for details of the specific requirements for reporting physician prolonged services in the office or outpatient setting.

- Direct prolonged services (**99356** and **99357**) may only be reported in conjunction with the following codes: **90837** (psychotherapy without E/M, 60 minutes), **99221–99223** (initial hospital care), **99218–99220** (initial observation care), **99234–99236** (admission/discharge same day), **99224–99226** (subsequent observation care), **99231–99233** (subsequent hospital care), **99251–99255** (inpatient consultations), and **99304–99310** (nursing facility services).
- Direct prolonged services (**99356** and **99357**) may not be reported in conjunction with observation or inpatient discharge management (**99217, 99238,** or **99239**), critical care (**99291, 99292; 99466, 99467; 99468–99476**), or intensive care (**99477–99480**) because none of these E/M services has an assigned typical time.
- Direct patient contact time in the inpatient facility is defined as floor or unit time dedicated to the patient. (*Note:* Medicare policy is that time spent reviewing charts or discussion of a patient with house medical staff and not with direct face-to-face contact with the patient, or waiting for test results, for changes in the patient's condition, for end of a therapy, or for use of facilities, cannot be billed as prolonged services. It is important to be aware of Medicaid and private payers that adopt Medicare policy.)
- When an E/M service is reported using time as the key or controlling factor, prolonged services can be reported only when the prolonged service exceeds 30 minutes beyond the highest level of E/M service (eg, **99220, 99223**).
- The medical record must reflect the total time of the service and medical need for the service.
- Non-direct prolonged physician services (**99358** and **99359**) may be reported on a different date than the related primary service. The related primary service may be an E/M service (with or without an assigned typical time), a procedure, or other service.
- Non-direct prolonged E/M services must relate to a face-to-face service that has occurred or will occur and must be relative to ongoing care.

Examples

➤ **The pediatrician spends 40 minutes reviewing extensive medical records that are received the day after a patient is admitted.**

Code **99358** would be reported. Prolonged service of less than 30 minutes' total duration would not be separately reported.

➤ **A 10-year-old patient is admitted to the care of a neurologist following a first-time seizure that occurred shortly after waking in the morning.** The neurologist completes a comprehensive history and physical examination. Results of an electroencephalogram are reviewed. The diagnosis is juvenile myoclonic epilepsy. Later that same day, the neurologist visits the patient and spends 60 minutes discussing the patient's test results and the anticipated plan of care with the parents and documents the total unit/floor time of 120 minutes in the medical record.

The neurologist reports her services with codes **99223** and **99356**.

Teaching Point: The neurologist reports initial inpatient hospital code **99223** based on the key components of comprehensive history and examination and high-complexity MDM. The typical time assigned to code **99223** is 70 minutes. This leaves an additional 50 minutes of unit/floor time that may be appropriately reported with prolonged services code **99356**.

Hospital-Mandated On-Call Services

99026   Hospital mandated on-call service; in-hospital, each hour
99027   out of hospital, each hour

* Codes **99026** and **99027** describe services provided by a physician who is on call per hospital mandate as a condition of medical staff privileges.

* Used to report on-call time spent by the physician when he or she is not providing other services.

* Time spent performing separately reportable services should not be included in time reported as mandated on-call services.

* Most payers do not cover these services because they consider this a contract issue between the hospital and physician. However, these codes may be used for tracking purposes.

Critical Care and Continuing Intensive Care Services

Specific guidelines for reporting hourly and inpatient neonatal and pediatric critical care are provided in Chapter 12, Critical and Intensive Care.

Medical Team Conferences

99366   Medical team conference with interdisciplinary team of health care professionals, face-to-face with patient and/or family, 30 minutes or more, participation by nonphysician qualified health care professional

99367   Medical team conference with interdisciplinary team of health care professionals, patient and/or family not present, 30 minutes or more; participation by physician

99368   Medical team conference with interdisciplinary team of health care professionals, patient and/ or family not present, 30 minutes or more; participation by nonphysician qualified health care professional

Codes **99366–99368** are used to report participation by physicians or nonphysician providers (NPPs) in conferences to coordinate or manage care and services for established patients with chronic or multiple health conditions (eg, cerebral palsy) or with congenital anomalies (eg, craniofacial abnormalities). Code **99367** is the only code that may be reported by a physician, and it can only be reported when the patient and/or family is not present at the team conference. When the physician or QHP who may report E/M services (eg, advanced practice nurse) participates in a medical team conference with the patient and/or family present, the appropriate-level E/M code (eg, **99231–99233**) will be reported based on the place of service and total face-to-face time spent in counseling and/or coordination of care.

See Chapter 8, Managing Chronic and Complex Conditions, for a complete summary of the reporting requirements.

Advance Care Planning

99497   Advance care planning, including the explanation and discussion of advance directives such as standard forms (with completion of such forms, when performed), by the physician or other qualified health care professional; first 30 minutes, face-to-face with the patient, family member(s) and/or surrogate

+99498   each additional 30 minutes (List separately in addition to code for primary procedure)

Codes **99497** and **99498** include

* Face-to-face service by a physician or QHP to a patient, family member, or surrogate spent in counseling and discussion of advance directives

* Completion of forms, when applicable (eg, Health Care Proxy, Durable Power of Attorney for Health Care, Living Will, and Medical Orders for Life-Sustaining Treatment)

Face-to-face time spent by the physician or QHP is required and the total time must be documented.

Active management of problems is not included in advance care planning. Other E/M services provided on the same date as advance care planning may be separately reported, with the exceptions of hourly critical care services (**99291** and **99292**), inpatient neonatal and pediatric critical care (**99468** and **99469**; **99471–99476**), and initial and continuing intensive care services (**99477–99480**). Do not report codes **99497** and **99498** in conjunction with codes **99291** and **99292**, **99468** and **99469**, **99471–99476**, or **99477–99480**.

Example

➤ **An adolescent with metastatic cancer wishes to discuss and be involved in planning her care.** Her oncologist spends 50 minutes face-to-face with the patient and her parent assessing their understanding of the diagnosis and prognosis, the continued hope that treatment is successful, and the patient's wishes to be included in decisions about her care. A plan of care is developed and documented and an appointment with the supportive care team at the hospital is scheduled to provide additional counseling and support services to the patient and family.

The oncologist may report codes **99497** and **99498** for the 50 minutes of face-to-face time spent providing the advance care planning. Because the *CPT®* prefatory language and code descriptors for advance care planning do not include other instruction on the time required for reporting, these services may be reported based on general *CPT* instruction to report when the midpoint is passed (eg, one unit of **99498** may be reported for 46–75 minutes). Exceptions may apply for payers with policy requiring that the time be met or exceeded.

Continuing Care After Hospitalization

A key goal of many quality improvement programs is avoidance of readmittance and/or ED visits following hospitalization. In recent years, *CPT* and payers have recognized a need for codes to capture services related to care coordination and management of chronic and episodic conditions that may lead to emergency and inpatient care. For physicians continuing patient care after hospital discharge, services such as transitional care management and chronic care management offer opportunities to provide and be compensated for care aimed at reducing the risk of decline, exacerbation, and/or functional decline.

See Chapter 8, Managing Chronic and Complex Conditions, for more information on transitional and chronic care management services.

Teaching Points: Progression of Care

Selecting the appropriate level of service from the appropriate family of codes will be dependent on the child's condition, type of service (observation vs inpatient), and intensity of the service provided and documented on a particular day of service. The following scenarios indicate the category of codes that should be reported based on the progression of care provided. Remember that the level of service reported is based on all the face-to-face care provided during the calendar day. See the progression of care when reporting daily hospital care and neonatal and pediatric critical care or neonatal intensive care in Chapter 12, Critical and Intensive Care.

One Physician or Physicians of the Same Specialty and Group

Examples

▶ **The patient receives E/M services in the office and is sent to the hospital on the same day.**

If the patient is examined in the office or outpatient setting, admitted to the hospital for observation or as an inpatient, and not seen in the hospital on the same day, report the appropriate office or outpatient code (**99201–99215**) or consultation code (**99241–99245**) as applicable.

If the patient is examined in the office or outpatient setting, admitted to the hospital for observation or as an inpatient, and seen in the hospital on the same day, report the appropriate initial observation or inpatient hospital code (**99218–99220** or **99221–99223**) based on all the E/M services provided on that calendar day.

If the patient is admitted by physician A and discharged on the same day by physician B (from same practice and of same specialty), a code for same-day admission and discharge observation or inpatient services (**99234–99236**) is reported based on the combined services.

▶ **The patient receives an initial face-to-face E/M service in the observation setting.**

If the patient is admitted to observation, the appropriate initial observation code (**99218–99220**) is reported.

If the patient is admitted and discharged on the same day, a code for admission and discharge observation or inpatient services (**99234–99236**) is reported.

If the patient is admitted for observation and subsequently formally admitted to the hospital on the same day, only the initial inpatient hospital code (**99221–99223**) is reported.

If the patient was admitted to observation care status and is seen the following day and not discharged, codes **99224–99226** are reported for the subsequent-day encounter.

If the patient is placed in observation status and then admitted as an inpatient the next day, initial observation (**99218–99220**) and initial hospital care (**99221–99223**) codes are reported with the appropriate dates of service. If the level of service performed during the initial hospital care does not meet the requirements for the initial hospital care (meet all 3 key components or time requirements), report the appropriate subsequent hospital care code (**99231–99233**).

If the patient is discharged from observation status on a day subsequent to the admission, observation care discharge management (**99217**) is reported.

▶ **The patient receives face-to-face E/M services in the inpatient hospital setting.**

If the patient is evaluated in the hospital, the appropriate initial hospital care code (**99221–99223**) is reported for the first face-to-face E/M service.

If the patient is followed on subsequent days, codes **99231–99233** are reported for each subsequent day of service.

If the patient's condition declines and he or she requires intensive care services, see Chapter 12, Critical and Intensive Care, for specific details about coding intensive care services for infants weighing 5,000 g or less.

If the patient's condition deteriorates and he or she requires critical care services, coding will be dependent on the age of the child. If the child is 6 years or older, hourly critical care services will be reported (**99291** and **99292**) in addition to codes **99231–99233**. See Chapter 12 for guidelines used to report critical care.

If the patient is discharged on a day subsequent to the initial service, discharge code **99238** or **99239** is reported.

Transfer of Service

If the patient is examined by physician A in the office or outpatient setting and sent to the hospital to be admitted by physician B from a different group or specialty (eg, hospitalist or other physician from a group with a different tax identification number than physician A), physician A will report all E/M and other services that he or she provided in the office (eg, **99201–99215**). Physician B will report the appropriate initial hospital observation or inpatient service code (**99218–99220**, **99221–99223**, or **99234–99236**).

If a patient is admitted by physician A and care is transferred to another physician from a different group or specialty (physician B), physician B will report subsequent hospital care services (**99231–99233**).

If physician A requests an opinion or advice from physician B, who may be from the same or different group or specialty, and the requirements for a consultation are performed, physician B will report the appropriate consultation code (**99241–99245** or **99251–99255**). If, subsequent to the consultation, both physicians provide E/M services, both will report subsequent observation or hospital care codes (**99224–99226** or **99231–99233**). If both physicians are from the same group, additional justification may be required to support payment for services by both physicians. See Chapter 12, Critical and Intensive Care, for guidelines for reporting concurrent critical care or transfer of care of the critically ill infant or child.

Split/Shared Billing

Example

> **A pediatrician and NPP from the same group practice see a patient on the same date.** The NPP provides and documents initial hospital care, including a comprehensive history, detailed examination, and MDM of moderate complexity. Later that day, the pediatrician is called to see the patient, who is exhibiting new symptoms, and to review new laboratory test results. Taking into account both services, which have been individually documented and signed, the examination and history are comprehensive and MDM is of high complexity.
>
> **Teaching Point:** Because both providers are from the same group practice and have signed off on their individually provided services, the services may be shared and billed under the physician as code **99223**.

A split/shared E/M service is one in which a physician and a QHP, such as a nurse practitioner or physician assistant, from the *same group practice* each personally perform a medically necessary and substantive portion of one or more face-to-face E/M encounters on the same date.

The following requirements apply to all split/shared services:

- A portion of the key components of the service must be provided face-to-face by the physician to report under the physician's National Provider Identifier.
- Split/shared services were defined and implemented for services to Medicare beneficiaries. Private payers may adopt the same or a similar policy.
- The physician and QHP must document and sign their portion of the service.
- A physician cannot merely sign off on the documentation of the NPP's work.
- If the E/M service is reported based on counseling and/or coordination of care, only the physician's time is used to select the level of service if billing under that physician.
    - The physician must document his or her total time, the portion of time (ie, >50%) spent in counseling and/or coordination of care, and a summary of the issues discussed or coordination of care provided.
- Shared services are not permitted if the QHP is a hospital employee.
- Services may be reported by the QHP or physician (if QHP may bill).
- Shared services are allowed when sick hospital care services are reported (combined physician and NPP time) and with discharge services.
- Critical care is never a split/shared service because critical care services reflect the work of only one individual.

Split/shared billing differs from incident-to billing, which is only allowed in the outpatient setting. See Chapter 14, Allied Health and Clinical Staff Services, for more information on incident-to rules.

Emergency Department Services

Contents

Reporting the Diagnosis Code for Emergency Department (ED) Visits

While several symptoms may be listed as the "chief complaint" as part of the emergency department (ED) triage process, the physician must designate only one sign, symptom, disease, or injury as the chief complaint. The hospital depends on the physician's designation of the chief complaint because only one diagnosis code may be reported for this category on the hospital claim form. This diagnosis is used to help support the urgency of the ED visit under prudent layperson guidelines. This may be different from conditions that are "present on admission" that must now be tracked by hospitals.

States may require EDs to report codes describing the circumstances of an injury. These codes are referred to as external cause codes in *International Classification of Diseases, 10th Revision, Clinical Modification (ICD-10-CM)*. These codes capture the cause, intent, place of occurrence, activity of the patient at the time of the event, and patient status (eg, employee, military, volunteer, student). External cause codes provide information that is valuable for research on the cause and occurrence of injuries and evaluation of injury prevention strategies (eg, reduced reporting of injuries due to automobile accidents following mandates to use seat belts and car seats).

Key points for reporting external cause codes include

* External cause codes may be reported in conjunction with any health condition that is related to an external cause (eg, adverse effect of medical treatment).
* External cause codes are never the principal or first-listed diagnosis code.
* In *ICD-10-CM*, only external cause codes for the cause and intent of an injury or illness are reported for the duration of treatment, with the seventh character of the code indicating whether an encounter is for initial care, subsequent care, or care for sequela (late effect) of the injury or illness.
* External cause codes indicating place of occurrence, activity, and patient status are reported only at the initial encounter for treatment.
* If the intent (eg, accident, self-harm, assault) of the cause of an injury or other condition is unknown or unspecified, code the intent as *accidental*.
* No external cause code should be assigned when the cause and intent of an illness or injury are included in another reported code (eg, **T58.11XA**, initial encounter for toxic effect of carbon monoxide from utility gas, accidental).

> ### ~ More From the AAP ~
>
> Learn more about seventh characters for external cause codes in "Maximizing 10: Initial, Subsequent, and Sequela Confusion" in the May 2016 *AAP Pediatric Coding Newsletter*™ at http://coding.aap.org (subscription required).

ED Evaluation and Management Codes

* Evaluation and management (E/M) codes **99281–99285** are only reported when care is provided in an ED. An ED is defined as an organized hospital-based facility for the provision of unscheduled episodic services to patients who present for immediate medical attention. The facility must be available 24 hours a day, 7 days a week.
* Services performed in an urgent care center, a nonhospital facility, or a facility that is not open for 24 hours a day should be reported with the appropriate *Current Procedural Terminology* (*CPT*®) office or outpatient visit codes (**99201–99215**) with the appropriate place of service code (eg, **20** for urgent care facility).
* Selection of the appropriate E/M code is primarily driven by the risk involved in the presenting problem, evaluation measures, and/or treatment options.
* Performance and documentation of all 3 key components (history, physical examination, and medical decision-making [MDM]) are used to select the level of an ED E/M code.
* Because of the unpredictability and inconsistency in the intensity of these services, there are no time values assigned to this family of codes. Therefore, time spent in counseling and/or coordination of care *cannot* be used as a key or controlling factor in the selection of the code, nor can prolonged services be reported with ED codes.

> ### ||||||| *Coding Pearl* |||||||
>
> Services provided in an urgent care center or nonhospital-based facility are not reported with codes **99281–99285**.

* There is no differentiation between new or established patients for ED encounters. All problems for encounters in the ED are considered new to the attending physician for purposes of determining MDM.

* The ED codes are not reported if the treating ED physician admits the patient to his or her service for observation or inpatient status on the same date of service as the ED encounter. Only the appropriate initial observation (**99218–99220**), initial hospital care (**99221–99223**), or initial observation or inpatient hospital admission and discharge same day (**99234–99236**) codes are reported instead of ED codes. All the E/M work performed in the ED should be combined with any additional work performed for admission (and, when appropriate, discharge) when selecting the correct code and level of care.

Emergency Department Caveat: Code 99285

The ED E/M code **99285** allows an exception to the "3 key components" rule (Level 5 caveat) for patients whose clinical condition, mental status, or lack of available history may not permit obtaining a comprehensive history and/or physical examination. Therefore, code **99285** may be reported in patients presenting with a high-severity condition that requires a high level of MDM when circumstances prevent the physician from obtaining a comprehensive history and/or completing a comprehensive physical examination. When such urgency exists, the physician must document the condition or reason why a comprehensive history and/or physical examination could not be obtained.

Table 11-1 summarizes the key components required for each ED E/M code based on the 1995 and 1997 Centers for Medicare & Medicaid Services *Documentation Guidelines for Evaluation and Management Services.* Also refer to Chapter 4, Evaluation and Management Documentation Guidelines, for more detail on E/M coding guidelines.

Examples

➤ **A 2-year-old girl presents with left ear pain, fever, and irritability.** Parents noticed that the child had a fever (temporal artery 39.5°C [103.1°F]) the prior evening and administered ibuprofen. Fever returned during the night, and the child has had 2 additional doses of ibuprofen, with the last dose provided 2 hours ago. The patient did not sleep well and has been alternately fussy and rather lethargic today. She has had some nasal congestion over the past week and shows little appetite today. The pediatrician diagnosed bilateral otitis media 1 month ago that was treated with amoxicillin. The patient has had no prior hospitalizations, has no known drug allergies, and no tobacco exposure. She attends child care. Her sibling has a history of ear infections requiring tube placement.

Review of systems (ROS): positive for fever, left ear pain, seasonal allergies, decreased appetite, and irritability. A review of the eyes is negative for purulent discharge; the parents deny cough, vomiting, diarrhea, and signs of abdominal pain. All other systems are reviewed and are normal.

Examination: The patient weights 12.2 kg (26.9 lb), is 86 cm (33.9") tall, and has a temperature of 38.2°C (100.8°F). She is alert and fussy but appears to be in no acute distress; she appears well developed and well nourished. The patient's eyelids and conjunctiva are normal; pupils are equal, round, and reactive to light and accommodation. Her ears are typical externally; otoscopic examination reveals the right tympanic membrane is slightly erythematous, and the left tympanic membrane is erythematous and bulging with decreased mobility. On examination of the nose, it is noted that the membranes are swollen and erythematous and there is opaque white mucous. The patient's throat is clear, her thyroid is normal, and neck is supple with no lymphadenopathy. Respiratory rate is typical, clear to auscultation; the patient's heart has typical rate and rhythm and no murmurs. She has typical cervical, axillary, supraclavicular, suboccipital, and periauricular nodes and no rashes.

The diagnosis is bilateral acute serous otitis media. The physician discusses the following plan with the parents: amoxicillin 400 mg/5 mL twice daily for 10 days, with follow-up with primary care in 10 days. A patient education handout is provided to the parents.

ICD-10-CM	CPT®
H65.03 (acute serous otitis media, bilateral)	99284

Table 11-1. Emergency Department Services

Key Components

3 of 3 key components must be performed to at least the degree specified for each code. All patients in the emergency department are considered new patients.

Code	MDM	History	Physical Examination
99281	**Straightforward** # diagnoses/options: Minimal Data: Minimal Risk: Minimal	**Problem focused** HPI: 1–3 elements ROS: 0 PFSH: 0	**Problem focused** **1995:** One body area/organ system **1997:** Performance and documentation of 1–5 elements identified by a bullet (●) in one or more areas or systems
99282	**Low complexity** # diagnoses/options: Limited Data: Limited Risk: Low	**Expanded problem focused** HPI: 1–3 elements ROS: 1 PFSH: 0	**Expanded problem focused** **1995:** Limited exam—affected body area/organ system and other related areas/systems **1997:** Performance and documentation of at least 6 elements identified by a bullet (●) in one or more areas or systems
99283	**Moderate complexity** # diagnoses/options: Multiple Data: Moderate Risk: Moderate	**Expanded problem focused** HPI: 1–3 elements ROS: 1 PFSH: 0	**Expanded problem focused** **1995:** Limited exam—affected body area/organ system and other related areas/systems **1997:** Performance and documentation of at least 6 elements identified by a bullet (●) in one or more areas or systems
99284	**Moderate complexity** # diagnoses/options: Multiple Data: Moderate Risk: Moderate	**Detailed** HPI: 4+ elements or status of 3 chronic or inactive conditions ROS: 2–9 PFSH: 1	**Detailed** **1995:** Extended exam—affected body area(s) and other symptomatic or related organ system(s) **1997:** Performance and documentation of at least 2 elements identified by a bullet (●) in at least 6 areas or systems or at least 12 elements identified by a bullet (●) in at least 2 areas or systems
99285	**High complexity** # diagnoses/options: Extensive Data: Extensive Risk: High	**Comprehensive** HPI: 4+ elements or status of 3 chronic or inactive conditions ROS: 10+ PFSH: 2 Or clinical condition or mental status did not permit performance of history (must document reason that comprehensive history could not be performed).	**Comprehensive** **1995:** 8+ organ systems or complete exam of a single organ system **1997:** <u>Multisystem exam</u>—At least 9 organ systems or body areas with performance of all elements identified by a bullet (●) in each area/system examined Documentation is expected for at least 2 elements identified by a bullet (●) of each area(s) or system(s). <u>Single organ system exam</u>—Performance of all elements identified by a bullet (●) and documentation of every element in each box with a shaded border and at least one element in a box with an unshaded border Or clinical condition or mental status did not permit performance of exam.

Abbreviations: HPI, history of present illness; MDM, medical decision-making; PFSH, past, family, and social history; ROS, review of systems.

Chapter 11: Emergency Department Services

Teaching Point: This example includes a chief complaint of ear pain, fever, and irritability. The history of present illness (HPI) includes location of left ear; timing of last evening; associated signs and symptoms of fever, not sleeping well, and little appetite; and a modifying factor of ibuprofen for fever. With 4 elements, the level of HPI is extended. The ROS is complete. Past (otitis media 1 month ago), family (sibling: otitis media), and social (child care; no tobacco exposure) history are documented. The level of history is comprehensive. Examination of constitutional (vitals, general appearance), eyes, ears, nose, mouth and throat, cardiovascular, respiratory, lymphatic, and skin is detailed. Medical decision-making is moderate with a new problem to the examiner, with no additional workup, and moderate risk. With all 3 key components required to support the level of ED service, this encounter is reported with code **99284**, which includes at least detailed history and examination and MDM of moderate complexity. (Mild presentation of otitis media may reduce MDM to low and support a lower level of service.)

➤ **A 7-year-old patient presents to the ED with acute exacerbation of asthma.** Parents report that the patient began wheezing and complained of chest tightness about 1 hour ago. His peak flow at initial onset of this attack was 50% of personal best. Treatment with rescue medication did not provide significant relief. The patient was hospitalized for severe exacerbation of asthma 1 year ago but, until now, has not required further emergency or hospital care. The patient has no known drug allergies. Father smokes but never in the home or near the child. Mother has seasonal allergies.

Examination: Patient appears ill and anxious. He is currently receiving oxygen by face mask. His respiratory rate is 28 breaths per minute, pulse is 110 beats per minute, and oxygen saturation is 86%. The patient weighs 22.5 kg (49.6 lb) and is 124 cm (48.8") tall. Pupils are equal, round, and reactive to light and accommodation. There is mild swelling of the nasal mucosa; tympanic membranes are clear; and oropharynx is dry but otherwise normal. The patient's neck is supple, with no lymphadenopathy. He is wheezing throughout expiration and speaks in partial sentences, with visible subcostal retractions. Patient has mild tachycardia and no rubs or murmur. His abdomen is soft and nontender, and he has no rashes.

Spirometry is successfully completed and results support moderate exacerbation. After 2 inhalation treatments over the course of an hour, the patient's symptoms are relieved and spirometry results are significantly improved. The patient is discharged to home, and his pediatrician is notified of the ED encounter and need for follow-up.

Discharge diagnosis is moderate persistent asthma with acute exacerbation.

ICD-10-CM	CPT®
J45.41 (moderate persistent asthma with acute exacerbation)	**99281**

Teaching Point: This example includes a chief complaint of acute exacerbation of asthma. The HPI includes location (chest tightness), signs and symptoms (wheezing, peak flow 50% of personal best), time (1 hour ago), and modifying factors (rescue medication did not provide relief). The HPI is extended. *No ROS is documented.* Past (hospitalized 1 year ago; no known drug allergies), social (father smokes), and family (mother has allergies) history is documented. The past, family, and social history (PFSH) is complete. With extended HPI, no ROS, and complete PFSH, the overall history is problem focused. The examination is comprehensive, with 8 organ systems, based on the 1995 guidelines. Medical decision-making is moderate with a new problem, with no additional workup, tests in the medicine section of *CPT* performed, and risk associated with an exacerbation of a chronic illness. The overall level of service is **99281**, which includes at least a problem-focused history, problem-focused examination, and MDM of straightforward complexity. If the history had included review of 2 to 9 systems, code **99284** would have been supported by a detailed history, comprehensive examination, and moderate-complexity MDM. While only medically necessary history should be counted when determining a level of E/M service, it is likely that an expanded ROS could be clinically justified.

Comanagement of ED Patients

Examples

Use **Table 11-1** to help you in the selection of the appropriate level of ED E/M service in the following examples:

➤ **The ED physician is treating a 6-year-old who was struck by a car while riding a bicycle on a neighborhood street.** The patient is brought in by emergency medical services (EMS) from the scene with concern for closed head trauma (no known loss of consciousness [LOC] is reported), a friction burn on her right shoulder, multiple abrasions on her forearm and elbow, and large contusions on her left hip and thigh. The child is not accompanied by a parent. While, initially, there was a concern that the child might be in imminent risk of a life-threatening condition, following further assessment, imaging studies, and consultation with a trauma surgeon, the ED physician determines there is no risk of deterioration and the child is clinically stable. No history, other than that obtained from EMS, is available prior to the *trauma service* evaluation. There was high-complexity MDM. No separately billable procedures were performed. The child is admitted for observation by a hospitalist for a concussion. On discharge, the patient is noted to have sustained a concussion.

Physician	ICD-10-CM	CPT®
ED physician	**S09.90XA** (head injury, no other symptoms, initial encounter) **T22.151A** (friction burn, first degree, right shoulder, initial encounter) **S50.811A** (abrasion, right forearm, initial encounter) **S50.311A** (abrasion, right elbow, initial encounter) **S70.02XA**, **S70.12XA** (contusions, left hip and thigh, initial encounter) **V13.4XXA** (pedal cycle driver injured in collision with car in traffic accident, initial encounter) **Y93.55** (activity, bike riding) **Y92.414** (local residential or business street as the place of occurrence of the external cause) **Y99.8** (other external cause status)	**99285** (ED visit code)
Trauma surgeon	**S09.90XA** **T22.151A** **S50.811A** **S50.311A** **S70.02XA**, **S70.12XA** **V13.4XXA**	**99241–99245** (office or other outpatient consultation [likely **99244** or **99245**])
Hospitalist	**S06.0X0A** (concussion with no LOC, initial encounter) **T22.151A**, **S50.811A**, **S50.311A**, **S70.02XA**, **S70.12XA**, **V13.4XXA**	**99218–99220** (initial observation care)

Teaching Point: The Level 5 caveat would apply because this patient's condition was initially felt to be unstable and no other history, other than that from EMS, was available. If included in the scenario, a diagnosis code indicating the place of occurrence of the accident would also be reported by each physician for the initial episode of care.

Chapter 11: Emergency Department Services

➤ **The ED physician evaluates a 10-month-old for fever, vomiting, and lethargy.** A comprehensive history and physical examination are performed and there is high-complexity MDM. Because of the concern for meningitis, the on-call pediatrician is consulted and is asked to perform the lumbar puncture and to determine the child's disposition. The pediatrician does the procedure, confirms the course of treatment by the ED physician, and admits the infant as an inpatient to his or her service.

ICD-10-CM	CPT®
Both physicians report **R50.9** (fever) **R11.10** (vomiting) **R53.83** (lethargy)	The ED physician reports **99285** (ED visit code)
	The pediatrician reports **99221–99223 25** (initial inpatient hospital care) **62270** (lumbar puncture)

Teaching Point: A code for meningitis is not reported because this condition has not been confirmed.

Only one physician should report an ED E/M service for a patient who receives care in the ED. In general, this will be the emergency physician or pediatric emergency medicine specialist who is staffing the ED. At times, other physicians (eg, generalists, specialists) may have to provide care for a patient in the ED. When this occurs, the code(s) used by each physician will depend on several factors.

* Is the physician managing the patient in the ED or was the physician called in by the ED physician?
* Did the physician personally perform any procedures in the ED or only direct the ED staff?
* Was the patient sent home, transferred to another facility, or kept at the hospital for observation or admission?
* Was the patient stable or critically ill or injured?

Follow these guidelines to determine which codes will be reported.

➤ **You are the primary physician managing the patient in the ED (ie, the ED physician or a physician meeting his or her patient in the ED).**
   Codes **99281–99285** (ED E/M service) will be reported.

➤ **You are the primary physician managing the patient in the ED (ie, the ED physician or a physician meeting his or her patient in the ED) and you call in another physician to see the patient.**
   The type of service reported will depend on whether the other physician is providing consultative services, a specific intervention (eg, diagnostic or therapeutic procedure), or primary management of the patient. The ED physician will typically report the ED E/M code and the other physician will report services as follows:
* *Consultation:* An outpatient consultation (**99241–99245**) may be reported when the ED physician requests the opinion of and/or advice from the other physician (and the request is documented in the medical record), the consulting physician provides an opinion and/or advice (including the initiation of diagnostic and/or therapeutic services), and a written report is documented (may be part of the ED medical record). If a payer follows Medicare guidelines and does not cover consultations, services should be reported using the office or outpatient E/M codes (**99201–99215**). See Chapter 6, Preventive Services, for detailed requirements for reporting consultations. No matter which code set you report, place of service code **23** (ED) would be used.
* *Procedure:* The second physician may report the diagnostic and/or therapeutic procedure requested by the ED physician that is provided to the patient in the ED (eg, fracture reduction by an orthopedic surgeon; wound repair by a plastic surgeon; echocardiogram performed by a cardiologist; imaging interpretation by a radiologist; lumbar puncture performed by a pediatrician, hospitalist, or neonatologist).
* *Assume management:* If the second physician is called in to take over management of the patient (not a consultation) and the patient is sent home, an office or outpatient code (**99201–99215**) would be reported with place of service code **23** (ED). This would also be the case when an insurance carrier does not recognize consultation codes and the patient is sent home.

- *Observation or inpatient admission:* If the other physician admits the child to the hospital for observation or inpatient services after stabilization and/or provision of care in the ED, he or she would report only the appropriate initial observation, hospital inpatient, or pediatric critical care or intensive care code (**99218–99220, 99221–99223, 99468, 99471, 99475, 99477**) as appropriate based on all the E/M services provided in the ED and as part of the initial service. That could also apply if
  - ❖ The admitting physician is a member of the same physician group as the ED physician, but the admitting physician is providing different services and is not considered the exact same specialty.
  - ❖ The other physician transferred the child to another facility where the child would be under his or her care (or a member of his or her group and same specialty).
- *Critical care:* If the patient is critically ill or injured, the physicians managing the patient's care may report their services using time-based critical care codes **99291** and **99292** (see Table 12-2 in Chapter 12, Critical and Intensive Care).

➤ **You are the primary physician managing the patient in the ED (ie, the ED physician or a physician meeting his or her patient in the ED) and you treat a patient and request an opinion and/or advice from another physician who provides consultative services. A third physician admits the child to the hospital.**

Each physician will report the appropriate service (ie, ED physician reports code **99281–99285**, consulting physician reports code **99241–99245** [or **99201–99215** if the payer follows Medicare rules], and admitting physician reports an appropriate initial code [eg, **99218–99220, 99221–99223**]) so long as the physicians are not in the same group practice and of the exact same specialty.

Directing Emergency Medical Technicians

99288   Physician or other qualified health care professional direction of emergency medical systems (EMS) emergency care, advanced life support

- Report code **99288** (physician direction of EMS) when
  - ❖ The physician directing the services is in the hospital and in 2-way communication with EMS personnel who are in the prehospital setting providing advanced life support that requires direct or online medical control.
  - ❖ The documentation includes the times of all contacts, any orders provided, and/or directions provided to the EMS team.
- Code **99288** may be reported on the same day as ED E/M or hourly critical care services. Modifier **25** would be appended to code **99288** to alert payers that this was a significant and separately identifiable service from ED E/M (**99281–99285**) or the critical care (**99291–99292**) service provided.
- The supervising physician cannot report the actual procedures and interventions performed by the EMS team because he or she is not physically present during the transport.
- Code **99288** is designated as a bundled procedure (included in the work value of other services) by Medicare. There are no relative values assigned under the Medicare Resource-Based Relative Value Scale. Check with your major payers and negotiate for coverage of this service.
- See codes **99485** and **99486** in Chapter 12, Critical and Intensive Care, for information on supervision of inter-facility transport of a critically ill or injured patient, 24 months or younger, via direct 2-way communication with a transport team.
- When a qualified health care professional (QHP) (eg, nurse practitioner) provides critical care services during transport and those services will be reported under the QHP's National Provider Identifier or by the employing hospital, the ED physician does not report **99288**.

Chapter 11: Emergency Department Services

Critical Care in the ED

99291   Critical care, E/M of the critically ill or critically injured patient; first 30 to 74 minutes

+99292   each additional 30 minutes (Use in conjunction with **99291**.)

A critical illness or injury is defined in *CPT*® as one that acutely impairs one or more vital organs such that there is a high probability of imminent or life-threatening deterioration of the patient's condition. Guidelines for reporting critical care codes **99291** (critical care, E/M of the critically ill or injured patient; first 30–74 minutes) and **99292** (each additional 30 minutes) are described in detail in Chapter 12, Critical and Intensive Care.

- Time-based critical care codes (**99291, 99292**) should be used to report the provision of critical care when performed in the ED. The patient's condition must meet the specific *CPT* definition of a critically ill or injured patient. The global codes for pediatric or neonatal critical care should not be reported by a physician providing critical care in the ED unless that physician (eg, an intensivist) will continue to provide critical care services in the inpatient setting.

- Critical care may be reported on the same day as an ED E/M code when provided by the same physician when 2 independent services are provided. Modifier **25** should be appended to the ED E/M code when this occurs. Here are examples of critical care and ED E/M services that may be separately reportable when provided on the same date.

  - ❖ A child injured in an accident arrives at the ED. The ED physician evaluates the child's injuries and orders a surgical consultation. While the surgeon is in route to the facility, the patient's condition deteriorates and the ED physician provides 40 minutes of critical care before the patient is transferred to the surgeon's care.

  - ❖ A child arrives to the ED in critical condition. The ED physician provides 45 minutes of critical care services. After the child's condition improves, the ED physician obtains a comprehensive history, completes a detailed examination, and arranges admission to the intensive care unit by a hospitalist.

- Time spent providing critical care does not need to be continuous and includes time at the bedside as well as time in the ED reviewing data specific to the patient, discussing the patient with other physicians, and discussing the patient's management or condition with the patient's family.

- Time reported for critical care must be devoted to the critically ill or injured patient. Therefore, the "critical care clock" stops when attention is turned to the care of another patient or the physician is not readily available in the ED.

- Those procedures not bundled with codes **99291** and **99292** and when personally performed by the reporting provider may be reported separately (eg, starting an intravenous line on a child younger than 3 years, placing an intraosseous or central venous line, endotracheal intubation, cardiopulmonary resuscitation [CPR], cardioversion). Time spent performing these separately reported services must be subtracted from the critical care time calculated and reported. See Table 12-1 in Chapter 12, Critical and Intensive Care, for a list of services and procedures that are included in hourly critical care codes.

Examples

➤ **The ED physician performs a comprehensive history and physical examination on a 13-month-old patient with severe stridor and respiratory distress believed to be secondary to croup.** Medical decision-making is highly complex. The patient's condition does not improve with nebulized epinephrine and then worsens, evidenced by progressive lethargy. The patient goes into respiratory failure and 75 minutes of critical care is provided. Ten minutes of the critical care time is spent performing endotracheal intubation.

ICD-10-CM	CPT
J96.00 (acute respiratory failure)	**99285 25** (ED visit code)
J05.0 (croup)	**99291 25** (critical care, first 30–74 minutes)
	31500 (emergency endotracheal intubation)

Teaching Point: Endotracheal intubation is not bundled with critical care; therefore, time spent in the provision of the service (10 minutes for this patient) is not considered in the total critical care time, so only the base code, **99291**, can be used. Modifier **25** is appended to codes **99285** and **99291** to indicate they were significant and separately identifiable services.

➤ **The ED physician saw a 10-year-old for moderate asthma exacerbation in the morning.** The child responded well to an aerosolized bronchodilator treatment and was discharged home. The child returns to the ED a few hours later with a more severe exacerbation and is seen by the same physician. The child now has respiratory failure with hypoxia. The child receives oxygen, a continuous bronchodilator nebulizer treatment, and, subsequently, a parenteral bronchodilation drug. The child improves enough to be admitted to a ED monitored medical ward bed with diagnosis of respiratory failure due to severe exacerbation of moderate persistent asthma. The ED physician spends a total of 60 minutes in patient-directed critical care.

ICD-10-CM	CPT®
J96.01 (acute respiratory failure with hypoxia) **J45.41** (moderate persistent asthma with acute exacerbation)	**99284 25** **99291**

Teaching Point: The patient received oxygen, continuous inhalation treatment, and parenteral bronchodilator in the ED. However, these services include no professional component. The facility will report the services because the cost of supplies and clinical staff time are an expense to the facility.

➤ **A 1-year-old with apparent sepsis and hypotension is brought to the ED.** The child requires placement of an intraosseous needle to achieve vascular access and, subsequently, receives parenteral fluids, antibiotics, and vasopressors. The child suffers cardiopulmonary arrest, prompting the ED physician to intubate the child. Cardiopulmonary resuscitation is performed for 20 minutes. The child is in the ED for a total of 45 minutes before transfer to the intensive care unit.

> If septic shock was specified as the cause of cardiac arrest, codes **A41.9**, sepsis, unspecified organism; **R65.21**, severe sepsis with septic shock; and **I46.8**, cardiac arrest due to other underlying condition, would be reported.

ICD-10-CM	CPT
I46.9 (cardiac arrest) If the physician included sepsis in the diagnosis, this would be reported.	**99285 25** **92950** (CPR) **36680** (placement of intraosseous needle) **31500** (emergency endotracheal intubation)

Teaching Point: Critical care time does not accrue during the performance of non-bundled, separately billable procedures. Because CPR is a separately billable, non-bundled procedure, the ED physician did not spend a minimum of 30 minutes providing critical care. Because the E/M service is reported rather than critical care, coding is based on documented key components of history, examination, and medical decision-making. However, the caveat for code **99285** allows reporting based on the extent of history and examination possible within the constraints imposed by the urgency of the patient's clinical condition and mental status.

Reporting Procedures in the ED

Many procedures performed in the ED have an associated global period assigned by payers. The global period affects reporting of pre- and post-procedural care. (See Chapter 15, Common Surgical Procedures and Sedation, for the definition of the *CPT* surgical package and Medicare global period.)

Table 11-2 contains a list of procedures (with assigned Medicare global periods) commonly performed in the ED.

Any separately identifiable procedure that is personally performed by the physician may be reported, with the exception of

* Procedures that are bundled in time-based critical care codes (See Table 12-1 for a list of services and procedures that are included in hourly critical care codes.)
* Services performed by hospital personnel because they are billed by the hospital facility (If a nurse or allied health care professional assists in part of a procedure, the ED physician may bill for the professional services if he or she provides the primary or key component of the procedure.)
* Hydration, infusion, and/or injection procedures (**96360–96379**) because the physician work associated with the procedures involves only confirmation of the treatment plan and not direct supervision of staff
* Procedures involving use of hospital-owned equipment (eg, pulse oximetry), unless the procedure includes a technical and professional component (The professional component may be reported if performed and documented with modifier **26** [professional component] appended to the procedure code.)

Table 11-2. Common Emergency Department Procedures

Procedure	*CPT*® Code	Global Period (d)ª
Arterial puncture	36600	NA
Bladder aspiration	51100	0
Burn care, >10% TBSA	16030	0
Burn care, 5%–10% TBSA	16025	0
Burn care, <5% TBSA	16020	0
Cardiopulmonary resuscitation	92950	0
Cardioversion	92960	0
Chest tube insertion	32551	0
Dislocation, shoulder, reduction	23650	90
Endotracheal intubation (open procedure)	31500	0
Foreign body removal, conjunctiva	65205	0
Foreign body removal, ear	69200	0
Foreign body removal, nose	30300	10
Foreign body removal with incision, subcutaneous, simple	10120	10
Fracture, clavicle	23500	90
Fracture, finger distal, each	26750	90
Fracture, finger shaft, each	26720	90
Gastric intubation and aspiration(s), therapeutic, including lavage (if performed)	43753	0
Gastrostomy tube change, percutaneous, without imaging guidance	43760	0
Incision and drainage, abscess, simple	10060	10
Incision and drainage, finger, complicated (eg, felon)	26011	10
Incision and drainage, perianal abscess	46050	10
Intraosseous needle placement	36680	0
Laceration repair, simple ≤2.5 cm, face/ears/lips	12011	0
Repair, simple ≤2.5 cm, scalp/trunk/extremities	12001	0
Repair, simple 2.6–5.0 cm, face/ears/lips	12013	0
Repair, simple 2.6–7.5 cm, scalp/trunk/extremities	12002	0

Table 11-2. Common Emergency Department Procedures (*continued*)		
Procedure	***CPT*® Code**	**Global Period (d)ᵃ**
Laceration repair, intermediate ≤2.5 cm, face/ears/lips	12051	10
Repair, intermediate ≤2.5 cm, hands/feet/neck	12041	10
Repair, intermediate ≤2.5 cm, scalp/trunk/arms/legs	12031	10
Repair, intermediate 2.6–5.0 cm, face/ears/lips	12052	10
Repair, intermediate 2.6–7.5 cm, hands/feet/neck	12042	10
Repair, intermediate 2.6–7.5 cm, scalp/trunk/extremities	12032	10
Lumbar puncture	62270	0
Nursemaid elbow reduction	24640	10
Pleural drainage, percutaneous, with insertion of indwelling catheter; without imaging guidance	32556	0
Pleural drainage, percutaneous, with insertion of indwelling catheter, with imaging guidance	32557	0
Puncture aspiration of abscess, hematoma, bulla, or cyst	10160	10
Repair, nail bed	11760	10
Splint, finger	29130	0
Splint, short arm	29125	0
Splint, short leg	29515	0
Strap, ankle	29540	0
Strap, knee	29530	0
Strap, shoulder	29240	0
Subungual hematoma evacuation	11740	0
Thoracentesis, needle or catheter, without imaging	32554	0
Thoracentesis, needle or catheter, with imaging	32555	0
Venipuncture, >3 y requiring physician skill	36410	NA
Venipuncture, requiring physician skill, femoral/jugular <3 y	36400	NA

Abbreviations: CPT, Current Procedural Terminology; NA, not applicable; TBSA, total body surface area.

ᵃ Procedures noted with global period NA have an X or M status in the Medicare Physician Fee Schedule.

Point-of-Care Ultrasound

Point-of-care ultrasound services performed by the ED physician (**Table 11-3**) are separately reportable in addition to the ED E/M service when *all 3 of the following conditions apply:*

- Thorough evaluation of organ(s) or anatomic region is performed.
- There is permanent image documentation.
- A written report equivalent to that typically produced by a radiologist is documented.

Without all of these elements, the examination is not separately reported and would be considered part of any E/M service provided. (*Exception:* Permanent image documentation is not required for ophthalmic ultrasound for biometric measurement.) Use of handheld or portable ultrasound that does not include all 3 of the previously listed elements is not separately reported.

> ||||||| **Coding Pearl** |||||||
>
> Use of handheld or portable ultrasound that does not include all 3 of the listed elements is not separately reported.

Table 11-3. Common Point-of-Care Procedures	
76536	Ultrasound, soft tissues of head and neck (eg, thyroid, parathyroid, parotid), real time with image documentation
76604	Ultrasound, chest (includes mediastinum when performed), real time with image documentation
76700	Ultrasound, abdominal, real time with image documentation; complete
76705	Ultrasound, abdominal, real time with image documentation; limited (eg, single organ, quadrant, follow-up)
76770	Ultrasound, retroperitoneal (eg, renal, aorta, nodes), real time with image documentation; complete
76775	Ultrasound, retroperitoneal (eg, renal, aorta, nodes), real time with image documentation; limited
76857	Ultrasound, pelvic (nonobstetric), real time with image documentation; limited or follow-up (eg, for follicles, presence of urine in bladder)
76870	Ultrasound, scrotum and contents[a]
76881	Ultrasound, extremity, nonvascular, real-time with image documentation; complete
76882	Ultrasound, extremity, nonvascular, real-time with image documentation; limited, anatomic specific
76885	Ultrasound, infant hips, real time with imaging documentation; dynamic (requiring physician or other qualified health care professional manipulation)
76886	Ultrasound, infant hips, real time with imaging documentation; limited, static (not requiring physician or other qualified health care professional manipulation)
76937	Ultrasound guidance for vascular access requiring ultrasound evaluation of potential access sites, documentation of selected vessel patency, concurrent real-time ultrasound visualization of vascular needle entry, with permanent recording and reporting (List separately in addition to code for primary procedure.)
93976	Duplex scan of arterial inflow and venous outflow of abdominal, pelvic, scrotal contents and/or retroperitoneal organs; limited study[a]

[a] Evaluation of vascular structures using both color and spectral Doppler is separately reportable. However, color Doppler alone, when performed for anatomic structure identification in conjunction with a real-time ultrasound examination, is not reported separately.

Bedside ultrasound services in the ED are reported by the physician with the professional service only modifier (26). (See Modifiers Used With ED Codes later in this chapter for more information.) The technical component (eg, equipment cost, facility overhead costs) is typically reported by the facility. (Payers may limit physicians to reporting of the professional component only for all facility-based services even if the physician performs the ultrasound and/or owns the equipment used for the service. The technical component includes all associated overhead costs. Check individual payer policies for reporting.)

One use of point-of-care ultrasound in the ED is the focused assessment with sonography for trauma (FAST) examination. This may consist of 2 distinct components: limited transthoracic echocardiogram and limited abdominal ultrasound. When 2 distinct procedures are performed, 2 codes are reported.

76705   Ultrasound, abdominal, real-time with image documentation; limited
93308   Echocardiography, transthoracic, real-time with image documentation (2D), includes M-mode recording, when performed, follow-up or limited study

When a limited ultrasound examination of the chest is included (eg, for pneumothorax), report code 76604 (ultrasound, chest [includes mediastinum when performed], real-time with image documentation). Limited studies are defined in CPT® as those that include examination of less than the required elements for a "complete" examination (eg, limited number of organs, limited portion of region evaluated). See your CPT reference for required components of complete examinations.

Ultrasound guidance for vascular access may be reported with code 76937. This service must include ultrasound evaluation of potential access sites, documentation of selected vessel patency, concurrent real-time ultrasound visualization of vascular needle entry, and permanent recording and reporting. This code is reported separately in addition to a code for primary vascular access procedure (eg, **36555**). Do not report **76937** if ultrasound guidance is not used for vascular needle placement (ie, vessel identification only), as this is not a separately reportable service. (If the same physician will provide neonatal or pediatric critical care on the same date, the vascular access procedure will not be separately reported. However, ultrasound guidance is not bundled to neonatal and pediatric critical care and may be separately paid.)

When ultrasound guidance is used for needle placement for procedures such as aspiration of an abscess, code **76942** is reported. Do not report code **76942** in conjunction with a service for which the code descriptor of the service includes ultrasound guidance (eg, joint aspiration). Code **76937** (ultrasound guidance for vascular access) is not reported in conjunction with code **76942**.

> ### ~ More From the AAP ~
>
> Read more about reporting ultrasound services in the November 2015 *AAP Pediatric Coding Newsletter*™ at http://coding.aap.org (subscription required).

Example

➤ **A child is seen in the ED for injuries sustained in a traffic accident.** The physician performs a trauma assessment, including a FAST examination. This examination may consist of 2 distinct components: limited transthoracic echocardiogram and limited abdominal ultrasound. When 2 distinct procedures are performed, 2 codes are reported.

The physician reports **76705 26** (ultrasound, abdominal, real-time with image documentation; limited) and **93308 26** (echocardiography, transthoracic, real-time with image documentation [2D], includes M-mode recording, when performed, follow-up or limited study). Modifier **26** signifies the physician is reporting the professional component of each service. The facility will report the same codes with modifier **TC** to indicate reporting of the technical component of each service. When applicable and all requirements for reporting are met, an ultrasound performed with physician-owned equipment is reported without a modifier (ie, modifier **26** is not applicable).

Modifiers Used With ED Codes

Physicians need to understand when it is appropriate to report modifiers in addition to E/M or procedural service codes. Modifiers **25** (significant, separately identifiable E/M service) and **57** (decision for surgery) may be appended to ED E/M codes to indicate E/M beyond the preservice work of a procedure. Procedures performed in the ED may require reporting of modifiers such as **26** (professional component) or **59** (distinct procedural service) or, when accepted by the payer in lieu of modifier **59**, modifier **XE** (separate encounter), **XP** (separate practitioner), **XS** (separate structure), or **XU** (unusual nonoverlapping service). **Table 11-4** lists modifiers commonly used in the ED. (See Chapter 3, Modifiers and Coding Edits, for more detail on the use of modifiers.)

Table 11-4. Common Modifiers Used in the Emergency Department

Modifier	When to Use
24	An unrelated E/M service is provided during the global period of a previously performed procedure by the same physician or group.
25	A significant, separately identifiable E/M service is performed by the same physician on the same day of the procedure or other service.
26	Reporting professional component only of a service for which payment includes equipment (or technical services) cost (eg, radiograph)
32	A service is mandated by third-party payer, regulation, or governmental entity.
51	Multiple procedures are performed on the same day other than E/M, physical medicine and rehabilitation services, or provision of supplies (eg, vaccines).
54	Only the surgical care component of a procedure was provided. Another physician will provide postoperative care.

Table 11-4. Common Modifiers Used in the Emergency Department (*continued*)

Modifier	When to Use
57	Decision for surgery was made. Some payers may require this modifier be appended to the E/M code only with procedures with 90-day global periods.
59	Distinct procedural service (non-E/M) was performed on the same day as another procedural service and was at a different encounter or a different surgery or procedure, or performed on a different body site or organ system.
63	Procedures (20000–69999) performed on an infant weighing <4 kg if the code descriptor does not include a descriptor of "young infant or neonate"
76	The same physician repeats a procedure or service on the same date of service.
77	Another physician repeats a procedure or service already performed by another physician on the same day of service.
79	An unrelated procedure is performed during the global period of a previously provided procedure by the same physician or group.
XE	The service was provided at a separate encounter on the same date.
XP	The non-E/M service or procedure was performed by a separate practitioner of the same group on the same date.
XS	The procedure or service was performed on a separate structure.
XU	Unusual nonoverlapping service

Abbreviation: E/M, evaluation and management.

Examples

➤ **A child is seen in the ED for left shoulder pain that occurred following a fall while playing soccer at a community sports field.** The child is examined for additional injuries (expanded problem-focused history, detailed examination). Radiograph reveals a mid-shaft clavicle fracture. The physician places the patient in a sling and refers the patient to another physician for follow-up care.

> A fracture not specified as displaced or non-displaced should be reported as displaced.

ICD-10-CM	CPT®
S42.022A (displaced fracture of left clavicle, initial encounter) **W18.30XA** (unspecified fall on same level, initial encounter) **Y93.66** (activity, soccer) **Y92.322** (soccer field as place of occurrence) **Y99.8** (external cause status, sport not for income)	**99283 25** **23500 54** (closed treatment of clavicular fracture, without manipulation)

Teaching Point: The use of modifier **54** (surgical care only) alerts payers that another physician will report postsurgical care. Alternatively, the ED physician may report the ED E/M code based on the level of service performed and documented and allow another physician to report the global fracture care.

► The ED physician evaluates a 6-year-old with a small (<2.5 cm) simple laceration on her right cheek that occurred when she fell, striking her face on the edge of a table at home. The wound is clean, there is no concern for other associated injury, and her immunization status is up-to-date. The parents are concerned about scarring and request a plastic surgeon to do the repair. The on-call surgeon is consulted and responds to the ED. The surgeon evaluates and repairs the wound with sutures in the ED. The ED physician documents a detailed history and physical examination with diagnoses of laceration right cheek and closed head injury without LOC. Instructions are provided to parents about home monitoring following a head injury.

Although the ED physician documented a detailed history and physical examination, the MDM would only rise to moderate complexity (new problem with no additional workup, potential for associated head injury). The surgeon does not report a consultation because the surgical service was at the request of the family and not the ED physician.

> Place of occurrence (**Y92.009**), activity, and external cause status codes are reported only at the initial encounter for treatment, so no seventh code character is required.

ICD-10-CM	CPT®
S01.411A (laceration without foreign body, right cheek, initial encounter) **S09.90XA** (unspecified injury of head) **W01.190A** (fall on same level from slipping, tripping, and stumbling with subsequent striking against furniture, initial encounter) **Y92.009** (occurred at home) **Y99.8** (other external cause status)	ED physician reports **99283 25** Surgeon reports **12011** (laceration repair)

Teaching Point: No modifiers are required for these services because the ED physician provided only the ED E/M service and not the procedure. The scenario does not indicate the surgeon provided any E/M service beyond the typical preservice work of the laceration repair.

► The ED physician is caring for a 9-year-old who has a 4-cm–long, deep laceration of the right calf and a separate 1-cm–long laceration of the right ankle from broken glass in his backyard. The physician performs a detailed history and physical examination. A radiograph of the extremity shows no retained radiopaque foreign bodies. The child's immunizations are current, with the last tetanus booster less than 5 years ago. The physician irrigates, carefully explores both wounds, and performs a 2-layer repair on the calf. The ankle laceration requires only single-layer closure. The child is discharged with appropriate follow-up plans.

ICD-10-CM	CPT
S81.811A (laceration without foreign body, right lower leg, initial encounter) **S91.011A** (laceration without foreign body, right ankle, initial encounter) **W25.XXXA** (contact with sharp glass, initial encounter) **Y92.007** (garden or yard of noninstitutional residence) **Y99.8** (other external cause status)	**99283 25** **12032** (intermediate repair of the extremities, 2.6–7.5 cm) **12001 59** or **XS** (simple repair of the extremity, ≤2.5 cm)

Teaching Point: Modifier **25** is used to indicate the ED E/M service was significant and separately identifiable from the preservice work of the laceration repairs. A modifier is required to indicate the simple repair was performed on a separate site from the intermediate or layered closure. Verify payer policy on reporting of modifier **59** (distinct procedural service) versus **XS** (separate structure). (See Chapter 3, Modifiers and Coding Edits, for more information on these modifiers.)

Chapter 11: Emergency Department Services

➤ A 14-year-old unconscious boy is brought to the ED after having ingested drugs at his father's apartment. The physician is unable to obtain additional history and documents this in the record. A comprehensive physical examination and high-level MDM are performed. The physician performs gastric intubation and lavage.

> *ICD-10-CM* codes for poisoning include intent. If intent is unknown, assign a code for accidental intent. No external cause code is required for poisonings, toxic effects, adverse effects, and underdosing codes.

ICD-10-CM	CPT®
T50.901A (poisoning, unspecified drug or medicinal substance, accidental intent)	**99285 25** **43753** (gastric lavage)

Teaching Point: The ED E/M service for this patient was comprehensive and involved high-level MDM that supports separate reporting of the E/M service in addition to the gastric lavage. Modifier **25** is used to indicate the same physician (or physician of the same group and specialty) provided the significant and separately identifiable E/M service and the procedure. Code **43753** would not be separately reported if critical care services had been provided.

Sedation

Moderate Sedation

Moderate sedation (**99151–99157**) (Table 11-5) is a drug-induced depression of consciousness during which patients may respond purposefully to verbal commands, alone or accompanied by light tactile stimulation. Moderate sedation may be necessary for the performance of certain procedures in the ED. Coding and documentation requirements for reporting this service are detailed in Chapter 15, Common Surgical Procedures and Sedation.

Table 11-5. Moderate Sedation		
Moderate Sedation	**First 10–22 min Intraservice Time**	**Each Additional 15 min Intraservice Time**
Moderate sedation services provided by the same physician or other qualified health care professional performing the diagnostic or therapeutic service that the sedation supports, requiring the presence of an independent trained observer to assist in the monitoring of the patient's level of consciousness and physiological status; initial 15 minutes of intra-service time, patient younger than 5 years of age	99151	+99153
5 years or older	99152	+99153
Moderate sedation services (other than those services described by codes **00100–01999**) provided by a physician other than the health care professional performing the diagnostic or therapeutic service that the sedation supports; younger than 5 years	99155	+99157
5 years or older	99156	+99157

Example

> **A 10-year-old presents to the ED with left forearm pain after falling from her bicycle.** She fell onto a concrete patio at her house but did not hit her head. The injury occurred 1 hour ago and was iced by the mother, but pain and swelling continued

Review of systems: Pain is limited to lower left arm and wrist; patient has no headache and no nausea or vomiting. She has had no past surgeries or hospitalizations; she has no known allergies; and her immunizations are up-to-date. The patient is active in gymnastics and dance. Family history is reviewed and is noncontributory. Detailed examination includes constitutional, head, eyes, neck, musculoskeletal, cardiovascular, and respiratory elements. Imaging shows a Salter-Harris type II physeal fracture of the left distal radius (interpreted by the radiologist). An orthopedic surgeon is consulted and requests that the ED physician provide moderate sedation for closed reduction in the ED. The ED physician documents 25 minutes of moderate sedation, beginning with administration of the sedating agent and ending when the patient is sufficiently recovered that the physician's continuous face-to-face monitoring is no longer necessary. The ED physician reports

ICD-10-CM	CPT
S59.222A (Salter-Harris Type II physeal fracture, lower left radius) **V18.000A** (pedal cycle rider injured noncollision transport accident, nontraffic accident) **Y92.018** (other place of single-family house) **Y99.8** (other external cause status)	**99283 25** **99156** (moderate sedation by other than physician performing procedure, first 15 minutes) **99157** (moderate sedation, each additional 15 minutes)

Teaching Point: The orthopedic surgeon will separately report the fracture reduction procedure (eg, **25605**, closed treatment with manipulation) and, if applicable, any medically necessary E/M service beyond the preservice work of the procedure (modifier **57** may be required to indicate that the physician determined the need for the procedure at this encounter).

Deep Sedation

Deep sedation or analgesia is a drug-induced depression of consciousness during which patients cannot be easily aroused but respond purposefully after repeated verbal or painful stimulation (eg, purposefully pushing away the noxious stimuli). The ability to independently maintain ventilatory function may be impaired. Patients may require assistance in maintaining a patent airway, and spontaneous ventilation may be inadequate. Cardiovascular function is usually maintained. A state of deep sedation may be accompanied by partial or complete loss of protective airway reflexes.

Although ED physicians may provide deep sedation, payment for these services is limited.

Deep sedation provided by a physician also performing the services for which the sedation is being provided is reported by appending modifier **47** (anesthesia by surgeon) to the procedure code for the service for which sedation is required. Many health plans do not pay separately for anesthesia by the physician or surgeon performing the procedure.

National Correct Coding Initiative (NCCI) edits do not allow payment of an ED visit (**99281–99285**) and deep sedation when provided by the same ED physician or 2 ED physicians of the same group practice. No modifier will override the NCCI edits. Payers that have adopted Medicare or Medicaid NCCI edits will deny the ED visit when reported on the same date as deep sedation.

Please see Chapter 15, Common Surgical Procedures and Sedation, for more information on deep sedation.

Chapter 11: Emergency Department Services

Special Service Codes

99053   Service(s) provided between 10:00 pm and 8:00 am at 24-hour facility, in addition to basic service

99056   Service(s) typically provided in office, provided out of office at request of patient, in addition to basic service

99060   Service(s) provided on an emergency basis, out of office, which disrupts other scheduled office services, in addition to basic service

Special service codes may be used to report services that are an adjunct to the basic service provided. *Current Procedural Terminology*® guidelines do not restrict the reporting of adjunct special service codes in the ED. However, third-party payers will have specific policies for coverage and payment. Communicate with individual payers to understand their definition or interpretation of the service and coverage and payment policies.

These codes are intended to describe services that are provided outside the normal time frame and location. Code **99053** would be reported when services are provided between the designated time limits in an ED.

Current Procedural Terminology does not restrict reporting of any procedure or service to any specific specialty. However, it would be inappropriate for an ED physician to report code **99056** or **99060** for services provided in the ED.

If appropriate, a non-ED physician could report *CPT* code **99056** or **99060** when he or she provides services in the ED in addition to an outpatient office or clinic visit, ED visit, or consultation E/M code.

> ||||||| *Coding Pearl* |||||||
>
> It would not be appropriate for an ED physician to report code **99056** or **99060** for services provided in the ED.

Continuum Models for Asthma, Head Injury, and Laceration

Three common conditions seen in the ED follow in a teaching tool called the Continuum Model. Each condition—asthma, head injury, and laceration—is described across the continuum of codes **99281–99285** plus critical care. Although the actual assignment of a code for an individual patient may vary from the examples, members of the American Academy of Pediatrics Committee on Coding and Nomenclature have generally agreed that these examples provide an accurate representation of how one condition typically flows across the family of codes.

Continuum Model for Asthma

CPT® Code Vignette	History	Physical Examination	Medical Decision-making

99281
Stable asthma, concern about potential, but not active problems 8 days later
	Problem focused
	1. Chief complaint
	2. Problem-focused HPI
	  a. Cough
	  b. Wheeze
		Problem focused
		1. Limited respiratory system
			Straightforward
			1. Anticipatory guidance.
			2. Recommend routine follow-up.

99282
Stable asthma, out of medication
	Expanded problem focused
	1. Chief complaint
	2. Brief HPI plus pertinent ROS
	  a. Cough
	  b. Wheeze
	  c. Respiratory distress
	  d. Home peak flow data
	  e. Frequency of rescue medication
	  f. Associated signs and symptoms
		Expanded problem focused
		1. Examination of respiratory system including lungs, ENT, and other pertinent organ systems
			Low complexity
			1. Review and evaluation of home medications
			2. Alteration in medication regimen
			3. Refills
			4. Criteria for urgent/emergent follow-up
			5. Plan for follow-up care

99283
Known asthmatic with URI symptoms or mild exacerbation
	Expanded problem focused
	1. Chief complaint
	2. Brief HPI plus pertinent ROS
	  a. Cough
	  b. Wheeze
	  c. Respiratory distress
	  d. Home peak flow data
	  e. Frequency of rescue medication
	  f. Associated signs and symptoms
		Expanded problem focused
		1. Examination of respiratory system including lungs, ENT, and other pertinent organ systems.
		2. A peak expiratory flow rate may be obtained.
			Moderate complexity
			1. Same as 99282 plus 1 respiratory treatment and reassessment (Pulse oximetry and peak flow may be included.)

99284 Known asthmatic with moderate exacerbation	**Detailed** 1. Chief complaint 2. Extended HPI and ROS 3. Problem-pertinent PFSH	**Detailed** 1. Constitutional, ENT, neck, respiratory, cardiovascular, and other pertinent systems. 2. A peak expiratory flow rate may be obtained.	**Moderate complexity** 1. Same as 99283 plus 1–3 respiratory treatments (or 1 continuous treatment). 2. Systemic (oral or parenteral) steroids 3. Multiple reassessments (pulse oximetry and peak flow may be included). 4. Chest radiograph may be obtained. 5. May be admitted for observation.

Chapter 11: Emergency Department Services

Chapter 11: Emergency Department Services

Continuum Model for Asthma (continued)

CPT® Code Vignette	History	Physical Examination	Medical Decision-making
99285 Known asthmatic with moderate to severe exacerbation	**Comprehensive** 1. Chief complaint 2. Extended HPI 3. Complete ROS 4. 2 of 3 PFSH	**Comprehensive** 1. Constitutional, eyes, ENT, respiratory, cardiovascular, gastrointestinal, neurologic, skin. 2. A peak expiratory flow rate may be obtained.	**High complexity** 1. Same as **99284** plus 4 respiratory treatments (or 2 continuous treatments or 1 continuous with 1 intermittent treatment). 2. Multiple reassessments (pulse oximetry and peak flow may be included). 3. Chest radiograph may be obtained. 4. Blood gas or end-tidal CO_2 monitoring may be obtained.
99291, 99292 Critical Care Known asthmatic unstable with marked distress and (impending) respiratory failure Critically ill, unstable patient; requires >30 min of directed patient care (bedside, review of data, consultation with other specialist, discussion with family members, documentation)			**High complexity** 1. Same as **99285**. Usually requires use of additional therapies such as ketamine, magnesium sulfate, parenteral adrenergic agents, and/or heliox; ET intubation; or BiPAP.

Abbreviations: BiPAP, bi-level positive airway pressure; CPT, Current Procedural Terminology; ENT, ear, nose, throat; ET, endotracheal; HPI, history of present illness; PFSH, past, family, and social history; ROS, review of systems; URI, upper respiratory infection.

Continuum Model for Head Injury

CPT® Code Vignette	History	Physical Examination	Medical Decision-making
99281 Repaired scalp laceration, well healed, presents for suture removal	**Problem focused** 1. Chief complaint 2. Problem-focused HPI a. Signs of infection, poor healing	**Problem focused** 1. Limited skin	**Straightforward** 1. Suture removal
99282 Minor head trauma without local bruising, swelling, or laceration, no neurologic changes	**Expanded problem focused** 1. Chief complaint 2. Injury mechanism a. Associated signs and symptoms	**Expanded problem focused** 1. Examination of skin and neurologic system and other pertinent organ systems	**Low complexity** 1. May recommend OTC analgesic or local care 2. Anticipatory guidance 3. Criteria for urgent/emergent follow-up 4. Plan for follow-up care
99283 Minor head trauma with local bruising, swelling, or laceration, no neurologic changes; GCS 15	**Expanded problem focused** 1. Chief complaint 2. Injury mechanism a. Associated signs and symptoms	**Expanded problem focused** 1. Eyes, ENT, skin, and neurologic system and other pertinent organ systems	**Moderate complexity** 1. Same as 99282 2. May require laceration repair 3. May require some ED observation
99284 Head trauma with signs of concussion including loss of recall, brief LOC (<5 min), and/or emesis but no focal neurologic changes; GCS ≥13	**Detailed** 1. Chief complaint 2. Extended HPI and ROS 3. Problem-pertinent PFSH	**Detailed** 1. Eyes, ENT, neck, respiratory, cardio-vascular, skin, neurologic, and other pertinent systems	**Moderate complexity** 1. Same as 99283 plus multiple reassessments. 2. Cervical spine radiographs may be obtained. 3. Head CT or MRI may be obtained. 4. Laboratory tests may be obtained. 5. Neurology or neurosurgical consulta-tion may be obtained.
99285 Head trauma with signs of concus-sion including LOC (>5 min), brief seizure, and/or persistent emesis; closed skull fracture and/or focal neurologic changes may be present; GCS 9–12	**Comprehensive** 1. Chief complaint 2. Extended HPI 3. Complete ROS 4. 2 of 3 PFSH	**Comprehensive** 1. Constitutional, eyes, ENT, respira-tory, cardiovascular, gastrointestinal, neurologic, skin	**High complexity** 1. Same as 99284 plus anticonvulsant(s) may be administered. 2. Head CT or MRI likely obtained.

Chapter 11: Emergency Department Services

Continuum Model for Head Injury (continued)

CPT® Code Vignette	History	Physical Examination	Medical Decision-making
99291, 99292 Critical Care Head trauma with persistent LOC and/or seizures; open or closed skull fracture and/or focal neurologic changes may be present; GCS ≤8 Critically ill, unstable patient; requires >30 min of directed patient care (bedside, review of data, consultation with other specialist, discussion with family members, documentation)			**High complexity** 1. Same as 99285 2. May require additional interventions, such as ET intubation

Abbreviations: CPT, Current Procedural Terminology; CT, computed tomography; ED, emergency department; ENT, ear, nose, throat; ET, endotracheal; GCS, Glasgow Coma Scale; HPI, history of present illness; LOC, loss of consciousness; MRI, magnetic resonance imaging; OTC, over the counter; PFSH, past, family, and social history; ROS, review of systems.

Continuum Model for Laceration

These codes reflect E/M services only and not any procedure the same physician may provide. The physician needs to be aware that the pre-procedural and intra-procedural global periods may include some of the medical decision-making indicated with each code, thus reducing the level of E/M service provided, and that any E/M service reported with a procedure must meet the requirement for a significant, separately identifiable service.

CPT® Code Vignette	History	Physical Examination	Medical Decision-making
99281 Patient with this condition in the ED usually does not meet the criteria for this level. Patient presenting for removal of sutures not placed at that facility			

99282
Uncomplicated laceration of single body area or organ system
	Expanded problem focused
	1. Chief complaint
	2. Mechanisms
	  a. Timing
	  b. Foreign body risk
	  c. Associated signs and symptoms
		Expanded problem focused
		1. Examination of affected body area and other pertinent organ systems
			Low complexity
			1. Laceration repair
			2. Criteria for urgent/emergent follow-up
			3. Plan for follow-up care

99283
Uncomplicated laceration of single body area or organ system with minor associated injury (eg, minor head injury)
OR
Uncomplicated lacerations of >1 body area or organ system
OR
Minimally complicated laceration (eg, small foreign body, delay in seeking care) of single body area or organ system
	Expanded problem focused
	1. Chief complaint
	2. Mechanisms
	  a. Timing
	  b. Foreign body risk
	  c. Associated signs and symptoms
		Expanded problem focused
		1. Examination of affected body area(s) and other pertinent organ systems
			Moderate complexity
			1. Same as 99282.
			2. Radiograph of affected area may be obtained.
			3. Oral pain medication may be administered.
			4. Antibiotics may be administered and/or prescribed.
			5. Moderate sedation with or without analgesia may be given.

Chapter 11: Emergency Department Services

Chapter 11: Emergency Department Services

Continuum Model for Laceration (continued)

These codes reflect E/M services only and not any procedure the same physician may provide. The physician needs to be aware that the pre-procedural and intra-procedural global periods may include some of the medical decision-making indicated with each code, thus reducing the level of E/M service provided, and that any E/M service reported with a procedure must meet the requirement for a significant, separately identifiable service.

CPT® Code Vignette	History	Physical Examination	Medical Decision-making
99284 Uncomplicated laceration of single body area or organ system with other associated injury (eg, mild concussion) OR Minimally complicated laceration (eg, small foreign body) >1 body area or organ system OR Complicated laceration (eg, infection, GSW, deep knife wound) of single body area or organ system without immediate threat to life or limb	**Detailed** 1. Chief complaint 2. Extended HPI and ROS 3. Problem-pertinent PFSH	**Detailed** 1. ENT, neck, respiratory, cardiovascular, musculoskeletal, neurologic, and other pertinent systems	**Moderate complexity** 1. Same as 99283. 2. Parenteral pain medication may be administered. 3. IV fluids may be administered. 4. Surgical consultation may be obtained. 5. Moderate to deep sedation with or without analgesia may be provided for another service. 6. May be admitted for observation.
99285 Uncomplicated laceration of ≥1 body area or organ system with significant associated injury (eg, multiple trauma) OR Complicated laceration (eg, GSW, deep knife wound) >1 body area or organ system without immediate threat to life or limb	**Comprehensive** 1. Chief complaint 2. Extended HPI 3. Complete ROS 4. 2 of 3 PFSH	**Comprehensive** 1. Constitutional, eyes, ENT, respiratory, cardiovascular, gastrointestinal, neurologic, skin	**High complexity** 1. Same as 99284 plus may require operating room for repair
99291, 99292 Critical Care Uncomplicated or complicated laceration of ≥1 body area or organ system with significant associated injury (eg, multiple trauma) with immediate threat to life or limb Critically ill, unstable patient; requires >30 minutes of directed patient care (bedside, review of data, consultation with other specialist, discussion with family members, documentation)			**High complexity** 1. Same as 99285 2. Usually requires use of additional therapies such as cardiovascular support

Abbreviations: CPT, Current Procedural Terminology; ED, emergency department; E/M, evaluation and management; ENT, ear, nose, throat; GSW, gunshot wound; HPI, history of present illness; IV, intravenous; PFSH, past, family, and social history; ROS, review of systems.

Critical and Intensive Care

Contents

This chapter focuses on the correct coding for critical and intensive care, including attendance at delivery, neonatal resuscitation, hourly critical care, critical care of the neonate and child younger than 6 years, and intensive care of the recovering or low birth weight infant. Services commonly reported before and after intensive or critical care services, such as care during emergency transport, consultations, and medical team care conferences, are included.

Evaluation and management (E/M) of the child who no longer requires intensive or critical care is discussed in Chapter 10, Noncritical Hospital Evaluation and Management Services.

Attendance at Delivery and Newborn Resuscitation

99464   Attendance at delivery (when requested by the delivering physician or other qualified health care professional) and initial stabilization of newborn

99465   Delivery/birthing room resuscitation, provision of positive pressure ventilation and/or chest compressions in the presence of acute inadequate ventilation and/or cardiac output

Attendance at delivery (**99464**) is only reported when the physical presence of the provider is requested by the delivering physician and indicated for a newborn who may require immediate intervention (ie, stabilization, resuscitation, or evaluation for potential problems). See coding examples in Chapter 9, Pre-birth Counseling and Care of the Newborn.

Code **99464** is not reported when hospital-mandated attendance is the only underlying basis for providing the service. When physician on-call services are not requested by the delivering physician but, rather, are mandated by the hospital (eg, attending specific types of deliveries without physician request, such as all repeat cesarean deliveries), report code **99026** (hospital-mandated on-call service; in hospital, each hour) or **99027** (hospital-mandated on-call service; out of hospital, each hour). See Chapter 10, Noncritical Hospital Evaluation and Management Services, for guidelines on the use of codes **99026** and **99027**.

Attendance at delivery (**99464**)

* Service is only reported when requested by the delivering physician.
* Medical record documentation must include the request for attendance at the delivery and substantiate the medical necessity of the services performed. If there is no documentation by the delivering physician for attendance at delivery, the verbal request and the reason for the request should be documented in the attendance note.
* Includes initial drying, stimulation, suctioning, blow-by oxygen, or continuous positive airway pressure (CPAP) without positive-pressure ventilation (PPV); a cursory visual inspection of the neonate; assignment of Apgar scores; and discussion of the care of the newborn with the delivering physician and parents. A quick look in the delivery room or examination after stabilization is not sufficient to support reporting of **99464**.
* Any medically necessary procedures to complete the resuscitation that are provided in the delivery room may be reported separately (eg, direct laryngoscopy without intubation).
* May be reported in addition to the initial normal newborn (**99460**), initial sick newborn (**99221–99223**), initial intensive care of the neonate (**99477**), or critical care (**99468**; **99291–99292**) codes.

When qualifying resuscitative efforts are provided, code **99465** (delivery/birthing room resuscitation) is reported instead. Codes **99464** and **99465** cannot be reported on the same day of service.

Attendance at delivery with neonatal resuscitation (**99465**)

* Includes bag-and-mask or bag-to-endotracheal tube ventilation (PPV) and/or cardiac compressions.
* Is reported when positive-pressure breaths are administered by the T-piece resuscitator in lieu of a manual bag-mask resuscitator (see Coding Conundrum: T-Piece Positive-Pressure Ventilation later in this chapter).
* Does not include other life support procedures that are performed as a necessary part of the resuscitation and may be reported separately (eg, **31500**, intubation, endotracheal, emergency procedure; **31515**, laryngoscopy, direct, for aspiration; **36510**, catheterization of umbilical vein for diagnosis or therapy, newborn; **94610**, surfactant administration).

Chapter 12: Critical and Intensive Care

- May be reported in addition to any initial care service, including initial critical care (**99468**; **99291**, **99292**), initial neonatal intensive care (**99477**), or normal newborn care (**99460**) if the resuscitation results in a stable term neonate.

- Medically necessary procedures (eg, intubation, umbilical line placement) essential to successful resuscitation (and not performed as a convenience before admission to the neonatal intensive care unit [NICU]) that are performed in the delivery room prior to admission may also be reported in addition to code **99468** or **99477**. Medical record documentation must clearly support that the services are provided as part of the preadmission or pre-global service.

Example

➤ **A neonatologist attends the cesarean delivery of a 27-weeks' gestation neonate at the request of an obstetrician, who suspects an abruption.** The neonate has no spontaneous activity. The resuscitation includes PPV, intubation, and placement of an umbilical vein catheter. The newborn is stabilized and admitted to the NICU, where the neonatologist administers surfactant and performs an umbilical artery catheterization.

The intubation and umbilical vein catheterization are separately reported procedures provided as part of the resuscitation and not as a convenience to the physician prior to admission.	**Current Procedural Terminology (CPT®)** **99465** (delivery/birthing room resuscitation) **31500** (endotracheal intubation) **36510** (catheterization of umbilical vein for diagnosis or therapy, newborn) **99468 25** (initial neonatal critical care)

Modifier **25** is appended to code **99468** to signify a significant, separately identifiable E/M service provided in addition to codes **31500** and **36510** because these services are bundled by National Correct Coding Initiative (NCCI) edits (for more on edits, see Chapter 3, Modifiers and Coding Edits). Codes **99465** and **99468** are not bundled by NCCI edits, but individual payers may require modifier **25** to designate separately identifiable critical care services on the same date. The surfactant administration and umbilical artery catheterization are not separately reported when performed in conjunction with neonatal critical care.

Coding Conundrum: T-Piece Positive-Pressure Ventilation

A frequently asked question is whether **99465** can be reported if the T-piece resuscitator is used to provide CPAP only. Clearly, from the definitions given previously, the answer is no. If CPAP is provided to the neonate and she responds with an adequate respiratory effort, **99464** should be reported. On the other hand, if the neonate is apneic or, in the judgment of the provider, exhibiting inadequate respiratory effort, positive-pressure breaths administered by the T-piece resuscitator in lieu of a manual bag-mask resuscitator would justify reporting **99465**. It would be important that the documentation explicitly state that the neonate demonstrated respiratory and/or cardiac instability requiring intervention, including apnea or inadequate respiratory effort to support gas exchange, the provider instituted PPV, and the neonate's response to the PPV.

Definition of Perinatal Period

The World Health Organization (WHO) defines the *perinatal period* as the time from the 22nd week of completed gestation through the 28th day following birth. Based on this definition, the perinatal period continues through the 28th day after birth, ending on the 29th calendar day after birth. The day of birth is considered day 0 (zero); therefore, the day after birth is considered day 1.

In addition to coding perinatal diagnoses, this definition affects reporting of the initial- and subsequent-day neonatal and pediatric critical care codes **99468–99472** and code **99477** for the initial hospital care of the neonate, 28 days or younger, who requires intensive observation, frequent interventions, and other intensive care services.

Critical Care Services

Critical Illness or Injury

- A *critical illness or injury* is defined by *CPT®* as one that acutely impairs one or more vital organs such that there is a high probability of imminent or life-threatening deterioration of the patient's condition.
- Critical care involves high-complexity medical decision-making (MDM) to assess, manipulate, and support vital organ system function(s); treat single or multiple organ system failure; and/or prevent further life-threatening deterioration of the patient's condition.
- Immaturity alone, or any of the specific procedures, equipment, or therapies associated with care of the immature neonate, does not define critical care.
- Coding critical care is not determined by the location in which the care is delivered but by the nature of the care being delivered and the condition of the patient requiring care.
- Services qualify as critical care *only if both* the injury or illness *and* the treatment being delivered meet the following criteria:
  - The illness or injury acutely impairs one or more vital organs as defined previously.
  - The treatment delivered involves high-complexity MDM to prevent life-threatening deterioration of the patient's condition.
- Critical care is not limited to an inpatient setting or a critical care area, and a physician of any specialty can provide these services. Services must be provided directly by the physician or other qualified health care professional (QHP).

Coding Conundrum: Applying the Critical Care Definition

The physician must use his or her experience and judgment in assigning the *CPT* definition of critical care. In summary, these are patients presently at clear risk of death or serious morbidity, requiring close observation and frequent interventions and assessments, and where the high-complexity MDM is apparent in the medical record documentation. No one criterion places or excludes a patient from this category, and the patient is not required to demonstrate all the characteristics listed in this chapter. The most convincing way to demonstrate the appropriate application of a critical care code is to clearly document in the medical record the child's condition, noting the risks to the patient, frequency of needed assessments and interventions, degree of and type of organ failure(s) the patient is presently experiencing, and complexity of the MDM. While immaturity commonly leads to many levels of organ dysfunction that will increase the risk of a critical illness in a newborn, neither immaturity alone nor any of the specific procedures or therapies associated with care of the immature neonate or infant qualifies alone for reporting critical care.

Hourly Critical Care

99291   Critical care, E/M of the critically ill or critically injured patient; first 30 to 74 minutes

+99292   each additional 30 minutes (Use in conjunction with **99291**.)

Guidelines for reporting codes **99291** and **99292**

- Reported when critical care is provided for 30 minutes or more
  - In the outpatient setting (eg, emergency department [ED], office, clinic) *regardless of age*
  - To an inpatient 6 years or older (Daily critical care of a child younger than 6 years is discussed later in this chapter.)
  - Concurrently by a second physician from a different specialty to a critically ill or injured child aged 5 years or younger
  - To an inpatient aged 5 years or younger when the patient is being transferred to another facility where the receiving physician of the same specialty but different medical group will be reporting the daily inpatient critical care service codes (**99468** and **99469**; **99471** and **99472**; and **99475** and **99476**)
  - By the physician physically transporting a critically ill child older than 2 years (Refer to codes **99466** and **99467** for face-to-face transport care of the critically ill or injured patient 24 months or younger.)

❋ These are bundled codes (include many procedures typically performed and included in the work valuation of the code that cannot be reported separately) (**Table 12-1**). (See also Procedures *Not* Bundled With Critical/ Intensive Care Services later in this chapter for commonly provided services not bundled with hourly and/or neonatal and pediatric critical care services.)

❋ Procedures not included as bundled may be reported separately (eg, lumbar puncture, endotracheal intubation, thoracentesis). The reported time of critical care *cannot* include any time spent performing procedures or services that are reported separately.

❋ Reporting is time-based. **Table 12-2** lists times and billing units. The total floor or unit time devoted to the patient in the provision of critical care is used in code selection. Critical care time includes physician– patient face-to-face time or time spent on the patient's *unit or floor* directly related to the patient's care (eg, hands-on care at the bedside, reviewing test results, discussing care with other medical staff or family, documenting services in the medical record).

❋ Time spent in the provision of critical care does not need to be continuous. The cumulative time of critical care provided on a single date of service is used to calculate the units of service provided. However, when a *continuous period* of critical care occurs before and after midnight, report the total time on the date that the period of care was initiated. Do not report a second initial hour of critical care for the period beginning at midnight.

❋ The physician must be immediately available to the patient during time reported as critical care. No time spent in activities that take place out of the unit, off the patient's floor, or consulting with other caregivers from home are included in critical care time.

❋ Code **99291** is reported once on a given date of service when 30 to 74 minutes of critical care is performed. If less than 30 minutes of critical care is provided, an appropriate E/M service (eg, **99201–99215** for office services, **99221–99233** for inpatient hospital care) is reported.

❋ Code **99292** is reported with one unit for each additional period up to 30 minutes beyond the previous period. See **Table 12-2** for reporting the correct codes based on the total duration of critical care. *Time spent providing critical care services must be documented in the medical record.*

❋ Critical care is not permitted to be reported as a split/shared service (ie, the times of a physician and QHP cannot be combined and reported as a single service). The time required to report code **99291** must be met by a single physician. If multiple providers from the same group practice and same specialty care for a patient after a single physician has provided the initial 30 minutes of critical care, combine the total time and report with code **99292** as appropriate. Do not report **99291** more than once per day.

❋ Time-based critical care services (**99291, 99292**) may be reported by an individual of a different specialty from either the same or different group on the same day that neonatal or pediatric critical care services are reported by another individual.

❋ A teaching physician may report time-based critical care services only when he or she was present for the entire period for which the claim is submitted and that time is supported in documentation of the service.

❋ When inpatient and outpatient critical care services are provided to a neonate, infant, or child younger than 6 years on the same date by the same physician (or physician of the same group and specialty), only the *inpatient* critical care codes are reported (**99468–99476**).

❋ Other significant, separately identifiable E/M services (eg, **99212–99215, 99281–99285**) can be reported in addition to time-based critical care services as appropriate. Do not count time spent in separately reported E/M services in critical care time.

Examples

➤ **A 3-week-old exposed to a sick sibling at home acquires respiratory syncytial virus and is seen in the ED for respiratory distress.** The ED physician provides an hour of critical care before the neonate is admitted to the NICU by the neonatologist.

Code **99291** with 1 unit of service (30–74 minutes) is reported by the ED physician. The neonatologist will report the appropriate level of daily hospital, intensive, or critical care.

Table 12-1. Critical Care Bundled Services

CPT® Code and Procedure	Hourly Critical Care 99291, 99292	Pediatric Transport 99466, 99467	Neonatal/Pediatric Critical and Intensive Care 99468–99476, 99477–99480
Interpretation and Monitoring			
71045 X-ray, chest; single view	×	×	×
71046 X-ray, chest, 2 views, frontal and lateral	×	×	×
93561 Cardiac output measurement	×		×
93562 subsequent measurement of cardiac output	×	×	×
94760 Pulse oximetry; single determination	×	×	×
94761 multiple determinations (eg, during exercise)			
94762 by continuous overnight monitoring			
99090 Analysis of clinical data stored in computers (eg, ECGs, BP, hematologic data)	×	×	×
Vascular Access Procedures			
36000 Introduction of needle or intracatheter, vein	×	×	×
36140 Catheterization extremity artery		×	
36400 Venipuncture, <3 years, requiring physician or QHP skill; femoral or jugular vein		×	×
36405 scalp vein			
36406 other vein			
36410 Venipuncture, ≥3 years, requiring physician or QHP	×		×
36415 Collection of venous blood by venipuncture	×	×	×
36420 Venipuncture, cutdown; younger than age 1 year			×
36430 Transfusion, blood or blood components			×
36440 Push transfusion, blood, 2 years or younger			×
36510 Catheterization of umbilical vein, newborn			×
36555 Insertion of non-tunneled CICC; <5 years of age			×
36591 Collection blood from venous access device	×	×	×
36600 Arterial puncture, withdrawal of blood for diagnosis	×	×	×
36620 Arterial catheterization, percutaneous			
36660 Catheterization, umbilical artery, newborn			×
Other Procedures			
31500 Endotracheal intubation			×
43752 Nasogastric/orogastric intubation, fluoroscopic guidance	×	×	×
43753 Gastric intubation including lavage if performed	×	×	×
51100 Aspiration of bladder; by needle			×

Chapter 12: Critical and Intensive Care

Table 12-1. Critical Care Bundled Services (*continued*)			
CPT® Code and Procedure	**Hourly Critical Care** 99291, 99292	**Pediatric Transport** 99466, 99467	**Neonatal/Pediatric Critical and Intensive Care** 99468–99476, 99477–99480
Other Procedures (*continued*)			
51701 Insertion of non-indwelling bladder catheter			×
51702 Temporary indwelling bladder catheter; simple			×
62270 Spinal puncture, lumbar, diagnostic			×
92953 Temporary transcutaneous pacing	×	×	×
94002 Ventilation initiation; inpatient/observation, initial day 94003 each subsequent day	×	×	×
94004 Ventilation initiation; nursing facility, per day	×		×
94375 Respiratory flow volume loop			×
94610 Intrapulmonary surfactant administration			×
94660 CPAP initiation and management	×	×	×
94662 CNP, initiation and management	×	×	×
94780 Car seat/bed testing, neonate; 60 minutes 94781 each additional full 30 minutes			×

Abbreviations: *BP, blood pressure; CICC, centrally inserted central venous catheter; CNP, continuous negative pressure ventilation; CPAP, continuous positive airway pressure; CPT, Current Procedural Terminology; ECG, electrocardiogram; QHP, qualified health care professional.*

➤ **A 4-month-old is admitted with fever, lethargy, and poor feeding. Laboratory work, cultures, and intravenous (IV) fluids are begun.** Later that afternoon, the infant decompensates, developing desaturation, apnea, and falling blood pressures. The pediatrician returns to the bedside; 3 hours are spent at the hospital stabilizing the infant, directing nursing staff, discussing management options with the tertiary care facility, speaking with the parents, and monitoring the infant while awaiting the transport team to take the infant to a hospital where the pediatrician does not practice.

Care is reported with an initial hospital care code (**99221–99223**) along with **99291** and **99292** with 4 units of service. It would be appropriate to report the critical care time in addition to the initial hospital care code by the transferring pediatrician, for 165 to 194 minutes of care on the same date of service.

➤ **A 3-year-old girl is seen in the physician's office with complaints of shortness of breath and wheezing.** She has a history of moderate persistent childhood asthma. The patient goes into respiratory distress and vital signs are deteriorating. The physician initiates critical care. After working for 10 minutes to stabilize the critical patient, an ambulance is called when the patient responds too slowly. The physician continues critical care services for another 25 minutes before the ambulance arrives. The total time for critical care services provided in the office was 35 minutes. The patient is admitted to the pediatric intensive care unit at the local university hospital under a pediatric intensivist. The pediatrician provides no more hands-on care for the patient that day and reports outpatient critical care services with a diagnosis of status asthmaticus.

Code **99291** with 1 unit of service (30–74 minutes) is reported. If the same physician or physician group of the same specialty provided outpatient and inpatient critical care services, due to the patient's age, only the pediatric critical care code (**99475**) would be reported. Had the patient been 6 years or older, the time spent in outpatient critical care by the same physician or group providing inpatient services would be combined. Keep in mind that **99291** is only reported once per day.

Table 12-2. Reporting Hourly Critical Care Services

Duration of Face-to-face Critical Care	CPT® Codes
<30 min	Do not report as critical care; included in the reported E/M service.
30–74 min	99291
75–104 min	99291 × 1 unit plus 99292 × 1 unit
105–134 min	99291 × 1 unit plus 99292 × 2 units

Abbreviations: CPT, Current Procedural Terminology; E/M, evaluation and management.

Procedures Not *Bundled With Critical/Intensive Care Services*

When reporting hourly critical or neonatal and pediatric critical and intensive care services, many services commonly provided with these codes are not bundled into the intensive or critical care services. However, claim edits may require appending a modifier to indicate the services were distinct. Examples of procedures that are not bundled with critical care services include (not all-inclusive)

- Thoracentesis (**32554, 32555**) (via needle or pigtail catheter)
- Percutaneous pleural drainage with insertion of indwelling catheter (**32556, 32557**)
  Tip: See Chapter 15, Common Surgical Procedures and Sedation, for more information on reporting thoracentesis, pleural drainage, and thoracostomy procedures.
- Complete (double volume) exchange transfusion (**36450, 36455**)
- Partial exchange transfusion (**36456**)
- Abdominal paracentesis (**49082, 49083**)
- Subdural or shunt tap (**61000, 61001, 61108**)
- Bone marrow aspiration (**38220**)
- Circumcision (**54150**)
- Cardioversion (**92960**)
- Cardiopulmonary resuscitation (**92950**)
- Extracorporeal membrane oxygenation (**33946–33949**)
- Peripherally inserted central catheter (PICC) (NCCI edits do bundle the PICC code [**36568, 36569**] with all neonatal and pediatric critical care codes. However, a modifier can override when appropriate. See Chapter 3, Modifiers and Coding Edits, for more information on NCCI edits.)
- Insertion of non-tunneled centrally inserted central venous catheter, older than 5 years (**36556**)
- Replacement (rewire) of non-tunneled centrally inserted central venous catheter (**36580**)
- Therapeutic apheresis (**36511–36514**)
- Insertion of cannula for hemodialysis, other purpose (separate procedure); vein to vein (**36800**)
- Placement of needle for intraosseous infusion (**36680**)
- Initiation of selective head or total body hypothermia in the critically ill neonate (**99184**) (Report only once at initiation of service.)

Payer edits may vary and certain services are bundled unless performed for diagnostic purposes rather than monitoring. The following instructions from the Medicaid NCCI manual demonstrate reporting of diagnostic services:

Lumbar puncture (**62270**) and suprapubic bladder aspiration (**51100**) are separately reportable with hourly critical care (**99291, 99292**) but are *not separately reportable* with the pediatric and neonatal critical care service codes (**99468–99472, 99475, 99476**) and the intensive care services codes (**99477–99480**).

Diagnostic rhythm electrocardiogram (ECG) codes **93040–93042** are reported only when there is a sudden change in a patient status associated with a change in cardiac rhythm that requires a diagnostic rhythm ECG and return to the critical care unit. When separately reporting a diagnostic ECG, do not include the time for this service in the time spent providing critical care. Modifier **59** is appended to the ECG code when indicated by patient status and performed on the same date as critical care services.

Many practice management and billing systems include claim scrubbers that provide an alert that claim edits apply and a modifier may be appropriate based on clinical circumstances.

Neonatal and Pediatric Daily Critical Care Codes

Codes are
* Reported for critical care of children younger than 6 years in the inpatient setting.
* Global—encompass all E/M services by a single provider (or provider of the exact same specialty in the same group) on one calendar date. (See exceptions under the Guidelines for Reporting Neonatal or Pediatric Inpatient Critical Care section.)
* Bundled—have commonly performed procedures included in the E/M codes.
* Not time-based. Prolonged services *may not* be reported in conjunction with neonatal or pediatric critical care services.
* Not based on typical E/M rules and the performance and documentation of key components (history, physical examination, MDM, and/or time).
* Reported based on postnatal age (see the Definition of Perinatal Period section earlier in this chapter) and initial or subsequent care (**Table 12-3**).

Table 12-3. Neonatal and Pediatric Global Critical Care

Inpatient Neonatal Critical Care	28 Days or Younger	29 Days Through 24 Months of Age	2 Through 5 Years of Age
Initial inpatient neonatal critical care	99468	99471	99475
Subsequent inpatient neonatal critical care	99469	99472	99476

Guidelines for Reporting Neonatal or Pediatric Inpatient Critical Care

* The physician primarily responsible for the patient on the date of service should report the neonatal or pediatric critical care codes. (A neonatal nurse practitioner [NNP] may be primarily responsible and report pediatric critical care if independent billing is allowed in a state, services are within scope of practice, and the NNP has hospital privilege credentials for the service.) When the physician and NNP provide critical care services to a patient only one may report the code.
* This includes most E/M services and bundled procedures provided on a calendar day. If critical care is provided in the outpatient and inpatient setting by the same physician or physician of the same specialty and group, only the inpatient code is reported.
* Codes may be reported in addition to normal newborn care (**99460** or **99462**) when the patient receives normal newborn care and then, at a subsequent separate encounter the same day, requires critical care. A neonatologist may also provide a consultation (**99251–99255**) at the request of the attending physician early in the day and later provide critical or intensive care services. However, the neonatologist would report only critical or intensive care services if a transfer of care occurs at the initial encounter.
* Codes are reported only once per day, per patient.
* When the same physician or physicians of the same specialty and group practice provide pediatric critical care during transport of a child 24 months or younger (**99466, 99467; 99485, 99486**) and critical care after admission to the receiving facility, both services are reported and modifier **25** is appended to the transport code.
* Initial critical care codes (**99468, 99471, 99475**) are only reported once per calendar day and once per hospital stay for a given patient. If the patient has to be readmitted to critical care during the same hospital stay, report a subsequent critical care code (**99469, 99472, 99476**).
* Subsequent critical care may be reported on multiple days even if there is no change in the patient's condition as long as the patient continues to meet the critical care definition and documentation supports this level of service.

- Procedures bundled in these codes must not be reported separately. The services and procedures that are included with neonatal critical care codes are identified in **Table 12-1**.
- Care may be provided on any unit in a hospital facility.
- Care must be provided by the reporting physician but also includes the services provided by the health care team functioning under the direct supervision of the physician or an advanced nurse practitioner who is employed by the physician or physician group and when allowed under state licensure requirements. See the Critical and Intensive Care Supervision Requirements section later in this chapter and Appendix V.
- Medical record documentation must support the need for and meet the definition of critical care (eg, complex MDM, high probability of imminent or life-threatening deterioration, organ system failure).

Subsequent-day neonatal and pediatric intensive care codes (**99478–99480**) are reported when critical care is no longer required, the neonate requires more intensive care than typically provided under routine subsequent hospital care (**99231–99233**), and the neonate weighs 5,000 g or less on the day the code is reported. Once the neonate weighs at least 5,001 g and critical care services are no longer required, report subsequent-day inpatient hospital visit codes (**99231–99233**).

Coding Conundrum: Selecting the Appropriate Code

Many diagnoses or conditions, such as respiratory distress, infection, seizures, mild to moderate hypoxic ischemic encephalopathy, and metabolic disorders, can be reported with codes **99468**, **99477**, or **99221–99223**. The patient's clinical status, required level of monitoring and observation, and present body weight will determine which of these code sets is chosen. Selection of the service must be justified by medical record documentation.

Critical and Intensive Care Supervision Requirements

The American Medical Association/Specialty Society Relative Value Scale Update Committee (RUC) makes valuation recommendations based on surveys in which physicians who perform services are presented with a vignette describing the typical patient and the face-to-face physician work associated with that service. The neonatal and pediatric critical and intensive care code vignettes describe hands-on care by the attending physician (intra-service work) as well as the preservice and post-service work associated with this service. Neither the vignette nor the intent of the codes was to imply that 24-hour in-house attendance was a requirement of this code set. However, the codes' values were established assuming the physician is physically present and participating directly in the patient's care for a significant portion of the reported service. Documentation in the patient's chart should reflect this active participation, including documentation of hands-on care, such as a personal physical examination. Supervision of all the care from a distance without face-to-face care is not reported as critical or intensive care. (Refer to Appendix V.)

The vignettes also include the phrase "repeated examinations over a 24-hour period," which was included to indicate that these neonates or infants do not receive "continuous" care but rather are typically evaluated during numerous intervals over a 24-hour period, depending on the clinical needs of the patient. In some cases, the neonate's or infant's level of illness requires in-house attending presence for extended periods, while in other situations, only daytime presence is required. While the critical care team is present with the neonate or infant for the full 24 hours, overnight in-house care by the reporting physician is determined by the complexity of the total population of neonates cared for in a nursery or the changes in a specific neonate's or infant's condition that cannot be adequately assessed or managed over the telephone.

Under the heading Inpatient Neonatal and Pediatric Critical Care Service, *CPT*® states that codes **99468**, **99469**, and **99471–99476** are used to report services provided by a physician "directing the inpatient care" of a critically ill neonate, infant, or child through 5 years of age. The medical record documentation must support the physician's presence and supervision of the team as well as the critical nature of the child's disease. As noted previously, the directing physician is not required to be present or in the facility for the total 24 hours of daily care. Rather, because neonatal and pediatric critical and intensive care may require numerous encounters to reevaluate and manage the patient each day, neonatal and pediatric critical and intensive care codes encompass all the sick care provided within a calendar day.

Neonatal Critical Care

99468   Initial inpatient neonatal critical care, per day, for the evaluation and management of a critically ill neonate, 28 days of age or younger

99469   Subsequent inpatient neonatal critical care, per day, for the evaluation and management of a critically ill neonate, 28 days of age or younger

Selection of the appropriate code will depend on the newborn's or infant's condition and the intensity of the service provided and documented on a particular day of service.

In some situations, the neonate will be normal at birth and, many hours later, will show signs of an illness. *Current Procedural Terminology*® guidelines specify that only one initial hospital service may be reported for the same patient on the same day of service by the same physician or physician of the same specialty within the same group. However, if 2 distinct, medically necessary services are provided, both services may be reported. Each service should be reported with the appropriate diagnosis code to support the service (eg, diagnosis codes for well newborn and the defined illness). In other situations, a newborn's illness or condition progresses during the hospital stay, requiring a higher intensity of service by the same physician or another physician from a different group or specialty. When all the neonate's care on the same date of service is related to the same condition or disease but the level of illness and required care progresses through the day, only a single code representing the highest level of service performed and documented is reported if all the care was provided by a single physician or physicians of the same specialty and group practice. However, when the intensity of care progresses over the day and services are provided by physicians from different groups or specialties or the patient is transferred to another facility, coding becomes more complicated.

> ||||||| **Coding Pearl** |||||||
>
> Report first a code from category **Z38** (liveborn infants according to place of birth and type of delivery) when care is provided by the attending physician during the birth admission. When a neonate is transferred to another facility after birth, the admission to the receiving facility is not a birth admission and **Z38** codes are not reported. Codes for abnormal conditions are reported secondary to the code for live birth.

Examples

➤ **A term 3,500-g neonate is born cyanotic following a vaginal delivery.** He has minimal respiratory distress and appears otherwise vigorous. He is brought to the NICU, where a chest radiograph shows dramatic cardiomegaly and a marked increase in pulmonary markings. An umbilical artery catheter and umbilical vein catheter are inserted to determine blood gases. An ECG is performed and a pediatric cardiologist is consulted to obtain an emergency echocardiogram.

It is important to remember that respiratory support (ie, mechanical ventilation) is not required to report critical care services. In this case, serious cyanosis and clear evidence of cardiac decompensation qualify as critical care. Code **99468** would be reported for initial date of neonatal critical care services. The umbilical vessel catheterizations are bundled with **99468**. Depending on the findings on the echocardiogram and a need for cardiac intensive care, the cardiologist may report hourly critical care for any additional time beyond the echocardiogram. If critical care is not provided, the cardiologist would report consultative services (**99251–99255**) or subsequent hospital care (if requirements for reporting a consultation are not met). (See Chapter 10, Noncritical Hospital Evaluation and Management Services, for more information on reporting consultations and reporting to payers who do not recognize consultation codes.) If the neonate were transferred to a cardiac center by the neonatologist, the neonatologist would report time-based critical care codes (**99291, 99292**) for the care provided prior to the transfer.

➤ **A 3-day-old recovering from respiratory distress syndrome with a present body weight of 1,600 g is still unstable but is weaned off the ventilator to CPAP.** He is continued on total parenteral nutrition by central vein and IV antibiotics.

Code **99469** is reported because the medical record continues to document the neonate's instability and the continued need for critical care services.

Coding Conundrum: Apnea in Neonates

Apnea in neonates may be an expected component of preterm birth and may be effectively managed by manual stimulation, pharmacological stimulation, high-flow nasal oxygen, or CPAP. At other times, this symptom will be associated with a serious underlying problem(s) and is a reflection of the instability of a critically ill neonate and will require one or more of the same interventions. The physician must employ his or her best clinical judgment and clearly document the factors that make the patient's present condition critical (or require intensive care). The same requirements for organ failure, risk of imminent deterioration, and complex MDM apply. With apnea and many other conditions, it is the total picture of the neonate with the diagnosis, clinical presentation, and immediate threat to life, amount of hands-on and supervisory care provided by the physician, as well as the level of intervention needed to manage that neonate's problems on a given day that drive the correct code selection. In all cases, when critical care codes are reported, the documentation must support the physician's judgment that the patient is critically ill and services provided are commensurate with the condition on that day of service on which critical care codes are reported.

Pediatric Critical Care

99471 Initial inpatient pediatric critical care, per day, for the evaluation and management of a critically ill infant or young child, 29 days through 24 months of age

99472 Subsequent inpatient pediatric critical care, per day, for the evaluation and management of a critically ill infant or young child, 29 days through 24 months of age

99475 Initial inpatient pediatric critical care, per day, for the evaluation and management of a critically ill infant or young child, 2 through 5 years of age

99476 Subsequent inpatient pediatric critical care, per day, for the evaluation and management of a critically ill infant or young child, 2 through 5 years of age

Codes **99471–99476** are used to report direction of the inpatient care of a critically ill infant or young child outside of the neonatal period. Services are provided to patients aged 29 days (postnatal age with day of birth being 0 [zero]) until the child reaches 6 years of age. Initial pediatric critical care for children of these ages is reported with code **99471** (29 days through 24 months of age—up to, but not including, the second birthday) or **99475** (2 through 5 years of age—up to, but not including, the sixth birthday). Initial pediatric critical care codes (**99471**, **99475**) are only reported once, per calendar day, per hospital stay for a given patient. If the patient has been sent to another inpatient unit for continued care and then requires readmission to critical care during the same hospital stay, report a subsequent critical care code (**99472**, **99476**) on the readmission date and each subsequent date the child remains critical. Subsequent days of care for the infant or child who remains critical are reported with code **99472** or **99476**. These subsequent-day codes may be reported only by a single individual and only once per day, per patient, in a given setting.

Example

➤ A 22-month-old with developmental delays and a seizure disorder is initially treated by the ED physician for status epilepticus (1 hour of critical care). Although seizures were initially controlled, the pharmacologic management led to irregular respiratory activity, lethargy, and hypotension. The patient was admitted to the pediatric intensive care unit at 11:00 pm that evening by the critical care attending physician, who intubated her, placed her on a ventilator, began fluid expansion, used dobutamine to control her blood pressure, and made arrangements for a bedside electroencephalogram (EEG).

The ED physician would report 1 hour of critical care (**99291**). The pediatrician or intensivist would report his or her services with the initial inpatient pediatric critical care code (**99471**) for that calendar day, even though only 1 hour of care was provided. One hour later, after midnight, a new date of service would begin. The intubation is bundled with **99471** and cannot be separately billed.

Chapter 12: Critical and Intensive Care

Patients Critically Ill After Surgery

Postoperative care of a surgical patient is included in the surgeon's global surgical package. For some neonatal surgical care (eg, codes **39503** [repair of diaphragmatic hernia], **43314** [esophagoplasty, thoracic approach; with repair of tracheoesophageal fistula], or **49605** [repair of large omphalocele or gastroschisis; with or without prosthesis]), some critical care days are included in the work values assigned to these surgical procedures.

However, if

* A second physician provides care for the routine postoperative patient, the surgeon must append modifier **54** (surgical care only) to the surgical code. (A formal transfer of care should be documented.)
* The surgeon provides and reports the complete surgical care package, a request for consultation from another specialist may be made.
* The patient's course is not typical and an unexpected complication occurs that requires the concurrent care of another specialist, both may report their service. For example, if the surgeon first requests a consultation, an initial consultation code (or other appropriate E/M code based on the payer's payment policy for consultations) would be reported. If the surgeon requests concurrent care for a specific medical problem, time-based critical care (**99291, 99292**) or subsequent hospital care (**99231–99233**) codes would be reported dependent on the child's condition and care provided. The diagnosis code representing the condition or symptom being treated should be reported with the concurrent *CPT* code. The rationale for the need for concurrent care must be documented in the surgeon's notes.

Remote Critical Care Services

★**0188T**   Remote real-time interactive video-conferenced critical care, evaluation and management of the critically ill or critically injured patient; first 30-74 minutes
★**0189T**   each additional 30 minutes (List separately in addition to code **0188T**)
95   Synchronous Telemedicine Service Rendered Via a Real Time Interactive Audio and Video Telecommunications System. Note: For a listing of codes that may be reported for telemedicine services, see *CPT* Appendix P. Additionally, stars have been added before the listing in the *CPT* manual for codes included in Appendix P.

Remote critical care is the direct delivery by a physician(s) of medical care for a critically ill or critically injured patient from an off-site location (ie, when a critically ill or injured patient requires additional critical care resources that are not available on-site). See Chapter 13, Telemedicine, for more information on reporting telemedicine services, including remote critical care.

Neonatal and Pediatric Intensive Care

99477   Initial hospital care, per day, for the evaluation and management of the neonate, 28 days of age or younger, who requires intensive observation, frequent interventions, and other intensive care services
99478   Subsequent intensive care, per day, for the evaluation and management of the recovering very low birth weight infant (present body weight less than 1500 grams)
99479   Subsequent intensive care, per day, for the evaluation and management of the recovering low birth weight infant (present body weight of 1500-2500 grams)
99480   Subsequent intensive care, per day, for the evaluation and management of the recovering infant (present body weight of 2501-5000 grams)

> |||||||| **Coding Pearl** ||||||||
>
> Continuing intensive care services provided to an infant weighing more than 5,000 g (approximately 11.02 lb) are reported with subsequent hospital care codes (**99231–99233**). Documentation of these services must support 2 of 3 key components or the total unit or floor time and time spent counseling and/or coordinating care.

Neonatal and pediatric intensive care codes (**99477–99480**) may be used to report care for neonates or infants who are not critically ill but have a need for intensive monitoring, observation, and frequent assessments by the health care team and supervision by the physician. This includes

- Neonates who require intensive but not critical care services from birth
- Neonates who are no longer critically ill but require intensive physician and health care team observation and interventions
- Recovering low birth weight infants who require a higher level of care than that defined by other hospital care services

These neonates often have a continued need for oxygen, parenteral or gavage enteral nutrition, treatment for apnea of prematurity, and thermoregulation from an Isolette or radiant warmer, and may be recovering from cardiac or surgical care. The intensive services described by these codes include intensive cardiac and respiratory monitoring, continuous and/or frequent vital sign monitoring, heat maintenance, enteral and/or parenteral nutritional adjustments, and laboratory and oxygen saturation monitoring when provided.

- Code **99477** is used to report the more intensive services that an ill but not critically ill neonate (28 days or younger) requires on the day of admission to inpatient care.
- Services are typically (but not required to be) provided in a NICU or special care unit and require a higher intensity of care than would be reported with codes **99221–99223** (initial hospital care of sick patient).
- Patients are under constant observation by the health care team under direct physician supervision.
- These are global codes and include all the E/M services (and bundled procedures) provided to the neonate on that date of service, excluding normal newborn care (**99460–99462**), when performed. Attendance at delivery (**99464**) or newborn resuscitation (**99465**) may be reported in addition to code **99477**, when performed. Append modifier **25** to code **99477** when reporting on the same date as **99460–99462**, **99464**, or **99465**. Note: Payers that have adopted the Medicare NCCI edits will not allow payment of codes **99460–99462** and **99477** for services by the same physician or physicians of the same specialty and group practice on the same date. Only code **99477** is reported under these circumstances. See more about NCCI edits in Chapter 3, Modifiers and Coding Edits.
- These are bundled services and include the same procedures that are bundled with neonatal and pediatric critical care services (**99468–99476**). See Table 12-1 for a list of all the services and procedures that are included.
- Code **99477** should also be used to report readmission to a facility (after initial discharge) of an ill neonate (aged 28 days or younger) if the neonate requires intensive (not critical) care services.
- If the infant is older than 28 days at admission but weighs less than 5,000 g, codes **99221–99223** should be used for intensive care on the date of hospital admission (typically **99233**, assuming documentation of comprehensive history and examination and high-level MDM) and **99478–99480** for subsequent days, as long as the infant continues to require intensive care.
- Table 12-4 contains code descriptions for subsequent-day neonatal and pediatric intensive care services (**99478–99480**).
- Codes **99478–99480** are reported once per calendar day of subsequent intensive (but not critical) care for the E/M of the recovering infant weighing 5,000 g or less. Selection of the code will be dependent on the *present* body weight of the infant, not the infant's age, on the date of service. Therefore, code selection may change from one day to the next depending on the infant's present body weight and condition.
- Once the baby's weight exceeds 5,000 g, subsequent hospital care codes (**99231–99233**) are reported until the date of discharge (**99238–99239**).

Table 12-4. Neonatal and Pediatric Subsequent-Day Intensive Care

Description	Present Weight <1,500 g	Present Weight 1,500–2,500 g	Present Weight 2,501–5,000 g	Present Weight 5,001 g+
Subsequent intensive care	99478	99479	99480	99231–99233

Examples

> **A 1,500-g neonate has mild respiratory distress.** She is on 30% oxygen by nasal cannula and on a cardio-respiratory monitor and continuous pulse oximetry. Laboratory tests and radiographs are ordered and IV fluids and antibiotics are started. Frequent monitoring and observation are required and ordered.
>
> Code **99477** (initial hospital care for the ill neonate, 28 days of age or less, who requires intensive observation and monitoring) would be reported by the admitting physician.

> **A 1,150-g neonate, now 5 days old, is receiving 30% oxygen and continues on IV fluids, small trophic feeds, and caffeine for apnea.**
>
> Code **99478** would be reported.

> **A 15-day-old, 1,600-g neonate remains in an Isolette for thermoregulation and is on methylxanthines for intermittent apnea and bradycardia, for which the neonate requires continuous cardiorespiratory and pulse oximetry monitoring.** The physician adjusts the neonate's continuous gavage feeds based on tolerance and weight.
>
> Code **99479** would be reported. In these examples, the neonate is not critically ill but continues to require intensive monitoring and constant observation by the health care team under direct physician supervision.

> **A baby requires intensive care and weighs 2,500 g on Monday.** The following day, she continues to require intensive care and her weight is 2,504 g.
>
> Code **99479** would be reported for the care provided on Monday. Code **99480** would be reported for the continuing intensive care provided the following day.

Emergency Medical Services Supervision and Patient Transport

Direction of Emergency Medical Services

99288   Physician or other qualified health care professional direction of emergency medical systems (EMS) emergency care, advanced life support

Guidelines for reporting code **99288** (direction of emergency medical systems emergency care, advanced life support) by physician or QHP include

* May be reported by any physician of any specialty or QHP when advanced life support services are provided via 2-way voice communications (eg, cardiac and/or pulmonary resuscitation; administration of IV fluids, antibiotics, or surfactant).

* This code reflects all the services provided by the directing physician and is not based on any time requirements. Code **99288** may be reported when less than 16 minutes is spent in physician non–face-to-face supervision of inter-facility transport of a critically ill or injured pediatric patient (ie, requirements for reporting **99485** are not met).

* The directing physician should maintain documentation of the times of all contacts, orders, and/or directions for treatment or management of the patient.

* Services or procedures performed by emergency medical services (EMS) personnel are not reported by the physician because he or she was not physically present.

* When an advance practice professional provides and reports face-to-face services during transport, the physician would not report **99288**.

* The appropriate diagnoses are linked to the service.

- If, after directing EMS personnel, the physician performs the initial critical care, code **99468** (initial inpatient neonatal critical care) would also be reported with modifier **25** appended to indicate that 2 separate and distinct E/M services were provided by the same physician on the same day of service.

There is no assigned Medicare relative value unit (RVU) to this service, so it is "carrier priced" and payments will vary by payer.

Medicare considers code **99288** a bundled service and does not pay separately for the service. Check with your state Medicaid program and other payers to determine their coverage policy.

See the Non–face-to-face Pediatric Critical Care Patient Transport section for discussion of physician non–face-to-face supervision of inter-facility transport of a critically ill or injured pediatric patient 24 months or younger (**99485, 99486**).

Pediatric Critical Care Patient Transport

Face-to-face Critical Care Patient Transport (99466 and 99467)

99466   Critical care face-to-face services, during an interfacility transport of critically ill or critically injured pediatric patient, 24 months of age or younger; first 30–74 minutes of hands-on care during transport

99467   each additional 30 minutes (List separately in addition to code **99466**)

Codes **99466** and **99467** are used to report the physical attendance and direct face-to-face care provided by a physician or QHP during the inter-facility transport of a critically ill or injured patient aged 24 months or younger.

- The patient's condition must meet the *CPT®* definition for critical care.
- Face-to-face time begins when the physician or practitioner assumes primary responsibility for the patient at the referring hospital or facility and ends when the receiving hospital or facility accepts responsibility for the patient's care. Only the time the physician spends in direct face-to-face contact with the patient during transport should be reported.
- Less than 30 minutes of face-to-face time cannot be reported.
- Code **99466** is used to report the first 30 to 74 minutes of physician face-to-face time with the critically ill or injured patient during the transport.
- Code **99467** is used to report each additional 30 minutes of physician face-to-face time of critical care provided on the same day of service.
- Codes include the bundled services listed in **Table 12-1**. Codes **99466** and **99467** may be reported separately from any other procedures or services that are not bundled and performed on the date of transfer. The time involved in performing any procedures that are not bundled and reported separately should not be included in the face-to-face transport time.
- Procedures or services that are performed by other members of the transport team with the physical presence, participation, and supervision of the accompanying physician may be reported by the physician. Documentation must support the physician's participation.
- Medical record documentation must include the total face-to-face time spent with the patient, the critical nature of the patient's condition, and any performed procedures that are not bundled.
- The pediatric critical care transport codes are preadmission codes and may be reported in addition to neonatal (**99468**) or pediatric (**99471**) initial-day critical care codes. For payers that have adopted NCCI edits, modifier **25** is required to indicate the significant and separately identifiable E/M services. Append modifier **25** to code **99466** when reporting in conjunction with daily critical care codes.
- Face-to-face critical care services provided during an inter-facility transport to a child older than 24 months are reported with hourly critical care codes (**99291** and **99292**).
- If an NNP employed by the neonatal group is on the transport team, the NNP may report codes **99466** and **99467** if independent billing by an NNP is allowed by the state and the activities are covered in the scope of practice. The neonatologist from that same group would not report codes **99485** and **99486** (physician direction of pediatric critical care transport) or **99288** (physician direction of EMS emergency care). The facility (hospital) could also report these services if the NNPs are employed by the hospital. In this case, the neonatologist would report codes **99485** and **99486**.

Chapter 12: Critical and Intensive Care

Example

➤ A 3,000-g, 38-weeks' gestation neonate born at a community hospital with meconium aspiration syndrome requires ventilator care and transport to a Level III unit where extracorporeal membrane oxygenation (ECMO) is also available. The receiving neonatologist accompanies the transport nurse and therapist. Ground transport takes 40 minutes one way. On arrival, the neonatologist spends 60 minutes face-to-face evaluating and stabilizing the newborn. The newborn is intubated, surfactant is administered, umbilical venous and arterial catheters are inserted, and parents are counseled. The neonatologist spends 5 minutes intubating and administering the surfactant and 10 minutes placing the umbilical venous and arterial catheters. The newborn is then transferred to the neonatal transport van and back to the receiving nursery. Total time from bedside back to the receiving nursery is 60 minutes. Frequent assessments and alterations in drugs, fluids, and ventilator settings are performed on the transport back. The neonatologist spent a total of 120 minutes of face-to-face critical care time with the neonate; 25 minutes is subtracted for the performance of non-bundled procedures. The neonatologist continues care of the newborn in the NICU.

99466 25

99467 25 × 1 unit

31500 (endotracheal intubation)

94610 (surfactant administration)

36510 (catheterization of umbilical vein)

36660 (catheterization of umbilical artery)

99468 25 (initial neonatal critical care)

Modifier **25** is appended to each of the services to designate a significant and separately identifiable E/M service provided by the same physician on the same date of service. Endotracheal intubation is bundled with daily neonatal critical care but is separately reported when provided during transport of the critically ill or injured neonate.

Non–face-to-face Pediatric Critical Care Patient Transport

#99485   Supervision by a control physician of interfacility transport care of the critically ill or critically injured pediatric patient, 24 months of age or younger, includes two-way communication with transport team before transport, at the referring facility and during the transport, including data interpretation and report; first 30 minutes

#99486   each additional 30 minutes (List separately in addition to code **99485**)

Code **99485** is used to report the first 30 minutes of a control physician's non–face-to-face supervision of inter-facility critical care transport of a patient 24 months or younger, which includes all 2-way communication between the control physician and the specialized transport team prior to transport, at the referring facility, and during transport to the receiving facility. Each additional 30-minute period of communication is reported with add-on code **99486**. These codes do not include communication between the control physician and referring facility before or following patient transport.

◉ The patient's condition must meet the *CPT®* definition of critical care.

◉ Only report for patients 24 months or younger who are critically ill or injured.

◉ The control physician does not report any services provided by the specialized transport team.

◉ The control physician only reports cumulative time spent communicating with the specialty transport team members during an inter-facility transport. Communication between the control physician and the referring facility before or following patient transport is not counted.

◉ Reportable time begins with the initial discussions with the transport team, including discussions of best mode of transport and strategies for therapy on arrival. Time ends when the patient's care is handed over to the receiving facility team.

◉ Code **99485** is used to report the first 16 to 45 minutes of direction on a given date and should only be used once even if time spent by the physician is discontinuous.

- Code **99486** is used in conjunction with **99485** for each additional 30 minutes.
- Do not report **99485** or **99486** for services of 15 minutes or less or any time when a provider from the same group is also reporting **99466** or **99467**.
- Time spent with the individual patient's transport team and reviewing data submissions should be recorded. Time spent discussing the patient with the referring physician or facility is not counted.
- Services represented by codes **99485** and **99486** are preadmission services and may be reported by the same or different individual of the same specialty and same group when neonatal or pediatric critical care services (**99468–99476**) are reported for the same patient on the same day.

Example

➤ **A community pediatrician asks to refer a newborn with cyanosis, tachycardia, and possible congenital cardiac disease.** The neonatologist dispatches the transport team, consisting of a hospital-employed transport nurse and a respiratory therapist. On the trip to the referring hospital, the neonatologist converses by telephone for 10 minutes with the team, explaining the newborn's condition and formulating an initial treatment plan. After arrival, the nurse evaluates the neonate and telephones the neonatologist to discuss the findings. The decision is made to provide prostaglandin to maintain ductal patency and avoid oxygen therapy. Because of the critical nature of the newborn, the neonatologist elects to remain on the telephone until therapy is completed (15 minutes). The team then leaves the referring hospital. On the return trip, telephone contact lasting 10 minutes is again made to update the physician on the neonate's condition, vital signs, and overall physical status. The team then completes the transport without further incident.

The neonatologist spent a total of 35 minutes in direct 2-way telephone communication with the team in 3 discrete episodes. The neonatologist carefully documents in the medical record the time spent and what decisions were made in each contact. Code **99485** is used to report this service.

Total Body Systemic and Selective Head Hypothermia

99184   Initiation of selective head or total body hypothermia in the critically ill neonate, includes appropriate patient selection by review of clinical, imaging and laboratory data, confirmation of esophageal temperature probe location, evaluation of amplitude EEG, supervision of controlled hypothermia, and assessment of patient tolerance of cooling
(Do not report **99184** more than once per hospital stay)

Examples

➤ **A term neonate born with evidence of hypoxic-ischemic encephalopathy is admitted to the NICU and receives critical care services.** Laboratory, EEG, blood gas, and imaging studies confirm the neonate meets objective criteria for *total body cooling.* Continuous total body cooling is undertaken.

Code **99184** is reported for total body systemic hypothermia in addition to **99468**, initial day of neonatal critical care.

➤ **A term neonate born with evidence of hypoxic-ischemic encephalopathy is admitted to the NICU and receives critical care services.** Laboratory, EEG, blood gas, and imaging studies confirm the neonate meets objective criteria for *selective head cooling.* Continuous selective head cooling is undertaken.

Code **99184** is reported for selective head hypothermia in addition to **99468**, initial day of neonatal critical care.

When total body systemic or selective head hypothermia is used in treatment of a critically ill neonate, code **99184** represents the work of initiating the service.

Chapter 12: Critical and Intensive Care

Chapter 12: Critical and Intensive Care

Documentation for use of total body systemic hypothermia and selective head hypothermia should include the neonatal criteria that support initiating this service.

- During either cooling approach, monitoring includes
  - Radiographic confirmation of core temperature probe
  - Continuous core temperature assessment and adjustment
  - Repeated assessment of skin integrity
  - Recurrent objective evaluation of evolving neurologic changes (eg, Sarnat score), which may also include assessment of continuous amplitude EEG monitoring
- In addition, cooling-related laboratory evaluations are required to monitor for cooling-specific complications, including metabolic and coagulation alterations.

Extracorporeal Membrane Oxygenation (ECMO) or Extracorporeal Life Support (ECLS) Services

Prolonged ECMO and extracorporeal life support (ECLS) services provide cardiac and/or respiratory support, allowing the heart and/or lungs to rest and recover when sick or injured. These services commonly involve multiple physicians and supporting health care personnel to manage each patient. Extracorporeal membrane oxygenation and ECLS codes differentiate components of initiation and daily management of ECMO and ECLS from daily management of a patient's overall medical condition.

These services include cannula(e) insertion (**33951–33956**), ECMO or ECLS initiation (**33946** or **33947**), daily ECMO or ECLS management (**33948** or **33949**), repositioning of the ECMO or ECLS cannula(e) (**33957–33964**), and cannula(e) removal (**33965–33986**). Each physician providing part of the ECMO/ECLS services may report the services they provide except when prohibited by *CPT®* instruction (eg, cannula repositioning is not reported by the same or another physician on the same date as initiation of ECMO/ECLS).

Example

➤ **Venoarterial ECMO is initiated for a patient with cardiac and respiratory failure.** Physician A inserts the cannulae. Physician B manages the initial transition to ECMO, including working with physician A, ECMO specialists, and others to initiate an ongoing assessment of anticoagulation, venous return, cannula positioning, and optimal flow. Physician B is also providing daily management of the patient's overall care. When ECMO is discontinued, physician A returns and removes the cannulae.

Physician A will report codes for insertion and removal of the ECMO cannulae (eg, **33952** and **33966**). Physician B will report initiation of venoarterial ECMO (**33947**), the appropriate hospital and/or critical care codes for overall management of the patient for each day provided (eg, **99291**, **99292** or **99231–99233**), and daily management of ECMO (**33949**) for each day provided.

ECMO/ECLS Initiation and Daily Management

33946	Extracorporeal membrane oxygenation (ECMO)/extracorporeal life support (ECLS) provided by physician; initiation, venovenous
33947	initiation, venoarterial
33948	daily management, each day, venovenous
33949	daily management, each day, venoarterial

Initiation of the ECMO or ECLS circuit and setting parameters (**33946**, **33947**) involves determining the necessary ECMO or ECLS device components, blood flow, gas exchange, and other necessary parameters to manage the circuit.

Daily care for a patient on ECMO or ECLS includes managing the ECMO or ECLS circuit and related patient issues. These services may be performed by one physician while another physician manages the overall patient medical condition and underlying disorders. Regardless of the patient's condition, the basic management of ECMO and ECLS is similar.

- Do not report modifier **63** (procedure performed on infants less than 4 kg) when reporting codes **33946–33949**.
- The physician reporting daily ECMO or ECLS oversees the interaction of the circuit with the patient, management of blood flow, oxygenation, carbon dioxide clearance by the membrane lung, systemic response, anticoagulation and treatment of bleeding, cannula(e) positioning, alarms and safety, and weaning the patient from the ECMO or ECLS circuit when heart and/or lung function has sufficiently recovered.
- Daily management of the patient may be separately reported using the relevant hospital observation services, hospital inpatient services, or critical care E/M codes (**99218–99220, 99221–99223, 99231–99233, 99234–99236, 99291, 99292, 99468–99480**).
- Daily management (**33948** or **33949**) or cannula repositioning (**33957–33959, 33962–33964**) may not be reported on the same date as initiation (**33946** or **33947**) by the same or different physician.

ECMO/ECLS Cannula Insertion, Repositioning, and Removal

Codes for insertion, repositioning, and removal of ECMO and ECLS are reported based on the patient's age, with separate codes for procedures on newborns through 5 years of age and on patients 6 years and older. Codes for these services are shown in **tables 12-5, 12-6,** and **12-7**. While typically only performed by surgeons, other pediatric providers may perform as well.

- Do not separately report repositioning of the ECMO or ECLS cannula(e) (**33957–33964**) at the same session as insertion (**33951–33956**).
- Fluoroscopic guidance used for cannula(e) repositioning (**33957–33964**) is included in the procedure when performed and should not be separately reported.
- Report replacement of ECMO or ECLS cannula(e) in the same vessel using the insertion code (**33951–33956**) only.
- If cannula(e) are removed from one vessel and new cannula(e) are placed in a different vessel, report the appropriate cannula(e) removal (**33965–33986**) and insertion (**33951–33956**) codes.
- Extensive repair or replacement of an artery may be additionally reported (eg, **35226, 35286, 35371, 35665**).
- Direct anastomosis of a prosthetic graft to the artery sidewall to facilitate arterial perfusion for ECMO or ECLS is separately reported with code **33987** in addition to codes **33953–33956**.

+33987 Arterial exposure with creation of graft conduit (eg, chimney graft) to facilitate arterial perfusion for ECMO/ECLS (List separately in addition to code for primary procedure)

Do not report **33987** in conjunction with **34833** (open iliac artery exposure with creation of conduit for delivery of aortic or iliac endovascular prosthesis, by abdominal or retroperitoneal incision, unilateral).

> ||||||||| **Coding Pearl** |||||||||
>
> Each physician providing a part of ECMO/ECLS services may report the part they provided except as prohibited by *CPT®* instruction.

Table 12-5. Insertion of ECMO or ECLS Cannula(e)			
ECMO/ECLS Provided by Physician	**Birth Through 5 Years of Age**	**6 Years and Older**	**Do Not Report With**
Insertion of peripheral (arterial and/or venous) cannula(e), percutaneous (includes fluoroscopic guidance when performed)	33951	33952	33957–33964
Insertion of peripheral (arterial and/or venous) cannula(e), open	33953	33954	33957–33964, 34812, 34820, 34834
Insertion of central cannula(e) by sternotomy or thoracotomy	33955	33956	33957–33964, 32100, 39010
Abbreviations: ECLS, extracorporeal life support; ECMO, extracorporeal membrane oxygenation.			

Chapter 12: Critical and Intensive Care

Chapter 12: Critical and Intensive Care

Table 12-6. Repositioning ECMO or ECLS Cannula(e)[a]

ECMO/ECLS Provided by Physician	Birth Through 5 Years of Age	6 Years and Older	Do Not Report With
Reposition peripheral (arterial and/or venous) cannula(e), percutaneous (includes fluoroscopic guidance when performed)	33957	33958	33946, 33947, 34812, 34820, 34834
Reposition peripheral (arterial and/or venous) cannula(e), open (includes fluoroscopic guidance when performed)	33959	33962	33946, 33947, 34812, 34820, 34834
Reposition of central cannula(e) by sternotomy or thoracotomy (includes fluoroscopic guidance when performed)	33963	33964	33946, 33947, 32100, 39010

Abbreviations: ECLS, extracorporeal life support; ECMO, extracorporeal membrane oxygenation.

[a] Repositioning of cannula(e) at the same session as insertion is not separately reported.

Table 12-7. Removal of ECMO or ECLS Cannula(e)[a]

ECMO/ECLS Provided by Physician	Birth Through 5 Years of Age	6 Years and Older	Do Not Report With
Removal of peripheral (arterial and/or venous) cannula(e), percutaneous	33965	33966	N/A
Removal of peripheral (arterial and/or venous) cannula(e), open	33969	33984	34812, 34820, 34834, 35201, 35206, 35211, 35216, 35226
Removal of central cannula(e) by sternotomy or thoracotomy	33985	33986	35201, 35206, 35211, 35216, 35226

Abbreviations: ECLS, extracorporeal life support; ECMO, extracorporeal membrane oxygenation; N/A, not applicable.

[a] Report only the insertion when cannula(e) is replaced in the same vessel.

Car Seat/Bed Testing

94780   Car seat/bed testing for airway integrity, neonate, with continual nursing observation and continuous recording of pulse oximetry, heart rate and respiratory rate, with interpretation and report; 60 minutes

+94781   each additional full 30 minutes (List separately in addition to 94780.)

Examples

➤ A neonate born at 35 weeks' gestation requires a car seat test on the date of discharge from the hospital.

Code 94780 is reported with hospital discharge management code 99238 or 99239.

➤ A neonate born at 35 weeks' gestation requires a car seat test prior to discharge from the hospital. The newborn has received 60 minutes of testing reported with 94780 and now receives an additional 30 minutes.

Codes 94780 and 94781 are reported with a subsequent hospital care code (99231–99233) or a discharge day management code (99238 or 99239).

Neonates who required critical care during their initial hospital stay are most often those patients who require monitoring to determine if they may be safely transported in a car seat or must be transported in a car bed. While these codes are bundled under neonatal and pediatric critical and intensive care codes, these services most often take place when a neonate is about to go home and, therefore, can be reported if hospital care services (**99231–99233**) or hospital discharge services (**99238**, **99239**) are being reported instead.

To report codes **94780** and **94781**, the following conditions must be met:

- The patient must be a neonate. Reassessment after the patient is 29 days or older is reported with unlisted code **94799**.
- Continual nursing observation with continuous recording of pulse oximetry, heart rate, and respiratory rate is required.
- Inpatient or office-based services are reported.
- Vital signs and observations must be reviewed and interpreted and a written report generated by the physician.
- Codes are reported based on the total observation time spent and documented.
- These codes may be reported with discharge day management (**99238**, **99239**), normal newborn care services (**99460**, **99462**, **99463**), or subsequent hospital care codes (**99231–99233**).
- Codes **94780** and **94781** may not be reported with neonatal or pediatric critical or intensive care services (**99468–99472**, **99477–99480**).
- If less than 60 minutes is spent in the procedure, code **94780** may not be reported.
- Each additional full 30 minutes (ie, not less than 90 minutes) is reported with code **94781**.
- Do not include the time of car seat/bed testing in time attributed to discharge day management services (**99238**, **99239**).

Sedation

Refer to Chapter 15, Common Surgical Procedures and Sedation, for specific guidelines for reporting sedation services, including moderate (conscious) sedation (**99151–99157**) and deep sedation.

Resources

Coding Education

American Academy of Pediatrics (AAP) Section on Neonatal-Perinatal Medicine coding trainers are available to provide coding education through local educational seminars and continuing education events. At least one coding trainer is appointed in each district. Each trainer is equipped with educational materials that can be used as an important resource for your state or hospital. Contact section manager Jim Couto (jcouto@aap.org) for additional information about these valuable services.

The AAP Section on Neonatal-Perinatal Medicine, in conjunction with state chapters and councils of the AAP, has developed strategies that have been successful in addressing payment concerns for neonatal care. Contact your state chapter, its pediatric council, your section district AAP Executive Committee representative, a neonatal trainer, or the AAP Committee on Coding and Nomenclature for assistance in addressing any payment inequities for neonatal services in your state.

Most of the codes used to report services for the intensive and critically ill neonate are reported based on the severity of the condition of the neonate and the intensity of the services that are required and performed. It is important to remember that specific therapies or diagnoses do not always equate to a specific level of care and, therefore, documentation of the critical status of the newborn is required.

Chapter 12: Critical and Intensive Care

Resource-Based Relative Value Scale

The 2017 RVUs for the services described in this chapter are included in the Resource-Based Relative Value Scale (RBRVS) brochure found at www.aap.org/cfp, or go to www.cms.gov to find the current year RVUs and Medicare conversion factor. At time of publication, the 2018 RVUs were not available; they are typically published in November for the upcoming year. The RBRVS brochure is updated accordingly.

Physician Work

The times for E/M services most commonly provided to newborns (typical time for neonatal services) based on RUC survey results for 2011 are provided in **Table 12-8**. Although not exact or applicable for every patient, they are the average times (in minutes) spent by neonatologists for the typical or average patient. This is an excellent and quick internal audit mechanism to judge the adequacy of your coding or nursery coverage.

Table 12-8. RUC Survey Times for Subsequent Hospital Care and Critical Care (min)

Code	Preservice	Intraservice	Post-service	Total RUC Time
99231	5	10	5	20
99232	10	20	10	40
99233	10	30	15	55
99291	15	40	15	70
99292	–	30	–	30
99468	45	180	48.8	274
99469	–	128	–	128
99471	30	180	30	240
99472	20	90	30	140
99475	30	105	30	165
99476	20	65	20	105
99477	30	77.5	40	147.5
99478	10	30	20	60
99479	10	30	15	55
99480	15	30	15	60

Abbreviation: RUC, American Medical Association/Specialty Society Relative Value Scale Update Committee.

Telemedicine

Contents

Telemedicine is the use of technology to bring a specialist in a distant location to a patient's bedside or to a setting right in the patient's own community without the need for either party to physically travel. *Telemedicine* is one term used to describe the provision of face-to-face services through the use of technology. Telemedicine may also be referred to as *telehealth*; definitions for each vary by state and payer, but telehealth is more commonly used to reference any health service provided via telecommunications. Telemedicine may be more appropriate to describe services of physicians and other qualified health care professionals and is the terminology used by *Current Procedural Terminology* (*CPT®*). Without any consideration of state law or payer policies, telemedicine services might be loosely defined as audiovisual technology-enabled, patient-specific services provided by a physician or practitioner in a distant geographic location to a patient who requires medical expertise not otherwise available at his or her location.

Interest in telemedicine services has grown significantly in recent years. In December 2016, the Expanding Capacity for Health Outcomes (ECHO) Act was signed into law. The ECHO Act requires the secretary of Health and Human Services, in collaboration with the Health Resources and Services Administration, to study and publish a report, within 2 years of enactment, on technology-enabled learning and capacity building models and their effect on

- Addressing mental and substance use disorders, chronic diseases and conditions, prenatal and maternal health, pediatric care, pain management, and palliative care
- Addressing health care workforce issues, such as specialty care shortages and primary care workforce recruitment, retention, and support for lifelong learning
- The implementation of public health programs, including those related to disease prevention, infectious disease outbreaks, and public health surveillance
- The delivery of health care services in rural areas, frontier areas, health professional shortage areas, and medically underserved areas and to medically underserved populations and Native Americans
- Addressing other issues the secretary determines appropriate

Findings from this study will likely serve as a catalyst for additional support of telemedicine in federally funded health programs.

In addition to increased federal interest in telemedicine services, most states have enacted or have pending legislation aimed at parity in payment of telemedicine services. The American Telemedicine Association offers state legislation and regulatory trackers online at https://www.americantelemed.org/policy-page/state-policy-resource-center.

Payer Coverage

Currently, payers may restrict utilization of telemedicine services to certain settings and to patients located in rural areas that Medicare designates as a Health Professional Shortage Area. However, demonstration projects, such as those for accountable care organizations, are expanding the provision of care via telemedicine and may provide evidence to support expansion to all patients in the future.

Although the federal Medicaid statute does not yet recognize telemedicine as a distinct service, states may choose to cover these services, and many do. However, there is wide variation in how private payers and state Medicaid plans define and cover telemedicine services, making it important to identify the applicable definition and payment policies prior to delivery of services. Many states limit coverage to that delivered via interactive systems using multimedia communications equipment that includes, at minimum, audio and video equipment permitting 2-way, real-time communication between the patient and the distant site practitioner. Asynchronous or store-and-forward technology may be allowed in some areas or for certain services.

From a coding perspective, telemedicine services are face-to-face services reported using the same evaluation and management (E/M) codes that would be appropriate for in-person encounters.

- Usually, these are consultation services (eg, **99251–99255**). Typically, key components or time spent in counseling and/or coordination of care may be used to select the level of E/M service provided.
- As with many services, there are combinations of *CPT* and Healthcare Common Procedure Coding System (HCPCS) codes and modifiers that may apply.

Chapter 13: Telemedicine

- An understanding of coverage, payment policies, and coding requirements is essential to establishing a successful telemedicine service. Coverage and reporting requirements will vary across payers, requiring verification of benefits prior to provision of services.
- The Medicare program limits payment for telemedicine services to a specific set of services.

A list of services designated as telemedicine services by *CPT*® and/or Medicare and the codes for reporting each are included in **Table 13-1**. Telemedicine services covered by Medicare are published each year as part of the update to the Medicare Physician Fee Schedule. Medicaid and/or private health plans may adopt Medicare's coverage policies and/or list of covered services.

Table 13-1. 2017 Telemedicine Services

CY 2017 Telehealth Services (Please see coding reference for code descriptors.)	HCPCS/*CPT* Code	*CPT* Allows[a]	CMS Allows
Advanced care planning	99497 and 99498		✓
Annual alcohol misuse screening, 15 min	G0442		✓
Annual behavioral therapy for cardiovascular disease, 15 min	G0446		✓
Annual depression screening, 15 min	G0444		✓
Annual wellness visit, first visit	G0438		✓
Annual wellness visit, subsequent visit	G0439		✓
Behavioral counseling for alcohol misuse, 15 min	G0443		✓
Behavioral counseling for obesity, 15 min	G0447		✓
Diabetes self-management training services	G0108 and G0109		✓
Electrocardiographic rhythm derived event recording	93268, 93270–93272	✓	
ESRD-related services[b]	90951, 90952, 90954, 90955, 90957, 90958, 90960, and 90961	✓	✓
ESRD-related services for home dialysis[b]	90963–90970		✓
External mobile cardiovascular telemetry with electro-cardiographic recording, concurrent computerized real-time data analysis	93228 and 93229	✓	
Genetic counseling	96040	✓	
Health and behavior assessment and intervention	96150–96154	✓	✓
High-intensity behavioral counseling to prevent sexually transmitted infection; 30 min	G0445		✓
Hospital subsequent care services (Payer may limit to 1 telehealth visit every 3 days.)	99231–99233	✓	✓
Inpatient consultation	99251–99255	✓	
Kidney disease education services	G0420 and G0421		✓
Medical nutrition therapy	G0270		✓
	97802–97804	✓	
Neurobehavioral status exam	96116	✓	✓
Nursing facility subsequent care services (Payer may limit to 1 telehealth visit every 30 days)	99307–99310	✓	✓
Office or other outpatient visits	99201–99215	✓	✓

Table 13-1. 2017 Telemedicine Services (*continued*)

CY 2017 Telehealth Services (Please see coding reference for code descriptors.)	HCPCS/*CPT* Code	*CPT* Allows[a]	CMS Allows
Office consultation	99241–99245	✓	
Pharmacologic management performed with psycho-therapy services	90863	✓	
Pharmacologic management, telehealth, inpatient	G0459		✓
Prolonged service in the inpatient or observation setting	99356 and 99357		✓
Prolonged service in the office or other outpatient setting	99354 and 99355	✓	✓
Psychiatric diagnostic interview examination	90791 and 90792	✓	✓
Psychoanalysis	90845	✓	✓
Psychotherapy, family	90846 and 90847	✓	✓
Psychotherapy, individual	90832–90834 and 90836–90838	✓	✓
Remote imaging for detection of retinal disease	92227	✓	
Remote imaging for monitoring and management of active retinal disease	92228	✓	
Remote interrogation implantable loop recorder	93298 and 93299	✓	
Self-management education and training	98960–98962	✓	
Smoking cessation services	G0436 and G0437		✓
	99406 and 99407	✓	
Structured assessment and intervention services for alcohol and/or substance (other than tobacco) abuse	G0396 and G0397		✓
	99408 and 99409	✓	
Telehealth consultations, emergency department or initial inpatient	G0425–G0427		✓
Telehealth consultation, critical care, initial, physicians typically spend 60 minutes	G0508		✓
Telehealth consultation, critical care, subsequent, physicians typically spend 50 minutes	G0509		✓
Telehealth consultations, follow-up inpatient hospital or SNF	G0406–G0408		✓
Transitional care management services	99495 and 99496	✓	✓

Abbreviations: CMS, Centers for Medicare & Medicaid Services; CPT, Current Procedural Terminology; CY, calendar year; ESRD, end-stage renal disease; HCPCS, Healthcare Common Procedure Coding System; SNF, skilled nursing facility.

[a] Append modifier 95 (telemedicine service rendered via a real-time interactive audio and video telecommunications system).

[b] For ESRD-related services, a physician, nurse practitioner, physician assistant, or clinical nurse specialist must furnish at least one "hands-on" visit (not telehealth) each month to examine the vascular access site.

Place and Site of Service

Effective January 1, 2017, a new place of service (POS) code (02) was added for reporting health services provided via a health communications system. This code applies to the location where health services and health-related services are provided or received through telecommunications technology. It may be necessary to work with your electronic system vendors to determine the best method for ensuring that telemedicine service claims contain this POS code. In most practice management systems, the POS may be manually entered for each charge entered.

Field 32 of the 1500 paper claim form and its electronic equivalent are used to report the site of service (eg, hospital name, address, National Provider Identifier). This is typically the physical location of the physician or other provider of service at the time of service when payment is influenced by geographic location. See individual payer policies for telemedicine services to determine if there are reporting requirements for the specific site of service (eg, physical location from which services were rendered or received).

Documentation of Services

Documentation of telemedicine services should be similar to that of services provided in traditional patient care settings. For E/M services, this means that documentation supports reporting of services based on the required key components (ie, history, examination, and/or medical decision-making [MDM]) or typical time of service (when >50% of the face-to-face time of the encounter is spent in counseling and/or coordination of care). See Chapter 4, Evaluation and Management Documentation Guidelines, and Chapter 5, Time-Based Coding, for more information on documentation of E/M services and instructions for reporting E/M services based on time spent in counseling and/or coordination of care.

Reporting Telemedicine With *CPT*®

Current Procedural Terminology® (*CPT*®) modifier **95** is appended to the appropriate procedure code to identify telemedicine services when rendered via real-time interactive audio and video telecommunications. This modifier is not applied if the communication is not real-time interactive audio and video. Telephone care is not telemedicine.

95   Telemedicine service rendered via a real-time interactive audio and video telecommunications system: Synchronous telemedicine service is defined as a real-time interaction between a physician or other qualified health care professional and a patient who is located at a distant site from the physician or other qualified health care professional. The totality of the communication of information exchanged between the provider or other qualified health care professional and the patient during the course of the synchronous telemedicine service must be of an amount and nature that would be sufficient to meet the key components and/or requirements of the same service when rendered via a face-to-face interaction. Modifier **95** may only be appended to the services listed in Appendix P. Appendix P is the list of *CPT* codes for services that are typically performed face-to-face but may be rendered via a real-time (synchronous) interactive audio and video telecommunications system.

In addition to modifier **95**, *CPT* includes Appendix P, listing all codes to which the **95** modifier is applicable, and adds a star symbol (★) to the listing of each code included in Appendix P in the main body of the manual. Appendix P codes that may be of particular interest to pediatricians include

- New and established patient office or other outpatient E/M services (**99201–99205**, **99212–99215**)
- Subsequent hospital care (**99231–99233**)
- Inpatient and outpatient consultations (**99241–99245**, **99251–99255**)
- Subsequent nursing facility care (**99307–99310**)
- Prolonged services in the office or outpatient setting (**99354**, **99355**)
- Individual behavior change interventions (**99406–99409**)
- Transitional care management services (**99495**, **99496**)
- Remote real-time interactive video-conferenced critical care codes (**0188T**, **0189T**)

Appendix P also includes codes for services such as psychotherapy, health and behavior assessment and intervention, medical nutrition therapy, and education and training for patient self-management, allowing for telemedicine services provided by certain qualified nonphysician health care professionals in addition to subspecialty physicians. See coding examples on page 347.

Critical Care via Telemedicine

★0188T   Remote real-time interactive video-conferenced critical care, evaluation and management of the critically ill or critically injured patient; first 30-74 minutes

★0189T   each additional 30 minutes (List separately in addition to code **0188T**)

Codes **0188T** and **0189T** are *CPT*® Category III codes (emerging technology). Not all payers accept Category III codes for payment. For payers that do not accept codes **0188T** and **0189T**, HCPCS codes **G0508** and **G0509** (discussed in the Reporting Telemedicine With HCPCS section) may alternatively be included as covered critical care services when provided via telemedicine.

Remote critical care is the direct delivery by a physician(s) of medical care for a critically ill or critically injured patient from an off-site location (ie, when a critically ill or injured patient requires additional critical care resources that are not available on-site). To report remote critical care, the following conditions must exist:

- The patient's condition must fall under the strict *CPT* definition of critically ill or critically injured.
- The physician(s) in the remote location must have real-time access to the patient's medical record, including progress notes, nursing notes, current medications, vital signs, clinical laboratory test results, other diagnostic test results, and radiographic images.
- The physician(s) must have real-time capability to enter electronic orders; document the remote care services provided in the hospital medical record; video-conference with the on-site health care team in the patient room; assess patients in their individual room using high-fidelity audio and video capabilities, including, but not limited to, clear observation of the patient, monitors, ventilators, and infusion pumps; and speak with the patient and family members.
- The total duration spent providing remote critical care on a given day should be reported, regardless of whether the time is continuous. The time reported includes time spent on work directly related to the patient's care (eg, time reviewing test results or imaging studies, discussing the patient's care with other medical staff, documenting remote critical care services in the medical record, talking with the patient and/or family or surrogate decision-makers to obtain history and/or discuss the management and prognosis of the patient). Any time spent away from the remote site when the physician does not have the real-time capabilities described previously or spent on activities that do not directly contribute to the treatment of the patient may not be reported.
- The first hour (**0188T**) of remote critical care can only be reported once on a given date of service and only if 30 minutes or more of critical care is performed. Remote critical care cannot be reported if less than 30 minutes of remote critical care is provided. Each additional 30 minutes beyond the first 74 minutes of remote critical care is reported with code **0189T** (Table 13-2).
- Medical record documentation must include the actual time spent providing remote critical care services and support the critical nature of the patient's condition and interactions with the patient, family, and other providers.
- For any given period, only one physician may report critical care services. If any physician is reporting in-person critical care services with hourly critical care codes (**99291**, **99292**) for the same period or daily critical care codes (**99468–99476**), codes **0188T** and **0189T** are not reported.
- Category III codes are not assigned relative values under the Medicare Resource-Based Relative Value Scale. Payment for remote critical care services is based strictly on payer policies. Work with your payers to determine their coverage, educate payers, and provide them with information that demonstrates the value of the service.

Codes **0188T** and **0189T** are listed in Appendix P and are appended with modifier **95** to indicate telemedicine services rendered via real-time interactive audio and video telecommunications. See coding example on page 348.

Chapter 13: Telemedicine

Table 13-2. Reporting Remote Critical Care Services

Duration of Remote Critical Care	CPT® Codes
<30 min	Do not report.
30–74 min	**0188T**
75–104 min	**0188T** × 1 unit plus **0189T** × 1 unit
105–134 min	**0188T** × 1 unit plus **0189T** × 2 units

Abbreviation: CPT, Current Procedural Terminology.

Reporting Telemedicine With HCPCS

Healthcare Common Procedure Coding System uses the term *telehealth* in code descriptors. HCPCS modifiers that identify telemedicine services are

GT   via interactive audio and video telecommunications system

GQ   via asynchronous telecommunications system (Medicare applies this modifier only to services provided as part of a telemedicine demonstration project in Alaska and Hawaii.)

These modifiers are appended to *CPT®* or HCPCS codes when required by the payer but are generally used by Medicare and some Medicaid programs.

Under some plans, additional codes may be reported for overhead expenses of providing telemedicine services.

Q3014   Telehealth originating site facility fee

T1014   Telehealth transmission, per minute, professional services bill separately

For Medicare purposes, an originating site is the location of an eligible Medicare beneficiary at the time the service is furnished via telemedicine occurs.

While *CPT* codes are accepted by most plans covering telemedicine services, payers may require HCPCS codes that are used in the Medicare program for consultations and other services with specific coverage policies (eg, inpatient telehealth pharmacologic management with no more than minimal psychotherapy). HCPCS codes are used for telemedicine consultations with Medicare beneficiaries because *CPT* consultation codes are not payable under the Medicare Physician Fee Schedule. Only specific services are eligible for Medicare payment when provided via telemedicine. The following codes do not apply in all potential settings where telemedicine might be provided (eg, Medicare does not cover telemedicine services to patients in observation settings). Exceptions apply for telemedicine services rendered as part of certain demonstration projects (eg, under telehealth waiver for patients associated with a Next Generation accountable care organization).

G0425   Telehealth consultation, emergency department or initial inpatient, typically 30 minutes communicating with the patient via telehealth

G0426   typically 50 minutes communicating with the patient via telehealth

G0427   typically 70 minutes or more communicating with the patient via telehealth

G0406   Follow-up inpatient consultation, limited, physicians typically spend 15 minutes communicating with the patient via telehealth

G0407   intermediate, physicians typically spend 25 minutes communicating with the patient via telehealth

G0408   complex, physicians typically spend 35 minutes communicating with the patient via telehealth

G0459   Inpatient telehealth pharmacologic management, including prescription, use, and review of medication with no more than minimal medical psychotherapy

G0508   Telehealth consultation, critical care, physicians typically spend 60 minutes communicating with the patient via telehealth (initial)

G0509   Telehealth consultation, critical care, physicians typically spend 50 minutes communicating with the patient via telehealth (subsequent)

When a payer uses Medicare program policies for telemedicine services, it is important to learn which services are and are not covered when delivered via telemedicine. A current listing of services covered under the Medicare program is available in Chapter 12 of the *Medicare Claims Processing Manual* (https://www.cms.gov/Regulations-and-Guidance/Guidance/Manuals/downloads/clm104c12.pdf).

Examples

➤ **A consultation is requested of a rheumatologist at a teaching facility for an inpatient in a rural hospital 75 miles away.** Through real-time interactive technology, the physician performs a consultation including a comprehensive history, comprehensive examination (assisted by clinical staff of the facility), and MDM of moderate complexity. The total time of the interactive communication is 30 minutes. A written report to the requesting physician is transmitted via secure electronic health information exchange.

MDM: Moderate History: Comprehensive Physical examination: Comprehensive	**CPT®** **99254 95** Or, if payer requires HCPCS codes, **G0425 GT** (telehealth consultation, emergency department or initial inpatient, typically 30 minutes communicating with the patient via telehealth)

Teaching Point: If payer policy allows payment for overhead expenses related to telemedicine services, also report **T1014**, telehealth transmission, per minute, professional services bill separately. Because this is billed per minute, 30 units are reported. The rural hospital, as the originating facility, may also report **Q3014**, telehealth originating site facility fee.

➤ **A child with a closed head injury is held in outpatient observation at a rural health facility until evaluated via interactive audiovisual technology by a neurosurgeon who is located 500 miles away.** The child, whose current injury is the result of a car crash, has history of a concussion sustained while playing football 1 year earlier. The neurosurgeon spends 35 minutes prior to initiation of the interactive telecommunications discussing the case with the attending physician and reviewing prior medical records pertaining to the previous concussion as well as the digital images of current and past computed tomography scans. Based on the neurosurgeon's findings after review of medical records, imaging, and consultation with the patient, the patient will remain in observation at the rural facility overnight and be discharged to home if no complications occur during observation. The neurosurgeon's total time of interactive communication is 30 minutes. A follow-up visit with the neurosurgeon via telemedicine is scheduled in 7 days.

Initial consultation	**CPT** **99242 95** (office consultation for a new or established patient, typical time of 30 minutes) (HCPCS codes for telemedicine services do not include services to patients in observation. Verification of benefits and reporting requirements for telemedicine services should be conducted prior to delivery of telemedicine services.) **99358** (prolonged E/M service before and/or after direct patient care; first hour)
Follow-up visit	Report the appropriate office or other outpatient visit (**99212–99215**) appended with modifier **95**.

Teaching Point: Because the physician spent more than 30 minutes in prolonged service related to the telemedicine service, code **99358** is reportable. Payers may or may not provide separate payment for indirect prolonged service. Modified **95** is not appended to **99358**, as this portion of the service was not face-to-face via interactive technology.

If the patient had been transferred and admitted to the neurosurgeon's care at the distant facility on the same date, all the neurosurgeon's E/M services provided on that date would be included in the initial hospital care.

➤ **An endocrinologist provides a follow-up visit for a patient who has uncontrolled diabetes mellitus type 1 and resides 3 hours away from the nearest pediatric endocrinology practice.** The patient is in her primary care physician's clinic, where clinical staff are present to assist with physical examination and other patient care that may be required during the telemedicine service. The endocrinologist spends 10 minutes prior to the visit reviewing the patient's medical records and 25 minutes face-to-face with the patient and caregivers via real-time audiovisual connection, obtaining more information and discussing options for better managing the patient's diabetes. Following the face-to-face encounter with the patient, the endocrinologist documents the service, indicating that 20 minutes of the 25-minute service were spent in counseling the patient and caregivers. A copy of the visit note is sent via secure electronic transmittal to the primary care physician. The patient's health plan accepts *CPT®* codes for telemedicine services. In addition, the health plan allows the primary care physician's clinic to report the practice expense of serving as the originating site for the encounter.

The endocrinologist reports	**99214 95** (office or other outpatient visit for the E/M of an established patient, which requires at least 2 of these 3 key components: ⊛ a detailed history; ⊛ a detailed examination; ⊛ MDM of moderate complexity) Counseling and/or coordination of care with other physicians, other qualified health care professionals, or agencies are provided consistent with the nature of the problem(s) and the patient's and/or family's needs. Usually, the presenting problem(s) are of moderate to high severity. Typically, 25 minutes are spent face-to-face with the patient and/or family.
The ordering physician reports	**Q3014** (telehealth originating site facility fee)

Teaching Point: Because the endocrinologist's visit was predominately spent counseling and/or coordinating care, the visit is reported based on time. The time spent before and after the real-time telemedicine service with the patient is included in the preservice and post-service work of the encounter just as it would be for an encounter in which the patient presented in the endocrinologist's office. Payment policies will vary regarding originating site fees. Practices choosing to offer telemedicine originating site services should verify the policies of plans commonly billed by the practice before initiating services.

➤ **A neonatologist is contacted via live audiovisual telecommunications to provide remote critical care to a neonate who was born in respiratory distress and continues to require critical care services.** The neonatologist views electrocardiograms and other data from monitoring devices in addition to performing visual and audio examination of the neonate. The attending physician at the hospital where the neonate was born performs necessary procedures as advised by the neonatologist to stabilize the neonate. The neonate remains at the same hospital under the care of the pediatrician. A total of 65 minutes of remote critical care service is provided.

The neonatologist reports	**0188T 95** (remote real-time interactive video-conferenced critical care, E/M of the critically ill or critically injured patient; first 30-74 minutes) Or, if the payer requires reporting via HCPCS codes, **G0508 GT** (telehealth consultation, critical care, physicians typically spend 60 minutes communicating with the patient via telehealth [initial])
The attending physician reports	*CPT* codes for services personally performed (eg, delivery/birthing room resuscitation, umbilical catheterization)

Teaching Point: Remote critical care is reported only if the neonate does not receive neonatal critical care services (**99468**) provided in-person by the same or different physician or other qualified health care professional on the same date.

Allied Health and Clinical Staff Services

Contents

Chapter 14: Allied Health and Clinical Staff Services

In the context of providing comprehensive and high-quality primary care to their patients, pediatric physicians are including more nonphysician providers (NPPs) in their practices. In addition to advanced practice providers, such as nurse practitioners and physician assistants, physicians are also including other allied health professionals (AHPs) in their practices to provide specialized services, such as nutrition counseling, condition-specific self-management education, and mental and behavioral health services.

This chapter focuses on services that are provided by health care professionals other than physicians. These services may be provided by AHPs within a physician's group practice based on a physician or other qualified health care professional's (QHP) orders.

Terminology

Of particular importance to correct reporting of nonphysician services is identifying the providers included when terms such as "physician or other qualified health care professional" or "qualified, nonphysician health care professional" are used in *Current Procedural Terminology (CPT®)* and/or payer instruction.

CPT Provider Definitions

Current Procedural Terminology provides definitions of providers as follows:
- **Physician or other qualified health care professional:** an individual who is qualified by education, training, licensure/regulation (when applicable), and facility privileging (when applicable) who performs a professional service within his or her scope of practice and independently reports that professional service
- **Clinical staff member:** a person who works under the supervision of a physician or other QHP and who is allowed by law, regulation, and facility policy to perform or assist in the performance of a specific professional service but does not individually report that professional service

Throughout the *CPT* code set, the use of terms such as "physician," "qualified health care professional," or "individual" is not intended to indicate that other entities may not report the service. In selected instances, specific instructions may define a service as limited to professionals or other entities (eg, hospital, home health agency).

Clinical staff member is used in *CPT* mostly in the context of staff who provide components of physician or QHP services, such as transitional care management (TCM) and chronic care management (CCM), and services that are always billed under incident-to guidelines (eg, nurse visit, medication administration), as discussed in the Medicare Incident-to Requirements: Supervision of Nonphysician Health Care Professionals section later in this chapter.

The *CPT* definition of physician or other QHP creates a broad category of providers (eg, advanced practice providers, therapists, social workers). The definition of *physician and other QHP* is used in relation to services such as evaluation and management (E/M) (**99201–99499**) and immunization administration with physician counseling (**90460, 90461**) and to codes *not reported* by physicians, such as genetic counseling (**96040**).

However, this definition may be confusing, as payer policies commonly differentiate QHPs such as advanced practice providers, who may perform and prescribe services much like a physician, from those who provide specialized services under the supervision and order of a physician or advanced practice provider. Payers may offer direct reporting by certain QHPs (eg, advanced practice provider, psychologist) while requiring others to report services in the name of the supervising physician or advanced practice QHP. To aid in differentiating how services are typically reported by these subcategories of QHPs, the following definitions will apply in discussions and examples in this chapter:

◉ **Qualified health care professional:** signifies advanced practice providers, such as advanced practice nurses and physician assistants, whose scope of practice includes E/M services beyond minimal services incident to a physician (ie, **99211**)

◉ **Clinical staff member** (as defined by *CPT* in differentiating from a physician or QHP): a health care team member who works under the supervision of a physician or other QHP and who is allowed by law, regulation, and facility policy to perform or assist in the performance of a specific professional service but *does not individually report that professional service.* These include, but are not limited to, registered nurses (RNs), licensed practical nurses (LPNs), and medical assistants (MAs).

⊛ **Allied health professional:** represents a broad category of health care professionals who typically would not independently prescribe and manage, whose professional services are typically performed under the order and supervision of a physician or QHP, and whose scope of practice does not include E/M services beyond **99211**. Sometimes they are able to bill under their own National Provider Identifier (NPI) and include providers such as clinical psychologists, dietitians/nutritionists, and lactation consultants.

Including Nonphysician Providers in Your Practice

Services such as medical nutrition therapy by a registered dietitian or nutritionist or behavioral health assessment by a licensed social worker or licensed psychologist may be provided within a physician group practice and can be an integral part of providing a full scope of care in the medical home. However, billing and coding of these services must align not only with coding guidelines but also state scope of practice (see the Scope of Practice Laws section later in this chapter) and individual payer policies on credentialing, contracting, and billing for services of the specific NPP. *Before including AHPs within your group practice,* it is important to seek expert advice on related state regulations for scope of practice and supervision requirements, enrollment and payment policies of the group's most common payers, and best practices in employment and/or contractual agreements. The number of services that may be provided can be estimated based on current patient diagnoses or history of referral for services. Reports from electronic health records or billing software may be used in this estimation (eg, report of number of unique patient accounts containing a diagnosis indicating mental or behavioral health conditions).

When physicians choose to arrange for services provided within their practice by AHPs who are not employed or contracted with their group practice, additional counsel should be obtained to avoid conflict with antikickback and/or self-referral regulations.

Payment for AHP services begins with negotiating and contracting with payers for coverage and payment of services as described by *CPT®* and/or Healthcare Common Procedure Coding System (HCPCS) codes. (A list of HCPCS codes that may be used to report nonphysician education services is included in the HCPCS Codes section later in this chapter.) Payers may pay separately for these services when your practice can demonstrate the overall cost savings (eg, decrease in physician or emergency department visits, decreased hospital care) that may be achieved through expanded care in the physician practice. If payers do not agree to directly compensate for individual services, consider opportunities for shared savings and other revenue that may be realized when AHP services support quality improvement initiatives (eg, per-member, per-month compensation for meeting certain quality measures) and redirection of physician and QHP time to services that are restricted to or best delivered within their scope of practice. (For more on quality and performance measurement, see Chapter 17, Coding to Demonstrate Quality and Value.)

Physicians should be especially aware of each payer's policy addressing use of E/M codes and, in particular, codes **99401–99404** (counseling and/or risk factor reduction for patient without symptom or diagnosed illness), as Medicare and payers that adopt Medicare policy do not allow reporting of E/M services other than **99211** (E/M visit not requiring physician face-to-face service) by AHPs or clinical staff. *Current Procedural Terminology* describes codes **99401–99404** as representing services provided face-to-face by a physician or other QHP for the purpose of promoting health and preventing illness or injury. However, other payers directly instruct that codes such as **99401** may be reported for specific services by specific AHPs, such as medical nutritionists or certified lactation consultants. See the Lactation Services section later in this chapter for an example of payer policy that includes reporting of codes **99401–99404** for lactation counseling by an RN. Always keep a printed or electronic copy of payer guidance that is in conflict with *CPT* or standard billing practices.

Scope of Practice Laws

Scope of practice is terminology that is used by state licensing boards for various professions to define the procedures, actions, and processes that are permitted for a licensed individual.

The level of medical responsibility or health services (boundaries within which a health care professional may practice) or range of activities that a practitioner is legally authorized to perform is based on his or her specific education and experience.

Physicians, RNs, clinical nurse practitioners, physician assistants, LPNs, physical therapists, and nutritionists are among some of the professions for which scope of practice laws are defined. However, it can vary by state.

Every state has laws and regulations that describe the requirements of education and training for health care professionals. However, some states do not have different scope of practice laws for every level of professional (eg, LPN).

National Provider Identifier

The NPI is a unique identification number for covered health care providers. The NPI is required on administrative and financial transactions under the Health Insurance Portability and Accountability Act (HIPAA) Administrative Simplification Standard. Anyone who directly provides health care services can apply for and receive an NPI. However, usually only those who will bill for services and/or order services or prescription drugs will need an NPI. The NPI is included on medical claims to indicate who ordered, provided, or supervised the provision of services.

Selecting Codes for Services of Allied Health Professionals

Certain codes are limited to reporting services performed by NPPs who cannot report E/M services under their own NPI. Thus, it is important to differentiate the QHP who may independently report E/M services from the AHP who reports other specific procedure codes rather than E/M services. The examples in **Table 14-1** illustrate the differences in reporting 30 minutes of asthma education by a certified asthma educator using a standardized curriculum based on the provider's scope of practice. Where payer policy directs to report differently, practices should maintain documentation of the payer's instruction and report codes accordingly.

As shown in **Table 14-1**, reporting the appropriate code may result in significantly different payment. This also indicates the value of allowing each provider to work within the full scope of practice as allowed by state regulations and for which he or she is trained. While payment to a QHP who may provide and independently report E/M services is higher, so also is the salary of these providers. Practices should consider the cost to benefit ratio for services by provider type when expanding services offered within the practice.

Table 14-1. Asthma Education Service Coding Examples	
Qualified Health Care Professional (eg, Nurse Practitioner, Physician Assistant) Providing 30 Minutes of Asthma Education Using Standardized Curriculum	**Allied Health Professional (eg, Respiratory Therapist, Registered Nurse With Asthma Education Certification) Providing 30 Minutes of Asthma Education Using Standardized Curriculum**
CPT **99214** (25 min typical time) Service may include additional elements of E/M service.	*CPT* **98960** Education and training for patient self-management by a qualified, nonphysician health care professional using a standardized curriculum, face-to-face with the patient (could include caregiver/family), each 30 minutes; individual patient
Payment example Total non-facility RVUs: 3.03 Conversion factor: $40 Payment: **$121.20**	*Payment example* Total non-facility RVUs: 0.79 Conversion factor: $40 Payment: **$31.60**
Abbreviations: CPT, Current Procedural Terminology; *E/M, evaluation and management; RVU, relative value unit.*	

Chapter 14: Allied Health and Clinical Staff Services

Medicare Incident-to Requirements: Supervision of Nonphysician Health Care Professionals

Billing for care provided by AHPs requires careful attention to state licensure and local payer requirements. Most state Medicaid programs and commercial payers follow the Medicare incident-to payment rules. Some have their own policies addressing incident-to provisions and certified AHP billing. Examples of incident-to policies that do not align with Medicare policy include

- One major payer bases incident-to billing on whether or not the nonphysician is credentialed with the payer. If the nonphysician provider is credentialed, he or she must report under his or her own NPI (ie, incident to does not apply). However, if the provider is not credentialed with the payer, all services are reported by the credentialed supervising physician or provider.
- Another major payer requires credentialing for all providers who may independently provide services under applicable state law for their commercial plans and provides a list of services that may not be reported under a physician's NPI.

Because of the variance in how payers treat the credentialing of NPPs and the related payment policies, it is important that practice administrators and/or billing managers verify payer policies prior to provision of services.

For those payers that align with Medicare policy, see the Medicare Requirements for Incident-to Services box for detailed requirements. See

> ||||||| **Coding Pearl** |||||||
>
> Incident-to provisions apply only in the office or other outpatient setting.

also Chapter 12, section 30.6, of the *Medicare Claims Processing Manual* and Chapter 15, section 60, of the *Medicare Benefit Policy Manual* at http://cms.gov/manuals for detailed information on incident-to services. Check with your payers and obtain a copy of their specific policies.

- The Centers for Medicare & Medicaid Services (CMS) defines *incident to* as "services incident to the service of a physician or other professional permitted by statute to bill for services incident to their services when those services meet all of the requirements applicable to the benefit."
- Incident-to services are always provided as a continuation of a physician's services and do not address new problems (eg, a nursing visit performed at patient or caregiver request and not based on a physician's recommendation is not an incident-to service).
- Although certain QHPs and AHPs otherwise may bill for their services under their own NPI when they provide medically necessary services (within their state's scope of practice), the incident-to provision allows for reporting under the name and NPI of a supervising physician when the requirements of incident-to billing are met. Payment for QHPs and AHPs billing under the incident-to provision may be 100% of the physician payment versus 85% when reporting under the QHP's and AHP's individual NPI.
- Nonphysician providers without their own NPI must report services incident to a physician and must meet all incident-to requirements, including physician presence in the office suite and continuation of a physician's previously established plan of care. Medicare makes an exception for the physician's presence in the office suite for CCM, TCM, and behavioral health integration activities by clinical staff. Private payers may also allow inclusion of time spent by clinical staff without direct supervision when reporting these services. For more information on CCM and TCM, see Chapter 8, Managing Chronic and Complex Conditions.
- Physicians and QHPs billing under their own NPI may
  - ❖ Bill directly for services they have personally performed.
  - ❖ Bill for the services that are performed by any employee, leased employee, or contracted employee (eg, nurse practitioners, physician assistants, therapists, nurses, MAs, technicians). Any services performed by an employee who does not have his or her own individual NPI must be reported as incident to (when provided within the incident-to requirements).

For example, an MA, as allowed under state scope of practice laws, administers a nebulizer treatment that was ordered, documented, and directly supervised by the physician. The treatment (**94640**) would be reported under the physician's NPI. If a certified pediatric nurse practitioner had ordered the treatment, the service would be reported under that practitioner's NPI.

Qualified health care professionals may also perform a split/shared E/M service with a physician. A *split/ shared* E/M service is one in which a physician and a QHP from the same group practice each personally perform a medically necessary and substantive portion of one or more face-to-face E/M encounters on the same date. A portion of the key components of the service must be provided face-to-face by the physician to report under the physician's NPI. For more on split/shared visits, see Chapter 10, Noncritical Hospital Evaluation and Management Services.

Documentation Requirements and Tips When Reporting Incident-to Services

- ☀ Physicians and QHPs must document their order for a service or treatment (eg, injection) that will be performed as incident to or document their plan for a follow-up visit in the treatment plan (eg, follow-up visit in 1 week for weight check).
- ☀ To demonstrate compliant incident-to billing, AHPs and clinical staff providing services in continuation of a physician's plan of care should, ideally, reference the date of the physician order for the service. This may be documented in the chief complaint for the encounter (eg, "Patient is seen today per Dr Green's 1/3/2017 order for dressing change to left arm wound in 10 days").
- ☀ Documentation of incident-to services should fully describe the services provided, including date of service, assessment, concerns noted and addressed, details of care provided (eg, wound cleansed and new bandage applied), and education and/or instructions for home care and follow-up. Inclusion of the supervising physician's name also supports that incident-to requirements were met. Medical record documentation must reflect the identity including credentials and legible signature of the person providing the service.

For Medicare purposes, the physician or QHP billing the service is not required to sign documentation prepared by the clinical staff. Other payer and state regulations may require physician authentication. Documentation may be as simple as "service performed/provided under the direct supervision of Dr X." When applicable, the supervising physician's signature must be legible.

Medicare Requirements for Incident-to Services[a]

- Services must be related to the physician service and must be of a type commonly furnished in a physician office or clinic (physician owned and independent of a hospital or other facility), commonly performed without charge, or included in the physician/QHP service (eg, vital signs, assistance with dressing change).
- Services performed must be reasonable and medically necessary.
- Services performed must be within the employee's state scope of practice and require direct physician supervision. Direct supervision of auxiliary personnel requires that the physician (ie, any physician in the group practice) be on the premises (eg, in the office or facility) and be immediately available to provide assistance or direction. The supervising physician who is reporting the service (his or her name is on the claim form) must be the one who was providing the direct supervision.
- Services can only be provided to an established patient after the physician has performed the initial visit, established the plan of care, and established the physician–patient relationship. The physician must evaluate and initiate the treatment of new problems. The physician is not required to be involved in each subsequent patient encounter. Subsequent patient encounters and services must be incidental and integral to the initial service. They do not require physician involvement, but the physician must remain actively involved in a patient's treatment and must personally see the patient. Review of the medical record alone does not constitute active management of the patient.
- Time cannot be used as the controlling factor when counseling and/or coordination of care is performed incident to the physician. Therefore, when an E/M service is provided as incident to the physician (physician is not involved in the service) and time is the key factor (ie, history, physical examination, and medical decision-making (MDM) requirements are not met), only code **99211** (minimal office/outpatient E/M service) may be reported.
- Services provided in a home are covered only if there is direct supervision by the physician.

Chapter 14: Allied Health and Clinical Staff Services

Medicare Requirements for Incident-to Services[a] (*continued*)

- Inpatient hospital services can be reported only if the physician sees the patient face-to-face. The physician must perform some portion of the required key components (history, physical examination, MDM) to report the encounter under his or her name. If the E/M encounter is reported based on time, only the physician face-to-face time is considered.
- Incident-to services cannot be billed for E/M services performed in the inpatient or outpatient hospital (unless a split/shared service is performed under the requirements of Transmittal 1776 for a nursing facility or home).
- Although diagnostic tests do not fall under incident-to provisions, the CMS requires certain levels of physician supervision for covered diagnostic tests. The Medicare Physician Fee Schedule database includes an indicator on each *CPT*® and HCPCS code to define the level of supervision required. The 3 levels of physician supervision include general supervision (ie, the procedure is performed under the physician's overall direction and control, but the physician's presence is not required during the performance of the test and the physician is responsible for personnel training and maintenance of the equipment and supplies), direct supervision (ie, the physician must be on the premises and immediately available to provide assistance or direction), or personal supervision (ie, the physician must be in the room while the test is being performed). Medicare regulations do not allow supervision of diagnostic tests by QHPs.
- Some payers may require the use of HCPCS codes and/or modifiers to identify services provided by AHPs.
- Medicare provides an exception to the requirement for direct physician supervision for clinical staff activities included in CCM, TCM, and behavioral health integration services. Clinical staff may perform these activities under general supervision. All other incident-to provisions apply.

[a] *Note that the term* physician *also includes QHPs billing under their own NPI.*

HCPCS Codes

Healthcare Common Procedure Coding System Level II codes may be reported when the narrative differs from the *CPT* code for the service. What follows is a small sample of HCPCS codes and modifiers that may be used for services by AHPs. Payer guidance for reporting HCPCS or *CPT* codes may vary.

Note that HCPCS codes may include the term NPP in lieu of AHP or QHP. These codes are only reported when services are provided by NPPs unless otherwise instructed by a payer. It is advisable to retain copies of a payer's written policies and guidance for reporting HCPCS codes.

G0108	Diabetes outpatient self-management training services, individual, per 30 minutes
G0109	Diabetes outpatient self-management training services, group session (2 or more), per 30 minutes
S0315	Disease management program; initial assessment and initiation of the program
S0316	Disease management program, follow-up/reassessment
S0317	Disease management program; per diem
S0320	Telephone calls by a registered nurse to a disease management program member for monitoring purposes; per month
S9441	Asthma education, NPP; per session
S9443	Lactation classes, NPP, per session
S9445	Patient education, not otherwise classified, NPP, individual, per session
S9446	group, per session
S9449	Weight management classes, NPP, per session
S9451	Exercise class, NPP, per session
S9452	Nutrition class, NPP, per session
S9454	Stress management class, NPP, per session
S9455	Diabetic management program, group session
S9460	nurse visit
S9465	dietitian visit
S9470	Nutritional counseling, dietitian visit

Payers may also instruct certain AHPs to report services by appending a HCPCS modifier to the *CPT®* or HCPCS code for services provided.

AE	Registered dietician
AH	Clinical psychologist
AJ	Clinical social worker
HA	Child/adolescent program
HN	Bachelor's degree level
HO	Master's degree level
HP	Doctoral level
HQ	Group setting
UN	Two patients served
UP	Three patients served
UQ	Four patients served
UR	Five patients served
US	Six or more patients served

Nonphysician Services

Nonphysician Evaluation and Management Services

Nursing Visit

99211   Office or other outpatient visit for the evaluation and management of an established patient, that may not require the presence of a physician or other qualified health care professional. Usually, the presenting problem(s) are minimal. Typically, 5 minutes are spent performing or supervising these services

When clinical staff and/or AHPs who do not independently report E/M services provide an E/M service that is not described by another procedure code, code **99211** is reported.

Report **99211** when

- ❉ Services meet the incident-to requirements of the payer.
- ❉ Problems addressed have previously been addressed by ordering physician or QHP and services are a continuation of care.
- ❉ The service is provided based on physician orders and within scope of practice and license.
- ❉ The service is rendered face-to-face with the patient/caregiver.

Never report **99211** when

- ❉ Another procedure code describes the service provided (eg, **36415**, venipuncture).
- ❉ The physician performs a face-to-face E/M service on the same date.
- ❉ The patient is new or the problem has not been addressed by the physician.

Examples

➤ A physician orders counseling by a nurse in the practice for a 16-year-old obese patient with borderline hypertension about diet and exercise (follow-up visit not on same day as physician visit). The follow-up visit is conducted by an RN who documents the patient's weight, body mass index (BMI), and blood pressure. The nurse spends 10 minutes face-to-face with the patient going over dietary guidelines, demonstrating proper portion sizes, and encouraging him to continue progress made in adopting an exercise routine and healthier diet.

The RN is not a registered dietitian or licensed medical nutritionist who may report medical nutrition therapy. This service was provided in continuation of the physician's plan of care and under direct (in-office) physician supervision. Code **99211** is reported.

➤ **A physician orders education and training on proper use of a metered-dose inhaler (MDI) for a patient seen in the emergency department and treated for new-onset asthma.** A respiratory therapist who works part-time in the physician's clinic providing asthma education sees the patient. The patient presents with an MDI and spacer. The therapist demonstrates proper use and evaluates the patient's use of the MDI. The patient is instructed to keep a follow-up appointment with the ordering physician in 10 days.

94664 (demonstration and/or evaluation of patient utilization of an aerosol generator, nebulizer, metered dose inhaler or IPPB device)

This service is not reported with code **99211** because code **94664** describes the service performed.

Prolonged Clinical Staff Service (99415 and 99416)

#+99415   Prolonged clinical staff service (the service beyond the typical service time) during an evaluation and management service in the office or outpatient setting, direct patient contact with physician supervision; first hour (List separately in addition to code for outpatient Evaluation and Management service)

#+99416   each additional 30 minutes (List separately in addition to code **99415**)

Codes **99415** and **99416** are used to report 45 minutes or more of prolonged clinical staff time spent face-to-face providing care to a patient under the supervision of a physician or other QHP who has provided an office or other outpatient E/M service at the same session. Report only prolonged service by a physician or other QHP (**99354–99355**) when provided on the same date as prolonged clinical staff services. The relative value units assigned to codes **99415** (0.25) and **99416** (0.13) represent only the intraservice time spent by clinical staff, as preservice and post-service times are valued in the related E/M service.

The following guidelines apply to reporting of prolonged clinical staff services:

- Prolonged clinical staff services are reported only in conjunction with E/M services in the office or other outpatient setting. Report **99415** and **99416** in addition to office or other outpatient E/M codes **99201–99215**. The related E/M service by the physician may be reported based on key components or time spent in counseling and/or coordinating care.

- Supervision must be provided by a physician or other QHP during the provision of prolonged clinical staff services.

- Prolonged clinical staff services are reported only when the face-to-face time spent by clinical staff is 45 minutes or more beyond the typical time of the related E/M service on the same date. Documentation of the physician's time spent in provision of the E/M service is not required when the level of service is selected based on key components. (See **tables 7-2** and **7-3** for typical times assigned to office and other outpatient services.)

- Do not report prolonged service of less than 45 minutes beyond the typical time of the related E/M service.

- The total time of and medical necessity for the service must be documented.

- Time spent providing separately reported services, such as intravenous medication administration or inhalation treatment, is not counted toward the time of prolonged service.

- It is not required that the clinical staff time be continuous, but each episode of face-to-face time should be documented.

- Report code **99416** for each additional 30 minutes of clinical staff time beyond the first hour and for the last 15 to 30 minutes of prolonged clinical staff service. Do not report **99416** for less than 15 minutes beyond the first hour or last 30-minute period.

See Chapter 7, Evaluation and Management Services in the Office, Outpatient, Home, or Nursing Facility Setting, for more information on prolonged clinical staff services.

Example

➤ **A child is seen for diarrhea and concerns of dehydration.** The physician diagnoses moderate dehydration due to viral gastroenteritis. Oral rehydration is ordered. The physician completes his or her documentation and selects code **99214** for service to this established patient based on the level of history, examination, and MDM. The physician remains in the office suite while a nurse delivers and monitors a time-based oral rehydration plan using an electrolyte solution. The nurse's total direct care time is 2 hours. The first 25 minutes are included in the practice expense of the physician service. The additional 95 minutes following the physician's service are reported as prolonged clinical staff service.

E/M service by physician Prolonged clinical staff time	**International Classification of Diseases, 10th Revision, Clinical Modification (ICD-10-CM)** **A08.4** (viral intestinal infection, unspecified) **E86.0** (dehydration)
	CPT® **99214** (typical time of 25 minutes) **99415** × 1 (first hour) and **99416** × 1 (final 35-minute period)

Teaching Point: *CPT* instructs that prolonged clinical staff time reporting begins 45 minutes after the typical time of the E/M service provided by the physician. In this scenario, the typical time of the physician service is 25 minutes, so prolonged clinical staff time is not reported until clinical staff have spent at least 70 minutes in face-to-face patient care. Code **99415** is reported for prolonged clinical staff service of 45 to 74 minutes beyond the typical time of the related E/M service. Code **99416** is reported with 1 unit of service for 75 to 104 minutes of service time. When reporting units of service for code **99416**, only time of 15 to 30 minutes beyond the previous period is reported. In this example, the final 5 minutes beyond the first 90 minutes is not separately reported.

Education and Training for Patient Self-management

98960   Education and training for patient self-management by a qualified, nonphysician health care professional using a standardized curriculum, face-to-face with the patient (could include caregiver/family) each 30 minutes; individual patient
98961   2–4 patients
98962   5–8 patients

Report codes **98960–98962** when

- The purpose of these services is to teach the patient and caregivers how to self-manage the illness or disease or delay disease comorbidities in conjunction with the patient's professional health care team.
- A physician prescribes the services and a standardized curriculum is used.
- Qualifications of the AHPs and the content of the program are consistent with guidelines or standards established or recognized by a physician or AHP society, association, or other appropriate source. For example, these codes apply to diabetic self-management training—an important category of patient self-management education and training. Such training can be provided by diabetic nurse educators—nurses who have received special education in addition to certification from accreditation societies or state licensing panels. In such scenarios, these services could be reported by the supervising physician when the services are rendered by the appropriately certified professional and acknowledged by the payer via the payer contract or published guidance of a government payer.
- Education and training services are provided to patients with an established illness or disease. Code **98960** is reported when services are provided to an individual patient; code **98961** is reported when services are provided to 2 to 4 patients; and code **98962** is reported when 5 to 8 patients receive the education and training.

Code selection is based on the general *CPT®* instruction for reporting services based on time. Time is met when the midpoint is passed (ie, report code **98960** for 16 or more minutes of face-to-face time and with units of service for each additional full 30 minutes and the last 16–30 minutes).

> **Coding Pearl** |||||||

Qualifications of the AHPs and the content of patient self-management education (**98960–98962**) must be consistent with guidelines or standards established or recognized by a physician or AHP society, association, or other appropriate source.

Example

➤ **A 7-year-old patient was recently diagnosed with asthma and is referred to the asthma educator for therapy and training under an approved curriculum.** This includes review of protocols for prevention, use of controller medications (eg, inhaler technique, use of holding chamber or spacer, self-monitoring), and handling potential exacerbations. The total documented time of service is 50 minutes.

The content, type, duration, and patient response to the training must be documented in the medical record. Two units of service are reported with code **98960**; one for the first 30 minutes of service and an additional unit for the last 20 minutes (16–30 minutes is reportable). Reporting of services under the name of the asthma educator or supervising physician or QHP will be determined by payer contract. If payer credentials educators, report under the name and NPI of the educator. If payer does not credential educators, report under the name of the supervising physician or QHP.

Genetic Counseling Services

96040   Medical genetics and genetic counseling services, each 30 minutes face-to-face with patient/family
* Trained genetic counselors provide services that may include obtaining a structured family genetic history, pedigree construction, analysis for genetic risk assessment, and counseling of the patient and family.
* Only face-to-face time with the patient or caregiver is used in determining the units of service reported. Do not report genetic counseling of 15 minutes or less. Report code **96040** with units of service for the first and each additional 30 minutes and the last 16 to 30 minutes.
* Services may be provided during one or more sessions and may include review of medical data and family information, face-to-face interviews, and counseling services.
* For genetic counseling and education on genetic risks by an AHP to a group, see codes **98961** and **98962**.
* Genetic counseling by physicians and other QHPs who may report E/M services are reported with the appropriate E/M service code.

Health and Behavior Assessments/Interventions

96150   Health and behavior assessment, each 15 minutes face-to-face with the patient, initial assessment
96151   reassessment
96152   Health and behavior intervention, each 15 minutes, face-to-face; individual
96153   group (2 or more patients)
96154   family (with patient present)
96155   family (without patient present)

Face-to-face health and behavior intervention services are reported per each 15 minutes of time spent. The total time must be documented in the medical record. Time is met when the midpoint is passed unless payer policy directs otherwise.

Codes **96150–96155**
* May be reported by psychologists, clinical social workers, licensed therapists, and other AHPs within their scope of practice who have specialty or subspecialty training in health and behavior assessment or intervention procedures.
* Physicians and other QHPs who may report E/M services are instructed to report E/M or preventive service codes.

- Are used when assessing or addressing psychosocial factors affecting patients who have an established medical illness or diagnosis and may benefit from assessments and interventions with a focus on the role that psychosocial adaptation may play on the clinical course of that condition (eg, services differ from preventive medicine counseling and risk-factor reduction interventions).

- Are not used in conjunction with a primary diagnosis of mental disorder. (Payers may deny when a diagnosis code indicating mental disorder is included on the claim for these services.)

- Are used to identify the psychological, behavioral, emotional, cognitive, and/or social factors needed for the prevention, treatment, or management of physical health problems, with a focus on treating the bio-psychosocial factors contributing to physical problems.

- Do not require a standardized curriculum.

- Are not reported with psychiatric codes (**90785–90899**) when provided on the same day. Only the primary service is reported (ie, either **96150–96155** or **90791–90899**).

- Are not reported with an E/M code (eg, **99201–99215**, **99401–99412**) on the same day.

- Are not reported in conjunction with adaptive behavior treatment (**0364T–0367T**, **0373T**, **0374T**).

- Do not include neuropsychological testing (**96116**), which can be reported separately.

- The initial assessment (**96150**) may include a health-focused clinical interview, behavioral observations, psychophysiological monitoring, and completion of health-oriented questionnaires.

- Code **96151** is used to report the reassessment of a patient's condition by interview and behavioral health instruments.

Examples

➤ **A 12-year-old girl undergoing treatment for acute lymphoblastic leukemia is referred to a social worker trained in health and behavior assessment or intervention procedures for assessment of pain, behavioral distress, and combativeness associated with repeated procedures and treatment.** The patient is assessed using standardized questionnaires (eg, Pediatric Pain Questionnaire, Coping Strategies Inventory). The child's parents are also interviewed.

Code **96150** would be reported with, for example, *ICD-10-CM* code **C91.00**, acute lymphoblastic leukemia, without remission. One unit of service would be reported for each 15 minutes of face-to-face time with the patient and/or parents. Time must be documented and does not include time spent before or after face-to-face services.

Results from the health and behavior assessment are used to develop a treatment plan. Thirty minutes is spent with the patient discussing the behavior and suggested coping skills. Code **96152** with 2 units of service would be reported with the same diagnosis as used in the initial assessment.

➤ **A 10-year-old boy diagnosed with attention-deficit/hyperactivity disorder 2 years ago has undergone health and behavior assessment after parents noted the boy was afraid to go to school, where he fears being in trouble and failing.** Based on the assessment conducted at a previous encounter, the clinical psychologist works with the boy to develop new coping skills and improve self-management. Parents are urged to meet with the boy's teacher about adherence to an existing behavioral intervention plan and recommended revisions. A total of 55 minutes is spent face-to-face with the boy and his parents.

Code **96154** is reported with 4 units of service (3 full 15-minute periods and 1 unit for the 10 minutes because the midpoint of 8 minutes beyond the last full period was passed).

Home Health Procedures/Services

99500	Home visit for prenatal monitoring and assessment to include fetal heart rate, non-stress test, uterine monitoring, and gestational diabetes monitoring
99501	Home visit for postnatal assessment and follow-up care
99502	Home visit for newborn care and assessment

Chapter 14: Allied Health and Clinical Staff Services

99503	Home visit for respiratory therapy care (eg, bronchodilator, oxygen therapy, respiratory assessment, apnea evaluation)
99504	Home visit for mechanical ventilation care
99505	Home visit for stoma care and maintenance including colostomy and cystostomy
99506	Home visit for intramuscular injections
99507	Home visit for care and maintenance of catheter(s) (eg, urinary, drainage, and enteral)
99509	Home visit for assistance with activities of daily living and personal care
99510	Home visit for individual, family, or marriage counseling
99511	Home visit for fecal impaction management and enema administration
99512	Home visit for hemodialysis
99600	Unlisted home visit service or procedure

Codes **99500–99600** are

* Typically reported for skilled nursing services ordered by a physician or QHP and are medically necessary services provided to a homebound patient. *Exception:* Nursing visit to a mother and newborn may be covered when provided within a specified time following hospital discharge (verify payer policy for coverage).

* Used to report services provided in a patient's residence (including assisted living apartments, group homes, nontraditional private homes, custodial care facilities, or schools). Physicians and QHPs providing E/M services in a patient's home report code **99341–99350**.

* Not reported if another code more accurately describes the service provided (eg, report home medical nutrition therapy with **97802–97804** rather than **99509**).

Coverage of home health procedures or services by QHPs who are authorized to use E/M home visit codes (**99341–99350**) may also be reported with codes **99500–99600** if both services are performed and the patient's condition requires a significant, separately identifiable service. Modifier **25** would be appended to codes **99341–99350**.

Lactation Services

S9443	Lactation classes, nonphysician provider, per session

Although code **S9443** is the code most specific to lactation services, it is not paid under many health plan contracts. Lactation consultation services do not have a specific *CPT®* code, and billing is a source of confusion for many providers. Less specific codes are often used to report these services. Options for reporting services by AHPs may include

S9445	Patient education, not otherwise classified, nonphysician provider, individual, per session
S9446	Patient education, not otherwise classified, nonphysician provider, group, per session
98960	Education and training for patient self-management by a qualified, nonphysician health care professional using a standardized curriculum, face-to-face with the patient (could include caregiver/family) each 30 minutes; individual patient
99401	Preventive medicine counseling and/or risk-factor reduction intervention(s) provided to an individual (separate procedure); approximately 15 minutes
96150	Health and behavior assessment, each 15 minutes face-to-face with the patient, initial assessment

Key considerations for reporting lactation services include

* Practices must verify coverage and reporting instructions for each payer prior to service. Examples of coding instructions from payers are included in the Examples of Payment Policies for Lactation Services box later in this chapter.

* Unless the newborn or infant has been diagnosed with a feeding problem, the mother is typically the patient and claims are filed to her health benefit plan. Although included as a covered preventive service under the Patient Protection and Affordable Care Act, breastfeeding services are linked to the mother's health coverage and often considered by payers to be included in E/M services provided to the mother by a physician.

Examples of Payment Policies for Lactation Services

- Lactation consultations (**98960**) are separately paid when filed by a licensed MD/DO or mid-level practitioner when the lactation consultation is the only service provided and performed by a certified lactation consultant under the general supervision of a licensed MD/DO or mid-level practitioner. Lactation consultations (**98960**) are considered not separately paid when provided at the same time as any E/M visit.
- Lactation counseling services may be billed directly by International Board Certified Lactation Consultants (IBCLCs) using codes **S9445** and **S9446**. A physician who employs an IBCLC physician assistant or RN may bill for lactation counseling provided by these health care professionals (**S9445** and **S9446**). Physicians providing lactation counseling must append modifier **AF** (specialty physician) to code **S9445** or **S9446**.
- Up to 6 individual outpatient breastfeeding or lactation counseling sessions (**99401–99404**), per birth event, may be covered. These counseling sessions are in addition to breastfeeding or lactation counseling that may be provided during an inpatient maternity stay, outpatient obstetrician visit, or well-child visit. However, these additional counseling sessions are only covered and separately paid when all the following conditions are met:
  - ❖ The breastfeeding or lactation counseling is billed using one of the preventive counseling *CPT* procedure codes **99401–99404**.
  - ❖ Breastfeeding or lactation counseling is the only service being provided.
  - ❖ The breastfeeding or lactation counseling is rendered by an authorized individual professional provider (eg, physician, physician assistant, nurse practitioner, nurse midwife, RN), outpatient hospital, or clinic.
- The following *CPT*/HCPCS codes are appropriate for lactation support and counseling services provided by an IBCLC: **99211, 99401, 99402, 99403, 99404**; for lactation classes, use codes **S9443, 99411**, or **99412**.

- Currently, no state licenses lactation consultants. This creates issues in credentialing and coverage by payers who cover only services provided by licensed health care professionals, although services provided incident to a physician or QHP may be allowed.
- When a medical condition (eg, feeding problem, low weight gain) has been previously diagnosed by the physician at an earlier date, an AHP may see the mother and patient to identify the psychological, behavioral, emotional, cognitive, and social factors important to the prevention, treatment, or management of physical health problems. Codes **96150–96155** may be reportable for these services.
- Codes **99401–99404** are described by *CPT* as services provided face-to-face by a physician or other QHP for the purpose of promoting health and preventing illness or injury. When payer policy instructs to report these codes for services by lactation consultants or other AHPs, a written copy of the payer policy should be kept on file.
- Lactation counseling provided in conjunction with a physician's or QHP's E/M service, though not separately reported, may reduce the physician's time spent on history taking, counseling, and education. This may also support quality initiatives.

ICD-10-CM code **Z39.1** is reported for encounter for care and examination of a lactating mother. When addressing lactation disorders, such as cracked nipple, suppressed lactation, or agalactia, see codes in category **O92**. It is important to verify benefits and bill for services to the mother separately from services to address a condition of the newborn. Feeding difficulty in the newborn is reported with codes in category **P92** (see **Table 9-4**). Remember that codes that define or describe maternal conditions cannot be reported for the baby.

Medical Nutrition Assessments

97802   Medical nutrition therapy; initial assessment and intervention, individual, face-to-face with the patient, each 15 minutes

97803   Reassessment and intervention, individual, face-to-face with the patient, each 15 minutes

97804   Group (2 or more individuals), each 30 minutes

Medical nutrition therapy is one of the services for which *CPT* instruction excludes reporting by a physician or QHP who may report E/M services. Many states restrict the provision of medical nutrition therapy to certain AHPs (eg, registered dietitian, licensed medical nutritionist). Practices providing medical nutrition therapy

Chapter 14: Allied Health and Clinical Staff Services

services should be aware of state licensing and scope of practice regulations. Coverage may be limited to patients with certain conditions (eg, diabetes, kidney disease) and a limited number of units of service or visits per year.

Payers that follow Medicare policy on reporting of E/M services will not accept codes **99201–99205**, **99212–99215**, or **99217–99499**. (Note: **99211** is reportable by AHPs and clinical staff. Payers may adopt Medicare incident-to policy requirements.)

- Codes are reported when provided by an AHP who may report medical nutrition therapy services under his or her individual state's scope of practice.
- When medical nutrition therapy is provided as a preventive service, modifier **33** may be appended to codes **97802–97804**. (For more on modifier **33**, see Chapter 3, Modifiers and Coding Edits, and Chapter 6, Preventive Services.)
- Services are reported based on time. Per *CPT* instruction, a unit of time is met when the midpoint is passed. Certain payers may require that the time in the code descriptor (eg, 15 minutes) be met or exceeded for each unit of service reported. Time must be documented. Report codes **97802** and **97803** with 1 unit for 8 to 22 minutes of service. An additional unit may be reported for each subsequent 15 minutes and the last 8 to 22 minutes of service.
- Healthcare Common Procedure Coding System codes may be required by certain payers when providing reassessment and subsequent intervention due to a change in diagnosis, medical condition, or treatment.

G0270   Medical nutrition therapy; reassessment and subsequent intervention(s) following second referral in same year for change in diagnosis, medical condition, or treatment regimen (including additional hours needed for renal disease); individual, face-to-face with the patient, each 15 minutes

G0271   group (2 or more individuals), each 30 minutes

- Documentation of services should include the physician or QHP order for services, information on the medical need for services, medical nutrition therapy evaluation and plan for intervention, time, correspondence with the referring provider, and date of service, name, credentials, and signature of the provider of medical nutrition therapy.

Examples

➤ **A 14-year-old girl was seen by her physician for a well-child visit 1 week ago.** Her BMI is at the 90th percentile, blood pressure was at upper limit of normal, and results of cholesterol screening indicate hypercholesterolemia. The patient is referred to the practice's registered dietitian for assessment and counseling on a diet to reduce the risk of cardiovascular and endocrine disorders. The dietitian meets with the child and her parents and spends 30 minutes discussing risk factors and developing a plan with goals to decrease weight, cholesterol, and blood pressure.

ICD-10-CM	CPT®
Z71.3 (dietary counseling and surveillance) **E78.00** (pure hypercholesterolemia) **Z68.53** (BMI pediatric, 85th percentile to less than 95th percentile for age)	If payer allows billing under registered dietitian's NPI **97802** × 2 (medical nutrition therapy, initial assessment and intervention, individual, face-to-face with the patient, each 15 minutes) If payer requires billing under the NPI of the supervising physician **97802 AE** × 2 (medical nutrition therapy as above by a registered dietitian)

Teaching Point: Some Medicaid plans and/or private payers may require that medical nutrition therapy in the physician practice be provided under a physician's order and general supervision. Services are reported as if provided by the physician, but modifier **AE** indicates the service was provided by a registered dietitian.

➤ **A 12-year-old girl has decided to become a vegetarian.** The patient's laboratory test results have shown iron deficiency, and she is referred by her pediatrician to a nurse practitioner in the same practice for consultation on a vegetarian diet that meets the patient's nutritional requirements. The nurse practitioner spends 30 minutes face-to-face with the patient and parents learning the patient's reasons for choosing a vegetarian diet, assessing the patient's current diet, and counseling on the importance of a plant-based diet that is balanced to provide adequate nutrition. A plan is developed to encourage food choices that support adequate nutrition, and a follow-up visit is scheduled in 2 weeks.

ICD-10-CM	CPT®
Z71.3 (dietary counseling and surveillance) **E61.1** (iron deficiency)	**99214** (25 minutes typical time)

   Teaching Point: While nutritional counseling is often provided by physicians and QHPs, use of medical nutrition therapy service codes is typically limited to other providers (eg, registered dietitian, certified nutritionist, clinical nutritionist) who are licensed or certified in the state where practicing. Physicians and other QHPs should verify payer policy prior to delivering services. Reporting with an E/M code based on time spent counseling and/or coordinating care is appropriate per *CPT* instruction.

Medical Team Conferences

99366   Medical team conference with interdisciplinary team of health care professionals, face-to-face with patient and/or family, 30 minutes or more; participation by nonphysician qualified health care professional

99368   Medical team conference with interdisciplinary team of health care professionals, patient and/or family not present, 30 minutes or more; participation by nonphysician qualified health care professional

   Medical team conference codes are used to report participation by a minimum of 3 health care professionals (includes physicians, QHPs, and AHPs) of different specialties in conferences to coordinate or manage care and services for established patients with chronic or multiple health conditions (eg, child who is ventilator dependent with developmental delays, seizures, and gastrostomy tube for nutrition).

❂ Codes differentiate provider (physician or QHP vs AHP) and between face-to-face and non–face-to-face (patient and/or family is not present) patient team conference services. Physicians or other QHPs who may report E/M services should report their time spent in a team conference *with the patient and/or family present* using E/M codes (and time as the key controlling factor for code selection when counseling and/or coordination of care dominates the service). Payer policy may vary.

❂ If QHPs (including clinical nurse specialists and clinical nurse practitioners) participated in the conference without direct physician supervision, they may report team conference participation *without the patient or caregiver present* as if provided by a physician (**99367**) if it is within the state's scope of practice and they use their own NPI. State Medicaid and commercial payers may follow these Medicare requirements or have their own specific rules.

❂ Medical team conferences may not be reported if the facility or organization is contractually obligated to provide the service, they are informal meetings or simple conversations between physicians and AHPs (eg, therapists), and less than 30 minutes of conference time is spent in the team conferences.

❂ Medical team conferences are not reported when provided during a month when the patient is receiving CCM or TCM services provided by the same individual. See Chapter 8, Managing Chronic and Complex Conditions, for more information on CCM and TCM services.

❂ Medicare assigns a bundled (B) status to team conference services in the Medicare Physician Fee Schedule and does not separate payment for participation in medical team conferences. Payment policies may vary among Medicaid and private health plans.

Medical team conferences require

- Face-to-face participation by a minimum of 3 health care professionals (any combination of AHPs, physicians, and/or QHPs) from different subspecialties or disciplines (eg, speech-language pathologists, dietitians, social workers), with or without the presence of the patient, family member(s), community agencies, surrogate decision-maker(s) (eg, legal guardian), and/or caregiver(s).

- Active involvement in the development, revision, coordination, and implementation of health care services needed by the patient by each participant.

- Face-to-face evaluations and/or treatments by the participant that are separate from any team conference within the previous 60 days.

- Only one individual from the same specialty may report codes **99366–99368** for the same encounter.

- Medical record documentation must support the reporting individual's participation, the time spent from the beginning of the review of an individual patient until the conclusion of the review, and the contributed information and subsequent treatment recommendations.

Examples

➤ **A 14-year-old girl with spinal muscular atrophy is wheelchair bound and receives her education at home.** Over the past 6 months, her respiratory compromise has progressed and she has required 2 inpatient admissions for pneumonia. She is on oxygen at night. She receives physical and occupational therapy services at home and twice-weekly visits from a respiratory therapist. She sees a pediatric pulmonologist every 4 months and a pediatric physiatrist every 6 months. You have started discussions with her parents about how aggressive the family wishes to be if she were to require assisted ventilation. The pediatrician, pulmonologist, physiatrist, occupational and physical therapists, respiratory therapist, home care coordinator, home educator, and social worker attend the conference to discuss the child's current medical status, prognosis for the short and long term, and the child's and family's wishes as her condition deteriorates. The conference lasts 60 minutes.

Each participating physician (if they are different specialties and/or from different practices [ie, separate tax identification numbers])	*ICD-10-CM* **G12.1** (other inherited spinal muscular atrophy) *CPT®* **99367**
Each AHP (eg, respiratory therapist, occupational therapist)	*CPT* **99368**

Code selection is, in part, determined by the type of provider reporting participation in a team conference. Allied health professionals report participation using code **99366** when the patient and/or caregivers are present at the conference or **99368** when the patient/caregivers are not present. However, physicians report an E/M code for the appropriate setting when the patient is present or code **99367** for physician participation in team conference when patient or caregivers are not present. *Current Procedural Terminology* allows reporting of codes **99366** and **99368** by QHPs. However, reporting an E/M code for participation when the patient or caregivers are present may be beneficial when allowed or required by individual payer policy.

➤ **A patient with cerebral palsy requires coordination with multiple health care professionals (eg, physical and occupational therapists, neurologist, pediatrician).** Each participant in the conference has completed his or her evaluation of the patient within 60 days prior to the conference, and a team conference of 40 minutes is held to assess the current plan of care and therapy. The patient's family is present at this conference.

Code **99366** would be reported by the physical and occupational therapists.

Medication Therapy Management Services

99605 Medication therapy management service(s) provided by a pharmacist, individual, face-to-face with patient, with assessment and intervention if provided; initial 15 minutes, new patient

99606 initial 15 minutes, established patient

+99607 each additional 15 minutes (List separately in addition to **99605** or **99606**)

Medication therapy management service(s)

- Are provided only by a pharmacist face-to-face with the patient or caregiver and usually in relation to complex medication regimens or medication adherence in conditions such as asthma and diabetes.
- Provided on request of the patient or caregiver, prescribing physician, other QHPs, or prescription drug benefit plan (not reported for routine dispensing-related activities).
- Are reported with codes selected based on whether the patient is new or established and by the pharmacist's face-to-face time with the patient.
- Includes review of pertinent patient history (not limited to drug history).
- Include documentation of review of the pertinent patient history, medication profile (prescription and nonprescription), and recommendations for improving health outcomes and treatment compliance.
- New patients are those who have received no face-to-face service from the pharmacist or another pharmacist of the same clinic or pharmacy within 3 years prior to the current date of service.
- Unless otherwise specified by the payer policy, time is met when the midpoint is passed. Report codes **99605** and **99606** for the first 8 to 22 minutes of face-to-face time with the patient. When time exceeds 22 minutes, code **99607** may be reported for subsequent 15-minute periods and the last 8 to 22 minutes.
- Under the Medicare program, pharmacists may also provide services incident to a physician or QHP and report E/M services with code **99211** when allowed under the scope of practice as defined by state licensure.

Online Medical Assessment

98969 Online assessment and management service provided by a qualified nonphysician health care professional to an established patient or guardian not originating from a related assessment and management service provided within the previous 7 days, using the Internet or similar electronic communications network

An online electronic medical evaluation (**98969**) is a non–face-to-face assessment and management service by an AHP to an established patient using Internet resources in response to a patient's online inquiry. This is in contrast to telemedicine services, which represent interactive audio and video telecommunications systems that permit real-time communication between the AHP, at the distant site, and the patient, at the originating site. Code **98969** is used by an AHP to report an online assessment and management service. One unit of service is reported for the sum of communications pertaining to the online encounter during a 7-day period.

The CMS has not assigned relative value units to online medical evaluation codes and considers them non-covered services. As a result, most third-party payers do not pay for them.

Before providing online medical services, understand local and state laws, ensure that communications will be HIPAA compliant, establish written guidelines and procedures, educate payers and negotiate for payment, and educate patients.

Online assessment and management includes

- Timely reply to the patient/caregiver's request for online service
- Permanent record of the service (hard copy or electronic)
- All related communications during a 7-day episode of care (eg, ordering laboratory or other testing, prescriptions, related phone calls)

Online assessment and management services *are not reported* when

- Related to a service provided by the AHP within the past 7 days regardless of whether the online service was planned or prompted by patient or caregiver concern
  - Result in an appointment within the next 24 hours or next available appointment
  - Within a global period of another service

- When provided during a month when the patient is receiving care plan oversight, CCM, or TCM services provided by the same individual (See Chapter 8, Managing Chronic and Complex Conditions, for more information on CCM and TCM services.)

Telephone Calls

98966   Telephone assessment and management services provided by a qualified nonphysician health care professional to an established patient, parent, or guardian not originating from related assessment and management service provided within the previous 7 days nor leading to an assessment and management service or procedure within the next 24 hours or soonest available appointment; 5–10 minutes of medical discussion

98967   11–20 minutes of medical discussion

98968   21–30 minutes of medical discussion

Codes **98966–98968** are used to report telephone assessment and management services by AHPs. Those QHPs who may independently provide and report E/M services report codes **99441–99443**. Report codes **98966–98968** when

- The patient or caregiver initiates a call that is not in follow-up to a service by the same AHP within the past 7 days.
- Five minutes or more is spent in assessment and management services. *Time must be documented.*
- No decision to see the patient within 24 hours or at the next available appointment is made during the telephone service.

Do not report telephone assessment and management services that

- Are related to a service provided by the AHP within the past 7 days, regardless of whether this service was planned or prompted by patient or caregiver concern.
- Result in an appointment within the next 24 hours or next available appointment. When telephone assessment and management results in scheduling the patient for an appointment within 24 hours or at the next available appointment, the service is considered preservice work to the face-to-face encounter.
- Is within a global period of another service.
- During a month when the patient is receiving CCM or TCM services provided by the same individual (see Chapter 8, Managing Chronic and Complex Conditions, for more information on CCM and TCM services).
- Most telephone services provided by clinical staff (eg, MA relaying physician instructions) are included in the practice expense value assigned to physician services and not separately reported. Telephone services by clinical staff may contribute to time of CCM or TCM when the services meet the description of the clinical staff activities included in CCM or TCM.

Example

➤ **The parents of a patient who has developed mealtime anxiety due to previous allergic reactions to multiple foods contact their child's registered dietitian for advice.** It has been 3 weeks since the dietitian provided education on food allergies and meeting the child's nutritional needs with a limited diet. The dietitian spends 18 minutes on the phone with the parents discussing techniques for encouraging a healthy diet while acknowledging and alleviating the child's anxiety.

The dietitian reports code **98967** based on the time spent addressing the parent's concerns. This service would not be reported if the call were provided within 7 days of a previous service by the same provider or if the call resulted in an appointment within 24 hours or next available face-to-face appointment.

Psychiatric Collaborative Care Management Services

●99492   Initial psychiatric collaborative care management, first 70 minutes in the first calendar month of behavioral health care manager activities, in consultation with a psychiatric consultant, and directed by the treating physician or other qualified health care professional, with the following required elements:

- ☀ outreach to and engagement in treatment of a patient directed by the treating physician or other qualified health care professional;
- ☀ initial assessment of the patient, including administration of validated rating scales, with the development of an individualized treatment plan;
- ☀ review by the psychiatric consultant with modifications of the plan if recommended;
- ☀ entering patient in a registry and tracking patient follow-up and progress using the registry, with appropriate documentation, and participation in weekly caseload consultation with the psychiatric consultant; and
- ☀ provision of brief interventions using evidence-based techniques such as behavioral activation, motivational interviewing, and other focused treatment strategies.

●99493   Subsequent psychiatric collaborative care management, first 60 minutes in a subsequent month of behavioral health care manager activities, in consultation with a psychiatric consultant, and directed by the treating physician or other qualified health care professional, with the following required elements:

- ☀ tracking patient follow-up and progress using the registry, with appropriate documentation;
- ☀ participation in weekly caseload consultation with the psychiatric consultant;
- ☀ ongoing collaboration with and coordination of the patient's mental health care with the treating physician or other qualified health care professional and any other treating mental health providers;
- ☀ additional review of progress and recommendations for changes in treatment, as indicated, including medications, based on recommendations provided by the psychiatric consultant;
- ☀ provision of brief interventions using evidence-based techniques such as behavioral activation, motivational interviewing, and other focused treatment strategies;
- ☀ monitoring of patient outcomes using validated rating scales; and
- ☀ relapse prevention planning with patients as they achieve remission of symptoms and/or other treatment goals and are prepared for discharge from active treatment.

●+99494   Initial or subsequent psychiatric collaborative care management, each additional 30 minutes in a calendar month of behavioral health care manager activities, in consultation with a psychiatric consultant, and directed by the treating physician or other qualified health care professional (List separately in addition to code for primary procedure)

(Use **99494** in conjunction with **99492, 99493**)

Psychiatric collaborative care management (PCCM) services are reported by a supervising physician or QHP for services by a behavioral health care manager (BHM) working under the supervision of the reporting physician or QHP. Psychiatric collaborative care management services are provided to patients who have a new or existing psychiatric disorder that requires a behavioral health assessment; care plan implementation, revision, or monitoring; and provision of brief interventions. These services require a team effort of 3 health care professionals: a treating physician or QHP, a BHM, and a psychiatric consultant. The treating physician or QHP reports codes **99492–99494** when all requirements for reporting are met. Evaluation and management and other services may be reported separately by the same physician or QHP during the same calendar month.

Each team member's role is defined in *CPT®* as follows:

- ☀ The treating physician or QHP directs the BHM and continues to oversee the patient's care, including prescribing medications, providing treatments for medical conditions, and making referrals to specialty care when needed. The treating physician or QHP engages the services of the psychiatric consultant who does not directly bill for PCCM services (ie, the treating physician or QHP's practice contracts with the psychiatric consultant for this component of the PCCM service).

Chapter 14: Allied Health and Clinical Staff Services

- The treating physician or QHP acts in a supervisory role to the BHM (may be a direct employee or contractual employee but should represent a practice expense similar to other clinical staff and AHPs). If the treating physician or QHP personally performs behavioral health care management activities and those activities are not used to meet criteria for a separately reported service, his or her time may be counted toward the required time for PCCM. As the reporting or billing provider for PCCM services, the treating physician or QHP is ultimately responsible for delivery, documentation, and billing of PCCM services in compliance with *CPT®* and payer policies.
- The BHM is an AHP or clinical staff member with master's or doctoral-level education *or* specialized training in behavioral health who provides behavioral health care management services under the treating physician's or QHP's supervision and in consultation with a psychiatric consultant. The BHM provides the following services, as needed:
  - Assessment of needs including the administration of validated rating scales
  - Development of a care plan
  - Provision of brief interventions face-to-face and non–face-to-face
  - Ongoing collaboration with the treating physician or QHP
  - Consultation with the psychiatric consultant at least weekly (typically non–face-to-face)
  - Maintenance of a registry
- The psychiatric consultant is a medical professional trained in psychiatry or behavioral health and qualified to prescribe a full range of medications. The psychiatric consultant typically does not see the patient nor prescribe medications, except in rare circumstances. The psychiatric consultant advises and makes recommendations to the treating physician or QHP (typically via consultation with the BHM). The psychiatric consultant's services include recommending the following services, as needed:
  - Psychiatric and other medical differential diagnosis
  - Treatment strategies addressing appropriate therapies
  - Medication management
  - Medical management of complications associated with treatment of psychiatric disorders
  - Referral for specialty services

    The psychiatric consultant may directly provide and separately report E/M or psychiatric services, such as psychiatric evaluation (**90791**, **90792**) to a patient within a calendar month when the same patient receives psychiatric collaborative care services. Activities for services reported separately are not included in the services reported with codes **99492–99494**.

  Reporting requirements for PCCM services include
- Psychiatric collaborative care management services are time-based services that are subject to the *CPT* midpoint rule for reporting time. Time of service is met when the midpoint is passed. Documentation must support provision of PCCM services for
  - 36 minutes or more to report a 70-minute service (**99492**)
  - 31 minutes or more to report a 60-minute service (**99493**)
  - 16 minutes or more beyond the last full service period to report an additional 30 minutes of service (**99494**)
- Time spent by the BHM coordinating care with the emergency department may be included in time attributed to PCCM services. However, time spent while the patient is an inpatient or in observation status at a hospital may not be included in time of PCCM services.
- Psychiatric collaborative care management services are provided for an episode of care defined as beginning when the treating physician or QHP directs the patient to the BHM and ending when
  - The attainment of targeted treatment goals, which typically results in the discontinuation of care management services and continuation of usual follow-up with the treating physician or other QHP
  - Failure to attain targeted treatment goals culminating in referral to a psychiatric care provider for ongoing treatment
  - Lack of continued engagement with no PCCM services provided over a consecutive 6-month calendar period (break in episode)
- A new episode of care starts after a break in episode of 6 calendar months or more.

- Medical necessity of PCCM services may be supported by documentation of a newly diagnosed condition, a patient's need for help engaging in treatment, a patient who has not responded to standard care delivered in a nonpsychiatric setting or who requires further assessment and engagement prior to consideration of referral to a psychiatric care setting. (These are typical patient scenarios. Other reasons for services may support medical necessity.) Where health plans implement specific coverage criteria and/or prior authorization for PCCM services, documentation of the patient's behavioral health conditions, psychosocial needs, and other factors influencing patient care may help support the necessity of services.

- Unlike CCM services, PCCM services do not require establishment of a care plan for all the patient's health care needs. Psychiatric collaborative care management services are directed to behavioral health needs. Patients may or may not have comorbid conditions that affect treatment and management.

- Provision of PCCM services may support quality initiatives such as use of an electronic clinical data system to track care and administration of a validated rating scale (eg, Patient Health Questionnaire-9) during a 4-month period for patients diagnosed with major depression or dysthymia.

Example

➤ **A pediatrician orders PCCM services for a 15-year-old patient diagnosed with moderate depression, single episode.** A licensed clinical psychologist acting as the BHM meets with the patient to discuss PCCM services and perform an initial assessment. Standardized assessment instruments are used to further assess the patient's health, and a treatment plan including psychotherapy is agreed on. After the meeting, the BHM enters the patient information into a registry, which will be used to track her medication compliance and progress. Later, the BHM has a regularly scheduled conference call with a consulting psychiatrist who reviews the patient's assessment and approves of the treatment plan. The supervising pediatrician is also consulted and approves the treatment plan. The BHM, whose scope of practice includes psychotherapy, provides 3 individual psychotherapy sessions within the calendar month in addition to PCCM services. The BHM will separately report the psychotherapy services in addition to PCCM. During the calendar month, the BHM documents 60 minutes of time spent in PCCM services.

PCCM 60 minutes in first calendar month of service Psychotherapy without E/M service	**ICD-10-CM** **F32.1** (major depressive disorder, single episode, moderate)
	CPT® **99492** (initial month PCCM service, first 70 minutes) **90832**, **90834**, or **90837** (psychotherapy based on time of service; 30, 45, or 60 minutes)

Teaching Point: *Current Procedural Terminology* instructs that time of service for PCCM services is met when the midpoint is passed. In this example, the 60 minutes spent by the BHM supports reporting of code **99492**, which includes the first 70 minutes of PCCM services in the initial month of service. No time spent in provision of psychotherapy may be attributed to the time of PCCM services. If psychotherapy services were not within the scope of practice for the BHM, the patient might be referred to another provider (eg, the consulting psychiatrist), who would report the services rendered.

General Behavioral Health Integration Care Management

●**99484** Care management services for behavioral health conditions, at least 20 minutes of clinical staff time, directed by a physician or other qualified health care professional, per calendar month, with the following required elements:
- Initial assessment or follow-up monitoring, including the use of applicable validated rating scales;
- Behavioral health care planning in relation to behavioral/psychiatric health problems, including revision for patients who are not progressing or whose status changes;

- Facilitating and coordinating treatment such as psychotherapy, pharmacotherapy, counseling and/or psychiatric consultation; and
- Continuity of care with a designated member of the care team

Current Procedural Terminology® does not define the education or credentials of clinical staff who may provide services described by code **99484**. Behavioral health care integration clinical staff are not required to have qualifications that would permit them to separately report services (eg, psychotherapy), but, if qualified and they perform such services, they may report such services separately, as long as the time of the service is not used in reporting **99484**.

Services must be provided under general physician supervision and in accordance with the licensing and scope of practice requirements of the state where services are provided. The individual supervising and reporting general behavioral health integration care management services must be able to report E/M services.

Use of validated rating scales is required and is not separately reported (ie, do not report code **96127** for rating scales administered during the period of behavioral health care management services).

See Chapter 8, Managing Chronic and Complex Conditions, for more information on reporting care management for behavioral health conditions.

Psychiatric Evaluation and Psychotherapy Without Evaluation and Management

+90785	Interactive complexity (List separately in addition to the code for primary procedure)
90791	Psychiatric diagnostic evaluation
90832	Psychotherapy, 30 minutes with patient and/or family member
90834	45 minutes with patient and/or family member
90837	60 minutes with patient and/or family member
90839	Psychotherapy for crisis; first 60 minutes
+90840	each additional 30 minutes (List separately in addition to code **90839**)
90846	Family psychotherapy (without the patient present)
90847	Family psychotherapy (conjoint psychotherapy) (with patient present)
90849	Multiple-family group psychotherapy
90853	Group psychotherapy (other than of a multiple-family group)
+90863	Pharmacologic management, including prescription and review of medication, when performed with psychotherapy services (List separately in addition to **90832**, **90834**, **90837**.)

> ||||||| **Coding Pearl** |||||||
> HCPCS modifiers identifying the type of provider may be necessary to override edits that bundle E/M and mental or behavioral health services on the same date.

Mental and behavioral health services may be covered through a provider network separate from other health care services. The scope of services may also be limited by payer policies allowing specific licensed providers, such as licensed clinical psychologists, to report certain services, while other AHPs (eg, licensed clinical social workers) may report a smaller scope of services. Verify coverage and billing options prior to provision of services.

A payer may apply bundling edits that do not allow separate payment for mental and behavioral health services and E/M services provided in the same practice on the same date. Follow payer instructions for reporting services such as psychotherapy by an AHP under the name and NPI of a supervising physician and E/M services by the physician on the same date. Healthcare Common Procedure Coding System modifiers identifying the type of provider (eg, **AJ**, clinical social worker) may be necessary to override edits that bundle E/M and mental or behavioral health services on the same date. See the HCPCS Codes section earlier in this chapter for HCPCS modifiers or your current HCPCS coding reference for additional modifiers.

See Chapter 16, Common Testing and Therapeutic Services, for information on codes for psychological and neuropsychological testing.

- Psychiatric diagnostic evaluation or reevaluation (**90791**) is reported once per day. Do not report psychotherapy codes (**90832–90839**) on the same date of service as **90791**.

- Psychotherapy times are for face-to-face services with a patient and/or family member. The patient must be present for all or some of the service except when reporting family psychotherapy without the patient present (**90846**). This allows for the participation of others in the psychotherapy session for the patient as long as the patient remains the focus of the intervention. The patient must be present for a significant portion of the session.

- Psychotherapy differs from family psychotherapy (**90846**, **90847**), which uses family psychotherapy techniques to benefit the patient (eg, attempting to improve family communication or alter family interactions that negatively affect the patient; encouraging interactions to improve family functioning). Family psychotherapy includes sessions with the entire family as well as sessions that may not include the patient.

- In reporting, choose the code closest to the actual time (**Table 14-2**). Do not report psychotherapy of less than 16 minutes' duration.

- Psychiatric services may be reported "with interactive complexity" (**90785**) when at least one of the following conditions is present:

  1. The need to manage maladaptive communication (related to, eg, high anxiety, high reactivity, repeated questions, disagreement) among participants that complicates delivery of care
  2. Caregiver emotions or behavior that interferes with the caregiver's understanding and ability to assist in the implementation of the treatment plan
  3. Evidence or disclosure of a sentinel event and mandated report to third party (eg, abuse or neglect with report to state agency) with initiation of discussion of the sentinel event and/or report with patient and other visit participants
  4. Use of play equipment, other physical devices, interpreter, or translator to communicate with the patient to overcome barriers to therapeutic or diagnostic interaction between the physician or other QHP and a patient who

     ❖ Is not fluent in the same language as the physician or other QHP
     ❖ Has not developed, or has lost, the expressive language communication skills to explain his or her symptoms and response to treatment or the receptive communication skills to understand the physician or other QHP if he or she were to use typical language for communication

- Do not report psychotherapy for crisis (**90839**, **90840**) for service of less than 30 minutes or on the same date as other psychiatry services (**90785–90899**).

- Code **90863** was created for medication management when provided on the same day as psychotherapy by QHPs who may not report E/M codes (ie, psychologists licensed to prescribe). This code is an add-on code and may only be reported in addition to one of the stand-alone psychotherapy codes (ie, **90832**, **90834**, **90837**). Time spent providing medication management is not included in the time spent in psychotherapy.

- Prolonged services in the office or other outpatient setting (**99354**, **99355**) or inpatient or observation setting (**99356**, **99357**) may be reported in addition to the psychotherapy service code **90837** when 90 minutes or longer of face-to-face time with the patient and/or family member is spent performing psychotherapy services, which are not performed with an E/M service.

- Do not report psychotherapy codes in conjunction with codes for adaptive behavior assessment or treatment services (**0359T–0374T**).

Table 14-2. Reporting Psychotherapy Services

Duration of Psychotherapy	CPT® Codes
<16 min	Do not report.
16–37 min	90832
38–52 min	90834
53–89 min	90837

Abbreviation: CPT, Current Procedural Terminology.

Chapter 14: Allied Health and Clinical Staff Services

Common Surgical Procedures and Sedation

Contents

Surgical Package Rules

Current Procedural Terminology (*CPT*®) surgical codes (**10021–69990**) are packaged or global codes.

- Surgical codes include certain anesthesia services and the associated preoperative and postoperative care.
- The *CPT* definition of a surgical package differs from the Centers for Medicare & Medicaid Services (CMS) definition of a global surgical period, as seen in **Table 15-1**.
- Most state Medicaid programs follow the CMS definition.
- Each commercial insurance company will have its own policy for billing and payment of global surgical care, and most will designate a specific number of follow-up days for surgical procedures.
- The CMS-designated global periods for each *CPT* procedure code can be found on the Medicare Resource-Based Relative Value Scale (RBRVS) Physician Fee Schedule at https://www.cms.gov/medicare/medicare-fee-for-service-payment/physicianfeesched.

When determining the postoperative period, the day after surgery is day 1 of a 10- or 90-day period.

> **Coding Pearl**
>
> Most state Medicaid programs follow the CMS surgical package guidelines.

Table 15-1. Comparison of the *CPT* and CMS Surgical Packages

CPT Definition of Surgical Package	CMS Medicare Global Surgery
Anesthesia Includes local infiltration, regional block, or topical anesthesia	Same
Preoperative Care • Includes E/M service(s) subsequent to the decision for surgery (eg, assessing the site and condition, explanation of procedure, obtaining informed consent) on the day before and/or on the date of the procedure (including history and physical). • When the initial decision to perform surgery is made on the day prior to or on the day of surgery, the appropriate-level E/M visit may be reported separately with modifier **57** (decision for surgery) appended. This modifier shows the payer that the E/M service was necessary to make the decision for surgery (ie, not the routine preoperative evaluation). • When an E/M service performed on the day of the procedure is unrelated to the decision to perform surgery and is significant and distinct from the usual preoperative care associated with the procedure, it may be reported with modifier **25** (significant, separately identifiable E/M service by the same physician on the same day of the procedure or other service) appended. • Medical record documentation must support that the service was significant, separately identifiable, and medically necessary or was performed prior to the decision to perform the procedure. • Different diagnoses are not required when reporting an E/M visit and procedure.	Same with following exceptions: • For "minor" procedures (ie, procedures assigned a 0- or 10-day global period or endoscopies), the E/M visit on the date of the procedure is considered a routine part of the procedure regardless of whether it is prior or subsequent to the decision for surgery. In these cases, modifier **57** is not recognized. • An E/M code may be reported on the same day as a minor surgical procedure only when a significant, separately identifiable E/M service is performed with modifier **25** appended to the E/M code. • When the initial decision to perform a major surgical procedure (ie, procedures assigned a 90-day global period) is made on the day prior to or on the day of a procedure, the E/M service may be reported appended with modifier **57**. Medical record documentation should support that the decision for surgery was made during the encounter and that additional time was spent in performing counseling of the risks, benefits, and outcomes.

Chapter 15: Common Surgical Procedures and Sedation

Table 15-1. Comparison of the *CPT* and CMS Surgical Packages (*continued*)

CPT Definition of Surgical Package	CMS Medicare Global Surgery
Postoperative Care ◉ Includes all associated typical postoperative care (dictation of progress notes; counseling with the patient, family, and/or other physicians; writing orders; evaluating the patient in the postanesthesia recovery area). ◉ Care for therapeutic surgical procedures includes only the care that is usually part of the surgical service. ◉ Care for diagnostic procedures (eg, endoscopies, arthroscopies, injection procedures for radiography) includes only the care that is related to the recovery from the diagnostic procedure. ◉ Care resulting from complications of surgery. ◉ Any complications, exacerbations, recurrence, treatment of unrelated diseases or injuries, or the presence of other diseases or injuries that require additional services may be reported separately.	Same ◉ Includes all additional medical or surgical services required of the surgeon during the postoperative period of the surgery because of complications that do not require additional trips to the operating room. ◉ Does not include treatment for the underlying condition or an added course of treatment that is not part of normal recovery from surgery. (See modifiers **24**, **58**, and **79**.)
Postoperative Days Does not include any specific number of postoperative days.	◉ Designates specific postoperative periods for certain procedure codes (0 days, 10 days, 90 days). Other codes are designated YYY, which means the postoperative period is set by the carrier. There are no associated postoperative days included in the payment for codes assigned with status codes XXX (the global concept does not apply) or ZZZ (assigned to an add-on code for a service that is always related to another service to which the global period is assigned). ◉ In addition to the *CPT* code, physicians use modifier **78** for return to the operating room for a related procedure during a postoperative period. This includes return to the operating room for treatment of complications of the first procedure. ◉ For return to the operating room for staged or more extensive procedures and therapeutic procedures following a diagnostic procedure, append modifier **58**. ◉ Report procedures during the postoperative period that are unrelated and not due to complications of the original procedure with modifier **79** and unrelated E/M services with modifier **24** (documentation is typically required prior to payment).

Abbreviations: CMS, Centers for Medicare & Medicaid Services; CPT, Current Procedural Terminology; *E/M, evaluation and management.*

Reporting Postoperative Care

◉ Report *CPT*® code **99024** (postoperative follow-up visit) for follow-up care provided during the global surgery period.
  ❖ Reporting code **99024** allows a practice to track the number of visits performed during the postoperative period of specific procedures, calculate office overhead expenses (eg, supplies, staff, physician time) associated with the procedure, and potentially use the data to negotiate higher payment rates.
  ❖ Payers track the postoperative care provided. If a physician is not providing or reporting the postoperative care typically performed for a procedure, payers may reduce payment for the surgical service because payment includes postoperative care as part of the procedure.
◉ When the physician who performed the procedure provides an unrelated evaluation and management (E/M) service during the postoperative period, modifier **24** (unrelated E/M service by the same physician during a postoperative period) should be appended to the E/M service code.
◉ When physicians from different practices perform part of a surgical package, the procedure should be reported with modifier **54** (surgical care only), **56** (preoperative management only), or **55** (postoperative management only). These situations require communication among the surgeon, the physician providing preoperative or postoperative care, and their respective billing personnel to ensure accurate reporting and payment. (See Chapter 3, Modifiers and Coding Edits, for a more detailed description of modifiers.)
◉ When a physician other than the surgeon provides unrelated services to a patient during the postoperative period, the services are reported without a modifier. Despite the use of different National Provider Identifiers and diagnosis codes, some payers with assigned follow-up surgical periods will deny the service. The claim should be appealed for payment with a letter advising the payer that the service was unrelated to any surgery.

> ‖‖‖‖‖ *Coding Pearl* ‖‖‖‖‖
>
> **Payers may reduce payment of a surgical procedure if the physician does not report code 99024.**

Supplies and Materials

99070   Supplies and materials provided by the physician over and above those usually included with the office visit or other services rendered

◉ Items such as elastic wraps, clavicle splints, or circumcision and suturing trays may be reported with this code. Remember that some supplies (eg, suturing trays, circumcision trays) may be included with the surgical procedure if the payer uses RBRVS as its basis for payment.
◉ Only the supplies purchased in an office-based practice may be reported.
◉ Some payers will require the use of Healthcare Common Procedure Coding System (HCPCS) codes. More specific HCPCS codes are available for a number of supplies (eg, codes **Q4001–Q4051** for cast and splint supplies). Use HCPCS codes when they are more specific.

> ‖‖‖‖‖ *Coding Pearl* ‖‖‖‖‖
>
> **If reporting code 99070, identify the supplies or materials on the claim form and be prepared to submit an invoice.**

Reporting Terminated Procedures

When a procedure is started but cannot be completed due to extenuating circumstances, physicians should consider the individual situation, including the reason for termination of the procedure and the amount of work that was performed, when determining how to report the service rendered.

When a procedure was performed but not entirely successful (eg, portion of foreign body removed), it may be appropriate to report the procedure code that represents the work performed without modification. Only report reduced services (modifier **52**) or discontinued procedure (modifier **53**) when the service was significantly reduced from the typical service. (See Chapter 3, Modifiers and Coding Edits, for more information on modifiers.) If the work performed prior to discontinuation was insignificant, it may

> ~ **More From the AAP** ~
>
> For more information on reporting discontinued or incomplete procedures, see "Reporting Terminated Procedural Services" in the November 2014 *AAP Pediatric Coding Newsletter*™ at http://coding.aap.org (subscription required).

Chapter 15: Common Surgical Procedures and Sedation

be appropriate to not report the procedure. When not reporting the procedure, consider whether the level of a related E/M service was increased due to the complexity of medical decision-making (MDM) associated with the attempted procedure, any complicating factors, and the revised management or treatment plan.

Physicians at Teaching Hospitals (PATH) Guidelines for Billing Procedures

Physicians at Teaching Hospitals (PATH) guidelines for billing procedures are less complex than those for billing E/M services. Guidelines specify that

* When a procedure is performed by a resident, teaching physician attendance and participation are required and must be documented.
* The level of participation required by the teaching physician depends on the type of procedure being performed.
* A resident, nurse, or teaching physician may document the teaching physician's attendance.

    The rules for supervising physicians in teaching settings can be obtained on the CMS Web site at http://cms.hhs.gov/manuals/downloads/clm104c12.pdf, section 100.

Minor Procedures

* The CMS defines a *minor procedure* as one taking 5 minutes or less to complete with relatively little decision-making once the need for the procedure is determined.
* Minor procedures are usually assigned a 0- to 10-day global period.
* Teaching physicians may bill for a minor procedure when they personally perform the service or when a resident performs the service and they are present for the entire procedure.
* The resident may document the procedure but must attest to the teaching physician's presence.

Interpretation of Diagnostic Radiology and Other Diagnostic Tests

* The teaching physician may bill for interpretation of the diagnostic service if he or she interprets tests or reviews findings with the resident.
* Documentation must support a personal interpretation or a review of the resident's notes with indication of agreement with the resident's interpretation.
* Changes to the resident's interpretation must be documented.

Endoscopy

* The teaching physician must be present for the entire viewing starting at the time of insertion and ending at the time of removal of the endoscope.
* Viewing the procedure through a monitor located in another room does not meet the requirements for billing.
* The presence of the teaching physician must be documented in the medical record. The teaching physician's presence must be stated.

Surgery Other Than Minor Procedures

* The teaching physician must assume the responsibility of preoperative, operative, and postoperative care of the patient. He or she must be present during all critical and key portions (as determined by the teaching physician) of the procedure. For example, if opening or closing is not considered to be key or critical, the teaching physician does not need to be present.
* The teaching physician must be immediately available to furnish services during the entire procedure.
* If circumstances prevent the physician from being immediately available, arrangements must be made with another qualified surgeon to be immediately available to assist with the procedure.
* The physician's presence for single surgical procedures may be demonstrated in notes made by the teaching physician, resident, or nurse.

* When the teaching physician is present for the entire procedure, only the written attestation of his or her presence is required.
* If the teaching physician is present during only the key or critical portions of the surgery, documentation must indicate his or her presence at those portions of the procedure (the resident may still document the operative report).
* When billing for 2 overlapping (concurrent) surgeries, the teaching physician must be present for the key or critical portions of both procedures and must personally document his or her presence. The surgeon cannot be involved in a second case until all key or critical portions in the first case have been completed.
* Arrangements may be made with another qualified surgeon to be present at one of the surgeries. The name of the other surgeon who was immediately available during overlapping surgeries must be documented.

Complex or High-risk Surgeries and Procedures

* A complex procedure or surgery is usually assigned a 90-day global period or, in the case of diagnostic procedures (eg, transesophageal echocardiography), requires the direct or personal supervision of a physician.
* A teaching physician must be present with a resident for the entire procedure when billing for a service identified by the CMS or local policy as complex and requiring personal supervision by a physician.
* Documentation must support that the teaching physician was present.

Postoperative Care

* The teaching physician determines which postoperative visits are considered key or critical and require his or her presence.
* If the teaching physician is not providing postoperative care included in the global surgery package, he or she will report the procedure(s) with modifiers **54** (surgical care only) and **56** (preoperative management only).
* Postoperative care is reported by another physician with the same surgical procedure code with modifier **55** (postoperative management only).
* The surgeon and physician providing postoperative care must keep a copy of a written transfer agreement in the patient's medical record.

PATH Guidelines: Examples of Appropriate Documentation	
Minor procedures	"Dr Teaching Physician was present during the entire procedure." –Nurse "Dr Teaching Physician observed me performing this procedure." –Dr Resident
Interpretation of diagnostic radiology and other diagnostic tests	"I personally reviewed the MRI with Dr Resident and agree with his findings." –Dr Teaching Physician "I personally reviewed the CAT scan with Dr Resident. Findings are indicative of (insert)." –Dr Teaching Physician
Endoscopy	"I was present during the entire viewing of this endoscopy." –Dr Teaching Physician
Surgery other than minor procedures	"Dr Teaching Physician was present during entire surgery." –Dr Resident "I was present and observed Dr Resident perform the key portion of this procedure." –Dr Teaching Physician
Complex or high-risk surgeries and procedures	"I was physically present during this entire procedure with the exception of the [opening and/or closing], as that overlapped with the key portion of another case." –Dr Teaching Physician "Dr Y was immediately available during the overlapping portions of this case, which included [cite specifics]." –Dr Teaching Physician

Minor Procedures

Minor Procedures That Do Not Have a Code

Some minor procedures are considered inherent to an E/M code or do not have separate *CPT*® codes. However, any supplies used may be reported. The following procedures are included in an E/M service:

- Insertion or removal of an ear wick.
- Removal of nonimpacted cerumen from the ear.
- Nasal aspiration.
- Nasogastric tube insertion without fluoroscopic guidance.
- Removal of an umbilical clamp.
- Removal of foreign bodies that do not require an incision.
- Puncture of abscess without aspiration.
- Wound closure with Steri-Strips only.
- The use of fluorescein dye and a Wood lamp to examine for a corneal abrasion or foreign body of the eye is included in the E/M service and is not reported separately. However, the work of a detailed eye examination and history may allow the reporting of a higher-level E/M code.

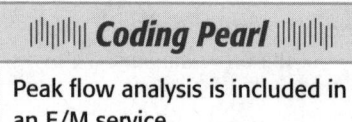

||||||| *Coding Pearl* |||||||

Peak flow analysis is included in an E/M service.

Common Minor Procedures

11200   Removal of skin tags, multiple fibrocutaneous tags, any area; up to and including 15 lesions

Code **11200** is used to report the removal of a sixth digit from a newborn. It is equivalent to a skin tag and would not fall under the coding of an actual digit removal. The *International Classification of Diseases, 10th Revision, Clinical Modification (ICD-10-CM)* codes for accessory digits would be **Q69.0**, accessory fingers; **Q69.1**, accessory thumb; **Q69.2**, accessory toes; or **Q69.9**, unspecified.

17110   Destruction (eg, laser surgery, electrosurgery, cryosurgery, chemosurgery, surgical curettement) of benign lesions other than skin tags or cutaneous vascular proliferative lesions; up to 14 lesions

17111   15 or more lesions

- To report destruction of common or plantar warts, flat warts, or molluscum contagiosum, report code **17110** or **17111** (with 1 unit of service), depending on the number of lesions removed. Do not report both **17110** and **17111** because they are mutually exclusive. Report *ICD-10-CM* using code **B08.1** for molluscum contagiosum, **B07.8** for common warts, or **B07.0** for plantar warts.

▲**17250**   Chemical cauterization of granulation tissue (ie, proud flesh)

- Code **17250** is revised in 2018 with removal of references to sinus or fistula. New parenthetical instructions advise against reporting **17250** with removal or excision codes for the same lesion, for achieving wound hemostasis, or in conjunction with active wound care management.

Example

➤ **A 1-month-old presents for her well-baby check.** On examination, a recently unseen umbilical granuloma is noted. The physician takes a very brief history and decides to cauterize. The routine well-baby check is completed.

ICD-10-CM	CPT
Z00.121 (encounter for routine child health examination with abnormal findings)	**99391 25**
P83.8XX (other granulomatous disorders of the skin and subcutaneous tissue)	**17250**

Teaching Point: Chemical cauterization (**17250**) to achieve wound hemostasis is included in active wound care procedures (**97597, 97598, 97602**) and should not be separately reported for the same lesion.

30901   Cauterization of nosebleed (control nasal hemorrhage, anterior, simple [limited cautery and/or packing], any method)

> If the cauterization is performed bilaterally, report code **30901** with modifier **50**.

41010   Incision in the lingual frenulum to free the tongue

51701   Urinary catheterization, straight

> Report code **51701** when you insert a urinary catheter to collect a clean-catch urine specimen, after which the catheter is removed.

51702   Urinary catheterization, temporary

> Code **51701** is reported when a non-indwelling bladder catheter (straight catheterization) is inserted (eg, for residual urine, for a urine culture collection). Code **51702** is reported when a temporary indwelling bladder catheter is inserted (ie, Foley).

Coding Conundrum: Procedure or E/M and Procedure?

The differences in the CMS and *CPT®* surgical package guidelines are somewhat open to interpretation, often leading to confusion. Try to answer the following questions when determining if you should report a procedure alone or a procedure with an E/M service:

- Did you address a problem or condition prior to making a decision to perform the procedure (above and beyond the usual preoperative care associated with the procedure) or a significant and separately identifiable problem? If yes, report an E/M service and procedure.
- Does the medical record documentation clearly support the performance of a medically necessary E/M service (required key components), the procedure (procedure note), the medical necessity for both, and the decision to perform the surgery? If yes, report an E/M service and procedure.
- Was the purpose of the visit for the procedure only? If yes, do *not* report an E/M service.
- Does the payer follow the *CPT* or CMS guidelines with regard to reporting surgical procedures? If the focus of an E/M service is related to the procedure, the history and physical examination are part of preoperative service and only the surgical procedure should be reported.

Table 15-2 details the number of global days for each of the commonly reported office procedures. Remember that when reporting any procedures containing 0, 10, or 90 global days, modifier **25** or **57** is required on any separately identifiable E/M service done on the same day (or, in some instances, the previous day prior to a planned major surgery). Also, those E/M services that are unrelated to the procedure that take place within the code's 10- or 90-day global period will require modifier **24**.

Table 15-2. Common Office Procedures and Global Days		
CPT Code	**Description**	**Global Days**
10120, 10121	FB removal, SQ	10
11200	Removal of skin tags	10
11760	Repair of nail bed	10
12001–12018	Laceration repair, simple	0
12031–12057	Laceration repair, intermediate	10
13100–13153	Laceration repair, complex	10
16000–16030	Burn care	0
17110, 17111	Destruction benign lesions	10
17250	Chemical cautery	0
28190	FB removal, foot	10
28192	FB removal, foot, complex	90
30300	Removal intranasal FB, office	10

Table 15-2. Common Office Procedures and Global Days (*continued*)

CPT Code	Description	Global Days
30310	Removal intranasal FB w/general anesthesia	10
30901	Nosebleed cautery/packing	0
40650	Repair of vermilion border of lip	90
41010	Incision in lingual frenulum	10
41250–41252	Laceration repairs of tongue	10
45915	Removal, fecal impaction or anal FB	10
51701, 51702	Bladder catheterization	0
57415	Removal FB vagina, general anesthesia	10
65205	Removal, superficial conjunctival FB	0
65220	Removal of a corneal FB w/o slit lamp	0
69200	Removal FB, ear	0
69209, 69210	Removal impacted cerumen	0

Abbreviations: FB, foreign body; CPT, Current Procedural Terminology; SQ, subcutaneous; w/, with; w/o, without.

Laceration Repairs

12001–12018	Simple repair
12031–12057	Intermediate repair
13100–13160	Complex repair

 Coding Pearl ||||||||

ICD-10-CM code **Z48.02** is not reported for removal of sutures placed to repair an injury. Code **Z48.02** is an aftercare code, and aftercare codes are not reported in relation to subsequent care of injuries or poisoning. Report the code for the injury or poisoning with seventh character **D** for aftercare of injury.

- Categories of difficulty of wound repairs are described as
  - *Simple:* Superficial wound and/or subcutaneous wound requiring a simple single-layer closure or tissue adhesives
  - *Intermediate:* Wound requiring layered closure of one or more of the deeper layers of subcutaneous tissue and non-muscle fascia in addition to skin closure or contaminated wound that requires extensive cleaning or removal of particulate matter
  - *Complex:* Wounds requiring reconstructive surgery, complicated closure, or grafting
- Codes **12001–13160** are used to report wound closure using sutures, staples, or tissue adhesives (eg, Dermabond), singly or in combination with adhesive strips.
- Wound closure using adhesive strips (eg, Steri-Strips, butterfly bandages) only is considered inherent to the E/M service. However, the supplies (eg, Steri-Strips, butterfly bandages) may be reported separately using code **99070** (supplies and materials) or **A4450** (tape, non-waterproof, per 18 sq in). There is not a specific HCPCS code for Steri-Strips or butterfly bandages.
- Some payers may accept HCPCS code **G0168** (wound closure using tissue adhesive[s]) in lieu of simple repair codes (eg, **12001, 12011**).
- Codes are reported based on the difficulty of the repair, measured length of the wound, and the location. To report wound repair, measure the length of the repaired wound(s) in centimeters.
  - If multiple wounds belong to the same category of difficulty and location, add the lengths and report with a single code.
  - If multiple wounds do not belong in the same category, report each repair separately with the more complicated repair reported as the primary procedure and the less complicated repair reported as the secondary procedure. Modifier **51** (multiple procedures) should be appended to the secondary code(s).
- Simple ligation of vessels is considered as part of the wound closure.

❋ Wound debridement and/or cleaning and the provision of topical or injected local anesthesia are considered to be included in the wound repair code. Debridement is considered a separate procedure only when gross contamination requires prolonged cleaning, excessive amounts of devitalized tissue are removed, or debridement is performed without immediate primary closure. To report extensive tissue debridement, see codes **11042–11047** for selective debridement of subcutaneous, muscle, fascial tissues and/or bone (includes debridement of dermis and epidermis when performed) or **97597** and **97598** for debridement of skin, epidermis and/or dermis.

Examples

➤ **A 10-year-old sustained a 1.5-cm laceration on his left knee requiring an intermediate repair after a fall from playground equipment.**

ICD-10-CM	CPT®
S81.012A (laceration without foreign body left knee, initial encounter) **W09.8XXA** (fall on or from other playground equipment, initial encounter) **Y92.838** (other recreation area)	**12031** (repair, intermediate, wounds of scalp, axillae, trunk, and/or extremities; 2.5 cm or less)

Teaching Point: External cause codes (eg, **W09.8XXA**) are assigned for each encounter for treatment with a seventh character indicating initial (**A**), subsequent (**D**), or sequela (**S**). Place of occurrence (eg, **Y92.838**) is reported only for the initial encounter for an injury and requires no seventh character.

➤ **A 10-year-old fell from playground equipment and sustained a 1.5-cm laceration on his left knee and a 1.5-cm laceration on his left forearm, with each laceration requiring an intermediate repair.**

ICD-10-CM	CPT
S81.012A **S51.812A** (laceration of left forearm without foreign body, initial encounter) **W09.8XXA** **Y92.838**	**12032** (intermediate repair, extremities, 2.6–7.5 cm)

Teaching Point: The measurement of both wounds (3 cm) is between 2.6 and 7.5 cm, both wounds are in the same family of anatomic sites, and both require the same level of repair.

➤ **An 8-year-old sustained a 0.5-cm laceration on her forehead.** The wound on her face requires a simple repair. She is seen in follow-up 7 days later. The wound is clean and sutures are removed.

ICD-10-CM	CPT
S01.81XA (laceration without foreign body of other part of head, initial encounter)	**Initial visit** **12011** (simple repair of the facial laceration 2.5 cm or less)
S01.81XD (laceration without foreign body of other part of head, subsequent encounter)	**Follow-up visit** **99212** (problem-focused E/M visit, office or outpatient)

Teaching Point: The seventh character **D** (ie, **S01.81XD**) is reported for encounters after the patient has received active treatment of the condition and is receiving routine care for the condition during the healing or recovery phase.

Other Repairs

Code **11760** (repair of nail bed) is reported when part or all of the nail plate is lifted and a laceration of the nail bed is repaired.

Report code **40650** (repair of vermilion border of the lip) when a laceration of the full thickness of the lip and vermilion is repaired.

Laceration repairs of the tongue (**41250–41252**) are reported based on size and location (eg, repair of laceration 2.5 cm or less, anterior two-thirds of the tongue is reported using code **41250**).

Coding Conundrum: Suture Removal

Suture removal can be coded in a variety of ways depending on the circumstances involved.

Sutures Placed by a Different Physician

When sutures are removed by another physician with a different tax identification number, an E/M office visit code may be reported for the suture removal. Some payers may allow reporting of HCPCS code **S0630**. Code **S0630** is for removal of sutures by a physician other than the physician who originally closed the wound. S codes are HCPCS Level II codes, designated by the CMS and recognized by national Blue Cross and Blue Shield payers, but coverage is on a payer-by-payer basis.

Sutures Placed by Same Physician or Physician of the Same Specialty in the Same Group (Same Tax Identification Number)

Simple Repair

The Medicare global surgery period for *CPT*® codes **12001–12018** (simple repair of superficial wound) is 0 days, meaning payment includes the procedure or service plus any associated care provided on the same day of service. Therefore, practices may report a separate E/M service for removal of sutures placed in the office.

Intermediate or Complex Repair

The Medicare global surgery period for intermediate (**12031–12057**) and complex (**13100–13153**) wound repairs is 10 days. Payment includes the procedure or service plus any associated follow-up care for a period of 10 days. Therefore, the charge for the procedure already includes suture removal by the same physician or physician of the same group and specialty as part of the global surgical package.

Burn Care

Current Procedural Terminology code **16000** (initial treatment, first-degree burn, where no more than local treatment is required) is reported when initial treatment is performed for the symptomatic relief of a first-degree burn that is characterized by erythema and tenderness.

16020	Dressings and/or debridement of partial-thickness burns, initial or subsequent; small or less than 5% total body (eg, finger)
16025	medium or 5%–10% total body surface area (eg, whole face or whole extremity)
16030	large or greater than 10% total body surface area (eg, more than 1 extremity)

Codes **16020–16030**

⁜ Are used to report treatment of burns with dressings and/or debridement of small to large partial-thickness burns (second degree), whether initial or subsequent.

⁜ Are reported based on the percentage of total body surface area (TBSA) affected.

⁜ The percentage of TBSA involved must be calculated and documented when reporting care of second- or third-degree burns. Physicians will use what is referred to as the Rule of 9s (ie, dividing the TBSA into 9% or multiples of 9% segments). There are 2 sets of rules: one for infants and another for adults. (The Rule of 9s diagram is located in *CPT 2018 Professional Edition*.) As you can see from the diagram, the rules differ because of the large area of an infant or child's torso and head.

⁜ An E/M visit with modifier **25** appended may be reported if a significant, separately identifiable E/M service is medically indicated, performed, and documented in addition to the burn care.

⁜ It is advisable to use *ICD-10-CM* category **T31**, burns classified according to extent of body surface involved, as an additional code for reporting purposes when there is mention of a third-degree burn involving 20% or more of the body surface.

Examples

➤ **A 9-year-old is seen by the physician complaining of sunburn on her shoulders.** There is redness and tenderness but no blistering. Topical treatment is applied and an over-the-counter treatment for the first-degree burn is ordered.

ICD-10-CM	CPT®
L55.0 (first-degree sunburn)	**16000** (first-degree burn requiring local treatment)

➤ **A 4-year-old is seen in the office after sustaining a burn on the first finger of her right hand.** The area is red and blistered. Following examination by the physician, the finger is treated with a topical cream and bandaged.

ICD-10-CM	CPT
T23.221A (second-degree burn of single finger, initial encounter) **X19.XXXA** (contact with other heat and hot substances, initial encounter)	**16020**

Removal of Impacted Cerumen (69209, 69210)

69209   Removal of impacted cerumen using irrigation/lavage, unilateral
69210   Removal of impacted cerumen requiring instrumentation, unilateral

For cerumen removal that is not impacted, report the appropriate E/M service code.

Modifier **25** should be appended to the significant, separately identifiable E/M service (eg, **99213**) provided on the same date as removal of impacted cerumen based on National Correct Coding Initiative (NCCI) edits. Payers that incorporate NCCI edits may deny the service when submitted without modifier **25**. For more information on NCCI edits, see Chapter 3, Modifiers and Coding Edits.

> **Coding Pearl** ||||||||
>
> Removal of cerumen that is not impacted is included in an E/M code regardless of how it is removed.

Code **69209** is used to report removal of impacted cerumen by ear wash without direct visualization and instrumentation. Do not report **69209** for removal of cerumen that is not impacted. This code is intended to capture the practice expense associated with the service and is not valued to include physician work. Separately report any significant and separately identifiable E/M service provided by a physician or other qualified health care professional (QHP) on the same date (modifier **25** may be appended to the E/M code when required by payers).

⁑ For bilateral procedure, report **69209** with modifier **50**.

⁑ Do not report **69209** in conjunction with **69210** when performed on the same ear (modifiers **LT** and **RT** may be used to identify contralateral procedures).

Code **69210** is *only* reported when the physician, under direct visualization, removes impacted cerumen using, at a minimum, an otoscope and instruments such as wax curettes or by using an operating microscope and suction plus specific ear instruments (eg, cup forceps, right angles).

⁑ Medical record documentation must support that the cerumen was impacted and removed by the physician and include a description of what equipment and method were used to perform the procedure.

⁑ Report code **69210** with modifier **50** when bilateral procedures are performed.

⁑ Removal of cerumen that is not impacted is included in an E/M code regardless of how it is removed.

Note: Medicare does not recognize modifier **50** when reported with code **69210** (impacted cerumen removal); therefore, those payers that follow Medicare payment policy will not recognize either and may deny the claim outright. Check with your payers.

Examples

➤ **A physician orders removal of impacted cerumen from the right ear by lavage.** Clinical staff perform the lavage, removing the impacted cerumen. Because the child is uncooperative, the procedure takes 10 minutes.

ICD-10-CM	*CPT®*
Appropriate diagnosis	**99201–99215 25** Report if appropriate and use modifier **25** if required by payer.
H61.21 (impacted cerumen, right ear)	**69209**

➤ **Physician documents, "Impacted cerumen removed from both ears using an otoscope and curette."**

ICD-10-CM	*CPT*
Appropriate diagnosis	**99201–99215 25** Report if appropriate and use modifier **25** if required by payer.
H61.23 (impacted cerumen, bilateral)	**69210 50**

Negative Pressure Wound Therapy

97605   Negative pressure wound therapy (eg, vacuum assisted drainage collection), utilizing durable medical equipment (DME), including topical application(s), wound assessment, and instruction(s) for ongoing care, per session; total wound(s) surface area less than or equal to 50 square centimeters

97606   total wound(s) surface area greater than 50 square centimeters

97607   Negative pressure wound therapy, (eg, vacuum assisted drainage collection), utilizing disposable, non-durable medical equipment including provision of exudate management collection system, topical application(s), wound assessment, and instructions for ongoing care, per session; total wound(s) surface area less than or equal to 50 square centimeters

97608   total wound(s) surface area greater than 50 square centimeters

It has become common in recent years for physicians to include use of negative pressure wound therapy (NPWT) or vacuum-assisted closure in the management of traumatic and surgical wounds. Codes **97605** and **97606** represent NPWT provided via a system that includes a *non-disposable* suction pump and drainage collection device. Codes **97607** and **97608** are used for NPWT that utilizes a *disposable* suction pump and collection system. Codes **97607** and **97608** are not reported in conjunction with codes **97605** and **97606**. Payer policies may limit coverage to care of specific types of wounds that require NPWT to improve granulation tissue formation and to certain types of NPWT equipment. Be sure to verify the coverage policy of the patient's health plan prior to provision of services.

Negative pressure wound therapy

◉ Requires direct (one-on-one) physician or QHP contact with the patient.
◉ May be initiated in a hospital or surgical center setting and continued in the home setting after discharge.
◉ Includes application of dressings.
◉ Is separately reported when performed in conjunction with surgical debridement (**11042–11047**).
◉ Documentation should include current wound assessment, including quantitative measurements of wound characteristics (eg, site, surface area and depth), any previous treatment regimens, debridement (when performed), prescribed length of treatment, dressing types and frequency of changes, and other concerns that affect healing. Encounters for ongoing NPWT may include documentation of progress of healing and changes in the wound, including measurement, amount of exudate, and presence of granulation or necrotic tissue.
◉ Supplies, including dressings, are reportable with HCPCS codes (eg, **A6550**, wound care set, for NPWT electrical pump, includes all supplies and accessories). Supplies for a disposable system are reported with code **A9272**, which also includes all dressings and accessories.

Removal of Foreign Bodies

Current Procedural Terminology® includes codes for reporting removal of foreign bodies from many different body sites. Removal of a foreign body from within the subcutaneous tissues above the fascia is reported with a code from the integumentary system regardless of the site (eg, hand, foot). Musculoskeletal codes are reported when a foreign body is removed from *within the fascia, subfascial, or muscle*. Always check the *CPT* index to direct you to the most accurate code.

❁ Code **10120** (removal of a foreign body from subcutaneous tissue via simple incision) includes the removal of splinters or ticks when the physician has to "break open" or incise the skin to retrieve the splinter.

❁ Code **10121** is used to report the complicated removal of a foreign body by incision.

The physician determines whether the procedure is simple or complex, but the significant difference in physician work relative value units (RVUs) for the procedures may be used as an indicator of the difference—1.22 for **10120** versus 2.74 for **10121**. Clearly, a procedure described by code **10121** would involve double the time and effort of the simple procedure.

> ||||||| **Coding Pearl** |||||||
>
> Do not report code **10120** or **10121** when a foreign body is removed using forceps alone with no incision.

Example

The removal of an embedded earring requiring an incision would be reported with code **10120** or **10121**, depending on the complexity of the procedure required to remove it. If the earring is removed by wiggling it out or other method that does not require incision, this work is included in the E/M service.

❁ Musculoskeletal foreign body: Codes in the musculoskeletal system *are not reported* for removal of foreign bodies within the skin and subcutaneous fat. Examples of codes for removal of foreign bodies within the musculoskeletal system are

  ❖ Foot: For foreign body removal *from within the fascia, subfascial, or muscle,* code **28190** is used to report the removal of a subcutaneous foreign body from the foot; code **28192** is used to report removal of a foreign body from the deep tissue of the foot.

  ❖ Upper arm or elbow: Report removal of foreign bodies from subcutaneous tissues within the fascia (**24200**) or deep, below the fascia or in the muscle (**24201**) of the upper arm or elbow area.

❁ Intranasal foreign body: Removal of intranasal foreign bodies is reported using code **30300** (removal of intranasal foreign bodies when performed in the office) or **30310** (removal of intranasal foreign bodies under general anesthesia).

❁ Fecal impaction or anal foreign body: Code **45915** is used to report removal of fecal impaction or foreign body when performed under anesthesia. When digital removal of fecal impaction or anal foreign body is performed by a physician without anesthesia, code **45999** (unlisted procedure, rectum) may be reported or the work credited toward the level of service for a related E/M service.

❁ Foreign body in vagina: Report code **57415** when a vaginal foreign body is removed when the child is under anesthesia (not local anesthesia). Code **58999** (unlisted procedure, female genital system, non-obstetrical) may be reported for removal of a vaginal foreign body without anesthesia.

Note: If an unlisted procedure code is reported, a written report must be submitted with the claim. It is more appropriate to report these procedures using an appropriate E/M service code or include the work in selecting the level of service for a related E/M service unless otherwise directed by payer policy.

❁ Foreign body in eye: When removing a superficial conjunctival foreign body, report code **65205**. Removal of a corneal foreign body without the use of a slit lamp is reported with code **65220**.

❁ External auditory canal: Report code **69200** when the foreign body is removed without general anesthesia.

Table 15-3 emphasizes the increase in revenue that results from reporting the appropriate code (eg, procedure vs low- and mid-level E/M codes).

Chapter 15: Common Surgical Procedures and Sedation

Table 15-3. Comparing RVUs: 2017 Medicare RBRVS[a]

Code	Description	Total Non-facility RVUs
99201	Level 1 office visit, new patient	1.24
99202	Level 2 office visit, new patient	2.11
99203	Level 3 office visit, new patient	3.05
99212	Level 2 office visit, established patient	1.23
99213	Level 3 office visit, established patient	2.06
99214	Level 4 office visit, established patient	3.03
30300	Foreign body removal from nose	5.04
10120	Foreign body removal from subcutaneous tissue	4.32

Abbreviations: RBRVS, Resource-Based Relative Value Scale; RVU, relative value unit.

[a] The 2018 Medicare RBRVS was not available at the time this manual was printed. For an online copy of the pediatric-specific 2017 Medicare RBRVS, go to www.aap.org/cfp, access code AAPCFP23.

Fracture and/or Dislocation Care

Casts/Strapping/Splints

- Codes for the application of casts, splints, or strapping (**29000–29590**) cannot be reported for the initial (first) application when fracture or dislocation care is reported because they are included as part of the global surgery package.
- May be reported when they are replacements for the initial application or performed as part of the initial E/M visit and fracture care is not reported.
  The following codes are commonly used when treating a fracture or dislocation:
- Application of splints
  - ❖ Short arm splint (forearm to hand): static (**29125**); dynamic (**29126**)
  - ❖ Finger splint: static (**29130**); dynamic (**29131**)
  - ❖ Short leg splint (calf to foot): **29515**
- Strapping
  - ❖ Shoulder: **29240**
  - ❖ Elbow or wrist: **29260**

Supplies

- Supplies associated with fracture care may be billed with every application, including the initial casting, splinting, or strapping performed in association with the global surgery procedure code when the service is performed in the private office setting.
- Healthcare Common Procedure Coding System codes **A4580**, **A4590**, and **Q4001–Q4051** may be reported for cast supplies; codes **E1800–E1841** may be reported for splints. Check with your major payers and/or review their payment policies for reporting these supplies.
- The HCPCS codes are accepted by many Medicaid and commercial payers and are very specific to the age of the patient and type of supply and/or material.
- A description of supplies may be required when reporting special supplies code **99070**.
- The following codes are commonly used:

99070	Supplies and materials (except spectacles)
A4565	Slings
A4570	Splint
L3650–L3678	Clavicle splints
Q4001–Q4051	Cast and splint supplies
S8450–S8452	Splint, prefabricated for finger, wrist, ankle, or elbow

Fracture and Dislocation Care Codes

Codes for fracture/dislocation care

* Are listed by anatomic location.
* Are provided (in most cases) for closed or open treatment, with or without manipulation, and with or without internal fixation.
* Most include a 90-day period of follow-up care under the Medicare global package.
* Include the initial casting, splinting, or strapping.
* Do not include radiographs.
* Fractures most commonly seen in a primary care pediatric practice include closed fractures (ie, fracture site is not surgically opened), and treatment is typically without manipulation (an exception is treatment of nursemaid elbow).
* Clavicular fracture: Report closed treatment without manipulation with code **23500**.
* Nursemaid elbow: Report closed treatment of radial head subluxation (nursemaid elbow) with manipulation with code **24640**. (This code has a 10-day global period.)
* Radial fracture: Report code **25500** for closed treatment of radial shaft fracture without manipulation and **25600** for closed treatment of distal radius fracture without manipulation.
* Phalanx fracture: Closed treatment of a proximal or middle phalanx, finger, or thumb (each) without manipulation is reported with code **26720**. Closed treatment of a distal phalangeal fracture (each) without manipulation is reported with code **26750**.
* Great toe fracture: Code **28490** is reported for the closed treatment of a fracture of the great toe, phalanx, or phalanges without manipulation.
* Metatarsal fracture: Report code **28470** for closed treatment of a metatarsal fracture without manipulation.
* Lesser toe fracture: Closed treatment of fracture, phalanx, or phalanges, other than great toe without manipulation, is coded with **28510**.

Tip: Unrelated services that are provided during the global surgery period by the same physician (or physician of the same group and specialty) may be reported. Modifier **24** would be appended to the unrelated E/M service. Refer to Chapter 3, Modifiers and Coding Edits, for instructions for reporting modifiers.

Examples

➤ An urgent care physician performs and documents a comprehensive evaluation on a child with multiple injuries, including a fracture of the shaft of the left clavicle and abrasions on the left upper arm and cheek, after a fall from the monkey bars.

ICD-10-CM	CPT®
S40.812A (abrasion upper arm, initial encounter) **S00.81XA** (abrasion face, initial encounter) **W09.8XXA** (fall from playground equipment, initial encounter)	**99201–99205 57**
S42.022A (displaced fracture shaft of clavicle, closed, initial encounter) **W09.8XXA**	**23500** (closed treatment clavicle fracture without manipulation)

Teaching Point: Fractures not specified as displaced or non-displaced are reported with an *ICD-10-CM* code for a displaced fracture. Fractures not specified as open or closed are reported with a code for a closed fracture. Because code **23500** is assigned a 90-day global period in the Medicare Physician Fee Schedule, many payers may require modifier **57** (decision for surgery) appended to the E/M code. Individual payers may have different policies.

Chapter 15: Common Surgical Procedures and Sedation

Coding Conundrum: Reporting Fracture Care

If a payer follows Medicare payment policy, the physician has the option of using the appropriate E/M codes and reporting each service separately in lieu of using procedure codes. The decision to use the global fracture code rather than E/M service codes requires an analysis of payment by payers for these codes.

Current Procedural Terminology® code **25600** (closed treatment of distal radial fracture, without manipulation) includes all associated preoperative care, application of the splint, and follow-up care for 90 days. If there was a significant, separately identifiable E/M service provided on the day of the fracture care (eg, child sustained sprain to other arm), an E/M service could also be reported with modifier **25** appended to the E/M service. Follow-up visits would be reported with code **99024** (postoperative follow-up visit included in surgical package). If a physician chooses not to bill fracture care, an E/M visit would be reported with code **29075** (application of short arm cast). You could also report code **Q4012** (cast supplies, short arm cast, pediatric, fiberglass). Any diagnostic procedures, such as radiographs, would be reported in either situation.

Before you decide how to bill the service, consider your total payments for the care associated with this fracture.

Reporting Fracture Care Codes		Reporting E/M and Follow-up	
Code	**2017 Medicare Non-facility RBRVS**[a]	**Code**	**2017 Medicare Non-facility RBRVS**[a]
25600	9.32	99213	2.06
73100	0.82	73100	0.82
		29075	2.48
Q4012[b]	—	Q4012[b]	—
99024	0.00	99212	1.23
Total	10.14		6.59

Abbreviations: E/M, evaluation and management; RBRVS, Resource-Based Relative Value Scale.

[a] The 2018 Medicare RBRVS was not available at the time this manual was printed. For an online copy of the pediatric-specific 2017 Medicare RBRVS, go to www.aap.org/cfp, access code AAPCFP23.

[b] Supplies are not valued on the RBRVS.

➤ A physician evaluates a 16-month-old girl whose parents report that she will not move her left arm. The child was playing in the yard when another child tried to pull her up the ladder of a playhouse. Mother thinks child fell, hitting her head and left side. Mother noted no bump or bruises but soon noticed she was not using her left arm. The fall was from no more than 3 feet off the ground. The patient is otherwise in good health, with no past hospitalizations or surgeries and no allergies or medications. Immunizations are up-to-date. The patient lives with her parents and 2 older siblings. Review of systems is negative for headache, vomiting, dizziness, or changes in behavior other than protection of left arm. On examination, the child is alert but apprehensive. She has no hematoma or skull defect, her face is symmetric, pupils are equal and responsive to light and accommodation, and her neck is supple. The child holds her left arm in front of her body with her right hand supporting her left forearm. Left upper extremity shows no visible signs of deformity or swelling, and skin is intact. Pain is elicited at the head of the radius. Subluxation of the radial head is reduced by manipulation. Reassessment after 10 minutes shows the child uses both arms now when presented with a balloon. The parents are counseled about potential for recurrent injury and avoidance. A follow-up with previously scheduled 18-month visit is arranged unless otherwise indicated.

ICD-10-CM	CPT
S53.032A (nursemaid's elbow, left, initial encounter) **W11.XXXA** (fall on and from ladder)	99214 25 24640 (closed treatment of radial head subluxation in child, nursemaid elbow, with manipulation)

Teaching Point: The physician provided a significant and separately identifiable E/M service to evaluate extent of injury in addition to treatment of nursemaid elbow. Although not specifically stated, the patient is established, as she is to return for an already scheduled 18-month preventive service. The history and examination are detailed and the MDM is of moderate complexity. Modifier **25** is required by most payers to indicate the E/M service was significant and separately identifiable from the preservice work of the minor procedure performed on the same date of service.

➤ **A 9-year-old established patient is seen with complaints of left and right arm pain following a fall while snowboarding.** An expanded problem-focused history and physical examination are performed. The radiograph demonstrates a left Colles fracture (distal radius with dorsal [posterior] displacement of the wrist and hand). A fiberglass cast is applied and the patient is advised to return for follow-up.

The physician can elect to report the fracture care or the E/M services provided over the course of the global surgery period (see the Coding Conundrum: Reporting Fracture Care box).

Respiratory

Intubation and Airway Management

31500   Intubation, endotracheal, emergency (and elective)

◉ Moderate sedation (**99151–99157**) may be reported in addition to the intubation if used to sedate the patient prior to and during the intubation procedure (eg, in rapid sequence intubation) and reporting criteria are met. See the Sedation section later in this chapter for more on moderate sedation.

31502   Tracheostomy tube change prior to establishment of fistula tract

◉ Report code **31502** when an indwelling tracheostomy tube is replaced. Routine changing of a tracheostomy tube after a fistula tract has been established is included in a related E/M service.

31505–31520   Indirect laryngoscopy

◉ Report code **31505** for indirect diagnostic laryngoscopy. If, while performing this procedure, a foreign body is removed, report code **31511** (laryngoscopy with removal of foreign body).

◉ Direct laryngoscopy with or without tracheoscopy: Code **31515** is reported when it is performed for aspiration.

◉ When a diagnostic direct laryngoscopy, with or without tracheoscopy, is performed on a newborn, report code **31520**. Do not report modifier **63** (procedure performed on infant less than 4 kg) in conjunction with code **31520**.

31525   Laryngoscopy, direct, with or without tracheoscopy; diagnostic except newborn

Thoracostomy, Thoracentesis, and Pleural Drainage

32551   Tube thoracostomy, includes connection to drainage system (eg, water seal), when performed, open (separate procedure)

32554   Thoracentesis, needle or catheter, aspiration of the pleural space; without imaging guidance

32555   Thoracentesis, needle or catheter, aspiration of the pleural space; with imaging guidance

32556   Pleural drainage, percutaneous, with insertion of indwelling catheter; without imaging guidance

32557   Pleural drainage, percutaneous, with insertion of indwelling catheter; with imaging guidance

◉ Thoracostomy (**32551**) represents an open procedure involving incision into a rib interspace with dissection extending through the chest wall muscles and pleura. Thoracentesis and percutaneous pleural drainage may be more commonly performed in pediatrics.

Chapter 15: Common Surgical Procedures and Sedation

- Percutaneous image guidance cannot be reported in conjunction with code **32551**, which represents an open procedure. Diagnostic ultrasound performed prior to thoracostomy to localize a collection in the pleural space is separately reportable only when the complete ultrasound study of the chest (**76441**) is performed with permanent recording of images.

- Thoracentesis codes **32554** and **32555** represent a procedure in which the surgical technique is puncture of the pleural space to remove fluid or air. Although a catheter (eg, pigtail catheter) may be used, it is not left in place at the end of the procedure.

- Percutaneous pleural drainage codes **32556** and **32557** represent procedures in which an indwelling catheter is inserted into the pleural space and remains at the end of the procedure. The catheter is secured in place and connected to a suction drainage system.

- Removal of chest tubes and non-tunneled indwelling pleural catheters is included in a related E/M service and not a separately reportable procedure.

- For insertion of a tunneled pleural catheter with cuff, see code **32550**. For removal of a tunneled pleural catheter with cuff, see **32552**.

Vascular Access

Central Venous Access

Insertion of central venous access device

36555	Insertion of non-tunneled centrally inserted central venous catheter; younger than 5 years of age
36556	age 5 years or older
36557	Insertion of tunneled centrally inserted central venous catheter, without subcutaneous port or pump; younger than 5 years of age
36558	age 5 years or older

- There is no distinction between venous access percutaneously or via cutdown.

- Report the code appropriate to the type of catheter (eg, non-tunneled vs tunneled), device (eg, with or without port), and age of child (**Table 15-4**).

- Moderate sedation services are separately reportable with codes **99151–99157**. For more information on reporting moderate sedation, see the Sedation section later in this chapter.

- Report code **76937** for ultrasound evaluation of potential access sites with documentation of selected vessel patency, concurrent real-time ultrasound visualization of vascular needle entry, and permanent recording and reporting. This code is reported separately in addition to a code for primary vascular access procedure (eg, **36555**). Do not report ultrasound for vessel identification only.

Table 15-4. Insertion of Central Venous Catheter		
Insertion of Central Venous Catheter	**Child <5 Years**	**Child ≥5 Years**
Non-tunneled centrally inserted central venous catheter	36555	36556
Tunneled centrally inserted central venous catheter, without subcutaneous port or pump	36557	36558
Tunneled centrally inserted central venous access device, with subcutaneous port	36560	36561
Peripherally inserted central venous catheter, without subcutaneous port or pump	36568	36569
Peripherally inserted central venous access device, with subcutaneous port	36570	36571

Arterial Access

36600 Arterial puncture, withdrawal of blood for diagnosis
36620 Arterial catheterization or cannulation for sampling, monitoring or transfusion (separate procedure); percutaneous
36625 cutdown

- An arterial puncture for diagnosis is reported with code **36600**.
- Code **36620** is reported when a percutaneous peripheral arterial catheterization is performed.
- Code **36625** is reported when a cutdown is performed.
  Removal of central venous access device
- Report repairs, partial catheter replacements, complete replacements, or removal of catheters with or without subcutaneous ports or pumps with codes **36578–36590**. Code **36589** is reported for removal of tunneled central venous catheter, without subcutaneous port or pump, and code **36590** for the removal of tunneled central venous catheter, with subcutaneous port or pump, central or peripheral.
- If a central venous access device is removed and replaced with a new one *through a separate venous access site,* the removal and insertion of the new device should be reported.

Transfusions

36430 Transfusion, blood or blood components
36440 Push transfusion; blood, 2 years or younger
36450 Exchange transfusion, blood, newborn
36455 other than newborn
36456 Partial exchange transfusion, blood, plasma, or crystalloid necessitating the skill of a physician or other qualified health care professional; newborn

- Indirect transfusion of blood or blood products (**36430**) should be used only if the physician personally infuses the substance, and not if the blood is administered by nursing personnel and allowed to enter the vessel via gravity or meter flow. Push transfusion (**36440**) is used only for patients younger than 2 years. This code should be used only if the physician personally performs the transfusion.

> ||||||| **Coding Pearl** |||||||
> The placement of catheters to support exchange transfusions may be reported separately with the appropriate vascular access codes.

- Complete exchange transfusions (double volume) performed during the neonatal period are reported using code **36450**; exchange transfusions for all other age groups are reported using code **36455**. The assumption is that the exchange for the neonate is performed via the umbilical vein, while an exchange for an older child or adult is performed via a peripheral vessel.
- The actual placement of catheters to support the exchange transfusion may be reported separately with the appropriate vascular access codes.
- Partial exchange transfusions (eg, for hyperviscosity syndrome in the neonate) should be reported using code **36456**.
- Do not report codes **36430**, **36440**, or **36450** with **36456**.

Hydration, Intravenous Infusions

Services included as inherent to an infusion or injection are the use of local anesthesia, starting the intravenous (IV) line, access to indwelling IV lines or a subcutaneous catheter or port, flushing lines at the conclusion of an infusion or between infusions, standard tubing, syringes and supplies, and preparation of chemotherapy agents.

These codes are intended for reporting by the physician or other QHP in an office setting. They are not reported by a physician or other QHP when performed in a facility setting because the physician work associated with these procedures involves only affirmation of the treatment plan and direct supervision of the staff performing the services. If a significant, separately identifiable E/M service is performed, the appropriate code may be reported with modifier **25** appended. The diagnosis may be the same for the E/M service and codes **96360–96379**.

Table 15-5 lists related primary and additional hydration, injection, and IV codes.

Table 15-5. Primary and Additional Hydration, Injection, and Intravenous Codes	
Primary Code	**Additional Codes**
96360 Intravenous infusion, hydration; initial, 31 minutes to 1 hour	**96361** Intravenous infusion, hydration; each additional hour
96365 Intravenous infusion, for therapy, prophylaxis, or diagnosis (specify substance or drug); initial, up to 1 hour	**96366, 96367, 96368, 96375** (each additional sequential intravenous push of a new substance/drug), **96376ª** (each additional sequential intravenous push of the same substance/drug provided in a facility)
96367 Intravenous infusion, for therapy, prophylaxis, or diagnosis (specify substance or drug); additional sequential infusion of a new drug/substance, up to 1 hour	**96366** Intravenous infusion, for therapy, prophylaxis, or diagnosis (specify substance or drug); each additional hour
96366	**96368** Intravenous infusion, for therapy, prophylaxis, or diagnosis (specify substance or drug); concurrent infusion
96369 Subcutaneous infusion for therapy or prophylaxis (specify substance or drug); initial, up to 1 hour, including pump set-up and establishment of subcutaneous infusion site(s)	**96370** Subcutaneous infusion for therapy or prophylaxis (specify substance or drug); each additional hour **96371** Subcutaneous infusion for therapy or prophylaxis (specify substance or drug); additional pump set-up with establishment of new subcutaneous infusion site(s)
96374 Therapeutic, prophylactic, or diagnostic injection (specify substance or drug); intravenous push, single or initial substance/drug	**96367, 96375, 96376ª**
96409 Chemotherapy administration; intravenous, push technique, single or initial substance/drug	**96367, 96375, 96376ª**
96413 Chemotherapy administration, intravenous infusion technique; up to 1 hour, single or initial substance/drug	**96367, 96368, 96375, 96376ª**
96415 Chemotherapy administration, intravenous infusion technique; each additional hour	**96368**
96416 Chemotherapy administration, intravenous infusion technique; initiation of prolonged chemotherapy infusion (more than 8 hours), requiring use of a portable or implantable pump	**96368**

ª Code is only to be reported in the facility setting.

Therapeutic, Prophylactic, and Diagnostic Injections

96372	Therapeutic, prophylactic, or diagnostic injection (specify substance or drug); subcutaneous or intramuscular
96373	intra-arterial
96374	intravenous push, single or initial substance/drug
+96375	each additional sequential intravenous push of a new substance/drug (List separately in addition to **96365**, **96374**, **96409**, or **96413**)
+96376	each additional sequential intravenous push of the same substance/drug provided in a facility (List separately in addition to **96365**, **96374**, **96409**, or **96413**)

Codes **96374** and **96375** are only used when the health care professional administering the substance or drug is in constant attendance during the administration *and* must observe the patient. The IV push must be less than 15 minutes. Short infusions of less than 15 minutes are reported as a push (eg, **96374**).

Codes **96372–96374**

- ⚙ Report code **96372** for the administration of a diagnostic, prophylactic, or therapeutic (eg, antibiotic) subcutaneous or intramuscular injection. Do not report for the administration of a purified protein derivative test.
- ⚙ Report code **96373** for an initial intra-arterial injection and **96374** for an initial injection administered by IV push. Sequential IV push of a new substance or drug is reported with add-on code **96375**. Code **96375** may be reported in addition to codes for IV infusion (**96365**), initial IV push (**96374**), or chemotherapy administration (**96409**, **96413**). Additional sequential IV push of the same substance or drug (**96376**) is reported only by a facility.

Each drug administered is reported separately with the appropriate infusion code.

Example

➤ A 3-year-old established patient is seen with a complaint of vomiting and fever for the past 24 hours. She has refused all food and liquids and last voided 12 hours prior to the visit. A detailed history and physical examination with moderate-level MDM are performed. Her diagnosis is bilateral acute suppurative otitis media and dehydration. Intravenous fluids are initiated with physiologic (normal) saline solution, and IV ceftriaxone (750 mg) is infused over 30 minutes for her otitis media. After 1 hour and 45 minutes of IV hydration, she urinates, begins tolerating liquids, and is released to home.

> **||||||||| Coding Pearl |||||||||**
>
> Short infusions of less than 15 minutes should be reported with code **96374**.

ICD-10-CM	CPT®
E86.0 (dehydration) **H66.003** (acute suppurative otitis media without spontaneous rupture of ear drum, bilateral)	**99214 25** (established patient office E/M) **96365** (IV infusion, for therapy) **96361** (IV infusion, hydration, each additional hour) **J0696** (ceftriaxone sodium, per 250 mg) × 3 units **J7030** (infusion, normal saline solution, 1,000 cc)

Link the appropriate diagnosis code to each procedure (eg, code **H66.003** is linked to code **J0696**). The medication and infusion solution may need to be reported with the National Drug Code if required by the payer. The fluid used to administer ceftriaxone is not reported because it is considered incidental hydration.

Hydration

Codes **96360** (IV infusion, hydration; initial, 31 minutes to 1 hour) and **96361** (each additional hour)

- ⚙ Are intended to report IV hydration infusion using prepackaged fluid and/or electrolyte solutions (eg, normal saline, D5½ normal saline with potassium).
- ⚙ Typically require direct physician supervision for purposes of consent, safety oversight, or supervision of staff with little special handling for preparation or disposal of materials.
- ⚙ Do not typically require advanced training of staff because there usually is little risk involved with little patient monitoring required.

Coding Conundrum: Multiple and Concurrent Infusions or Injections

When administering multiple infusions, injections, or combinations, only one "initial" service code should be reported for a given date, unless protocol requires that 2 separate IV sites must be used. Do not report a second initial service on the same date due to an IV line requiring a restart, an IV rate not being able to be reached without 2 lines, or accessing a port of a multi-lumen catheter. If an injection or infusion is of a subsequent or concurrent nature, even if it is the first such service within that group of services, a subsequent or concurrent code from the appropriate section should be reported. For example, the first IV push given subsequent to an initial 1-hour infusion is reported using a subsequent IV push code.

When services are performed in the physician's office, report as follows:

Initial Infusion

Physician reporting: Report the code that best describes the *key* or *primary* reason for the service regardless of the order in which the infusions or injections occur. Only one initial service code (eg, **96365**) should be reported unless the protocol or patient condition requires using 2 separate IV sites. The difference in time and effort in providing this second IV site access is also reported using the *initial* service code with modifier **59**, distinct procedural service, appended (eg, **96365, 96365 59**).

Facility reporting: An initial infusion is based on the hierarchy. Only one initial service code (eg, **96365**) should be reported unless the protocol or patient condition requires using 2 separate IV sites. The difference in time and effort in providing this second IV site access is also reported using the *initial* service code with modifier **59**, distinct procedural service, appended (eg, **96365, 96365 59**).

Sequential Infusion

This is an infusion or IV push of a new substance or drug following a primary or initial service. For example, if an IV push was performed through the same IV access subsequent to an IV infusion for therapy, the appropriate codes to report would be **96365** and **96375**. If an IV push was performed through a different IV access route, the services would be reported using codes **96365** and **96374**. Sequential infusions are reported only one time for the same infusate. However, if additional hours were required for the infusion, the appropriate "each additional hour" add-on code would be reported. Different infusates can be reported using the same code as the original sequential code. Hydration may not be reported concurrently with any other service. All sequential services require that there be a new substance or drug, except that facilities may report a sequential IV push of the same drug using **96376**.

Concurrent Infusion

This is an infusion of a new substance or drug infused at the same time as another drug or substance. This is not time-based and is only reported once per day regardless of whether a new drug or substance is administered concurrently. Hydration may not be reported concurrently with any other service. A separate subsequent concurrent administration of another new drug or substance (the third substance or drug) is not reported.

If IV hydration (**96360, 96361**) is given from 11:00 pm to 2:00 am, code **96360** would be reported once with **96361** with 2 units of service. However, if instead of a continuous infusion, a medication were given by IV push at 10:00 pm and 2:00 am, both administrations would be reported as initial (**96374**) because the services are not continuous. For continuous services that last beyond midnight, use the date in which the service began and report the total units of time provided continuously. Although in conflict with *CPT*® guidelines, some payers may require that the primary infusion code be reported for each day of service.

- ☀ Are reported based on the actual time over which the infusion is administered and do not include the time spent starting the IV and monitoring the patient after infusion. Medical record documentation must support the service reported.

- ☀ Code **96360** may be reported for hydration infusion lasting more than 31 minutes and up to 1 hour. Code **96361** is reported for each additional hour of hydration infusion and for a final interval of greater than 30 minutes beyond the last hour reported.

- ☀ Are not reported when IV infusions are 30 minutes or less.

- ☀ Are not used to report infusion of drugs or other substances; nor are they reported when it is incidental to non-chemotherapeutic/diagnostic or chemotherapeutic services.

- ☀ Code **96361** is reported if an IV hydration infusion is provided secondary or subsequent to a therapeutic, prophylactic, or diagnostic infusion and administered through the same IV access.

Chapter 15: Common Surgical Procedures and Sedation

Therapeutic, Prophylactic, and Diagnostic Infusions

96365 Intravenous infusion, for therapy, prophylaxis, or diagnosis (specify substance or drug); initial, up to 1 hour

+96366 each additional hour (List separately in addition to **96365** or **96367**.)

+96367 additional sequential infusion of a new drug/substance, up to 1 hour (List separately in addition to **96365**, **96374**, **96409**, **96413**.)

+96368 concurrent infusion (List separately in addition to **96365**, **96366**, **96413**, **96415**, or **96416**.)

Codes **96365–96368**

* Are for infusions for the purpose of administering drugs or substances.
* Typically require direct physician supervision and special attention to prepare, calculate dose, and dispose of materials.
* If fluid infusions are used to administer the drug(s), they are considered incidental hydration and are not reported.
* Each drug administered is reported separately with the appropriate infusion code.

Other Injection and Infusion Services

96523 Irrigation of implanted venous access device for drug delivery systems

Code **96523** is used to report irrigation required for implanted venous access devices for drug delivery systems when services are provided on a separate day from the injection or infusion service. Do not report **96523** in conjunction with other services.

Ear, Nose, and Throat Procedures

30901 Central nasal hemorrhage, anterior, simple (cautery or packing)
If performing cautery or packing on both sides, report **30901** with modifier **50**.

69420 Myringotomy

92511 Nasopharyngoscopy with endoscope (separate procedure)
Code **92511** is designated as a "separate procedure" and should not be reported in addition to the code for the total procedure or service of which it is considered an integral component. However, if carried out independently or considered to be unrelated or distinct from other procedures or services provided at that time, it may be reported by itself or in addition to other procedures or services by appending modifier **59** to the specific separate procedure code.

Laryngoplasty

#31551 Laryngoplasty; for laryngeal stenosis, with graft, without indwelling stent placement, younger than 12 years of age

#31552 age 12 years or older

#31553 Laryngoplasty; for laryngeal stenosis, with graft, with indwelling stent placement, younger than 12 years of age

#31554 age 12 years or older

31580 Laryngoplasty; for laryngeal web, with indwelling keel or stent insertion

31584 Laryngoplasty; with open reduction and fixation of (eg, plating) fracture, includes tracheostomy, if performed

* Do not report graft separately if harvested through the laryngoplasty incision (eg, thyroid cartilage graft).
* Report only one of the following codes for a single operative session: **31551–31554** and **31580**.

- Codes for treatment of laryngeal stenosis by laryngoplasty with graft are selected based on whether or not the procedure includes indwelling stent placement and by the age of the patient (<12 years old or ≥12 years).
- Open treatment of a hyoid fracture is reported with code **31584** (repair procedure on the larynx).
- To report tracheostomy, see code **31600, 31601, 31603, 31605,** or **31610.**
- Report laryngoplasty, not otherwise specified or for removal of a keel or stent, with code **31599.**

Cardiovascular Procedures

Valvuloplasty

33390   Valvuloplasty, aortic valve, open, with cardiopulmonary bypass; simple (ie, valvotomy, debridement, debulking, and/or simple commissural resuspension)

33391   complex (eg, leaflet extension, leaflet resection, leaflet reconstruction, or annuloplasty)
            (Do not report **33391** in conjunction with **33390**)

Codes for open valvuloplasty of the aortic valve
- Are more descriptive of currently performed valvuloplasty procedures.
  - ❖ Code **33390** is specifically for reporting valvotomy, debridement, debulking, and/or simple commissural resuspension.
  - ❖ Code **33391** represents more complex procedures not limited to the examples in the code descriptor.
- May be reported in conjunction with the code for transmyocardial revascularization (**33141**), operative tissue ablation and reconstruction of atria (**33255–33259**), and reoperation, valve procedure, more than 1 month after original operation (**33530**), when appropriate.

Codes for aortic valve replacement (**33405, 33406, 33410**) were revised to reflect that these are open procedures.

Transcatheter Pulmonary Valve Implantation

33477   Transcatheter pulmonary valve implantation, percutaneous approach, including pre-stenting of the valve delivery site, when performed

The key instructions for reporting code **33477** are
- Should only be reported once per session
- Includes, when performed,
  - ❖ Percutaneous access
  - ❖ Placing the access sheath
  - ❖ Advancing the repair device delivery system into position
  - ❖ Repositioning the device as needed and deploying the device(s)
  - ❖ Angiography, radiologic supervision, and interpretation performed to guide transcatheter pulmonary valve implantation (TPVI)
  - ❖ All cardiac catheterization(s), intraprocedural contrast injection(s), fluoroscopic radiologic supervision and interpretation, and imaging guidance performed to complete the pulmonary valve procedure
  - ❖ Percutaneous balloon angioplasty of the conduit or treatment zone, valvuloplasty of the pulmonary valve conduit, and stent deployment within the pulmonary conduit or an existing bioprosthetic pulmonary valve
  - ❖ Contrast injections, angiography, road mapping, and/or fluoroscopic guidance for TPVI
  - ❖ Pulmonary conduit angiography for guidance of TPVI
  - ❖ Right heart catheterization for hemodynamic measurements before, during, and after TPVI for guidance of TPVI
- Does not include (Report separately, when performed.)
  - ❖ Codes **92997** and **92998** when pulmonary artery angioplasty is performed at a site separate from the prosthetic valve delivery site

❖ Codes **37236** and **37237** when pulmonary artery stenting is performed at a site separate from the prosthetic valve delivery site

❖ Same-session/same-day diagnostic cardiac catheterization services (See your *CPT*® reference for further instruction and append catheterization code with modifier **59**.)

❖ Diagnostic coronary angiography performed at a separate session from an interventional procedure

❖ Percutaneous coronary interventional procedures

❖ Percutaneous pulmonary artery branch interventions

❖ Percutaneous ventricular assist device procedure codes (**33990–33993**), extracorporeal membrane oxygenation/extracorporeal life support procedure codes (**33946–33989**), or balloon pump insertion codes (**33967, 33970, 33973**)

❖ Percutaneous peripheral bypass (**33367**), open peripheral bypass (**33368**), or central bypass (**33369**)

Digestive System Procedures

Gastric Intubation and Aspiration

43752   Naso- or oro-gastric tube placement, requiring physician's skill and fluoroscopic guidance (includes fluoroscopy, image documentation and report)

43753   Gastric intubation and aspiration(s), therapeutic (eg, for ingested poisons), including lavage if performed

Do not report **43752** or **43753** in conjunction with critical care codes (**99291, 99292**), neonatal critical care codes (**99468, 99469**), pediatric critical care codes (**99471–99476**), or pediatric intensive care service codes (**99477–99480**).

Note that code **43752** is reported when a physician's skill is required for placement of a nasogastric or oro-gastric tube using fluoroscopic guidance. This service is not separately reported when a physician's skill is not required or placement is performed without fluoroscopic guidance. Replacement of a nasogastric tube requiring physician's skill and fluoroscopic guidance may also be reported with code **43752**.

Examples

➤ **A 10-year-old is brought to the emergency department (ED) after having ingested drugs.** Gastric intubation and lavage are performed.

Code **43753** would be reported in addition to the appropriate E/M service (eg, ED services **99281–99285**) but is not separately reported when performed in conjunction with critical care (eg, **99291, 99292; 99468–99476**) or by a physician during pediatric patient transport (**99466, 99467**).

➤ **A patient requires placement of a nasogastric tube.** Attempts by nursing staff are unsuccessful, so placement by the physician is required. The physician places the tube using fluoroscopic guidance.

Code **43752** would be reported in addition to the appropriate E/M service but is not reported when the service is performed by the physician out of convenience rather than necessity for a physician's skill. Use of fluoroscopic guidance is required and must be documented (ie, image documentation and report).

Gastrostomy Tube Replacement

43760   Change of gastrostomy tube, percutaneous, without imaging or endoscopic guidance

Code **43760** is reported for gastrostomy tube change without imaging or endoscopic guidance. See codes **49450** and **43246** for placement with imaging or endoscopic guidance. A significant, separately identifiable E/M service on the same date may be reported with modifier **25** appended to the E/M code (eg, **99213 25**). An E/M service should not be reported when the encounter is solely for replacement of the gastrostomy tube. Code **43760** includes the gastrostomy tube kit.

Enterostomy/Cecostomy With Colonic Lavage

A new parenthetical instruction follows code **44300** in *CPT® 2018* to allow reporting of this code in conjunction with tube placement except when tube placement is for intraoperative colonic lavage. In addition, the instruction below add-on code **44701** (intraoperative colonic lavage) is revised to allow reporting of codes **44300** and **44701** except in instances when the tube placement is for intraoperative colonic lavage.

44300 Placement, enterostomy or cecostomy, tube open (eg, for feeding or decompression) (separate procedure)

(Do not report **44300** in conjunction with **44701** for cannulation of the colon for intraoperative colonic lavage)

(For percutaneous placement of duodenostomy, jejunostomy, gastro-jejunostomy or cecostomy [or other colonic] tube including fluoroscopic imaging guidance, see **49441–49442**)

+44701 Intraoperative colonic lavage (List separately in addition to code for primary procedure)

(Use **44701** in conjunction with **44140, 44145, 44150**, or **44604** as appropriate)

(Do not report **44701** in conjunction with **44950–44960**)

Genitourinary System Procedures

Lysis/Excision of Labial or Penile Adhesions

54450 Foreskin manipulation including lysis of preputial adhesions and stretching

54162 Lysis or excision of penile post-circumcision adhesions

56441 Lysis of labial adhesions

If lysis of labial or penile adhesions is performed by the application of manual pressure without the use of an instrument to cut the adhesions, it would be considered part of the E/M visit and not reported separately.

Code **54450** does not require general anesthesia. It has an RVU of 2.00 when performed in a non-facility setting (eg, office). Medicare has assigned it a 0-day global surgery period. This procedure is performed on the uncircumcised foreskin and the head of the penis. Adhesions are broken by stretching the foreskin back over the head of the penis onto the shaft or by inserting a clamp between the foreskin and the head of the penis and spreading the jaws of the clamp.

Code **54162** is only reported when lysis is performed under general anesthesia or regional block, with an instrument, and under sterile conditions. This code has an RVU of 7.31 when performed in a non-facility setting (eg, office) and a Medicare 10-day global surgery period, which payers may or may not use. If post-circumcision adhesions are manually broken during the postoperative period by the physician or physician of the same group and specialty who performed the procedure, it would be considered part of the global surgical package. Report the service with *ICD-10-CM* code **N47.0**, adherent prepuce in a newborn, or **N47.5**, adhesions of prepuce and glans penis (patients older than 28 days).

Code **56441** is performed by using a blunt instrument or scissors under general or local anesthesia. The total RVUs for this procedure in a non-facility setting are 4.09. This procedure also includes a Medicare 10-day global surgery period, which may or may not be used by payers. *ICD-10-CM* code **Q52.5** (fusion of labia) would be reported with *CPT* code **56441**. When provided without anesthesia, modifier **52** may be appended to indicate reduced services. Payer guidance may vary with regard to use of modifier **52**.

Anogenital Examination

99170 Anogenital examination, magnified, in childhood for suspected trauma including image recording when performed

Moderate sedation may be separately reported when performed by the same physician performing the anogenital examination. Moderate sedation service of less than 10 minutes of intraservice time is not separately reported.

Example

➤ **A 6-year-old girl is brought to the ED by her mother after the mother noted blood in the child's underpants and was concerned about sexual molestation.** The physician performs a comprehensive history and physical examination. Because of the findings on general examination, the physician elects to further examine the child's genitalia with magnification to document findings that may be consistent with abuse or trauma.

ICD-10-CM	CPT®
Report confirmed abuse with **T74.22XA** (child sexual abuse, confirmed, initial encounter); an appropriate injury code (eg, **S39.848A**, other specified injuries of external genitals, initial encounter); a code from categories **X92–Y06** or **Y08** for assault; and a code from category **Y07** to identify the perpetrator of assault. If abuse is suspected but not confirmed, report **T76.22XA** (child sexual abuse, suspected, initial encounter) and a code for injury. If there are no findings, report **Z04.42** (encounter for examination and observation following alleged child rape or sexual abuse).	**99285** (comprehensive ED examination) **99170** (anogenital examination) If the same physician performs moderate (conscious) sedation, also report code **99152**. See more on moderate sedation in the Sedation section, which follows.

Sedation

Moderate Sedation

Moderate sedation codes **99151–99153** and **99155–99157** are used for reporting moderate sedation when intraservice time is 10 minutes or more. **Table 15-6** contains sedation codes and descriptors.

Moderate sedation is a drug-induced depression of consciousness. No interventions are required to maintain cardiovascular functions or a patent airway, and spontaneous ventilation is adequate. Moderate sedation codes are not used to report administration of medications for pain control, minimal sedation (anxiolysis), deep sedation, or monitored anesthesia care (**00100–01999**).

Moderate sedation in the office or outpatient setting is typically performed by the same physician or QHP who is performing the diagnostic or therapeutic service and requires the presence of an independent trained observer. An *independent trained observer* is an individual qualified to monitor the patient during the procedure but who has no other duties (eg, assisting at surgery) during the procedure. In the facility setting, a physician or QHP other than the person performing the diagnostic or therapeutic service may provide moderate sedation services.

Codes **99151**, **99152**, and **99153** are reported when

❋ The administration of moderate sedation is provided by the physician who is simultaneously performing a procedure (eg, fracture reduction, vessel cutdown, central line placement, wound repair).

❋ An independent trained observer is present to assist the physician in the monitoring of the patient during the procedure or diagnostic service.

Codes **99155**, **99156**, and **99157** are reported when

❋ A second physician or QHP other than the health care professional performing the diagnostic or therapeutic services provides moderate sedation.

❋ Codes **99153–99157** are reported for each additional 15 minutes of intraservice time. The midpoint between the end of the previous 15-minute period must be passed to report an additional unit of intraservice time (ie, intraservice time must continue for at least 8 minutes beyond the last full 15 minutes of intraservice time).

Note: Documentation must include the description of the procedure, name and dosage(s) of the sedation agent(s), route of administration of the sedation agent(s), and who administered the agent (physician or independent observer); the ongoing assessment of the child's level of consciousness and physiological status (eg, heart rate, oxygen saturation levels) during and after the procedure; and the presence, name, and title of the independent observer and total time from administration of the sedation agent(s) (start time) until the physician's face-to-face service is no longer required (end time).

- Codes are selected based on intraservice time. Intraservice time
  - Begins with the administration of the sedating agent(s)
  - Ends when the procedure is completed, the patient is stable for recovery status, and the physician or other QHP providing the sedation ends personal continuous face-to-face time with the patient
  - Includes ordering and/or administering the initial and subsequent doses of sedating agents
  - Requires continuous face-to-face attendance of the physician or other QHP
  - Requires monitoring patient response to the sedating agents, including
    - Periodic assessment of the patient
    - Further administration of agent(s) as needed to maintain sedation
    - Monitoring of oxygen saturation, heart rate, and blood pressure
- Moderate sedation service of less than 10 minutes intraservice time is not separately reported.
- Preservice work of moderate sedation services is not separately reported and not included in intraservice time. Preservice work includes
  - Assessment of the patient's past medical and surgical history with particular emphasis on cardiovascular, pulmonary, airway, or neurologic conditions
  - Review of the patient's previous experiences with anesthesia and/or sedation
  - Family history of sedation complications
  - Summary of the patient's present medication list
  - Drug allergy and intolerance history
  - Focused physical examination of the patient, with emphasis on
    - Mouth, jaw, oropharynx, neck, and airway for Mallampati score assessment
    - Chest and lungs
    - Heart and circulation
    - Vital signs, including heart rate, respiratory rate, blood pressure, and oxygenation, with end-tidal carbon dioxide when indicated
  - Review of any pre-sedation diagnostic tests
  - Completion of a pre-sedation assessment form (with American Society of Anesthesiologists [ASA] physical status classification)
  - Patient informed consent
  - Immediate pre-sedation assessment prior to first sedating doses
  - Initiation of IV access and fluids to maintain patency
- Do not separately report or include the time of post-service work in the intraservice time. Post-service work of moderate sedation includes
  - Assessment of the patient's vital signs, level of consciousness, neurologic, cardiovascular, and pulmonary stability in the post-sedation recovery period
  - Assessment of patient's readiness for discharge following the procedure
  - Preparation of documentation for sedation service
  - Communication with family or caregiver about sedation service
- Oxygen saturation (**94760–94762**) cannot be reported separately.
- Codes **99151–99157** are distinguished by service provider, patient age, and time spent (see **Table 15-6**).
- If a medically necessary, significant, and separately identifiable E/M service had also been performed, an E/M visit with modifier **25** appended could be reported.
- The agent itself may also be reported.

Table 15-6. Moderate Sedation		
Moderate Sedation	**First 10–22 Minutes of Intraservice Time**	**Each Additional 15 Minutes of Intraservice Time**
Moderate sedation services provided by the same physician or other qualified health care professional performing the diagnostic or therapeutic service that the sedation supports, requiring the presence of an independent trained observer to assist in the monitoring of the patient's level of consciousness and physiological status; initial 15 minutes of intra-service time, patient younger than 5 years of age	99151	+99153
5 years or older	99152	+99153
Moderate sedation services (other than those services described by codes 00100–01999) provided by a physician other than the health care professional performing the diagnostic or therapeutic service that the sedation supports; younger than 5 years	99155	+99157
5 years or older	99156	+99157

Examples

➤ **A 24-month-old requires a layered closure of a 2.5-cm laceration of the right knee.** Moderate sedation is required and is performed by the Pediatric Advanced Life Support–trained physician with an independent trained observer who has been trained in pediatric basic life support. The physician supervises the administration of the sedating agent and assesses the child until an effective, safe level of sedation is achieved and continues to assess the child's level of consciousness and physiological status while also performing the laceration repair. The procedure, from the time of administration of the agent until the physician completes the repair and determines the child is stable and face-to-face physician time is no longer required, takes a total of 28 minutes.

ICD-10-CM	*CPT®*
S81.011A (laceration without foreign body, right knee, initial encounter) Codes for external cause, activity, and place of injury are reported when documented.	**12031** (intermediate repair of wound of extremities, 2.5 cm or less) **99151** (moderate [conscious] sedation, patient younger than 5 years, first 15 minutes) **+99153** (moderate [conscious] sedation, each additional 15 minutes of intraservice time)

➤ **A 5-year-old hospitalized child needs insertion of a tunneled central venous catheter (36558).** A second physician will provide the moderate sedation while the first physician performs the procedure. The sedating physician administers the agent(s) and assesses the patient continuously until a safe level of moderate sedation is achieved. He or she monitors the child closely and administers additional doses of sedating and/or analgesic agent(s) as needed. The service, from the time of administration of the agent until determination that the child is stable and face-to-face physician time is no longer required, takes a total of 35 minutes. The physician providing the moderate sedation will report

ICD-10-CM	*CPT*
Appropriate diagnosis code	**99156** (moderate [conscious] sedation services by second physician or QHP, patient 5 years or older, first 15 minutes) **+99157** (moderate [conscious] sedation, each additional 15 minutes of intraservice time)

Chapter 15: Common Surgical Procedures and Sedation

Deep Sedation

Deep sedation/analgesia is a drug-induced depression of consciousness during which patients cannot be easily aroused but respond purposefully after repeated verbal or painful stimulation (eg, purposefully pushing away the noxious stimuli). The ability to independently maintain ventilatory function may be impaired. Patients may require assistance in maintaining a patent airway, and spontaneous ventilation may be inadequate. Cardiovascular function is usually maintained. A state of deep sedation may be accompanied by partial or complete loss of protective airway reflexes.

Pediatricians who provide deep sedation services for procedures performed outside the operating suite should follow the same anesthesia policies and coding instructions as other providers of anesthesia services. *Current Procedural Terminology*® codes for reporting anesthesia services, including deep sedation, monitored anesthesia care, or general anesthesia, are **00100–01999**. These codes are not as specific as codes for other services and generally identify a body area or type of procedure.

00102	Anesthesia for procedures involving plastic repair of cleft lip
01820	Anesthesia for all closed procedures on radius, ulna, wrist, or hand bones

Add-on codes may be reported to identify special circumstances that increase the complexity of providing anesthesia care, including

99100	Patient under 1 year or older than 70 years (not reported in conjunction with codes **00326**, **00561**, **00834**, or **00836**)
99116	Anesthesia complicated by total body hypothermia
99135	Anesthesia complicated by controlled hypotension
99140	Emergency conditions

Emergency is defined by *CPT* as a situation in which delay in treatment of the patient would lead to a significant increase in the threat to life or body part.

Modifiers are reported in addition to anesthesia codes to indicate the physical status of the patient. The ASA classification of the patient's physical status is represented by the following HCPCS modifiers:

> ### ~ More From the AAP ~
> For more information on coding for deep sedation services, see articles in the April and May 2014 *AAP Pediatric Coding Newsletter*™ at http://coding. aap.org (subscription required).

P1	Normal healthy patient
P2	Patient with mild systemic disease
P3	Patient with severe systemic disease
P4	Patient with severe systemic disease that is a constant threat to life
P5	Moribund patient who is not expected to survive without the operation
P6	Declared brain-dead patient whose organs are being removed for donor purposes

Other modifiers that may be required by payers for anesthesia services by pediatric physicians are those identifying the type of anesthesia or anesthesia provider.

AA	Anesthesia services performed personally by anesthesiologist
	◉ Payers may require this modifier for services personally rendered by physicians other than anesthesiologists. This signifies that services were not rendered by a nonphysician provider, such as a certified registered nurse anesthetist.
G8	Monitored anesthesia care for deep complex, complicated, or markedly invasive surgical procedure
G9	Monitored anesthesia care for patient who has history of severe cardiopulmonary condition
QS	Monitored anesthesia care service
	◉ Medicare considers deep sedation equivalent to monitored anesthesia care. Private payers may vary.
GC	This service has been performed in part by a resident under the direction of a teaching physician

Base units for anesthesia services are published in the ASA *Relative Value Guide* and by the CMS for each anesthesia procedure code. Payers typically do not require reporting of base units on the claim for services.

◉ Many private payers will allow additional base units for physical status modifiers **P3** (1 unit), **P4** (2 units), and **P5** (3 units).

◉ Anesthesia time is reported in minutes unless a payer directs to report units (1 unit per 15 minutes). Start and stop times must be documented, including multiple start and stop times when anesthesia services are discontinuous.

Common Testing and Therapeutic Services

Contents

Chapter 16: Common Testing and Therapeutic Services

Allergy and Clinical Immunology

Allergy Testing

Allergy testing is coded by type of test (percutaneous, immediate type reaction [**95004**], or any combination of percutaneous and intracutaneous, sequential and incremental tests with venoms [**95017**] or with drugs or biologicals [**95018**]) and requires specification of the number of tests applied.

- Codes **95004**, **95017**, **95018**, **95024**, and **95027** include test interpretation and report.
  - Patch and photo patch testing are reported with code **95044–95056**.
  - Specific challenge testing (**95060–95079**) is coded according to target organ (eg, ophthalmic mucous membrane, nasal, inhalation bronchial challenges without pulmonary function testing, ingestion).
  - An evaluation and management (E/M) service should not be reported for interpretation and report. However, if a significant, separately identifiable E/M service is performed and documented, it may be reported with modifier **25** appended to the appropriate E/M code.
  - Nasal cytology, a test for allergy-type cells (eosinophils) or infection-type cells (neutrophils) on a nasal scraping, is reported with code **89190**.
  - Nitric oxide expired gas determination is reported with *Current Procedural Terminology* (*CPT*®) code **95012**. Nitric oxide determination by spectroscopy should be reported with code **94799**.

Allergen Immunotherapy

95115	Professional services for allergen immunotherapy not including provision of allergenic extracts; single injection
95117	2 or more injections
95144	Professional services for the supervision of preparation and provision of antigens for allergen immunotherapy, single-dose vials(s) (specify number of vials)
95145	Professional services for the supervision of the preparation and provision of antigens for allergy immunotherapy (specify number of doses); single stinging insect venom

Allergen Immunotherapy, Extract Provided

Immunotherapy administered by the prescribing physician is listed by number of antigens or venoms and by antigen or venom type.

Administration of Extract Only

- Codes **95115** and **95117** are used to report administration of the allergenic extract only. Code **95115** or **95117** (not both) is reported when another health care professional (eg, the patient's allergist) prepares and supplies the allergenic extract or when a physician (usually an allergist) administers the prospectively prepared extract (ie, prepared with the intent to administer on a planned schedule).
- Codes **95144–95170** are used to report preparation and provision of antigens for allergen immunotherapy without administration of the allergenic extract.
  - Codes **95144–95170** describe the preparation of the antigen, the antigen extract itself, the physician's assessment and determination of the concentration and volume to use based on the patient's history and results of previous skin testing, and the prospective planned schedule of administration of the extract.
  - The number of doses or vials must be specified when reporting these codes.
  - Services may be reported at the time the allergenic extract is prepared because injections occur on later dates (prospectively planned) or may not occur at all.
  - Administration of the allergenic extract is not included.
- Codes **95146–95149** are reported for more than one single stinging venom (eg, code **95146** is reported for 2, **95147** for 3).

Chapter 16: Common Testing and Therapeutic Services

Same Encounter Provision of Allergenic Extract With Administration

- Codes **95120–95134** are reported when the entire service of preparing, providing, and administering (injection) allergenic extract is performed at one patient encounter.

95120   Professional services for allergen immunotherapy in the office or institution of the prescribing physician or other qualified health care professional, including provision of allergenic extract; single injection

95125   2 or more injections

95130   single stinging insect venom

- Codes **95131–95134** are reported for more than one single stinging venom.

95131   2 stinging insect venoms

95132   3 stinging insect venoms

95133   4 stinging insect venoms

95134   5 stinging insect venoms

- Codes **95115** and **95117** *cannot* be reported with codes **95120–95134**.
- *Current Procedural Terminology*® recommends codes **95120–95134** be reported only when specifically required by the payer.
- Codes **95120** and **95125** are reported based on the number of injections administered (ie, a single injection or ≥2 injections). Codes **95130–95134** are reported per injection. Therefore, if 2 separate injections of 2 stinging insect venoms (eg, wasp and bee) are provided, code **95131** would be reported 2 times.
- An appropriate office/outpatient code may be reported with allergen immunotherapy codes. Modifier **25** is appended to the E/M service when it is performed and documented.
- For rapid desensitization per hour, see code **95180**.

Examples

➤ **An allergist prepares a 10-dose vial of allergen extract and administers 1 dose at the time of the visit (allergenic extract was prepared with the intent to administer on a planned schedule).**

The allergist will report code **95165** with 10 units of service and **95115** with 1 unit of service and the specific diagnosis code. Allergic rhinitis due to pollen would be reported with *International Classification of Diseases, 10th Revision, Clinical Modification* (ICD-10-CM) code **J30.1** or, if due to food, code **J30.5**.

➤ **The patient has a reaction to the allergenic extract. The physician injects epinephrine using an auto-injector device (eg, EpiPen Jr).**

The injection using an auto-injection device would be reported as an intramuscular injection with code **96372**. Although code **J0171** is used to report provision of epinephrine, the auto-injector is not described by this code. Prior to claim submission, it is advisable to verify payer policy addressing submission of code **J0171** (epinephrine 0.01 mg) versus **J3490** (unspecified drug) with the product National Drug Code (NDC) to specify the exact product provided. (See the HCPCS Codes section later in this chapter for more information on NDCs.)

➤ **The pediatrician administers 3 injections of allergen extract for a patient with allergic rhinitis due to pollen. The extract was prepared and supplied by the allergist.**

The pediatrician will report code **95117** with *ICD-10-CM* code **J30.1**.

Coding Conundrum: CMS Allergen Immunotherapy Guidelines

The Centers for Medicare & Medicaid Services (CMS) Medicare program will only accept codes **95115**, **95117**, and **95144–95170** and will not allow payment for codes **95120–95134**. State Medicaid and commercial payers may follow the CMS Medicare guidelines or may have their own established guidelines. Therefore, before reporting these services, research the reporting policies of your major payers.

Immune Globulins

When reporting codes **90281–90399**, remember that they are only for the cost of the immunoglobulin and the appropriate separate administration code should also be reported (eg, **96372**, **96374**). A significant, separately identifiable E/M service performed during the same visit may also be billed if indicated. *ICD-10-CM* diagnosis codes to support immunoglobulin services include codes from categories **D80–D84** for certain disorders involving the immune mechanism or codes for specific conditions, such as mucocutaneous lymph node syndrome (**M30.3**).

> When reporting administration of immune globulin, report the diagnosis code for the condition for which immune globulin administration is performed (eg, pulmonary hypertension, exposure to disease).

Note: This information does not apply to immunization services. Immunization services and vaccines are discussed in length in Chapter 6, Preventive Services.

Example

➤ **An infant with moderate pulmonary hypertension is seen for administration of the second of 5 monthly doses of palivizumab.** A nurse administers the immunoglobulin under direct physician supervision.

Code **96372** (intramuscular injection) is reported in addition to code **90378** (respiratory syncytial virus, monoclonal antibody, recombinant, for intramuscular use, 50 mg, each). The appropriate number of units reported for the dose given is 1 unit per 50 mg. The NDC for each vial should be included on claims for most payers. (See the HCPCS Codes section later in this chapter for more on NDC reporting.)

Blood Sampling for Diagnostic Study

Venipuncture

36400	Venipuncture, younger than age 3 years, necessitating the skill of a physician or other qualified health care professional, not to be used for routine venipuncture; femoral or jugular vein
36405	scalp vein
36406	other vein
36410	Venipuncture, age 3 years or older, necessitating the skill of a physician or other qualified health care professional (separate procedure), for diagnostic or therapeutic purposes (not to be used for routine venipuncture)
36415	Collection of venous blood by venipuncture
36416	Collection of capillary blood specimen (eg, finger, heel, ear stick)
36591	Collection of blood specimen from a completely implantable venous access device

Codes **36415** and **36416** are used for any age child when the physician is not needed to perform the procedure.

☀ When a physician's skill is required to perform venipuncture (eg, access is too difficult for other staff to attain) on a child younger than 3 years, codes **36400–36406** are reported based on the anatomic site of the venipuncture. Report code **36400** when performed on the femoral or jugular vein, code **36405** when performed on the scalp vein, or code **36406** when another vein is accessed.

☀ When a physician's skill is required to perform venipuncture on a child 3 years and older, code **36410** is reported.

❖ If the physician performs the venipuncture as a convenience or because staff is not trained in the procedure, code **36415** is reported because the physician's skill was not required.

❖ Although typically not required, some payers will require that modifier **25** be appended to the E/M code if an E/M service is reported on the same day of service.

||||||||| *Coding Pearl* |||||||||

Report code **36415** when the physician performs a venipuncture as a convenience.

❋ It is not appropriate to report *CPT*® code **99211** along with code **36415** if the nurse only collects the blood specimen and no medically necessary and separately identified E/M service is provided.

❋ Code **36591** (collection of blood specimen from a completely implantable venous access device) is reported only when in conjunction with a laboratory service.

Other Percutaneous Vessel

36510 Catheterization of umbilical vein for diagnosis or therapy, newborn

36660 Catheterization, umbilical artery, newborn, for diagnosis or therapy

Catheterization of the umbilical vein will be reported with code **36510**; catheterization of the umbilical artery is reported with code **36660**.

Arterial access

36600 Arterial puncture, withdrawal of blood for diagnosis

36620 Arterial catheterization or cannulation for sampling, monitoring or transfusion (separate procedure); percutaneous

36625   cutdown

❋ An arterial puncture for diagnosis is reported with code **36600**.

❋ Code **36620** is reported when a percutaneous peripheral arterial catheterization is performed.

❋ Code **36625** is reported when a cutdown is performed.

Bone Marrow Aspiration and/or Biopsy

▲**38220** Diagnostic bone marrow; aspiration(s) only

▲**38221**   biopsy(ies)

(Do not report **38221** in conjunction with **38220**)

(For diagnostic bone marrow biopsy[ies] and aspiration[s] performed at the same session, use **38222**)

●**38222**   biopsy(ies) and aspiration(s)

To clarify that codes **38220** and **38221** (bone marrow aspiration and biopsy) represent diagnostic services, these codes are revised in 2018. In addition, new code **38222** is added for reporting biopsy and aspiration at the same encounter. Parenthetical instructions are revised and/or added following all codes for diagnostic and therapeutic biopsy or aspiration to direct to appropriate codes for each.

❋ Codes **38220** and **38221** are not reported for services at the same encounter. Report code **38222** in lieu of the individual codes.

❋ Do not report **38222** in conjunction with **38220** and **38221**.

❋ For bilateral procedure, report **38220**, **38221**, **38222** with modifier **50**.

❋ For bone marrow biopsy interpretation, use code **88305**.

❋ For aspiration of bone marrow for bone graft, spine surgery only, use **20939**.

❋ Bone marrow aspiration(s) for platelet rich stem cell injection is reported with Category III code **0232T**.

Specimen Handling

99000 Handling and/or conveyance of specimen for transfer from the office to a laboratory

99001 Handling and/or conveyance of specimen for transfer from the patient in other than an office to a laboratory (distance may be indicated)

❋ Codes **99000** and **99001** are used to report packaging and sending medical specimens (eg, blood, throat swabs, urine specimens, stool samples) to an off-site laboratory.

❋ Code **99000** may be reported for each specimen for which the practice incurs costs in the handling and/or transportation.

Respiratory Tests and Treatments

Pulmonary Function Tests

National Correct Coding Initiative (NCCI) edits exist between office-based E/M services and all pulmonology services (**94010–94799**). Append modifier **25** to the E/M service as appropriate when also reporting a pulmonology service on the same claim. Refer to Chapter 3, Modifiers and Coding Edits, for more information on coding edits.

There is no code for peak flow analysis. It is considered part of the E/M service and/or a component of pulmonary function testing.

❋ Codes include laboratory procedure(s) and interpretation of test results. If a separately identifiable E/M service is performed, the appropriate E/M service code may also be reported.

❋ When spirometry is performed before and after administration of a bronchodilator, report code **94060** (bronchodilation responsiveness, spirometry as in **94010**, pre- and post-bronchodilator administration) only. Code **94640** (nebulizer treatment) is inherent to (ie, included as part of) code **94060**. Code for supplies and medication separately as appropriate.

❋ Measurement of vital capacity (**94150**) is a component of spirometry and is only reported when performed alone.

❋ Measurement of spirometric forced expiratory flows in an infant or child through 2 years of age is reported with code **94011**.

❋ Code **94012** is used to report measurement of bronchodilation spirometric forced expiratory flows (before and after bronchodilator) in an infant or child.

❋ Code **94013** is used to report measurement of lung volumes (eg, functional residual capacity, expiratory reserve volume, forced vital capacity) in an infant or child through 2 years of age.

❋ Report pulse oximetry (**94760** [noninvasive ear or pulse oximetry for oxygen saturation; single determination] and **94761** [multiple determinations]) because *CPT*® guidelines allow reporting the services, services may be paid if they are the only service received (according to the NCCI), some payers do allow payment, and a practice needs to be aware of all services that are performed and monitor associated costs. See Chapter 3, Modifiers and Coding Edits, for a detailed explanation of NCCI edits.

> ||||||| **Coding Pearl** |||||||
>
> *CPT* code **94060** includes spirometry and pre- and post-bronchodilation. Do not report code **94060** with **94010** or **94640** when they are a component of code **94060**.

Inhalation

94640 Pressurized or nonpressurized inhalation treatment for acute airway obstruction for therapeutic purposes and/or for diagnostic purposes such as sputum induction with an aerosol generator, nebulizer, metered dose inhaler (MDI) or intermittent positive pressure breathing (IPPB) device

94644 Continuous inhalation treatment with aerosol medication for acute airway obstruction; first hour
(For services of less than 1 hour, use **94640**)

+94645 each additional hour (List separately in addition to code for primary procedure)

Report **94640**

❋ When treatment such as aerosol generator, nebulizer, MDI, or IPPB device is administered.

❋ With modifier **76** (repeat procedure) with the number of units when more than one treatment is given on a date of service. Some payers require reporting with the number of units only and no modifier. Follow payer guidelines for reporting these services.

❋ When any treatment of less than 30 minutes is performed.

At the time of publication, NCCI edit policy does not allow for code **94640** to be reported more than once per patient encounter. The American Academy of Pediatrics (AAP) is working with NCCI edit staff to change this policy.

Report codes **94644** and **94645** when

⊛ A treatment lasts 31 minutes or longer.

⊛ The total time spent in the provision of continuous inhalation treatments is documented in the medical record.

Codes **94644** and **94645** are not reported by physicians when services are provided in a facility setting because no physician work value is assigned to these codes.

Report code **94664** (demonstration and/or evaluation of patient utilization of an aerosol generator, nebulizer, MDI, or IPPB device) when an initial or subsequent demonstration and/or evaluation is performed and documented. This code is intended to be reported only once per day.

Note that peak flow analysis and administration of oxygen do not have *CPT*® codes. They are inherent to E/M services.

Examples

➤ **A 6-year-old established patient with asthma arrives to the office in acute exacerbation.** Pulse oximetry is performed and one nebulizer treatment given via a small-volume nebulizer (SVN); physical examination after first treatment shows decreased wheezing and work of breathing. The nurse documents her evaluation of use and education for home use of the MDI. An order is written for continuing treatments at home, evaluation and education in use of MDI, and return to the office as needed. Later the same day, the patient returns, again in acute exacerbation. A second nebulizer treatment is given by SVN. Physical examination after the second treatment shows no improvement and the patient is hypoxic. He is sent to the hospital to be admitted to observation by the hospitalist. Diagnosis is acute exacerbation of mild persistent asthma with hypoxemia.

ICD-10-CM	CPT
J45.31 (mild persistent asthma with acute exacerbation) **R09.02** (hypoxemia)	**99212–99215 25** (office/outpatient E/M, established patient) **94640 76** × 2 units or **94640** × 2 (nebulizer treatments × 2) **94664 59** (MDI demonstration) Medication (See HCPCS codes listed in **Table 16-1**.) **94760** (pulse oximetry)

Teaching Point: Modifier **59** appended to **94664** indicates the MDI demonstration is reported in addition to nebulizer treatments provided via a different device. See the Coding Conundrum: Reporting **94664** With **94640** box for more information.

➤ A 12-year-old with severe exacerbation of mild persistent asthma is seen in the physician's office. The patient is placed on continuous bronchodilator therapy for an hour and a half. The patient is monitored closely during the procedure. Medical record documentation supports the total time of the treatment and frequent assessments.

ICD-10-CM	CPT
J45.31	**99212–99215 25** (office/outpatient E/M, established patient) **94644** (continuous inhalation treatment with aerosol medication for acute airway obstruction; first hour) **94645** (each additional hour) Medication (See HCPCS codes listed in **Table 16-1**.)

Table 16-1. Common J Codes

Inhalation Solution	Brand Name[a]	J Code	Administration
Albuterol, inhalation solution, FDA-approved final product, noncompounded, administered through DME, concentrated form, 1 mg	Proventil, Ventolin	J7611	94640 or 94644 (for first hour)
Levalbuterol, inhalation solution, FDA-approved final product, noncompounded, administered through DME, concentrated form, 0.5 mg	Xopenex	J7612	94640 or 94644 (for first hour)
Albuterol, inhalation solution, FDA-approved final product, noncompounded, administered through DME, unit dose, 1 mg	AccuNeb, Proventil, Ventolin	J7613	94640 or 94644 (for first hour)
Levalbuterol, inhalation solution, FDA-approved final product, noncompounded, administered through DME, unit dose, 0.5 mg	Xopenex	J7614	94640 or 94644 (for first hour)
Levalbuterol, inhalation solution, compounded, administered through DME, unit dose, 0.5 mg	Levalbuterol HCl	J7615	94640 or 94644 (for first hour)
Albuterol, up to 2.5 mg, and ipratropium bromide, up to 0.5 mg, FDA-approved final product, noncompounded, administered through DME	Albuterol, DuoNeb, Ipratropium bromide	J7620	94640 or 94644 (for first hour)
Budesonide, inhalation solution, FDA-approved final product, noncompounded, administered through DME, unit dose form, up to 0.5 mg	Pulmicort	J7626	94640 or 94644 (for first hour)
Budesonide, inhalation solution, compounded product, administered through DME, unit dose form, up to 0.5 mg	Pulmicort Respules	J7627	94640 or 94644 (for first hour)
Epinephrine, 0.1 mg	Adrenalin chloride Sus-Phrine	J0171	96372
Ampicillin, 500 mg	Omnipen-N Totacillin-N	J0290	96372 (IM) (IV)[b]
Atropine sulfate, 0.01 mg	AtroPen	J0461	96372
Penicillin G benzathine and penicillin G procaine, 100,000 units	Bicillin CR	J0558	96372
Penicillin G benzathine, 100,000 units	Bicillin LA	J0561	96372
Ceftriaxone, per 250 mg	Rocephin	J0696	96372 (IM) (IV)[b]
Cefotaxime, per gram	Claforan	J0698	96372 (IM) (IV)[b]
Betamethasone acetate, 3 mg, and betamethasone sodium phosphate, 3 mg	Celestone Soluspan	J0702	96372
Dexamethasone acetate, 1 mg	Decadron LA	J1094	96372
Dexamethasone sodium phosphate, 1 mg	Decadron	J1100	96372 (IM) (IV)[b]
Phenytoin sodium, per 50 mg	Dilantin	J1165	96374
Diphenhydramine HCl, up to 50 mg	Benadryl	J1200	96372
Gamma globulin, IM, 1 cc	Gammar	J1460	96372
Gamma globulin, IM, more than 10 cc	Gamastan	J1560	

Chapter 16: Common Testing and Therapeutic Services

Table 16-1. Common J Codes (*continued*)

Inhalation Solution	Brand Name[a]	J Code	Administration
Immunoglobulin, 500 mg	Gammar-IV	J1566	96374
Gentamicin, up to 80 mg	Garamycin	J1580	96372 (IM) (IV)[b]
Glucagon, per 1 mg	GlucaGen	J1610	96374
Heparin sodium (heparin lock flush), per 10 units	Hep-Lock	J1642	96374
Hydrocortisone sodium succinate, up to 100 mg	Solu-Cortef	J1720	96374
Promethazine HCI, up to 50 mg	Phenergan	J2550	96372
Other	**Brand Name**[a]	**J Code**	**Administration**
Dexamethasone, oral, 0.25 mg	Decadron	J8540	None
Antiemetic drug, rectal/suppository, not otherwise specified	Phenergan	J8498	None

Abbreviations: DME, durable medical equipment; FDA, US Food and Drug Administration; HCPCS, Healthcare Common Procedure Coding System; IM, intramuscular; IV, intravenous.

[a] Brand names are furnished for identification purposes only. No endorsement of the manufacturers or products is implied.

[b] For IV administration codes, see **Table 15-5**.

The 2018 HCPCS codes were released subsequent to the publication of this book. Refer to www.aap.org/cfp for HCPCS updates.

Coding Conundrum: Reporting 94664 With 94640

When the physician or nurse (of the same group and specialty) performs demonstration and/or evaluation of patient use of a nebulizer (**94664**) on the same day as a nebulizer treatment (**94640**), modifier **59** (distinct procedural service) should be appended to code **94664** to indicate to the payer that the services were separate and distinct and that both were clinically indicated. Per the 2017 Medicaid NCCI manual, the demonstration and/or evaluation described by code **94664** is included in code **94640** if it utilizes the same device (eg, aerosol generator) that is used in the performance of *CPT*® code **94640**. The NCCI edits pair code **94664** with **94640** but allow an override of the edit with modifier **59** when the services are indicated. However, as currently written, some payers may not allow the use of modifier **59** in this instance because the 2 services did not occur at separate encounters. Check with your Medicaid payers.

Modifier **25** should be appended to the E/M service to signify a separately identifiable service. All services must be documented in the medical record as significant, separately identifiable, and medically necessary.

Neonatal Car Seat/Bed Testing for Airway Integrity

94780	Car seat/bed testing for airway integrity, neonate, with continual nursing observation and continuous recording of pulse oximetry, heart rate, and respiratory rate, with interpretation and report; 60 minutes
+94781	each additional full 30 minutes (List separately in addition to code for primary procedure.)

Pediatric Home Apnea Monitoring

94772	Circadian respiratory pattern recording (pediatric pneumogram), 12-24 hour continuous recording, infant
94774	Pediatric home apnea monitoring event recording including respiratory rate, pattern and heart rate per 30-day period of time; includes monitor attachment, download of data, review, interpretation, and preparation of a report by a physician or other qualified health care professional
94775	monitor attachment only (includes hook-up, initiation of recording and disconnection)

| 94776 | monitoring, download of information, receipt of transmission(s) and analyses by computer only |
| 94777 | review, interpretation and preparation of report only by a physician or other qualified health care professional |

- ☀ Report code **94772** when circadian respiratory pattern recording (pediatric pneumogram), 12- to 24-hour continuous recording, is performed on an infant.
- ☀ Codes **94774–94777** are reported once per 30-day period.
- ☀ Codes **94774** and **94777** are reported by the physician.
  - ❖ Code **94774** is reported by the physician when he or she orders home monitoring, chooses the monitor limits, and arranges for a home health care provider to teach the parents. It includes reviewing and interpreting data and preparation of the report.
  - ❖ Code **94777** is reported when the physician receives the downloaded information on disc or hard copy, reviews the patterns and periods of abnormal respiratory or heart rate, and summarizes, in a written report, the findings and recommendations for continuation or discontinuation of monitoring. This information is provided to the primary care physician and/or the family.
- ☀ Codes **94775** and **94776** are reported by the home health agency because there is no physician work involved.
  - ❖ Code **94775** is reported by the home health agency and includes connecting the child to the monitoring equipment, teaching the family how to connect and disconnect the leads, checking the proper function of the equipment, responding to alarms, and resetting the monitor.
  - ❖ Code **94776** is reported when the monitor is downloaded by the home health care agency and converted to a hard copy or CD-ROM and provided to the interpreting physician.
  - ❖ Codes **94774–94777** are not reported in conjunction with codes **93224–93272** (electrocardiographic monitoring). The apnea recording device cannot be reported separately. When oxygen saturation monitoring is used in addition to heart rate and respiratory monitoring, it is not reported separately.

Example

➤ **An infant born at 23 weeks' gestation, now 2 months old, has chronic lung disease and requires prolonged low-flow oxygen.** She continues to have occasional episodes of self-stimulated apnea lasting less than 15 seconds. Her physicians and parents are concerned about the possibility of unwitnessed prolonged apnea requiring intervention but agree to have her go home with heart rate and respiratory monitoring during unattended periods and sleep. The physician orders the monitor, contacts the home health agency for its provision, and instructs the home health agency to teach the parents about cardiopulmonary resuscitation, proper attachment of the monitor leads, and resetting of the monitor. The home health agency provides the physician with the downloaded recordings. The first month's data are interpreted by the physician and a written report generated. The physician counsels the parents about the need to continue monitoring.

Report code **94774** and the appropriate *ICD-10-CM* code (eg, **G47.35** for congenital central alveolar hypoventilation/hypoxemia).

In subsequent months, the physician receives the downloaded recordings, interprets them, and generates reports with recommendations for continued or discontinuation of monitoring. These services are reported with code **94777**.

Ventilation Assist and Management

94002	Ventilation assist and management, initiation of pressure or volume preset ventilators for assisted or controlled breathing; hospital inpatient/observation, initial day
94003	hospital inpatient/observation, each subsequent day
94004	nursing facility, per day
94005	Home ventilator management care plan oversight of a patient (patient not present) in home, domiciliary or rest home (eg, assisted living) requiring review of status, review of laboratories and other studies and revision of orders and respiratory care plan (as appropriate), within a calendar month, 30 minutes or more

Chapter 16: Common Testing and Therapeutic Services

- Ventilation assist and management, with initiation of pressure or volume preset ventilators for assisted or controlled breathing, is reported based on the location of the service and whether performed on an initial or subsequent day of service.
- When performed in the hospital or observation setting, report code **94002** for the initial day of care and code **94003** for subsequent day of care.
- Report code **94004** for the initial or subsequent daily care provided in the nursing home.
- Services include determining ventilator settings, establishing a plan of care, and providing ongoing monitoring.
- Ventilator management includes all the E/M services (physical examination, review of the medical record or diagnostic tests performed, counseling the patient and/or parents, coordinating care with other health care professionals, and documenting the medical record) performed by the physician responsible for providing the ventilation management.
  - ❖ Codes **94002–94004** are not reported when performed in conjunction with an E/M service (**99201–99499**).
  - ❖ Concurrent care may be reported by physicians from different practices (usually, but not always, different specialties) when services are medically necessary. Each physician should only submit the diagnosis(es) for which he or she is managing the patient. The diagnosis code reported should reflect the need for the services and the physician's role in the care and management of the patient.
- Code **94005** is used to report home ventilator management care plan oversight. It may only be reported when 30 or more minutes of care plan oversight is provided within a calendar month. See Chapter 8, Managing Chronic and Complex Conditions, for a full description of requirements for reporting care plan oversight services.
- Initiation and management of continuous positive airway pressure (CPAP) is reported with code **94660** (CPAP ventilation, initiation and management); initiation and management of continuous negative pressure ventilation is reported with code **94662**, not codes **94002–94005**.
- Ventilation assist and management is a bundled component of all critical care and neonatal and pediatric intensive care services (codes **99291** and **99292**, **99466–99476**, and **99477–99480**).
- Endotracheal intubation (**31500**) may be reported separately when performed in addition to ventilation assist and management.

Examples

➤ **A 4-year-old is admitted in acute respiratory distress.** The pediatric pulmonologist is called and performs a history and physical examination, reviews the diagnostic study results, counsels the parents, discusses the case with the pediatrician, and initiates ventilator support.

ICD-10-CM	CPT®
J80 (acute respiratory distress syndrome)	**94002** (initial ventilator management)

➤ **A pediatric pulmonologist is providing ventilator management care plan oversight of a 2-year-old with spinal muscular atrophy who is cared for at home.** The patient's pediatrician also provides care plan oversight services to manage the patient's overall health conditions. Each physician maintains a care plan oversight service log that includes documentation of the activities performed and time spent on each activity. The pulmonologist spent 35 minutes providing ventilator management oversight in December. The pediatrician spent 25 minutes providing home care plan oversight services.

The pediatric pulmonologist would report code **94005** for his 35 minutes of oversight services. The pediatrician would report code **99339** (care plan oversight, home, 15–29 minutes). Each physician would report the appropriate ICD-10-CM code(s) for the diagnosis and/or conditions that were treated.

Tip: It may be appropriate for the pediatrician managing the patient's overall health care needs to report care management services (eg, **99490**). Care management services combine time spent by physicians and clinical staff working under physician supervision, giving potential for a higher frequency of reporting. See Chapter 8, Managing Chronic and Complex Conditions, for more information, including required practice capabilities and patient populations.

Hearing Screening and Other Audiologic Function Testing Codes

*(For central auditory function evaluation, see **92620**, **92621**.)*

Audiometric tests require the use of calibrated electronic equipment, recording of results, and a written report with interpretation. Services include testing of both ears. If the test is applied to one ear only, modifier **52** (reduced services) must be appended to the code.

❊ Code **92551** (screening test, pure tone, air only) is used when earphones are placed on the patient and the patient is asked to respond to tones of different pitches and intensities. This is a limited study to identify the presence or absence of a potential hearing problem. Code **92551** is not used to report hearing screenings performed on newborns and infants.

❊ Code **92552** (full pure tone audiometric assessment) is used when earphones are placed on the patient and the patient is asked to respond to tones of different pitches and intensities. The threshold, which is the lowest intensity of the tone that the patient can hear 50% of the time, is recorded for a number of frequencies. Bone thresholds are obtained in a similar manner. Air and bone thresholds (**92553**) may be obtained and compared to differentiate among conductive, sensorineural, or mixed hearing losses.

❊ Code **92558** is reported for evoked otoacoustic emissions, screening (qualitative measurement of distortion product or transient evoked otoacoustic emissions), automated analysis. This is used when the results are obtained automatically. Coverage for this is typically limited to newborn screening, including follow-up newborn screening from a failed screen in the hospital and screening on younger children. Check with your payers, however.

❊ Code **92583** (select picture audiometry) is typically used for younger children. The patient is asked to identify different pictures with the instructions given at different intensity levels.

❊ Auditory evoked potentials for evoked response audiometry and/or testing of the central nervous system, comprehensive, is reported with code **92585**. A limited study is reported with code **92586**.

❊ Distortion product evoked otoacoustic emissions codes are reported based on the number of frequencies used. Code **92587** is used to report testing for confirmation of the presence or absence of a hearing disorder, 3 to 6 frequencies. Code **92588** is reported when a comprehensive (quantitative analysis of outer hair cell function by cochlear mapping) diagnostic evaluation with a minimum of 12 frequencies is performed. A written interpretation and report are required. Do not report these codes for automated analysis.

❊ Other commonly performed procedures include codes **92567** (tympanometry [impedance testing]) and **92568** (acoustic reflex testing, threshold portion). Code **92550** is reported when tympanometry and reflex threshold measurements are performed.

❊ Category III codes for optical coherence tomography of the middle ear with interpretation and report are added to *CPT®* in 2018. Report procedures as unilateral (**0485T**) or bilateral (**0486T**).

> |||||||||| **Coding Pearl** ||||||||||
>
> Automated audiometry testing is reported with Category III codes **0208T–0212T**. See Chapter 1, New and Revised *CPT®* Codes for 2018, for a listing of these codes.

Example

➤ A 3-year-old with bilateral acute recurrent otitis media undergoes optical coherence tomography of the middle ears to evaluate the presence and purulence of effusion in the middle ears. After sufficient images are collected and areas of interest identified, a printout of selected data is obtained and reviewed by the physician or other qualified health care professional (QHP), who creates a report of the findings. Diagnosis is bilateral acute recurrent otitis media with effusion.

ICD-10-CM	CPT
H66.006 (acute suppurative otitis media without spontaneous rupture of ear drum, recurrent, bilateral)	**0486T** (Optical coherence tomography [OCT] of middle ear, with interpretation and report; bilateral)

Chapter 16: Common Testing and Therapeutic Services

Teaching Point: If a unilateral procedure were performed, code **0485T** would be reported in lieu of **0486T**. Note that the printout produced in testing is not the physician or QHP interpretation and report but provides information for the interpretation and report.

Central Nervous System Services

Assessment Tests/Developmental Services Codes

96110 Developmental screening (eg, developmental milestone survey, speech and language delay screen), with scoring and documentation, per standardized instrument

96111 Developmental testing, (includes assessment of motor, language, social, adaptive, and/or cognitive functioning by standardized developmental instruments) with interpretation and report

96120 Neuropsychological testing [eg, Wisconsin Card Sorting Test], administered by a computer, with QHP interpretation and report

96125 Standardized cognitive performance testing (eg, Ross Information Processing Assessment) per hour of a qualified health care professional's time, both face-to-face time administering tests to the patient and time interpreting these test results and preparing the report

96127 Brief emotional/behavioral assessment (eg, depression inventory, attention-deficit/hyperactivity disorder [ADHD] scale), with scoring and documentation, per standardized instrument

96160 Administration of patient-focused health risk assessment instrument (eg, health hazard appraisal) with scoring and documentation, per standardized instrument

96161 Administration of caregiver-focused health risk assessment instrument (eg, depression inventory) for the benefit of the patient, with scoring and documentation, per standardized instrument

Standardized (ie, validated) screening instruments are used for testing and screening purposes as reported by codes **96110**, **96111**, and **96127**. Examples of assessment and screening tools by code are available in Appendix I. Health risk assessments that are patient-focused (**96160**) are differentiated from those such as maternal depression screening that are caregiver-focused (**96161**) for the benefit of the patient.

Code **96110**

* Is reported for standardized developmental screening instruments. It is not reported when the pediatrician conducts an informal survey or surveillance of development as part of a comprehensive preventive medicine service (which is considered to be part of the history and is not separately billed).
* May be reported for each standardized developmental screening instrument administered.
* Includes standardized screening tools, such as the Ages & Stages Questionnaire, Australian Scale for Asperger's Syndrome, Modified Checklist for Autism in Toddlers, or Parents' Evaluation of Developmental Status (PEDS). Other tools are also used for developmental screening.
* Is not reported for brief emotional or behavioral assessment; see code **96127**.

Code **96111**

* Is used by pediatricians with a special interest or special training in developmental and behavioral pediatrics.
* Allows reporting of developmental testing in which the child is observed doing standardized tasks that are then scored, with interpretation and report.
* Includes assessment of motor, language, social, adaptive, and/or cognitive function by standardized developmental instruments, such as the Bayley Scales of Infant Development.
* When reported in conjunction with an E/M service, the time and effort to perform the developmental testing itself should not count toward the key components (history, physical examination, and medical decision-making) or time for selecting the accompanying E/M code level.
* Medicare NCCI edits pair code **96111** with E/M services but allow both services when modifier **25** is appended to the medically necessary E/M service. See Chapter 3, Modifiers and Coding Edits, for more information on NCCI edits.

> **~ More From the AAP ~**
>
> For more information on coding for central nervous system testing services, see the January 2016 *AAP Pediatric Coding Newsletter*™ at http://coding.aap.org (subscription required).

- For more information on reporting codes **96110** and **96111**, refer to the Developmental Screening/Testing Fact Sheet at www.aap.org/cfp, access code AAPCFP23.

Code **96125** includes standardized cognitive performance testing performed by a QHP (eg, speech-language pathologists, occupational therapists). Note that a minimum of 31 minutes must be provided when reporting the per-hour codes (ie, **96101**, **96116**, **96118**, and **96125**). Services of 30 minutes or less may be reported with modifier **52**. The time reported includes face-to-face time with the patient and time spent interpreting and preparing the report.

Code **96120**

- May be reported for computerized testing requiring a technician's oversight (instructs patient on test procedures, provides access to each ordered test, administers pretest trials, and periodically monitors patient progress)
- Includes physician or other QHP interpretation and report
- Is reported once per session regardless of the number of tests administered

Code **96127**

- Like developmental screening (**96110**), represents the practice expense of administering, scoring, and documenting each standardized instrument. No physician work value is included. Physician interpretation is included in a related E/M service.
- May be used for screening but also for assessment in monitoring treatment efficacy and to support clinical decision-making.
- Not reported in conjunction with **99401–99404**, **96101–96103**, or **96118–96120**.
- Two separate completions (eg, by teacher and parent) of the same form may be separately reported (ie, 2 units of service). When reporting multiple units of service, it is advisable to learn if the payer has specific guidance for reporting as a single line item with the total number of units or requires splitting to multiple claim lines. Medically Unlikely Edits may apply. (See Chapter 3, Modifiers and Coding Edits, for more information on Medically Unlikely Edits.)
- Administration of a brief emotional/behavioral assessment to and about a caregiver for the benefit of a patient (eg, maternal depression) is reported with code **96161**.

Code **96160** is intended for reporting administration of a structured health risk assessment instrument other than those for developmental screening or brief emotional/behavioral assessment.

Code **96161** is used to report administration of a standardized health risk assessment that is focused on the caregiver (eg, screening for maternal depression or caregiver strain index for parents).

Examples

➤ **The mother of a 5-year-old expresses her concern about her child's language delay.** The PEDS (a standardized developmental screening instrument) is ordered, completed by the mother, and scored by the nurse. Results indicate concerns only limited to expressive language delay.

The appropriate E/M service code (preventive medicine visit, new or established patient office visit, or consultation) would be reported in addition to code **96110**. The diagnosis, expressive language disorder, would be reported with *ICD-10-CM* code **F80.1**.

➤ **The mother of an 8-year-old girl expresses concerns about the child daydreaming and not paying attention at school.** The parent version of a behavior assessment system for children is administered to the mother and scored for the physician's review. The physician recommends that an additional behavioral assessment be completed by the girl's teacher to confirm or rule out predominantly inattentive ADHD.

The appropriate E/M service code (preventive medicine visit, new or established patient office visit, or consultation) would be reported in addition to code **96127**. Because the physician did not diagnose ADHD, assign *ICD-10-CM* code **R41.840** for symptoms of attention and concentration deficit.

Chapter 16: Common Testing and Therapeutic Services

➤ **A 10-year-old established patient has shown a progressive pattern of academic struggles since the first grade.** He says the fourth-grade work is "too hard." His parents wonder if he is "lazy" or if he may not be "smart enough." His school psychologist says there is no reason for her to do any psychoeducational testing. The physician administers a Kaufman Brief Intelligence Test, Second Edition, and a Wide Range Achievement Test 4 to briefly assess overall cognitive level and academic achievement levels. The tests are scored, interpreted, and discussed with the family in a 40-minute visit with more than 50% spent in counseling. A concise written report is created for them to take to the school psychologist.

This service is reported with code **99215** (office/outpatient E/M, established patient, based on 40 minutes with more than 50% counseling time) and **96111** (developmental testing, extended). Modifier **25** is appended to the E/M code to signify that it was significant and separately identifiable.

➤ **As part of an established patient preventive health visit for a newborn, the physician directs clinical staff to administer a screening for postpartum depression.** Clinical staff explain the purpose of the instrument to the newborn's mother. After the mother has completed the screening instrument, clinical staff score and document the result in the patient record. The physician completes the preventive medicine service. Included is anticipatory guidance to the mother advising that her screening indicates no current signs of postpartum depression and advising of symptoms that should prompt a call to her physician.

ICD-10-CM	CPT®
Z00.129 (encounter for routine child health examination without abnormal findings) **Z13.89** (encounter for screening for other disorder)	**99391** (preventive medicine visit) **96161** (administration of caregiver-focused health risk assessment [eg, depression inventory] for the benefit of the patient, with scoring and documentation, per standardized instrument)

Teaching Point: The screening for postpartum depression is caregiver-focused (sign/symptoms of depression in mother) but performed in this setting for the benefit of the newborn. This service is reported as a service provided to the newborn with code **96161**. Check payer policy on adoption of code **96161** versus a requirement to report as a service to the mother (ie, to mother's health plan) with code **96127** (brief emotional/behavioral assessment [eg, depression inventory, ADHD scale], with scoring and documentation, per standardized instrument).

Psychological and Neuropsychological Testing

96101 Psychological testing (includes psychodiagnostic assessment of emotionality, intellectual abilities, personality and psychopathology, eg, MMPI, Rorschach, WAIS), per hour of the psychologist's or physician's time, both face-to-face time administering tests to the patient and time interpreting these test results and preparing the report

96102 Psychological testing (includes psychodiagnostic assessment of emotionality, intellectual abilities, personality and psychopathology, eg, MMPI and WAIS), with qualified health care professional interpretation and report, administered by technician, per hour of technician time, face-to-face

96103 Psychological testing (includes psychodiagnostic assessment of emotionality, intellectual abilities, personality and psychopathology, eg, MMPI), administered by a computer, with qualified health care professional interpretation and report

96116 Neurobehavioral status exam (clinical assessment of thinking, reasoning and judgment, eg, acquired knowledge, attention, language, memory, planning and problem solving, and visual spatial abilities), per hour of the psychologist's or physician's time, both face-to-face time with the patient and time interpreting test results and preparing the report

96118 Neuropsychological testing (eg, Halstead-Reitan Neuropsychological Battery, Wechsler Memory Scales and Wisconsin Card Sorting Test), per hour of the psychologist's or physician's time, both face-to-face time administering tests to the patient and time interpreting these test results and preparing the report

96119 Neuropsychological testing (eg, Halstead-Reitan Neuropsychological Battery, Wechsler Memory Scales and Wisconsin Card Sorting Test), with qualified health care professional interpretation and report, administered by technician, per hour of technician time, face-to-face

96120 Neuropsychological testing (eg, Wisconsin Card Sorting Test), administered by a computer, with qualified health care professional interpretation and report

These codes are used to report services provided during testing of the cognitive function of the central nervous system. They include use of standardized instruments to screen for and/or assess cognitive, mental status, speech/language, and other areas of development. A written report is required (or written documentation that is made available to other health care professionals). Although any QHP may report these codes, payers may restrict payment to psychiatrists or other mental health specialists based on the code descriptor and their payment policy for mental health–related services when reported using mental health diagnosis codes.

Note that a minimum of 31 minutes must be provided when reporting the per-hour codes (ie, **96101**, **96116**, **96118**, and **96125**). Services of 30 minutes or less may be reported with modifier **52**. The time reported includes face-to-face time with the patient and time spent interpreting and preparing the report.

Codes **96101** and **96118**

* Are used in those circumstances when additional time is necessary to integrate other sources of clinical data, including previously completed and reported technician- and computer-administered tests, with psychologist/physician testing done as described by **96101** and **96118**.
* Should not be reported for interpreting or reporting tests administered by a technician (**96102** and **96119**) or computer (**96103** and **96120**) when the psychologist/physician does not perform separate testing. Services reported with codes **96102**, **96103**, **96119**, and **96120** include any additional necessary time for integration of the test data acquired from the computer or technician testing or other data into the report.
* Are reported based on time spent in the provision of the service. Additional units of the code may be reported when time exceeds the average time listed for the service.

Code **96116**

* Is used to report a neurobehavioral status examination. This might also include assessment for serious communication/social developmental disorders, such as autism spectrum disorder (ASD) through the use of the Autism Diagnostic Observation Schedule (ADOS).
* Mini-mental status examination performed by a physician would be included as part of the nervous system physical examination of an E/M service and not separately reportable.
* Documentation of these services includes scoring, observation of behavior, and interpretation and report. It should include the date and time of testing, reason for the test, and titles of all instruments used.

Examples

➤ **A 4-year-old boy is being evaluated for possible ASD.** The ADOS is administered, scored, and interpreted in a written report. The diagnosis is ASD. The total time for testing, scoring, and report writing is 3 hours.

This service is reported with code **96116** (neurobehavioral status examination).

The diagnosis code would be *ICD-10-CM* code **F84.0** (autistic disorder). Depending on payer requirements, the service may be reported as **96116** with 3 units of service or on 3 service lines with modifier **59** appended (**96116, 96116 59, 96116 59**).

➤ A 15-year-old girl is seen in follow-up for a concussion caused by hitting her head against another player's during a soccer match 5 days ago. The patient requested a release to participate in soccer. Her physician has ordered computerized neuropsychologic testing for comparison to a baseline performed at the start of the school year. A technician instructs the patient about the test program, conducts pretest trials for each test, and monitors the patient's progress as she completes the series of tests. After the tests are completed, the physician interprets the test results and creates a report. Results are discussed with the patient and her caregivers as part of an E/M service that takes place later that day.

This service is reported with code **96120** (neuropsychological testing administered by a computer) and an appropriate E/M code (eg, **99213**). Modifier **25** indicates the E/M was a significant, separately identifiable service from the physician interpretation and report of the neuropsychologic testing.

HCPCS Codes

Medications

A9150	Nonprescription drugs
J7030–J7121	Infusions (eg, normal saline solution)
J8498	Antiemetic drug, rectal/suppository (not otherwise specified [NOS])
J8499	Prescription drug, oral, non-chemotherapeutic (NOS)
J8540	Dexamethasone, oral, 0.25 mg
J8597	Oral antiemetic drug (NOS)

See **Table 16-1** for a list of the most commonly used J codes.
- The practice must have incurred a cost for the medication reported.
- Most payers do not cover services reported with nonspecific codes.
- Check with payers to determine if they accept these Healthcare Common Procedure Coding System (HCPCS) codes or if they require reporting with code **99070**.
- Drugs are listed with a base dosage. When the dosage exceeds the amount listed, report additional units for the total dosage administered.
- Some payers require use of the NDC instead of or in addition to J codes. The NDC should always be reported in addition to code **99070** or **J3490** (unclassified drug).

The NDCs are universal product identifiers for prescription drugs and insulin products. Codes are 10-digit, 3-segment numbers that identify the product, labeler, and trade package size. The Health Insurance Portability and Accountability Act of 1996 (HIPAA) standards require an 11-digit code. If you are not currently reporting injectables with NDCs, be sure to coordinate the requirements with your billing software company. For more information on NDCs, visit www.fda.gov/drugs/informationondrugs/ucm142438.htm or link through www.aap.org/cfp, access code AAPCFP23.

> |||||||| **Coding Pearl** ||||||||
> You can find a list of NDCs at www.fda.gov/drugs/informationondrugs/ucm142438.htm.

> **~ More From the AAP ~**
> For more information on reporting NDCs, see "Reporting the National Drug Code: A Refresher" in the August 2014 *AAP Pediatric Coding Newsletter* at http://coding.aap.org (subscription required).

Professional and Technical Components

26	Professional component: When the physician or other qualified health care professional is reporting only the professional component of a service, append modifier **26** to the procedure code.
TC	Technical component: When reporting only the technical component of a service, append modifier **TC** to the procedure code.

Certain procedures (eg, electrocardiograms [ECGs], radiographs, surgical diagnostic tests, laboratory tests) include a professional and technical component. The professional component includes the physician work (eg, interpretation of the test, written report). The technical component includes the costs associated with providing the service (eg, equipment, salaries of technical personnel, supplies, facility expense). Some codes were developed to distinguish between the technical and professional components (eg, routine ECG codes **93000–93010**); however, many are not. If a physician is performing a service or procedure with equipment owned by a facility or another entity and the codes are written as a global service, services are reported with modifier **26** (professional component). *Current Procedural Terminology*® does not include a modifier for reporting the technical component. However, most payers recognize HCPCS modifier **TC**. Facilities or an office providing use of its equipment only would report the same service using modifier **TC**. When the physician owns the equipment and is performing the technical and professional services, a modifier should not be appended to the code.

No modifier is appended when the code descriptor for the service identifies whether the professional, technical, or global service is being reported.

> **~ More From the AAP ~**
>
> For more information on reporting professional and technical components of service, see "Professional Component Services: More Than Codes" in the July 2014 *AAP Pediatric Coding Newsletter*™ at http://coding.aap.org (subscription required).

Examples

➤ **A pediatrician orders a 2-view chest radiograph on a child.** The child is sent to a neighboring physician's office (or outpatient department) for the x-ray. The films are then brought back to the office and the pediatrician interprets them.
>   Pediatrician: ●**71046 26** (radiologic examination, chest; 2 views)
>   Other office or outpatient department: **71046 TC**

➤ **A pediatrician orders a 12-lead ECG on an adolescent patient.** The patient is sent to another office with the ECG machine to perform the ECG. The tracings are taken back to the pediatrician for review and written interpretation and report.
>   Pediatrician: **93010** (routine ECG with at least 12 leads; interpretation and report only)
>   Other office: **93005** (routine ECG with at least 12 leads; tracing only, without interpretation and report)

Radiology Services

The following general guidelines are for reporting radiology services:
* Report only the service provided. See the Professional and Technical Components section earlier in this chapter for appropriate reporting when the physician does not provide the global service.
* An authenticated (signed) written report of the physician's or QHP's interpretation of imaging is an integral part of the professional component of a radiologic service.
* A reference to *image* in *CPT* may refer to that which is acquired on film or in digital format.
* Certain health plans, including Medicaid plans, may require use of modifier **FX** (x-ray taken using film) when reporting the technical component or global radiology service (ie, combined professional and technical components). Verify health plan requirements, as payment may be reduced for radiographs taken using film.

Several categories of codes for radiology services have been revised in recent years. The following sections highlights some of these changes. Please see your coding reference for a full listing of codes and reporting instructions.

Abdominal Radiographs

●**74018**   Radiologic examination, abdomen; 1 view

●**74019**   2 views

●**74021**   3 or more views

74022   complete acute abdomen series, including supine, erect, and/or decubitus views, single view chest

The types of views (eg, frontal and lateral) obtained no longer affect coding of chest radiographs.

Chest Radiographs

●**71045**   Radiologic examination, chest; single view

●**71046**   2 views

●**71047**   3 views

●**71048**   4 or more views

❖ The types of views (eg, frontal and lateral) obtained no longer affect coding of chest radiographs.

❖ Do not separately report a single-view chest radiograph when obtained in conjunction with an acute abdomen series (**74022**).

Hip Radiographs

73501   Radiologic examination, hip, unilateral, with pelvis when performed 1 view

73502   Radiologic examination, hip, unilateral, with pelvis when performed 2-3 views

73503   Radiologic examination, hip, unilateral, with pelvis when performed minimum of 4 views

73521   Radiologic examination, hips, bilateral, with pelvis when performed 2 views

73522   Radiologic examination, hips, bilateral, with pelvis when performed 3-4 views

73523   Radiologic examination, hips, bilateral, with pelvis when performed minimum of 5 views

73525   Radiologic examination, hip, arthrography, radiological supervision and interpretation

73592   Radiologic examination lower extremity, infant, minimum of 2 views

Codes **73501–73523** include radiograph of the pelvis when performed. Do not separately report a single-view radiograph of the pelvis (**72170**) when performed in conjunction with a radiograph of the hip.

Total Spine Radiographs

72081   Radiologic examination, spine, entire thoracic and lumbar, including skull, cervical and sacral spine if performed (eg, scoliosis evaluation); one view

72082   2 or 3 views

72083   4 or 5 views

72084   minimum of 6 views

❖ Previously reported with a single code regardless of the number of views, examination of the entire thoracic and lumbar spine is now reported based on the number of views obtained.

❖ Codes **72081–72084** describe imaging of the entire thoracic and lumbar spine and, when performed, the skull, cervical, and sacral spine. Do not separately report codes for views of the individual spinal segments or skull when performed in conjunction with radiologic examination of the spine. Rather, select the code that represents the number of views obtained of the hip and/or pelvis.

Pathology and Laboratory Procedures

Current Procedural Terminology® laboratory codes may be generic for a particular analyte that is independent of testing method or else have a specific *CPT* code, depending on the method used for the particular analysis.

Reporting guidelines

- A test performed in the office's laboratory should be billed using the appropriate laboratory code and, if performed, the appropriate blood collection code (**36400–36416**).
- If the specimen (eg, blood, urine, stool, cerebrospinal fluid) is collected in the office and sent to an outside laboratory, the office visit (if applicable) plus any specimen acquisition procedure code (eg, venipuncture, capillary blood collection, spinal tap) and a handling fee (**99000**) should be billed.
- If the laboratory bills the pediatrician for the test, bill the patient using the appropriate laboratory analysis code with modifier **90** to indicate the procedure was performed in an outside laboratory.
- Link the appropriate diagnosis code to the laboratory procedure and/or venipuncture and handling fee. The diagnosis must support the medical necessity or reason for the test or service.
- If the only service provided is a urinalysis or obtaining a blood specimen, only the laboratory test and/or venipuncture or capillary stick is reported. It is not appropriate to report a nurse visit (**99211**) in these cases.
- Do not report any laboratory test that is *not performed* in the office (eg, thyroid, laboratory panels, phenylketonuria). Instead, report the appropriate blood-drawing code (**36415** or **36416**).
  - ❖ For example, the physician orders a lead test and the nurse obtains the blood via venipuncture. The specimen is sent to an outside laboratory for processing. Only the venipuncture (**36415**) and handling fee (**99000**) would be reported in addition to the E/M service and other procedures performed on that day.

Laboratory Tests Frequently Performed in the Office

Clinical Laboratory Improvement Amendments–Waived Tests

The Clinical Laboratory Improvement Amendments (CLIA) establish quality standards for all laboratory testing to ensure the accuracy, reliability, and timeliness of patient test results regardless of where the test was performed.

A *laboratory* is defined as any facility that performs laboratory testing on specimens derived from humans for the purpose of providing information for the diagnosis, prevention, and treatment of disease or impairment or assessment of health.

- The term *CLIA waived* refers to tests commonly done in a laboratory or office. One typical test in the *CPT* **80000** series that is CLIA waived is the rapid streptococcus group B test (**87802**).
- Laboratories and physician offices performing waived tests may need to append modifier **QW** to the *CPT* code for CLIA-waived procedures. Some of the CLIA-waived tests are exempt from the use of modifier **QW** (eg, **81002**, **82272**). The use of modifier **QW** is payer specific. To review the list of CLIA-waived procedures, go to www.cms.hhs.gov/CLIA.

Urinalysis

81000	Urinalysis, by dipstick or tablet reagent for bilirubin, glucose, hemoglobin, ketones, leukocytes, nitrite, pH, protein, specific gravity, urobilinogen, any number of these constituents; nonautomated, with microscopy
81001	as per **81000** but automated
81002	as per **81000** but without microscopy
81003	as per **81000** but automated, without microscopy

For urinalysis, infectious agent detection, semiquantitative analysis of volatile compounds, use **81099**.

CPT copyright 2017 American Medical Association. All rights reserved.

Urine Pregnancy Test

81025   Urine pregnancy test, by visual color comparison method

> Report code **81025** with *ICD-10-CM* codes **Z32.00–Z32.02**, depending on the findings of the test (ie, unconfirmed result, positive result, or negative result).

Glucose Tests

82947   Glucose, quantitative, blood (without a reagent strip)

82948   blood, reagent strip

82951   Glucose tolerance test (GTT), 3 specimens

82952   each additional beyond 3 specimens

Continuous glucose monitoring of interstitial tissue fluid via a subcutaneous sensor with sensor placement, hookup, calibration of monitor, patient training, removal of the sensor, and printout of the recording is reported with code **95250**. Monitoring must be a minimum of 72 hours. Physician interpretation and report of the continuous glucose monitoring is reported with code **95251**.

82962   Glucose, blood by glucose monitoring device(s) cleared by the US Food and Drug Administration specifically for home use

Code **82962** describes the method when whole blood is obtained (usually by finger-stick device) and assayed by glucose oxidase, hexokinase, or electrochemical methods and spectrophotometry using a small portable device designed for home blood glucose monitoring use. The devices are also used in physician offices, during home visits, or in clinics.

Infectious Agent Detection by Immunoassay With Direct Optical Observation (ie, Rapid Tests)

87802   Streptococcus group B

87804   Influenza

If tests performed separately detect the influenza A and B antigen, providing 2 distinct results, report code **87804** twice with modifier **59** appended to the second service. This applies whether the test kit uses 1 or 2 analytic chambers to deliver 2 distinct results. Check with your payers because some do not recognize modifier **59** and may require reporting with 2 units of service and no modifier.

87807   Respiratory syncytial virus

87880   Streptococcus, group A

Tuberculosis Skin Test (Mantoux)

86580   Tuberculosis, intradermal

◈ The tuberculosis (TB) skin test (Mantoux) using the intradermal administration of purified protein derivative (PPD) is the recommended diagnostic skin test for TB. This is not the BCG TB vaccine. The AAP supports the use of the Mantoux test (TB, intradermal) for TB screening when appropriate.

◈ Code **99211** is the appropriate code to report the reading of a PPD test when that is the only reason for the encounter. The appropriate *ICD-10-CM* code is **Z11.1** (encounter for screening for respiratory TB). In the case of a positive test result when the physician sees the patient, the complexity may lead to a higher-level code. There is not a separate administration code reported when the PPD is placed.

Lead Testing

83655   Lead, quantitative analysis

◈ This test does not specify the specimen source or the method of testing. Alternative tests sometimes (though now rarely) used for lead screening are **82135** (aminolevulinic acid, delta), **84202** (protoporphyrin, red blood cell count, quantitative), and **84203** (protoporphyrin, red blood cell count, screen).

- ❋ Some states provide the lead testing at no cost to patients covered under the Medicaid Early and Periodic Screening, Diagnosis, and Treatment program. Check your state Medicaid requirements for reporting this service.
- ❋ Report *ICD-10-CM* code **Z13.88** (encounter for screening for disorder due to exposure to contaminants) when performing lead screening. Some payers require **Z77.011**, contact with and (suspected) exposure to lead, in lieu of **Z13.88**.

Cultures

- ❋ Use code **87086** (culture, bacterial; quantitative colony count, urine) once per encounter for urine culture to determine the approximate number of bacteria present per milliliter of urine. Use of a commercial kit with defined media to identify isolates in a positive urine culture is reported with **87088** (culture, bacterial; quantitative colony count, urine with isolation and presumptive identification of each isolate).
- ❋ Code **81007** (urinalysis; bacteriuria screen, except by culture or dipstick) can be used for a bacteriuria screen by non-culture technique using a commercial kit. The type of commercial kit must be specified.
- ❋ Code **87070** (culture, bacterial; any other source except urine, blood, or stool) is reported for throat cultures.
- ❋ Use code **87045** to report culture, bacteria of the stool, aerobic, with isolation and preliminary examination (eg, Kligler iron agar, lysine iron agar) for *Salmonella* and *Shigella* species. Additional pathogens are reported with code **87046** with 1 unit per plate.
- ❋ Report services with the symptoms (eg, microscopic hematuria) or the confirmed diagnosis (eg, urinary tract infection).

Respiratory Syncytial Virus Test

●**87634**   Infectious agent detection by nucleic acid (DNA or RNA); respiratory syncytial virus, amplified probe technique

For assays that include respiratory syncytial virus with additional respiratory viruses, see **87631**, **87632**, and **87633**.

Streptococcal Test

87081   Culture, presumptive pathogenic organisms, screening only
87430   Enzyme immunoassay, qualitative, streptococcus, group A

- ❋ Report the code based on the test method rather than on the site of specimen collection.
- ❋ Culture plates using sheep blood agar with bacitracin disks should be coded with **87081**.

Zika Virus Testing

●**86794**   Zika virus, IgM
●**87662**   Zika virus, amplified probe technique

- ❋ The IgM test described by code **87662** is used when suspected patient exposure to the Zika virus was less than 2 weeks before testing.
- ❋ The amplified probe technique (**86794**) is used when potential exposure occurred 2 weeks or more prior to testing.

Testing Stool for Occult Blood

82272   Blood, occult, by peroxidase activity (eg, guaiac), qualitative, feces, 1–3 simultaneous determinations, performed for other than colorectal neoplasm screening

Code **82272** is reported when a single sample is obtained from a digital rectal examination or a multi-test card is returned from the patient and is tested for blood. Report **82272** with 1 unit when up to 3 cards are returned.

Hematology

85013	Spun microhematocrit
85018	Hemoglobin
85025–85027	Complete blood cell count, automated

- If using a complete blood cell count (CBC) machine to perform only a hemoglobin test, follow these guidelines.
- If the CBC result is normal, only the hemoglobin may be reported because that was the medically necessary test ordered.
- If the CBC reveals an abnormality and it is addressed during the course of the visit, the CBC result may be reported. The abnormality would be linked to the procedure, and the medical record would need to include documentation for the ordering of the test and to support the medical necessity of the procedure.

Laboratory Panel Coding

All laboratory test panels in *CPT*® were specifically developed for coding purposes only and should not be interpreted as clinical parameters. (See codes **80047–80076** for a component listing of these panels.) For example, the lipid panel (**80061**) includes total cholesterol (**82465**), high-density lipoprotein cholesterol (**83718**), and triglycerides (**84478**). Any additional tests performed can be coded separately from the panel code. Do not unbundle individual laboratory tests if a laboratory panel code is available.

Serum and Transcutaneous Bilirubin Testing

82247	Total bilirubin
82248	Direct bilirubin
88720	Transcutaneous total bilirubin

Papanicolaou Tests

- The laboratory performing the cytology and interpretation reports Papanicolaou (Pap) tests with codes **88141–88155**, **88164–88167**, or **88174** and **88175**.
- Obtaining a Pap test specimen is inherent to the physical examination performed during a preventive medicine visit or a problem-oriented office visit.
- Medicare does require reporting HCPCS code **Q0091** (screening Papanicolaou, obtaining, preparing, and conveyance of cervical and vaginal smear to laboratory) in addition to the E/M service for preventive medicine and problem-oriented office visits.
  - Some state Medicaid programs and commercial payers may also recognize obtaining a Pap test as a separate service.
  - Code **Q0091** cannot be reported when a patient must return for a repeat Pap test due to inadequate initial sampling.
  - If not reporting **Q0091**, a handling fee (**99000**) can be reported in addition to an E/M service if the Pap test was obtained.
- The appropriate *ICD-10-CM* code to link to the E/M code or code **Q0091** is either **Z01.411** (encounter for gynecological examination [general] [routine] with abnormal findings) or **Z01.419** (encounter for gynecological examination [general] [routine] without abnormal findings). For screening cervical Pap test not part of a gynecologic examination, report *ICD-10-CM* code **Z12.4** (encounter for screening for malignant neoplasm of cervix). For high-risk patients, you may also use code **Z92.89** or **Z77.9**. These diagnosis codes may be used as secondary when linked with a routine preventive medicine code or problem-oriented sick visit.

Administrative Services and Supplies

Administrative Services

Codes in this section cover some of the administrative aspects of medical practice.

99071   Educational supplies, such as books, tapes, and pamphlets, for the patient's education at cost to physician or other qualified health care professional

99075   Medical testimony

99082   Unusual travel (eg, transportation and escort of patient)

99090   Analysis of clinical data stored in computers (eg, ECG, blood pressure, hematologic data)

99091   Collection and interpretation of physiological data (eg, ECG, blood pressure, glucose monitoring) digitally stored and/or transmitted by the patient and/or caregiver to the physician or other qualified health care professional, requiring a minimum of 30 minutes of time (Do not report more than once in a 30-day period.)

Codes **99071–99091** are for administrative services.

- Code **99071** may be reported when the physician incurs costs for educational supplies and provides them to the patient at his or her cost.
- Code **99075** may be reported when a physician presents medical testimony before a court or other administrative body.
- With the exception of code **99091**, none of these services are assigned Medicare relative value units.
- Healthcare Common Procedure Coding System code **S9981** (medical records copying fee, administrative) or **S9982** (medical record copying fee, per page) may be reported when it is appropriate to charge for copies of medical records. Commercial payers and some Medicaid programs may accept S codes.
- State medical insurance departments or medical associations determine the amount a practice can charge for copying medical records. Be sure to know the state charge limitations and do not overcharge. The HIPAA regulations, where more stringent, will override state regulations. For information on charges to patients for copying health records, see www.hhs.gov/hipaa/for-professionals/privacy/guidance/access/index.html#newlyreleasedfaqs.

Physician Group Education Services

99078   Physician or other qualified health care professional qualified by education, training, licensure/regulation (when applicable), educational services rendered to patients in a group setting (eg, prenatal, obesity, or diabetic instructions)

Code **99078** is used to report physician educational services provided to established patients in group settings (eg, obesity classes, diabetes classes).

- There are no time requirements.
- Modifier **25** (significant, separately identifiable E/M service) should *not* be appended to the E/M service because **99078** is an adjunct service.
- Documentation in each medical record includes the education and training provided, follow-up for ongoing education, and total time of the education.
- Services are reported on each participating child.
- Payers may require that these services be reported differently.

Chapter 16: Common Testing and Therapeutic Services

Supplies and Materials

99070   Supplies and materials provided by the physician over and above those usually included with the office visit or other services rendered

* Items such as elastic wraps, clavicle splints, or circumcision and suturing trays may be reported with this code. Remember that some supplies (eg, suturing trays, circumcision trays) may be included with the surgical procedure if the payer uses the Resource-Based Relative Value Scale as its basis for payment.

* Only the supplies purchased in an office-based practice may be reported.

* Some payers will require the use of HCPCS codes. More specific HCPCS codes are available for a number of supplies (eg, codes **Q4001– Q4051** for cast and splint supplies). Use HCPCS codes when they are more specific.

> **||||||| Coding Pearl |||||||**
>
> If reporting code **99070**, identify the supplies or materials on the claim form and be prepared to submit an invoice.

Coding to Demonstrate Quality and Value

Contents

Quality and performance measurement are important aspects of the pediatric medical home and the movement from payment by fee for service alone to value-based payment. Physicians who have successfully participated in quality measurement may see incentive payments, such as per-member/per-month payments, annual incentives, or a percentage of savings.

Physicians, payers, and accreditation organizations may use codes or claims data as a first line of quality measurement. When diagnosis or procedure codes provide necessary information for reviewing quality performance data, more time-consuming and costly medical record review may be avoided. In January 2017, the American Academy of Pediatrics (AAP) published a policy statement, "A New Era in Quality Measurement: The Development and Application of Quality Measures" (available online at http://pediatrics.aappublications.org/content/139/1/e20163442). This policy statement includes a recommendation to national policy makers as follows:

"Quality measures, as much as possible, should be reportable by either *International Classification of Diseases, 10th Revision, Clinical Modification*, or *Current Procedural Terminology®* category II codes to reduce burden on pediatric health care providers. However, the inclusion of measures that also capture patient-centered perspectives on care is essential."

Clinical registries and other electronic data may also be used in quality measurement. This chapter discusses 2 ways that correct coding may support performance measurement: codes that may support Healthcare Effectiveness Data and Information Set (HEDIS) quality measurement and *Current Procedural Terminology* (*CPT®*) Category II codes.

For more information on value-based payment and other emerging payment models, see Chapter 19, The Business of Medicine: Working With Current and Emerging Payment Systems.

Healthcare Effectiveness Data and Information Set (HEDIS)

The National Committee for Quality Assurance (NCQA) describes HEDIS as a tool used by more than 90% of American health plans to measure performance on important dimensions of care and service. It is intended to allow purchasers and consumers to compare quality between health plans. The HEDIS measures are often incorporated in physician quality initiatives. Altogether, HEDIS consists of 81 measures across 5 domains of care (effectiveness of care, access/availability of care, experience of care, utilization and relative resource use, and health plan descriptive information). To insure HEDIS stays current, the NCQA has established a process to update the measurement set annually.

The HEDIS measures address a broad range of important health issues. Among them are

- Asthma Medication Use
- Antidepressant Medication Management
- Childhood and Adolescent Immunization Status
- Childhood Weight/BMI Assessment

Each health plan reviews a select set of measures each year. Because so many plans collect HEDIS data and the measures are so specifically defined, it is important to become familiar with the HEDIS system as it relates to quality measures and pay for performance (P4P).

Why HEDIS Matters to Pediatricians

The Centers for Medicare & Medicaid Services (CMS) has directly linked payment for health care services to patient outcomes. Consequently, health plans and providers, including physicians, are being asked to close gaps in care and improve overall quality. This focus on quality outcomes can help patients and members get the most from their benefits, which ultimately means better use of limited resources.

There are large sums of money at stake for health plans. For example, for a health plan with just 100,000 members being evaluated by HEDIS, each quality measure could mean millions in payments from federal or state agencies. When you consider that there are 20 to 25 measures directly tied to payment (depending on the health plan and population served), these are significant amounts of money! Now consider what that might look like for larger managed care organizations who have 1 million or more members enrolled. This is what keeps health care plans running. However, they cannot do it without physicians, and this is the fundamental concept behind P4P quality initiatives. The plans will pay the physicians to help them attain these funds from the CMS.

What Is a Pediatrician's Role in HEDIS?

You and your office staff can help facilitate the HEDIS process improvement by

* Providing the appropriate care within the designated time frames.
* Not all patients will be included in a physician's patient count for HEDIS purposes, as continuous enrollment in the health plan without a gap of more than 45 days may be required for inclusion. However, attention to the time frames for providing recommended screenings and services across the patient population is important. For instance, practices should have a reminder system to track immunizations for children younger than 24 months to avoid failure to provide the recommended immunizations prior to 25 months of age. If patients reach 25 months of age without receiving the recommended vaccines, this negatively affects the HEDIS score for the physician until the child turns 3 years old (ie, is no longer included in the patient count for the measure).
* Documenting all care in the patient's medical record.
* Accurately coding all claims. Providing information accurately on a claim may reduce the number of records requested.
* Responding to a health plan's requests for medical records timely (typically within a week).

    The time frames are set each year.
* January to May 15: Medical record requests will come in from the plans. All data have to be gathered by the plan by May 15, with no exceptions.
* June: The plans have to report their results to NCQA.
* July to October: NCQA releases the new Quality Compass nationwide—commercial plans in July; Medicaid and Medicare in September and October.

Medical Record Requests

Some information cannot be captured through claims data, so requests for medical records related to health plan HEDIS surveys are necessary. The Health Insurance Portability and Accountability Act of 1996 allows disclosure of protected health information to a health plan for the plan's HEDIS purposes, so long as the period for which information is needed overlaps with the period for which the patient is or was enrolled in the health plan. Health plans may contract with outside vendors to conduct HEDIS record reviews.

* Providers are notified of record requests (often by fax but may vary by plan).
* The request will include a member list, the measure that is being evaluated, and the minimum necessary chart information needed.
* Data collection may vary by plan but may include fax, mail, on-site visits for large requests, remote electronic health record (EHR) access, and electronic data interchange via a secure Web portal.

HEDIS Measures and Codes

In **Table 17-1**, some of the pediatric HEDIS measures for 2017 are listed, including the codes that may be used in HEDIS review (HEDIS 2018 measures were not finalized at time of publication). These include *International Classification of Diseases, 10th Revision, Clinical Modification (ICD-10-CM)*; Healthcare Common Procedure Coding System; and *CPT®* codes. **Table 17-1** does not contain all measures applicable to the pediatric population. Note that each measure includes a defined patient population (eg, children who turn 2 years of age during the measurement year).

Physicians and group practices may also report HEDIS measures as part of a pediatric medical home or other quality improvement initiative using data pulled from internal administrative data (eg, number of preventive medicine service *CPT* codes reported for population of patients 3–6 years old). Pediatric medical home and quality improvement initiatives vary by state or region and may include a combination of HEDIS and other nationally recognized quality measures.

Table 17-1. HEDIS Pediatric Performance Measure Codes

Measure/Description	Codes
Weight Assessment and Counseling for Nutrition and Physical Activity for Children and Adolescents (WCC) Description: Percentage of members 3–17 years of age who had an outpatient visit with a PCP or an OB/GYN that included evidence of BMI documentation with corresponding height and weight, counseling for nutrition, and/or counseling for physical activity	**Diagnosis** *(ICD-10-CM)* BMI percentile: **Z68.51–Z68.54** Counseling: nutrition (**Z71.3**) Counseling for physical activity (no specific code but some plans accept **Z02.5**, encounter for sports physical) **Procedure** Nutrition counseling—*CPT*®: **97802–97804** HCPCS: **S9470**, **S9452**, **S9449**, **G0270**, **G0271**, or **G0447** Physical activity counseling—HCPCS: **S9451** *or* **G0447**
Immunizations for Adolescents (IMA) Description: Percentage of adolescents 13 years of age (during the year) with appropriate immunizations	**Procedure** (vaccine products) Meningococcal—*CPT:* **90734** Tdap—*CPT:* **90715** Td—*CPT:* **90714** or **90718** Tetanus—*CPT:* **90703** Diphtheria—*CPT:* **90719** Human papillomavirus—*CPT:* **90651**
Follow-up Care for Children Prescribed ADHD Medications Percentage of children newly prescribed ADHD medication who had at least 3 follow-up care visits within a 10-month period, one of which was within 30 days of when the first ADHD medication was dispensed. Two rates are reported. 1. Initiation phase: The percentage of members 6–12 years of age as of the IPSD with an ambulatory prescription dispensed for ADHD medication, who had one follow-up visit with practitioner with prescribing authority during the 30-day initiation phase. 2. Continuation and maintenance phase: The percentage of members 6–12 years of age as of the IPSD with an ambulatory prescription dispensed for ADHD medication, who remained on the medication for at least 210 days and who, in addition to the visit in the initiation phase, had at least 2 follow-up visits with a practitioner within 270 days (9 months) after the initiation phase ended. One of the 2 visits (during the 31–300) may be a telephone visit with any practitioner.	**Procedure** *CPT* Stand-alone visits: **90804–90815**, **96150–96154**, **98960–98962**, **99078**, **99201–99205**, **99211–99215**, **99217–99220**, **99241–99245**, **99341–99345**, **99347–99350**, **99381–99384**, **99391–99394**, **99401–99404**, **99411**, **99412**, **99510** Telephone visits: **98966–98968**, **99441–99443** HCPCS: **G0155**, **G0176**, **G0177**, **G0409–G0411**, **G0463**, **H0002**, **H0004**, **H0031**, **H0034–H0037**, **H0039**, **H0040**, **H2000**, **H2001**, **H2010–H2020**, **M0064**, **S0201**, **S9480**, **S9484**, **S9485**, **T1015** **Follow-up visits identified by the following *CPT* codes must be with a mental health practitioner:** *CPT* in most outpatient and partial hospitalization settings: **90791–90792**, **90801**, **90802**, **90816–90819**, **90821–90824**, **90826–90829**, **90832–90834**, **90836–90840**, **90845**, **90847**, **90849**, **90853**, **90857**, **90862**, **90875–90876** *CPT* in partial hospitalization or community mental health centers only: **99221–99223**, **99231–99233**, **99238**, **99239**, **99251–99255**

Abbreviations: ADHD, attention-deficit/hyperactivity disorder; BMI, body mass index; CPT, Current Procedural Terminology; HCPCS, Healthcare Common Procedure Coding System; HEDIS, Healthcare Effectiveness Data and Information Set; ICD-10-CM, International Classification of Diseases, 10th Revision, Clinical Modification; IPSD, Index Prescription Start Date; OB/GYN, obstetrician/gynecologist; PCP, primary care physician; Td, tetanus, diphtheria; Tdap, tetanus, diphtheria toxoid, and acellular pertussis.

Examples

➤ **A physician sees a 12-year-old girl for a new patient office visit with a chief complaint of acne.** The physician identifies that the girl is not up-to-date with immunizations and has not received preventive care in the last year. The physician recommends and provides a preventive medicine service. The encounter includes documentation of the services recommended by the AAP *Bright Futures: Guidelines for Health Supervision of Infants, Children, and Adolescents,* 4th Edition, and counseling and administration of age-appropriate immunizations. Documentation does not support a separately identifiable evaluation and management (E/M) service but includes a diagnosis of mild acne vulgaris.

ICD-10-CM	CPT®
Z00.121 (encounter for routine child health examination with abnormal findings) **L70.0** (acne vulgaris) **Z71.3** (dietary counseling and surveillance) **Z68.52** (body mass index [BMI] pediatric, 5th percentile to <85th percentile for age) **Z13.89** (encounter for screening for other disorder [alcohol or drug use, depression])	**99384** (initial comprehensive preventive medicine E/M, new patient; age 12–17 years old) **90460** × 4 units (immunization administration, each initial component) **90461** × 2 units (immunization administration, each additional component) **90686** (IIV4 vaccine) **90651** (9-valent human papillomavirus [9vHPV]) **90734** (MenACWY) **90715** (tetanus, diphtheria, acellular pertussis [Tdap]) **96160** (administration and interpretation of health risk assessment instrument [alcohol and drug assessment]) **96127** (brief emotional/behavioral assessment, with scoring and documentation, per standardized instrument [depression screening])

The physician in this scenario has proactively provided preventive care that is recommended for this patient and, in doing so, is able to report diagnosis and procedure codes demonstrating that quality measures have been met. For instance, HEDIS includes measurements for immunization for meningococcus; tetanus, diphtheria, and pertussis; and human papillomavirus for all adolescents prior to their 13th birthday, in addition to measures for adolescent well-care visits, BMI measurement, and counseling on nutrition and physical activity (may be assessed by chart review). There is no specific *ICD-10-CM* code for reporting counseling about physical activity. However, some health plans recommend **Z02.5** (encounter for sports physical).

➤ **A physician sees an established patient for complaints associated with upper respiratory infection (URI).** The caregiver requests an antibiotic but is instructed that the condition is viral and to use over-the-counter medicine as necessary for the child's comfort. No antibiotic is ordered.

ICD-10-CM	CPT
J06.9 (acute URI, unspecified)	**99213** (office or other outpatient visit for the E/M of an established patient, which requires at least 2 of these 3 key components: ☀ An expanded problem focused history; ☀ An expanded problem focused examination; ☀ Medical decision-making of low complexity.) Counseling and coordination of care with other physicians, other qualified health care professionals, or agencies are provided consistent with the nature of the problem(s) and the patient's and/or family's needs. Usually, the presenting problem(s) are of low to moderate severity. Typically, 15 minutes are spent face-to-face with the patient and/or family.

Because no antibiotic was ordered at this encounter, the HEDIS measure for appropriate treatment of children 3 months to 18 years old with URIs was met. The diagnosis of URI indicates this measure may apply. The health plan may measure this through comparison of medical claims data with prescription drug plan claims data. Similar measures may apply for antibiotics appropriately prescribed for diagnosis of streptococcal pharyngitis following positive laboratory test for group A streptococcal infection.

Category II *CPT*® Codes: Pay for Performance Measures

Category II codes were developed and are used by physicians and hospitals to report performance measures and certain aspects of care not yet included in performance measures. The performance measures are developed by national organizations, including the NCQA and the American Medical Association (AMA) Physician Consortium for Performance Improvement (PCPI), and based on quality indicators currently accepted and used in the health care industry. As a member of the AMA PCPI, the AAP is involved with the development of performance measures for pediatric diseases or conditions. The AAP policy statement, "A New Era in Quality Measurement: The Development and Application of Quality Measures" (available online at http://pediatrics. aappublications.org/content/139/1/e20163442) includes recommendations to physicians and policy makers on adoption and use of quality measures. Any updated information on quality improvement can be found at www2.aap.org/visit/qualityimppublic.htm.

Reporting Category II codes allows internal monitoring of performance, patient compliance, and outcomes.

Performance Measure Codes

Performance measure codes
* Are intended for reporting purposes only.
* Describe clinical conditions (including complete performance measurements sets) and screening measures.
* Have no relative values on the Medicare Physician Fee Schedule (Resource-Based Relative Value Scale).
* Are reported on a voluntary basis.
* Are reported in addition to, *not in place of,* Category I *CPT* codes.
* Describe the performance of a clinical service typically included in an E/M code or the result that is part of a laboratory procedure/test.

Category II code development and maintenance take place on an as-needed basis. Category II code changes since the printing of the last *CPT* manual are posted to https://www.ama-assn.org/practice-management/cpt-category-ii-codes. The online document, "CPT Category II Codes Alphabetical Clinical Topics Listing" (ACTL), includes the latest code changes with revision, implementation, and publication dates.

Codes are grouped within categories based on established clinical documentation methods (ie, history, physical findings, assessment, and plan). Each code identifies the specific clinical condition and performance measured.

Categories are defined in **Table 17-2.**

Category II Modifiers

Category II modifiers (**1P, 2P, 3P,** and **8P**) are used to report services that were considered but not provided because of a medical reason(s), patient choice, or system reason. Modifier **8P** is equivalent to "action not performed, reason not otherwise specified." **Table 17-3** contains modifiers and examples.

Category II modifiers
* Are used only when allowed based on the specific reporting instructions for each performance measure.
* Are appended only to Category II *CPT* codes.
* Serve as a denominator exclusion from a performance measure (when measure allows).

The medical record should include written documentation of the reason that the service was ultimately not provided. Category II modifiers are only appended to Category II codes.

Chapter 17: Coding to Demonstrate Quality and Value

Table 17-2. Performance Measure Codes

Category of Codes	Examples
Composite Measures—0000F Series Codes in the 0000F range comprise several measures that are grouped to facilitate reporting of a clinical condition when all included components are performed.	Code 0012F is reported when the assessment on an 18-year-old with community-acquired bacterial pneumonia includes all the following components: **1026F** Comorbid conditions assessed **2010F** Vital signs recorded **2014F** Mental status assessed **2018F** Hydration status assessed
Patient Management—0500F Series Codes in the 0500F range are used to describe utilization measures or measures of patient care provided for specific clinical purposes (eg, prenatal care, presurgical and postsurgical care, referrals).	Code 0545F is used to report that a plan for follow-up care was documented on a 15-year-old with a diagnosis of major depressive disorder.
Patient History—1000F Series Codes in the 1000F range are used to describe measures for aspects of patient history and review of systems.	Code 1031F is used to report that the smoking status and exposure to secondhand smoke in the home were assessed in patients with asthma. Code 1050F is used to report a patient history of new or changing moles.
Physical Examination—2000F Series Codes in the 2000F range describe aspects of the physical examination or clinical assessment.	Code 2030F is reported when the hydration status is documented as normally hydrated on a 2-month-old with acute gastroenteritis.
Diagnostic/Screening Processes or Results—3006F Codes in the 3006F range are used to report results of clinical laboratory tests and radiologic or other procedural examinations.	When the most recent hemoglobin A_{1c} level is less than 7.0% on an 18-year-old with diabetes mellitus, code 3044F is reported.
Therapeutic, Preventive, or Other Interventions—4000F Codes in the 4000F range are used to report pharmacologic, procedural, or behavioral therapies, including preventive services such as patient education and counseling.	Code 4058F is reported when gastroenteritis education is provided to the mother of a 6-month-old with acute gastroenteritis and documented in the medical record.
Follow-up or Other Outcomes—5005F Codes in the 5005F range are used to describe the review and communication of test results to patients, patient satisfaction and experience with care, patient functional status, and patient morbidity and mortality.	Code 5050F is reported when a treatment plan is communicated to the provider(s) managing continuing care within 1 month of the diagnosis of melanoma.
Patient Safety—6005F Codes in the 6005F range are used to describe patient safety practices.	Code 6005F is used to report the rationale (eg, severity of illness and safety) for the recommended level of care (eg, home, hospital) for a patient with community-acquired bacterial pneumonia.
Structural Measures—7010F Codes in the 7010F range are used to identify measures that address the setting or system of the delivered care and address aspects of the capabilities of the organization or health care professionals providing the care.	Code 7010F is reported when patient information is entered into a recall system that includes a specified target date for the next examination of a patient with melanoma and a process to follow up with patients about missed or unscheduled appointments.
Non-measure Claims-Based Reporting—9001F Codes in the 9001F range are used to identify certain aspects of care not currently represented by recognized performance measures but which may later be associated with measures approved by an appropriate quality improvement organization.	Code 9001F is reported to identify the size of an abdominal aortic aneurysm less than 5.0 cm maximum diameter on centerline-formatted computed tomography (CT) or minor diameter on axial-formatted CT.

Table 17-3. Category II Modifiers	
Category II Modifier	**Examples**
Modifier 1P (performance measure exclusion modifier due to medical reasons) Used to report that one of the performance measures was not performed because it was not indicated (eg, already performed) or was contraindicated (eg, due to a patient's allergy)	Modifier **1P** is appended to code **6070F** (documentation that patient was queried and counseled about antiepileptic drug [AED] side effects) because the patient is not receiving an AED.
Modifier 2P (performance measure exclusion modifier due to patient choice) Used to report that the performance measure was not performed due to a patient's religious, social, or economic reasons; the patient declined (eg, noncompliance with treatment); or other specific reasons	Modifier **2P** is appended to code **3210F** (group A streptococcus test performed) when a physician considered the testing for streptococcus but the parent refused testing.
Modifier 3P (performance measure exclusion modifier due to system reasons) Used to report that the performance measure was not performed because the payer does not cover the service, the resources to perform the service are not available, or other reasons attributable to the health care delivery system Keep in mind that in the emergency department setting, appropriate medical screening and stabilization must be provided regardless of any consideration of payment. Providers are prohibited by federal statute from making treatment decisions in these circumstances based on payer coverage.	Modifier **3P** is appended to code **4062F** (patient referral for psychotherapy documented) when a 15-year-old with a diagnosis of major depressive disorder is not referred for psychotherapy because it is not available.
Modifier 8P (performance measure reporting modifier—action not performed, not otherwise specified) Used to allow the reporting of circumstances when an action described in a measure's numerator is not performed and the reason is not otherwise specified	Modifier **8P** would be appended to code **2001F** (weight recorded) when a 2-year-old with acute gastroenteritis is not weighed and, therefore, does not meet the performance measurement requirement.

Performance Measures Applicable to Pediatrics

Many performance measures apply to the pediatric population. In addition, pediatric practices caring for patients 18 years or older may report Category II codes for conditions such as hypertension, diabetes mellitus, chronic kidney disease, gastroesophageal reflux disease, and community-acquired bacterial pneumonia and screening codes for tobacco use and cessation. Refer to the ACTL at www.ama-assn.org/practice-management/cpt-category-ii-codes for updated measures and reporting instructions.

Acute Otitis Externa

These codes apply to patients aged 2 years and older with a diagnosis of acute otitis externa (AOE). Clinical components are reported to denote if pain was assessed, if topical therapy was prescribed, and if systemic antimicrobial therapy was avoided.

Category II Codes: Acute Otitis Externa	Guidelines
1116F Auricular or periauricular pain assessed	Report at each encounter. Append modifier 1P when the appropriate performance exclusion exists.
4130F Topical preparations (including over the counter) prescribed for acute otitis externa	If topical preparations are not prescribed, medical record documentation must indicate the medical and/or patient reasons, and modifier 1P or 2P would be appended to code 4130F or drug allergy or other adverse effects would be indicated by diagnosis codes.
4131F Systemic antimicrobial therapy prescribed 4132F Systemic antimicrobial therapy not prescribed	Report code 4132F when systemic antimicrobial therapy is not prescribed. Report code 4131F with modifier 1P when there is a valid medical reason for prescribing systemic antimicrobial therapy. Exclusion modifiers cannot be reported with code 4132F.

Acute Otitis Media With Effusion

These codes apply to patients aged 2 months through 12 years with a diagnosis of acute otitis media with effusion. Clinical components reported as part of this measure signify that an assessment of tympanic membrane mobility was performed using pneumatic otoscopy or tympanometry, that hearing testing was performed within 6 months prior to a tympanostomy tube insertion, and whether or not antihistamines, decongestants, or systemic steroids were avoided.

Category II Codes: Acute Otitis Media With Effusion	Guidelines
2035F Tympanic membrane mobility assessed with pneumatic otoscopy or tympanometry	Reported at each encounter. Modifier 1P or 2P is appended when appropriate.
3230F Documentation that hearing test was performed within 6 months prior to a tympanostomy tube insertion	Reported at the time the tympanostomy tube insertion is performed. Medical record documentation must reflect the performance and results of the test or, if the test is performed by another physician or provider, should include a copy of the test results. Modifiers 1P or 3P may be appended to code 3230F as appropriate.
4131F Systemic antimicrobial therapy prescribed 4132F Systemic antimicrobial therapy not prescribed 4133F Antihistamines or decongestants prescribed or recommended 4134F Antihistamines or decongestants neither prescribed nor recommended 4135F Systemic corticosteroids prescribed 4136F Systemic corticosteroids not prescribed	Used to report the absence or overuse of medications for each patient. Modifier 1P is used with codes 4131F, 4133F, and 4135F when appropriate. Modifiers 1P, 2P, and 3P may not be reported with codes 4132F, 4134F, or 4136F.

Asthma

This measure is applicable to all patients 5 to 50 years of age with a diagnosis of asthma.

Category II Codes: Asthma	Guidelines
2015F Asthma impairment assessed 2016F Asthma risk assessed	Used for each patient who was evaluated at least once for asthma control. Evaluation of asthma impairment and asthma risk must occur during the same medical encounter. There are no exclusions to the measures. Code 2016F is also reported independently for each emergency department encounter or inpatient admission (with a diagnosis of acute asthma exacerbation). There are no performance exclusions for this measure.

Category II Codes: Asthma	Guidelines
1031F Smoking status and exposure to secondhand smoke in the home assessed	Report for each patient whose smoking status and exposure to secondhand smoke in the home was assessed. There are no performance exclusions.
1032F Current tobacco smoker OR currently exposed to secondhand smoke **1033F** Current tobacco non-smoker AND not currently exposed to secondhand smoke **4000F** Tobacco use cessation intervention, counseling **4001F** Tobacco use cessation intervention, pharmacologic therapy	Report code **1032F** or **1033F** to indicate tobacco use status. If reporting code **1032F**, report **4000F** OR **4001F** to indicate type of tobacco use cessation intervention. There are no performance exclusions for this measure. Tobacco cessation interventions may be reported when provided to the patient's primary caregiver even if the caregiver is not the source of secondhand smoke in the home.
1038F Persistent asthma, mild, moderate, or severe **1039F** Intermittent asthma **4140F** Inhaled corticosteroids prescribed **4144F** Alternative long-term control medication prescribed	Report code **1038F** or **1039F** to indicate asthma severity. For patients with persistent asthma (**1038F**), report code **4140F**, **4144F**, or both. For patients with appropriate exclusion criteria, report code **4140F** or **4144F** with modifier **1P** or **2P**.
5250F Asthma discharge plan provided to patient	Report for each emergency department encounter or inpatient admission (with a diagnosis of acute asthma exacerbation) when an asthma discharge plan is provided to patient at time of discharge. There are no performance exclusions for this measure.

Pediatric Acute Gastroenteritis

The pediatric acute gastroenteritis measure applies to patients aged 1 month through 5 years with a diagnosis of acute gastroenteritis.

Category II Codes: Pediatric Acute Gastroenteritis	Guidelines
4056F Appropriate oral rehydration solution recommended **4058F** Pediatric gastroenteritis education provided to caregiver	Used to report that the patient's caregiver was given a recommendation on an appropriate oral rehydration solution, diet education was performed, and the patient's caregiver was advised when to contact the physician. There are no performance exclusions.
2030F Hydration status documented, normally hydrated **2031F** Hydration status documented, dehydrated	Report when hydration status is documented in the medical record. When the patient is dehydrated and appropriate oral rehydration solution is recommended, report codes **4056F** and **2031F**. There are no performance exclusions.
2001F Weight recorded	Report when weight measurement is documented in the medical record. Modifiers **1P**, **2P**, and **3P** may not be reported. Modifier **8P** may be reported.

Pediatric Pharyngitis and Upper Respiratory Infection

The pediatric pharyngitis measure applies to patients 2 through 18 years of age (inclusive) with a diagnosis of pharyngitis who were dispensed or prescribed antibiotic treatment and/or received a group A streptococcus test.

The URI measure applies to patients 3 months through 18 years of age (inclusive) who were seen with a diagnosis of only URI and were appropriately not prescribed or dispensed an antibiotic.

Category II Codes: Pediatric Pharyngitis and Upper Respiratory Infection	Guidelines
3210F Group A streptococcus test performed	Report when a patient is diagnosed with pharyngitis, is dispensed or prescribed an antibiotic, and received a group A streptococcus test. Modifier 1P for medical exclusions or 2P for patient exclusions may be used.
4120F Antibiotic prescribed or dispensed 4124F Antibiotic neither pre-scribed nor dispensed	Report as appropriate for both performance measures (pediatric pharyngitis and URI). Modifier 1P, 2P, or 3P may not be reported with code 4120F or 4124F for pharyngitis. Modifier 1P is reported with code 4124F when appropriate for URI. If a patient was dispensed or prescribed an antibiotic and received the group A streptococcus test, codes 3210F and 4120F would be reported.

Pediatric End-stage Renal Disease

This measure applies to patients aged 17 years and younger with a diagnosis of end-stage renal disease receiving hemodialysis, having clearance of urea/volume (Kt/V) measurements as per the criteria listed in the codes, having received an influenza vaccine, and having a plan of care documented. This measure is reported during each calendar month that the patient is receiving hemodialysis.

Category II Codes: End-stage Renal Disease	Guidelines
0505F Hemodialysis plan of care documented	Report when the hemodialysis plan of care is documented in the medical record on a patient aged 17 years or younger.
3082F Clearance of urea/volume (Kt/V) less than 1.2 3083F Kt/V greater than or equal to 1.2 and less than 1.7 3084F Kt/V greater than or equal to 1.7	Report code applicable to the corresponding Kt/V measurement. If the Kt/V is less than 1.2 (3082F) and the patient has a plan of care for inadequate hemodialysis, also report code 0505F. There are no performance exclusions for this measure.
4274F Influenza immunization adminis-tered or previously received	Report when a patient aged 6 months through 17 years (with a diagnosis of end-stage renal disease and receiving dialysis) is seen between November 1 and February 15 and receives the influenza immunization or has received the influenza immunization from another provider. The medical record must support that the vaccine was administered. Modifier 1P, 2P, or 3P may be used when appropriate.

Epilepsy

This measure will be reported by the physician providing care to children and adults with a diagnosis of epilepsy.

Category II Codes: Epilepsy	Guidelines
1200F Seizure type(s) and current seizure frequency(ies) documented **1205F** Etiology of epilepsy or epilepsy syndrome(s) reviewed and documented	Report when the seizure type(s) and current seizure frequency for each seizure type are documented in the medical record. Modifier **1P** or **2P** may be reported if appropriate. When the medical record documentation includes the etiology of epilepsy or the epilepsy syndrome(s) is reviewed and documented (if known) or documented as unknown or cryptogenic, code **1205F** is reported. There are no performance exclusions for code **1205F**.
3650F Electroencephalogram (EEG) ordered, reviewed, or requested **1119F** Initial evaluation for condition **1121F** Subsequent evaluation for condition	Code **3650F** is used to report whether or not the patient with a diagnosis of epilepsy seen for an initial evaluation had at least one EEG ordered or, if an EEG was performed previously, results were reviewed or requested. If code **3650F** is reported on the same day as a new patient E/M service (**99201–99205**), neither code **1119F** nor **1121F** is reported. If code **3650F** is reported on the same day as an established patient E/M visit (**99211–99215**) or office or outpatient consultation (**99241–99245**), code **1119F** is also reported to denote an initial evaluation for the condition or code **1121F** is reported to denote a subsequent evaluation. Modifier **1P**, **2P**, or **3P** may be reported with code **3650F** when appropriate.
3324F Magnetic resonance imaging (MRI) or computed tomography (CT) scan ordered, reviewed, or requested **1119F** Initial evaluation for condition **1121F** Subsequent evaluation for condition	When a patient with the diagnosis of epilepsy has MRI (preferred imaging) or CT ordered or if results are reviewed or requested of an MRI or CT previously obtained, code **3324F** is reported. If code **3324F** is reported on the same day as a new patient E/M service (**99201–99205**), neither code **1119F** nor **1121F** is reported. If code **3324F** is reported on the same day as an established patient E/M visit (**99211–99215**) or office or outpatient consultation (**99241–99245**), code **1119F** is also reported to denote an initial evaluation for the condition or code **1121F** is reported to denote a subsequent evaluation. Modifier **1P**, **2P**, or **3P** may be reported with code **3324F**.
6070F Patient queried and counseled about antiepileptic drug (AED) side effects	Report when the patient is queried and counseled about AED side effects and the counseling is documented in the medical record. Modifier **1P** may be reported. This includes patients who are not taking an AED.
5200F Consideration of referral for a neurologic evaluation of appropriateness for surgical therapy for intractable epilepsy within the past 3 years	Report when a patient with a diagnosis of intractable epilepsy was considered for referral for a neurologic evaluation of appropriateness for surgical therapy within the past 3 years. There are no performance exclusions applicable.
4330F Counseling about epilepsy-specific safety issues provided to patient (or caregiver[s])	Report when counseling is provided to a patient and/or their caregiver(s) about context-specific safety issues, appropriate to the patient's age, seizure type(s) and frequency(ies), and occupation and leisure activities (eg, injury prevention, burns, appropriate driving restrictions, bathing), at least once a year and is documented in the medical record. Modifier **3P** may be reported when appropriate.
4340F Counseling for women of childbearing potential with epilepsy	Report whether or not a female of childbearing potential (12–44 years old) was counseled about how epilepsy and its treatment may affect contraception and pregnancy and the counseling is documented in the medical record. Modifier **1P** may be reported.

Chapter 17: Coding to Demonstrate Quality and Value

Major Depressive Disorder—Child and Adolescent

This measure is applicable for reporting care to all patients aged 6 through 17 years with a diagnosis of major depressive disorder (MDD).

Category II Codes: Major Depressive Disorder	Guidelines
2060F Patient interviewed directly by evaluating clinician on or before date of diagnosis of MDD **1040F** *Diagnostic and Statistical Manual of Mental Disorders*, 5th Edition (*DSM-5*) criteria for MDD documented at the initial evaluation **3085F** Suicide risk assessed	Report code **2060F** when a patient is interviewed directly by the evaluating clinician on or before the date of diagnosis. Report code **1040F** when there is documented evidence that the patient met the *DSM-5* criteria—at least 5 elements with symptom duration of 2 weeks or longer, including depressed mood (can be irritable mood in children and adolescents) or loss of interest or pleasure—during the visit in which the new diagnosis or recurrent episode was identified. Code **3085F** is reported when an assessment for suicide risk is performed and documented. Modifiers **1P, 2P, 3P**, and **8P** may not be reported.
4060F Psychotherapy services provided **4062F** Patient referral for psychotherapy documented	Report code **4060F** when a patient receives psychotherapy during an episode of MDD and the service is documented in the medical record. Report code **4062F** when a patient is referred for psychotherapy and the referral is documented in the medical record. Modifier **1P, 2P**, or **3P** may be reported.
4063F Antidepressant pharmacotherapy considered and not prescribed **4064F** Antidepressant pharmacotherapy prescribed	Used to report whether the patient was considered or prescribed an antidepressant medication during an episode of MDD. Modifier **1P, 2P**, or **3P** may not be reported.
0545F Plan for follow-up care for MDD, documented	Report when a plan for follow-up care is documented in the medical record. There are no performance exclusions for this measure.

HIV/AIDS

This measure is reported by the physician providing ongoing HIV care to children and adults. There are 29 Category II codes used in this measure. Each measure has a different denominator that is specific to the patient's age. Measures include reporting cell counts, use of antiretroviral therapy, screening for opportunistic infections and high-risk behaviors, administration of vaccines, and use of *Pneumocystis jiroveci* pneumonia prophylaxis. Refer to the ACTL at https://www.ama-assn.org/practice-management/cpt-category-ii-codes for details on the requirements for reporting these codes.

Reporting Category II Codes

The ACTL should be used in coordination with the Category II section in *CPT*®.

Alphabetical Clinical Topics Listing

* Includes an alphabetic index of performance measures by clinical condition or topic
* Includes the measure developer (eg, PCPI), the performance measure, a description of the measure, and the associated Category II code
* Directs the reader to the measure developer's Web site to access the complete description of the measure (eg, specifications and requirements for reporting performance measures for asthma are located at www.aaaai.org/practice-resources/practice-tools/quality-measures)

Access the measure developer's Web site for the specification documents (ie, clinical measurement set, measurement set numerators and denominators, measure specifications, specifications for paper and EHRs, an algorithm for measure calculation, data abstraction definitions, a medication table, and a retrospective data abstraction tool) of the performance measure.

The following Web sites provide information and resources:

- www.qualitymeasures.ahrq.gov
- https://www.ama-assn.org/practice-management/cpt-category-ii-codes
- www.thepcpi.org

> |||||||||| **Coding Pearl** ||||||||||
>
> A patient must meet the criteria specified in the denominator (diagnosis code) to be included in the numerator (Category II code) for a particular performance measure. Only the diagnosis code for the condition or disease will be linked to Category II *CPT* codes.

Each performance measure includes a symptom or activity assessment, numerator, denominator, percentage, and reporting instructions. A patient must meet the criteria specified in the denominator (diagnosis code) to be included in the numerator (Category II code) for a particular performance measure.

Reporting measures to a payer (electronically or with a CMS-1500 claim form) is done the same way as reporting any *CPT*® code. Report the appropriate E/M code (eg, **99201–99215**, **99241–99245**) based on the level of service performed and documented with all the appropriate *diagnosis* codes that were addressed during the course of the visit. Report the Category II *CPT* code that relates to the performance measure with any applicable Category II modifier. Only the diagnosis code for the condition or disease will be linked to Category II *CPT* codes.

Examples

➤ **A 4-year-old presents with acute onset of right ear pain.** An expanded-level history and physical examination are performed. The diagnosis is AOE. The patient is sent home on topical antimicrobial and anti-inflammatory medication. All the criteria in the AOE measurement set as specified by the developer of the performance measurement are met. The applicable codes identified under the Category II *CPT* code section are reviewed and the ACTL is consulted for current measure criteria.

ICD-10-CM	CPT
H60.501 (AOE noninfective right ear)	**99213** (established patient; expanded history and physical examination with low-complexity medical decision-making) **1116F** (auricular or periauricular pain assessed) **4130F** (topical preparations [including over the counter] prescribed for AOE) **4132F** (systemic antimicrobial therapy not prescribed)

➤ **A 15-year-old new patient is seen with complaints of sleep disturbance and depressed mood.** The adolescent has not been eating well and has been increasingly irritable. A comprehensive history and detailed physical examination are performed. The patient is determined to meet *DSM-5* criteria for moderate MDD. Treatment options, including psychotherapy and antidepressant medications, are discussed. The patient chooses to pursue psychotherapy but refuses medication and a referral is provided. The patient is scheduled for follow-up by phone call from nurse in one week and appointment in 6 weeks.

ICD-10-CM	CPT
F32.1 (MDD single episode, moderate)	**99203** (new patient; comprehensive history, detailed physical examination with moderate-complexity medical decision-making) **2060F** (patient interviewed directly by evaluating clinician on or before date of diagnosis of MDD) **1040F** (criteria for MDD documented at the initial evaluation) **3085F** (suicide risk assessed) **4062F** (patient referral for psychotherapy documented) **4063F** (antidepressant pharmacotherapy considered and not prescribed) **0545F** (plan for follow-up care documented)

Chapter 17: Coding to Demonstrate Quality and Value

➤ **A 10-year-old is seen with exacerbation of asthma.** His last exacerbation was 3 months ago. An expanded history and detailed physical examination are performed. A nebulizer treatment with albuterol is ordered and administered. Examination following treatment shows decreased wheezing. He is sent home on albuterol and steroids administered by metered-dose inhaler with plan to follow up as necessary. Assessment of asthma status is documented as mild persistent. Category II codes for evaluation of asthma symptoms, persistent asthma, assessment of asthma status, and prescription of inhaled corticosteroids are reported. If documentation supports asthma risk (**2016F**), smoking status and exposure to secondhand smoke in the home (**1031F–1033F**), or tobacco use cessation intervention (**4000F–4001F**), these may be additionally reported.

ICD-10-CM	CPT®
J45.31 (mild persistent asthma with exacerbation)	**99214 25** (established patient; expanded history, detailed physical examination with moderate-complexity medical decision-making) **94640** (aerosol treatment) **J7611** (albuterol, inhalation solution, US Food and Drug Administration–approved final product, non-compounded, administered through durable medical equipment concentrated form, 1 mg) **1005F** (asthma symptoms evaluated) **1038F** (persistent asthma, mild, moderate, or severe) **2015F** (assessment of asthma status) **4140F** (inhaled corticosteroids prescribed)

||||||||

Preventing Fraud and Abuse:
Compliance, Audits, and Paybacks

||||||||

This chapter was contributed by the American Academy of Pediatrics Committee on Medical Liability and Risk Management.

Contents

Chapter 18: Preventing Fraud and Abuse: Compliance, Audits, and Paybacks

Although most physicians work ethically, provide high-quality care, and submit appropriate claims for payment, unfortunately, there are some providers who exploit the health care system for personal gain. These few have necessitated an array of laws to combat fraud and abuse and protect the integrity of the health care payment system. Just as patients put enormous trust in physicians, so do payers. Medicare, Medicaid, other federal health care programs, and private payers rely on physicians' medical judgment to treat patients with appropriate services. They depend on physicians to submit accurate and truthful claims for the services provided to their enrollees. And most physicians intend to do just that. However, the process is made more difficult by the complex and dynamic nature of payer coding and billing procedures, which, despite efforts to standardize variations, persist from carrier to carrier, policy to policy, state to state, and month to month.

This chapter outlines the importance of safeguarding the health care system from fraud and abuse, describes how compliance programs can protect medical practices from unintentional billing errors, and provides general considerations on how to respond to overpayment notices and inquiries from auditors.

Defining Medical Fraud and Abuse

The federal government has more than a dozen laws in its antifraud and abuse arsenal. The 5 most important laws that apply to physicians are the False Claims Act, Anti-Kickback Statute, Physician Self-Referral Law, Exclusion Authorities, and Civil Monetary Penalties Law. Abiding by these laws is not only the right thing to do; violating them, even (for some) unwittingly, could result in criminal penalties, civil fines, exclusion from federal health care programs, or loss of medical license from a state medical board. It all begins with understanding the definition of *fraud and abuse* in health care.

Fraud

Fraud is obtaining something of value through intentional misrepresentation or concealment of material facts. Examples of fraud in the physician's office may include
* Requiring that a patient return for a procedure that could have been performed on the same day
* Billing Medicare or Medicaid for services not provided, including no-shows
* Billing one member for services provided to another (non-covered) member
* Billing more than one party for the same service
* Billing services under a different National Provider Identifier (NPI) (except as allowed by payer guidance)
* Taking a kickback in money, in-kind, or other valuable compensation for referrals
* Completing a certificate of medical necessity for a patient who does not need the service or who is not professionally known by the provider

Abuse

Abuse includes any practice that is not consistent with the goals of providing patients with services that
* Are medically necessary
* Meet professionally recognized standards
* Are fairly priced

Some examples of actions that will likely be considered to be abuse are
* Charging in excess for services or supplies
* Billing Medicare or Medicaid based on a higher fee schedule than for other patients
* Providing medically unnecessary services
* Submitting bills to Medicare or Medicaid that are the responsibility of another insurance plan
* Waiving co-payments or deductibles (except as permitted for financial hardship)
* Advertising for free services
* Coding all visits at the same level
* Unbundling claims—ie, billing separately for services that are correctly billed under one code
* Billing claims under the wrong NPI

CPT copyright 2017 American Medical Association. All rights reserved.

Kickbacks, Inducements, and Self-referrals

Business arrangements in which physician practices refer business to an outside entity (eg, hospitals, hospices, nursing facilities, home health agencies, durable medical equipment suppliers, vendors) should be on a fair market value basis. Whenever a physician practice intends to enter into a business arrangement that involves making referrals, legal counsel familiar with antikickback and physician self-referral laws should review the arrangement.

Risk areas that may need to be addressed in policies and procedures include

- Offering inappropriate inducements to patients (eg, waiving coinsurance or deductible amounts without a good-faith determination that the patient is in financial need, failing to make reasonable efforts to collect the cost-sharing amount)
- Financial arrangements with outside entities to which the practice may refer federal health care program business
- Joint ventures with entities supplying goods or services to the physician practice or its patients
- Participation in an accountable care organization and/or compliance in the context of participation in a Medicaid shared savings program
- Consulting contracts or medical directorships
- Laboratory payments based on volume of referred services
- Payments for services already covered by a federal health insurer (double-dipping)
- Office and equipment leases with entities to which the physician refers business
- Soliciting, accepting, or offering any gift or gratuity of more than nominal value to or from those who may benefit from a physician practice referral of federal health care program business

When considering whether to engage in a particular billing practice, enter into a particular business venture, or pursue an employment, consulting, or other personal services relationship, it is prudent to evaluate the arrangement for potential compliance problems. Use experienced health care lawyers to analyze the issues and provide a legal evaluation and risk analysis of the proposed venture, relationship, or arrangement. The state bar association may have a directory of local attorneys who practice in the health care field. The American Health Lawyers Association is another resource (www.healthlawyers.org).

> **||||||| Coding Pearl |||||||**
>
> Use experienced health care lawyers. To locate one, contact your state bar association or the American Health Lawyers Association (www.healthlawyers.org).

Antifraud and Anti-abuse Activities

The battle against health care fraud and abuse is being waged on many fronts—federal and state governments as well as private payers. More and more, these groups are sharing information, so that a provider under investigation by one government health care program will likely be contacted by another and possibly by private payers. The Department of Health and Human Services (HHS) Office of Inspector General (OIG) has several antifraud campaigns underway. In addition to federal antifraud and abuse laws, many states have enacted antifraud and anti-abuse legislation, and state Medicaid programs have established Medicaid fraud control units. That means physician practices are subject to several levels of scrutiny for possible fraudulent activity. The Patient Protection and Affordable Care Act (PPACA) introduced new Medicaid program integrity provisions, such as increased fraud detection methods, terminating providers previously terminated from other government health care programs, suspending future payments based on credible allegations of fraud, and adopting the National Correct Coding Initiative edits (see Chapter 3, Modifiers and Coding Edits, for more information on edits). All this means that the momentum and resources for rooting out fraud and abuse at the federal and state level have intensified.

In addition, Medicaid auditors have a financial incentive to find fraud. The Medicaid Recovery Audit Contractors (RAC) program allows states to hire private contractors to audit Medicaid payments and keep a percentage of what they collect. Contingency fees for these contractors vary by state and range from 5.25% to 17%, with most between 9% and 13%. Under some circumstances, there can be bonuses paid that increase these fees to greater than 20%. Because it is Medicaid, pediatricians may be included in RAC audits. The RAC program was established in provisions of the PPACA and modeled on a similar successful Medicare program. So far, the

Medicare and Medicaid RAC programs have gone after larger organizations, but it is not inconceivable that they will eventually turn their attention to physician practices. It's always better to be prepared. Information on the status of state Medicaid RAC programs is available through the Centers for Medicare & Medicaid Services (CMS) Medicaid site, www.medicaid.gov. This site includes the name and contact information for each state's RAC and medical directors and look-back period for audits.

Areas of Specific Concern

The Department of Health and Human Services and the Department of Justice Health Care Fraud and Abuse Control Program Annual Report for Fiscal Year 2016, published in February 2017, highlights some of the newer initiatives and findings of the Health Care Fraud and Abuse Program coordinated through the OIG. Many findings and initiatives put physician practices under high scrutiny for miscoded services, failure to adequately document services, and operating in a manner that conflicts with antikickback and self-referral laws. Examples of audit and evaluation findings in fiscal year (FY) 2016 include

- The FY 2016 national Medicaid improper payment rate is 10.48%, representing $36.3 billion in gross improper payments, compared with the FY 2015 improper payment rate of 9.8% or $29.1 billion in improper payments. The FY 2016 national Children's Health Insurance Program (CHIP) improper payment rate is 7.99%, representing $0.7 billion in gross improper payments, compared with a FY 2015 national CHIP improper payment rate of 6.8%, representing $0.6 billion in estimated improper payments. As these error rates are well above targets set by the OIG, expect continued aggressive efforts to discover and reduce improper payments.
- Specific areas of concern that affect physicians include billing for a higher level of service than was provided, billing for services by clinical staff that do not meet incident-to provisions, and physician self-referral violations.
- Several cases in 2016 involved inappropriate payments or other incentives to physicians for using particular medical devices or medications.
- Analysis of claims data is increasingly combined across payers and care settings to identify physicians and other providers who are outliers in their billing and referral patterns to identify potential fraud and abuse. The fraud and abuse control units of HHS and the US Department of Justice also continue to cross-reference enrollment information for the same physicians and providers when there is history of enrollment in multiple states and/or programs. By cross-referencing enrollment data, conflicting information and/or evidence of prior revocation of eligibility to participate in federal programs may be discovered.

Compliance Programs

Does your practice have a fraud and abuse prevention compliance program? For many years, compliance programs for small practices were voluntary. This is no longer the case; they are now required, even for small practices, but they can be scalable.

What is a compliance program? A compliance program establishes strategies to prevent, detect, and resolve conduct that does not conform to

- Federal and state law
- Federal, state, and private payer health care program requirements
- The practice's own ethical and business policies

Pediatric practices benefit from having compliance initiatives because they tighten billing and coding operations and documentation. Practices with written compliance programs report having better control on internal procedures, improved medical record documentation, and streamlined practice operations.

Section 6401(a) of the PPACA requires physicians and other providers and suppliers who enroll in Medicare, Medicaid, or CHIP to establish a compliance program with certain "core elements."

Chapter 18: Preventing Fraud and Abuse: Compliance, Audits, and Paybacks

The 7 Elements of the OIG Compliance Program

Although the OIG has yet to publish the official guidance for required compliance programs, it is helpful to look at the 7 core elements described in the OIG guidance on voluntary compliance program for small physician practices published in 2000.

- Conduct internal monitoring and auditing.
- Implement written compliance and practice standards.
- Designate a compliance officer, contact, or committee.
- Conduct appropriate training and education.
- Respond appropriately to detected offenses and develop corrective action.
- Develop open lines of communication.
- Enforce disciplinary standards through well-publicized guidelines.

It's also useful to consult the *United States Sentencing Commission Guidelines Manual,* which makes it clear that an organization under investigation may be given more sympathetic treatment if a good compliance program is in place. Compliance programs not only help to prevent fraudulent or erroneous claims, but they also show that the physician practice is making a good-faith effort to submit claims appropriately. However, that would require the program to be integrated into the daily operations of the practice. It cannot be a set of policies and procedures merely kept in a binder or on a computer unrelated to actual business operations.

Here are some reasons the *United States Sentencing Commission Guidelines Manual* identifies to implement an effective compliance program.

- It may save the practice money if it prevents costly civil suits and criminal investigations.
- It sends an unambiguous message to employees: Fraud and abuse will not be tolerated.
- It decreases the risk of employees bringing suit against the practice under the False Claims Act because employees will have an internal communication system for reporting questionable activities and resolving problems.
- It helps if an investigation occurs. Investigators may be more inclined to resolve the problem as a civil rather than a criminal matter, or it may lead to an administrative resolution rather than a formal false claim action.
- It may help reduce the range used for imposing fines under federal sentencing guidelines.
- It may influence an OIG decision whether to exclude a provider from participation in federal health care programs.
- It frequently results in improved medical record documentation.
- It improves coding accuracy, reduces denials, and makes claims and payment processes more effective.
- It educates physicians and employees on their responsibilities for preventing, detecting, and reporting fraud and abuse.
- It should meet governmental requirements for practices to have a formal compliance plan.

Steps to Developing a Compliance Program

The CMS has described the steps to create an effective compliance and ethics program. A key aspect is that the organization exercises due diligence to prevent and detect criminal conduct and promotes a culture that encourages ethical conduct and a commitment to compliance with the law.

The CMS specifies that in creating the compliance program, the practice

1. Develop and distribute written policies, procedures, and standards of conduct to prevent and detect inappropriate behavior.
2. Designate a chief compliance officer and other appropriate bodies (eg, a corporate compliance committee) charged with the responsibility of operating and monitoring the compliance program and who report directly to high-level personnel and the governing body.
3. Use reasonable efforts not to include any individual in the substantial authority personnel whom the organization knew, or should have known, has engaged in illegal activities or other conduct inconsistent with an effective compliance and ethics program.
4. Develop and implement regular, effective education and training programs for the governing body; all employees, including high-level personnel; and, as appropriate, the organization's agents.

5. Maintain a process, such as a hotline, to receive complaints and the adoption of procedures to protect the anonymity of complainants and protect whistle-blowers from retaliation. (In a small practice, a hotline could be replaced with an "anonymous fraud report box.")
6. Develop a system to respond to allegations of improper conduct and the enforcement of appropriate disciplinary action against employees who have violated internal compliance policies, applicable statutes, regulations, or federal health care program requirements.
7. Use audits and/or other evaluation techniques to monitor compliance and assist in the reduction of identified problem areas.
8. Investigate and remediate identified systemic problems, including making any necessary modifications to the organization's compliance and ethics program.

Written Policies and Procedures

A compliance program should have written compliance standards and procedures that the practice follows. They should specifically describe the lines of responsibility for implementing the compliance program. Those standards and procedures should reduce the likelihood of fraudulent activity while also helping to identify any incorrect billing practices. Policies and procedures should be updated periodically to address newly identified areas of risk, new regulations, or process changes in the practice. All staff should receive periodic education on policies and procedures to maintain up-to-date knowledge.

Coding and Billing

The following billing risk areas have been frequent areas of investigations and audits by the OIG and should be addressed in a good compliance program:
* Billing for items or services not provided or not provided as claimed
* Submitting claims for equipment, medical supplies, and services that are not reasonable and necessary
* Double billing
* Billing for non-covered services as if covered
* Known misuse of NPIs, which results in improper billing
* Billing separately for bundled services
* Misuse of modifiers
* Consistently under-coding or over-coding services
* Using only one evaluation and management (E/M) service code within a category of service

  Other areas that may trigger an audit include
* Profile of services reported differs from payer profiles of physicians of your specialty.
* Repeated use of unspecified diagnosis codes or use of codes that are not consistent with the service or your specialty.
* Surgical services not consistent with claims submitted by a facility.
* Number of procedures or services reported exceed the hours in a day.
* High numbers of denials.

> ||||||||| **Coding Pearl** |||||||||
>
> Place of service errors are a targeted area of review for the OIG. See Chapter 19, The Business of Medicine: Working With Current and Emerging Payment Systems, for more information on reporting correct place of service codes.

Medical Record Documentation

One of the most important physician practice compliance issues is the appropriate documentation of diagnosis and treatment. Patients and other providers must be able to trust that information within shared records is accurate and actionable for the care of the patient. With most pediatricians now using electronic health records (EHRs) to document office-based services, compliant documentation must now encompass not only what should be documented but also what must be safeguarded from inaccuracies and potential noncompliant access to or disclosure of information.

The CMS has published guidance for physicians on detecting and responding to fraud, waste, and abuse associated with the use of EHRs (https://www.cms.gov/Medicare-Medicaid-Coordination/Fraud-Prevention/Medicaid-Integrity-Education/electronic-health-records.html). The CMS instructs that physicians should apply the compliance program components previously discussed to take preventive action to deter the inappropriate use of EHR system features or inappropriate access to patient information. This includes a written compliance plan. The written compliance plan should specify that medical record documentation should comply with the following documentation principles and guidelines:

- The medical record should be complete (and legible, when handwritten) and individualized for each patient encounter. Do not allow cut-and-paste functionality in the EHR. Any use of copy and paste, copy forward, macros, or auto-population should be regulated by office policies that address maintenance of record integrity and supplementation via free text, where indicated. (Guidance from the CMS includes a decision table for ensuring proper use of EHR features and capabilities.)
- Retain all signatures when there are multiple authors or contributors to a document, so that each individual's contribution is unambiguously identified.
- All staff should receive initial and periodic education on compliant medical record documentation, including, as applicable, use of EHR functionality, use of individual sign-on, and appropriate access to records.
- Documentation should be completed at the time of service or as soon as possible afterward.
- The documentation of each patient encounter should include the reason for the encounter; any relevant history; physical examination findings; prior diagnostic test results, when pertinent; assessment, clinical impression, or diagnosis; plan of care; and date and legible identity of the observer.
- If not documented, the rationale for ordering diagnostic and other ancillary services should be easily inferred by an independent reviewer or third party. Past and present diagnoses and history should be accessible to the treating and/or consulting physician.
- Appropriate health risk factors should be identified. The patient's progress, patient's response to and any changes in treatment, and any revision in diagnosis should be documented.
- All pages in the medical record should include the patient name and an identifying number or birth date.
- Prescription drug management should include the name of the medication, dosage, and instructions.
- Clinically important telephone calls should be documented, including date, time, instructions, and follow-up.
- Anticipatory guidance, patient education, and counseling are best documented when performed.
- Any addenda should be identifiable with the author's signature and dated with the date the addendum was made. The compliance plan should address what circumstances justify making changes to the EHR record and identify who can make changes, requirements for amendments and corrections to an EHR, and what information cannot be changed (ie, author, date, and time of original note).
- Consent forms should be dated, the procedure documented, and the form signed by the patient or his or her legal representative. Documentation should include a summary of the discussion of the procedure and risks.
- All abbreviations used should be explicit.
- Patient noncompliance, including immunization refusal, should be documented as well as discussion of the risks and adverse consequences of noncompliance.
- Allergies and adverse reactions should be prominently displayed.
- Immunization and growth charts must be maintained and current.
- Problem and medication lists should be completed and current, including over-the-counter medications.
- The EHR audit log should be enabled at all times so it creates an accurate chronological history of changes to the EHR. Practice procedures should describe any exceptions, including who can disable the log and under what circumstances this may be appropriate.

> **~ More From the AAP ~**
>
> See also "What Does Your EHR Documentation Say?" in the March 2017 *AAP Pediatric Coding Newsletter*™ at http://coding.aap.org (subscription required).

See the Coding Conundrum: Pitfalls of EHR Coding box later in this chapter for other considerations specific to EHR documentation.

Retention of Records

Policies and procedures should be written to include the creation, distribution, retention, and destruction of documents. In designing a record-retention system, privacy concerns and federal and state regulatory requirements should be taken into consideration. In addition to maintaining appropriate and thorough medical records on each patient, the OIG recommends that the system include the following types of documents:

* All records and documentation (eg, billing and claims documentation) required for participation in federal, state, and private-payer health care programs
* All records necessary to demonstrate the integrity of the physician practice's compliance process and to confirm the effectiveness of the program

   The following record-retention guidelines should be used:

* The length of time that a physician's medical record documentation is to be retained should be specified. Federal and state statutes should be consulted for specific time frames.
* Consulting with an attorney or risk management department of a medical liability insurer is prudent to determine the appropriate retention period. At a minimum, pediatricians may want to retain records until patients obtain the age of majority plus the statute of limitations in their jurisdiction. Longer retention periods may be prudent, depending on the circumstances.
* Medical records, including electronic correspondence, should be secured against loss, destruction, unauthorized access, unauthorized reproduction, corruption, and damage.
* Policies and procedures should stipulate the disposition of medical records in the event the practice is sold or closed.

   The American Academy of Pediatrics (AAP) provides free Health Insurance Portability and Accountability Act of 1996 (HIPAA) privacy and security manuals with downloadable templates, policies, and procedures at https://www.aap.org/en-us/professional-resources/practice-transformation/managing-practice/Pages/HIPAA-Privacy-and-Security-Compliance-Manuals.aspx.

Document Advice From Payers

A physician practice should document its efforts to comply with applicable federal, state, and private health care program requirements. For example

* When requesting advice from a government agency charged with administering a federal or state health care program or from a private payer, document and retain a record of the request and of all written or oral responses.
* Maintain a log of oral inquiries between the practice and third parties.
* Keep copies of all provider manuals, provider bulletins, and communications from payers about coding and submission of claims.

Designate a Compliance Officer

To administer the compliance program, the practice should designate an individual responsible for overseeing the program. More than one employee may be designated with the responsibility of compliance monitoring, or a practice may outsource all or part of the functions of a compliance officer to a third party. Attributes and qualifications of a compliance officer include

* Independent position to protect against any conflicts of interest from "regular" position responsibilities and compliance officer duties
* Attention to detail
* Experience in billing and coding
* Effective communication skills (oral and written) with employees, physicians, and carriers

   The primary responsibilities of a compliance officer include

* Overseeing and monitoring the implementation of the compliance program.
* Establishing methods, such as periodic audits, to improve the practice's efficiency and quality of services and reduce the practice's vulnerability to fraud and abuse.

Chapter 18: Preventing Fraud and Abuse: Compliance, Audits, and Paybacks

Coding Conundrum: Pitfalls of EHR Coding

One of the advantages of using EHRs is enhanced documentation of services. Documentation of an E/M service may be easier because of the use of templates or drop-down options, and legibility is not an issue. However, there are disadvantages to EHRs when it comes to documentation. When completing an audit, be aware of

- The use of templates may not accurately describe pertinent patient history or abnormal findings on examination. Some EHRs do not allow free texting, thereby prohibiting more detailed, appropriate documentation. If a system does not allow free texting, work with the vendor to add this capability, or add any and all abnormal findings that might be pertinent in the template so documentation can be complete and accurate.

- Avoid templates and documentation tools that feature predefined text that may include information that is not relevant to the patient presentation and/or services rendered. Review and edit all defaulted data to ensure only patient-specific data is recorded for that visit, while removing all other irrelevant data pulled in by the default template.

- Users should be familiar with the manner in which the EHR constructs a note from the data entered into each field and how the system may be customized to enhance the final note.

- Only the history and physical examination that are pertinent to the problem or condition should be used in selection of an E/M code. Therefore, physicians should code each E/M service and override the EHR-assigned E/M code when appropriate.

- The physician must document history of present illness (HPI). The EHR will usually capture all documentation, whether performed by ancillary staff or the provider. Make certain it is clear who documented each portion of the service. For example, if HPI is documented by a nurse or medical assistant, the physician *must* document his or her HPI. (Electronic health record systems include audit trails that may be used to prove who entered specific elements of documentation. It is important to understand how the practice's EHR system creates and produces an audit trail.)

- The use of a scribe to enter information relayed by a physician or provider must be clearly entered in each record, when applicable. Most payers require identification of the scribe that includes a statement such as "acting as a scribe for Dr X." The physician or provider must review the note for accuracy and cosign indicating his or her words and actions were accurately recorded.

- If an EHR system automatically transfers the documented review of systems (ROS) and past, family, and social history from one encounter to the next or lists every medication that has been prescribed in the past, make certain the physician reviews the information to be certain it is still accurate and documents his or her review of the pertinent copied information to support the level of history that was necessary and performed.

- Physicians may document the same comment in the ROS that was obtained and documented in the HPI (eg, HPI, "fever of 102°F"; ROS, "fever"). The repeated comment should only be used as HPI or ROS, not both, based on the context for which it was obtained (eg, description of problem, question to better define problem). The EHR system may not differentiate and will count the redundant information twice (or more), leading to a higher level of history.

- Most EHR systems have integrated an E/M coding system using the CMS 1995 or 1997 *Documentation Guidelines for Evaluation and Management Services.* Systems measure or count the elements of each of the required key components (ie, history, physical examination, and medical decision-making) without regard to the nature of the presenting problem, severity of illness, or medical necessity. Therefore, if a physician elects to perform a detailed or comprehensive-level history and physical examination on every established patient, the reported E/M code will always be a potentially inappropriate higher-level E/M service.

- If previous diagnoses are carried over from one encounter to the next, make sure only those that are pertinent to the current visit are considered when determining the complexity of the service provided.

- List the primary diagnosis first because the EHR may report the diagnoses in the order in which they are documented.

- To support management options, it may be necessary to document the diagnoses being considered. These suspected or ruled-out diagnoses should not be reported by the EHR system in the outpatient setting.

- Make certain that any separately reportable procedure or service has documentation to support that it was performed.

- Don't depend on the software vendor to add *Current Procedural Terminology (CPT®)*; *International Classification of Diseases, 10th Revision, Clinical Modification (ICD-10-CM)*; or Healthcare Common Procedure Coding System (HCPCS) codes to the system. Review all new, deleted, and revised codes each year. Notify the vendor if codes have not been revised and educate physicians and billing staff on their appropriate use.

- Revising the compliance program in response to changes in the needs of the practice or changes in the law and in the policies and procedures of government and private payer health plans.
- Developing, coordinating, and participating in a training program that focuses on the elements of the compliance program and seeks to ensure that training materials are appropriate.
- Checking the HHS OIG List of Excluded Individuals and Entities and the federal System for Award Management to ascertain whether any potential new hires, current employees, medical staff, or independent contractors are listed; advising management of findings; and seeing that appropriate action is taken as described in the compliance program.
- Informing employees and physicians of pertinent federal and state statutes, regulations, and standards and monitoring their compliance.
- Investigating any report or allegation concerning suspected unethical or improper business practices and monitoring subsequent corrective action, compliance, or both.
- Assessing the practice's situation and determining what best suits the practice in terms of compliance oversight.
- Maintaining records of compliance-related activities, including meetings, educational activities, and internal audits. Particular attention should be given to documenting violations found by the compliance program and documenting the remedial actions.

The Audit/Review Process

1. Obtain and review a productivity report from your billing system.
2. Calculate the percentage distribution of E/M codes within each category of service (new and established office or outpatient visits, initial observation or inpatient services, use of modifier **25**) for each physician in the practice. (Most billing software provides these calculations.) You might also use the AAP Coding Calculator, found at https://www.aap.org/en-us/professional-resources/practice-transformation/getting-paid/Coding-at-the-AAP/Pages/Coding-Calculator.aspx, to help you profile your E/M code use and distribution.
3. Use data from a 12-month period because they include seasonal trends and are more reflective of practice patterns.
4. Perform a comparative analysis of the distribution with each physician in the practice. Remember that data only reflect the billing patterns, and not if one is more correct than another. More frequent oversight and monitoring is necessary for services provided by physicians who are new to the practice and may use documentation or coding guidance that conflicts with practice policy.
5. Review the report to ensure that all procedures performed are being captured and reported appropriately. For example, are discharge visits (**99238** and **99239**) being billed and is the number proportionate to the number of newborn and other hospital admissions performed?
6. Review the practice encounter form or code selection application to ensure that *CPT®* and *ICD-10-CM* codes are correct and match the corresponding description.
7. Review the actual encounter and claim form with the medical record to ensure the claim is submitted with the appropriate codes and/or modifiers. (See the Documentation and Coding Audits section later in this chapter.)
8. Review medical records to ensure they are compliant with national standards and office policies. Standards for maintenance of medical records can be found on the National Committee for Quality Assurance Web site (www.ncqa.org).
9. Review each medical record and encounter form (as applicable) with these questions in mind.
   - Are the patient's name, identification number, and/or date of birth on every page in the medical record?
   - Does the medical record contain updated demographic information?
   - Are allergies noted and prominently displayed?
   - Is the date of service documented?
   - Was the service medically necessary?
   - Does the documentation support the level of E/M service based on the required key components and/or type of service (eg, consultation, preventive medicine service)?
   - Are all the services and/or procedures documented/captured on the encounter form?

- Does the documentation for the preventive medicine visit meet the requirements of the Medicaid Early and Periodic Screening, Diagnosis, and Treatment program when applicable?
- Does the documentation support the procedure billed (eg, administration of injection, catheterization, impacted cerumen removal)?
- Does the documentation support the diagnosis code(s) billed?
- If using an EHR, does the documentation support physician review and personal documentation? For example, if the EHR always brings up the patient's history, is there a notation that the physician reviewed it? If not, it should not be counted as part of the service.
- Is there a completed growth chart and immunization record?
- Is the documentation legible?
- Does any order for medication include the specific dosage and use?
- Is there documentation of a follow-up plan?
- Are diagnostic reports (eg, laboratory tests, radiograph) signed and dated to reflect review?
- Does documentation include the name and credentials of each contributing author in a manner that reflects each author's individual contributions?
- Was an appropriate modifier reported with sufficient documentation?
- Is the documentation in compliance with Physicians at Teaching Hospitals (PATH) guidelines and/or incident-to provisions as appropriate?

Documentation and Coding Audits

Medicare, state Medicaid programs, and commercial payers will audit claims as well as monitor E/M coding profiles. While the specialty-specific E/M profiles published by the CMS provide helpful information, keep in mind that these distributions only reflect code use and not code accuracy. An atypical distribution of codes may be the result of care for a more complex patient population than average, including patients with chronic diseases or with social and economic challenges. Correct coding appropriately identifies the risk stratification for your patients and may directly affect your payments.

Also, just because you got paid does not mean that payers will not retrospectively audit and demand repayment or withhold future payments, particularly if claims were processed incorrectly or it was in error according to your contract. Practices are advised to become familiar with state laws addressing retrospective audits and repayments and with payer procedures for repayment. Your AAP chapter or state medical society may be able to help you understand your state-specific laws.

- Focus audits on documentation and coding of the most commonly performed services, adherence to medical record standards, appropriate reporting of diagnosis codes, use of modifiers, and adherence to coding and federal guidelines (eg, PATH guidelines, physician self-referral laws).
- Make certain all physicians in the practice are in agreement with how any review will be conducted and how results will be used.
- The person performing the audit (eg, physician, physician extender, coder or other administrative employee, outside consultant, a combination thereof) must be proficient at coding, understand payer guidelines and requirements, and know medical terminology. Consider a team approach (eg, nurse and coder). If a physician is not actually performing record reviews, one should be available to assist as necessary.
- Determine if audits should be performed under the direction of a health care attorney who may offer assistance with developing an audit process and provide guidance on any internal compliance concerns discovered in the process. Attorney–client privilege may apply when audits are directed by an attorney.
- Determine if your review will be retrospective (ie, performed on paid claims and services) or prospective (ie, performed on services and claims that have not yet been billed). It is recommended that practices conduct a prospective review because any necessary corrections can be made before a claim is filed. Although a prospective review will delay claims submission and introduce additional practice expense, this practice may have a net positive financial effect.

- Select the types of services or procedures that will be included in the review. For example, if the review will include only office or outpatient services, include those services most frequently reported (eg, a sampling of new and established patient problem-oriented and preventive medicine visits, documentation of nebulizer treatments). When performing a review of hospital services, include newborn care, critical care, initial and subsequent observation, and inpatient services.
- Determine the number of records or encounters that will be included in the audit. Most coding consultants recommend that a minimum of 10 records per physician or provider be reviewed in a baseline or subsequent review. However, if a more focused review is required, the sample size may need to be increased. Medical records should be randomly selected for each E/M level of service and from different dates of service.
- Determine the frequency of audits. Large practices might consider conducting audits on one physician or provider per week during a quarter or one physician or provider per month throughout the year.
- Make certain that the reviewer has all appropriate and necessary tools, which may include
  - ❖ The CMS *Documentation Guidelines for Evaluation and Management Services* (1995 and/or 1997) that are used by the practice or physician.
  - ❖ Current *CPT*®, *ICD-10-CM*, and HCPCS manuals.
  - ❖ Access to or copies of all payer newsletters or information bulletins that outline coding and/or payment policies.
  - ❖ An audit worksheet. This may be one designed by your practice, or one of many published templates may be used. Note that the CMS has never endorsed any specific audit form or coding template. Make certain the audit form used includes appropriate requirements for selection of an E/M service.
  - ❖ A log to document findings for each provider. This log should include a summary detail of findings for each encounter reviewed. The log and E/M audit worksheets can be used as teaching tools at the conclusion of the audit.

Sample Audit Log[a]

Physician:		Date:		Auditor:	
Patient Name	**Patient ID/DOB**	**Date of Service**	**Reported Code**	**Audited Code**	**Comments**
Jane	5/1/09	6/3/13	99214	99213	Total and counseling time not documented; key components = 99213; plan for return not documented
			J45.31; R06.2	J45.31	Wheezing is inherent to asthma (J45.31).
Zach	2/4/10	6/4/13	69210	0	Cerumen not documented as impacted
Gracie	11/12/08	6/4/13	99213	99214	Key components = 99214

Abbreviations: DOB, date of birth; ID, identification.

[a] Also available at www.aap.org/cfp; use access code AAPCFP23.

Following the Audit

- Discuss audit findings with each provider.
- Educate providers and staff as necessary.
- If a problem is encountered (eg, inappropriate use of modifiers, miscoding), a more focused retrospective review should be conducted to determine how long the error has been occurring and its effect. This is especially important when reviewing claims for physicians new to the practice or when a particular coding guideline or code has changed.
- Use an audit tool for verifying E/M levels, such as the *Pediatric Evaluation and Management Coding Card*.

- If overpayments have occurred due to miscoding or billing errors, the errors should be corrected and education of appropriate staff performed. The errors may need to be disclosed and incorrect payments refunded. Always refer to payer contracts and agreements to understand their requirements and policies for overpayments and disclosure. Always seek advice from the practice's attorney prior to disclosure or repayment.

- Schedule follow-up audits, if indicated, to determine if problems have been resolved (eg, improved documentation, capturing procedures, correct use of modifiers).

- Determine if audits need to be performed on a quarterly or annual basis and follow through with audits on a routine basis.

- If changes need to be made to the EHR system, contact the vendor and discuss how these might be accomplished. Educate physicians and providers on the changes made or need for additional physician documentation.

- Establish or update written policies and procedures.

- Maintain records of your compliance efforts and training.

Don't Get Caught Without a Plan

Most practices will never have to deal with demands for paybacks or fraud audits. Nevertheless, all practices should have a plan just in case they occur. Because time is of the essence in responding to these communications, it would be a calamity to have a letter sit on someone's desk while precious days tick away. Often, a response must be received within 30 days of the date of the request, and the paperwork demanded is not insignificant.

The first communication may be a request for repayment based on payer software analysis of claims history to detect claims paid in conflict with payment policies. It is important for all staff to be trained to recognize these requests and know to get them to the compliance officer immediately. Then, qualified staff tasked with receiving all requests for paybacks can determine the veracity of the request and, if inaccurate, act in accordance with the payer's rebuttal and appeal processes in a timely manner. Likewise, requests for records must be handled carefully and expeditiously.

Responding to Repayment Demands

In an effort to control costs and stamp out fraud, carrier claims processing and special investigative units use sophisticated software programs to identify providers with atypical coding patterns that could indicate erroneous coding and potential overpayments. For example, some carriers may flag providers considered outliers in frequently reporting high-level E/M codes or frequent use of modifiers. They then extrapolate the alleged overpayments over several years and demand across-the-board repayments. Worse, carriers will reduce payments on future claims to correct alleged overpayments on past claims. These requests require a swift and skilled response. Usually, several thousand dollars are involved. Given the compressed timeline and dollars at stake, seeking legal advice is invaluable in these situations.

Here is some general guidance for your consideration.

- If it is truly due to a billing error by the practice, take action to correct the problem and demonstrate to the carrier how it has or will be corrected and the measures implemented to avoid the problem in the future.

- Reply in writing to inform the carrier you are willing to work with it, and ask that it identify each of the claims in question as well as the specific criteria or standards it is applying to the audit.

- Make sure the practice and the carrier consistently apply current *CPT* guidelines. Reference *CPT* coding guidelines and have appropriate documentation for support. The AAP Coding Hotline can be a resource to you as well; inquiries can be made to aapcodinghotline@aap.org.

- Review your carrier contract's clauses on audits and dispute resolution as well as applicable state laws on audits and repayments with your attorney.

- Focus any overpayment recovery efforts on a case-by-case basis. Avoid unilateral take-backs by not allowing the carrier to extrapolate repayments on any or all future claims.

- Have the carrier provide documentation as proof of overpayment for each contested claim.

- Obtain and secure written documentation of all contacts with the carrier on this issue. Should a carrier payment policy require reporting that varies from *CPT*® guidelines, obtain written, dated documentation from the carrier to verify that is the case. Keep this documentation permanently.
- Use legal counsel skilled in carrier contracting when negotiating contracts and confronted with repayment demands.

The AAP Private Payer Advocacy Advisory Committee has a resource for AAP members on responding to retrospective audit and carrier take-back. To access it, go to www.aap.org/cfp (use access code AAPCFP23).

What if Your Practice Is Audited?

- Contact legal counsel as soon as possible. Make sure the attorney or legal practice has experience with audits. If it is a Medicaid audit, it is preferable to have an attorney with Medicaid audit experience. An audit is a complex legal process with significant consequences. It is unwise to attempt to maneuver through this process without sound legal advice.
- Designate one physician or staff member to serve as the primary contact with the attorney and auditors. However, keep in mind that all physicians and staff members may need to work with auditors to some extent.
- Request that the auditor provide you with an opening and closing conference. At the initial meeting, ask for the individual's credentials and job title and ask him or her to summarize the purpose of the review or audit.
- Know how far back auditors may conduct reviews, the number of records a contractor may request, the amount of time allowed to respond to each request, any rebuttal process in place, and steps necessary to appeal adverse findings.
- If the time requirements for producing copies or gathering medical records are unmanageable, contact the auditing entity and request an extension in writing. Provide a clear justification for the extension request.
- Keep copies of all written communication (eg, letters, directives, memos, e-mails). Keep the postmarked envelopes of all letters, including the original notice.
- Fully document all verbal communication, including time, date, persons involved, substance of the discussion, and conclusions and agreements.
- In response to requests for information, provide only the information requested and maintain copies of what you provide auditors. Before providing files, remove any information unrelated to the audit. For example, in a Medicaid audit, you could exclude information related to services provided when the patient was covered under a commercial plan or was uninsured.
- Do not alter any documents or medical records.
- Respond only to questions from the auditors; do not try to engage them in any conversations. If the auditors are conducting the review in your office, try to place them in a separate office away from patients, staff, and business operations.
- Be prepared to respond promptly to each request received. Keep a log of requests received by date, response due date, requesting party, any communication with the requestor, date of response, and outcome.
- Know HIPAA privacy regulations, documentation principles, coding guidelines, and payment policies, and verify that all supporting documentation is included in each response.
- If legibility of the record is questionable, include a transcribed copy with attestation by the author of the original document stating that the transcription is accurate and provided to ensure legibility. Any unsigned entry should also be accompanied by a separate attestation by its author.
- Copied or scanned medical records should be carefully reviewed to be sure that all pages were legibly copied (front and back, if applicable) and are straight and within the margins on the page.
- Any questions about the sufficiency of medical record documentation should be addressed with the physician or provider who ordered or documented the service prior to responding to the request for records. Any corrections to an entry should be performed in a manner that maintains legibility of the original content (eg, single-line strike-through) and should be signed and dated. A summary of the service provided may be included to provide more information but should be distinctly labeled as such and not as part of the original record.

- Include any policy or correspondence from the payer that was used to guide your billing and coding practices related to the service. (Archived payer manuals supportive of claims from previous years may be available on state Medicaid Web sites.) Clinical practice guidelines, policy statements, textbooks, and manuals may also be supportive of medical necessity.
- Send records in a manner that allows for confirmation of receipt.
- Secure a copy of auditors' contact information in case you need to follow up.
- Obtain, in writing, the expected date of a written summary of findings.

Can This Really Happen?

Conventional wisdom says that auditors will probably go after big organizations when it comes to investigating fraud and abuse, but the OIG has said repeatedly that it has zero tolerance for fraud, so, technically, everyone is at risk. Because most of the software programs used to detect unusual coding and billing patterns are based on adult services, pediatricians may be identified as outliers because their coding does not conform to adult-based parameters. Unfortunately, valid pediatric coding may be tagged as improper and honest providers may have to respond to inappropriate recoupment requests or audits. The AAP works hard to minimize these problems and help chapters respond when state Medicaid programs target pediatric coding as inappropriate. This is an ongoing challenge.

Sadly, there are instances of fraud involving pediatricians. A review of past OIG reports to Congress revealed the following cases:

- In March 2016, an owner of several mental and behavioral health clinics (who had previously been excluded from the Medicaid program) was sentenced to the statutory maximum of 20 years for health care fraud and money laundering. The owner worked with a fraudulent biller concocting numerous schemes to bill the Medicaid program by stealing the identities of a physician and numerous practitioners and children.
- In August 2015, in Newark, NJ, 3 physicians were sentenced to a combined 7 years and 2 months in jail and ordered to pay a combined $434,300 in restitution after pleading guilty to charges related to a test-referral kickback scheme. As part of the kickback scheme, a laboratory entered into sham consulting agreements and sham rental and service agreements and offered cash and other inducements, such as third-party businesses, credit card payments, and valuable items (cars and electronics). The laboratory used the patient blood specimens to submit more than $100 million in claims to Medicare and private insurers. In April and May 2015, the physicians admitted to accepting approximately $1,500 or more per month in return for referring patient blood specimens. The laboratory's owner pleaded guilty to conspiracy to commit bribery and money laundering and is awaiting sentencing.
- Operation Free Shot focuses on health care providers who bill Medicaid and other insurance programs for childhood vaccines the providers received free of charge from the Vaccines for Children (VFC) program, a joint federal and state program that provides childhood immunizations. Under the VFC program, doctors and other health care providers receive free vaccines distributed by HHS and agree not to bill Medicaid or any other third party for the cost of the vaccines. The provider may recover a minimal fee for administrative costs associated with inoculating a child. Fraudulent claims have led to civil and criminal convictions with millions of dollars recovered and civil settlements as high as $430,000 against one practice.
- In one state, an investigation of the VFC program resulted in 4 settlements against a pediatrician in the amount of $53,000 over a 3-year period.
- A pediatrician who operated an immunization program utilizing federal VFC program funds agreed to pay the government $65,000. The pediatrician allegedly administered 3,851 vaccine doses to children who were not eligible to receive the free immunizations. He also allegedly administered expired vaccines to children in at least 2 cases.

Explore the Need for Additional Insurance

Many medical liability insurers and insurance brokers offer products to provide additional coverage for the consequences of billing errors and omissions. Pediatric practices may want to contact their insurers to see whether their current medical liability policies cover any of the following problems. If they don't, it might be worthwhile to explore insurance options for obtaining that additional protection.

- Defense coverage for a Medicaid audit
- Qui tam action (False Claims Act)
- Unintentional billing errors and omissions
- Physician Self-Referral Law (Stark) violations
- Unintentional release of medical or financial data
- Breach of computers or network security
- Data recovery
- Health Insurance Portability and Accountability Act fines or investigation costs

Summary

These are interesting times for pediatric practices that require thoughtful preparation and ongoing concern. Learn about the fraud and abuse enforcement climate in your state. Implement an effective compliance program and follow it. Be sure your staff knows what a demand for repayment or audit notice looks like and what they need to do with it just on the off chance that something should happen. Have a response plan in place should an auditor knock on your door or a recoupment letter come in the mail. Consult with an attorney when needed. Think about the need for insurance for billing errors and omissions. Keep current with coding and billing updates.

Chapter 18: Preventing Fraud and Abuse: Compliance, Audits, and Paybacks

CHAPTER 19

The Business of Medicine: Working With Current and Emerging Payment Systems

Contents

To maintain a viable practice, physicians and their staff must continually refine their practice management skills as they respond to changing payment systems. The first section of this chapter provides an overview of how services are currently valued and how assigned values may be used to guide practice management. The second section reviews guidelines and tools that may be used to monitor and manage charge accumulation, claims filing, review of payments, the appeals process, contract negotiations, and the use of audits to protect against lost revenue and incorrect billing practices. The third section provides an introduction to emerging payment methodologies and how these may affect traditional and newer practice models, such as accountable care organizations (ACOs).

Connecting Codes to Payment and Budget

Before a claim is generated, a physician practice must establish fees for services that are greater than the cost of providing the service. A simple fee schedule methodology involves use of the Medicare Resource-Based Relative Value Scale (RBRVS). In 2018, most pediatric services are still valued and paid by Medicare, Tricare, and commercial payers using a fee-for-service methodology based on the RBRVS. An understanding of how values are assigned to the codes for services, how the values relate to payment, and how this information contributes to a practice's finances is critical for the practice's financial viability and success.

The 3 components of the RBRVS are as follows:

1. *Physician work:* Physician work represents approximately 50% of the total relative value units (RVUs) assigned to most services. Work is described as time required to perform the service, mental effort and judgment, technical skill, physical effort, and psychological stress associated with concern about iatrogenic risk to the patient. Work is further broken down to preservice, intraservice, and post-service components. Understanding these components of work is important to code correctly, as preservice and post-service components should not be separately reported.

   * Preservice work: For nonsurgical services, this preparatory non–face-to-face work includes typical review of records and communicating with other professionals. (Prolonged preservice work, such as extensive record review, may be separately reportable.) For surgical services, this includes physician work from the day before the service to the procedure but excludes the encounter that resulted in the decision for surgery or unrelated evaluation and management (E/M) services. (For more on the global period for surgery, see Chapter 15, Common Surgical Procedures and Sedation.)

   * Intraservice work: For nonsurgical services, this includes time spent by the physician or other qualified health care professional in direct patient care activities, such as obtaining history, examining the patient, and counseling the patient and/or caregivers. Surgical intraservice work begins with incision or introduction of instruments (eg, needle, scope) and ends with closure of the incision or removal of instruments.

   * Post-service work: For nonsurgical services, post-service work includes arranging for further services, reviewing and communicating test results, preparing written reports, and/or communicating by telephone. Separately reportable services, such as chronic care management or care plan oversight, are not included in post-service work. For surgical services, post-service work includes typical work in the procedure or operating room after the procedure has ended, stabilization of the patient in the recovery area, communications with family or other health care professionals, and visits on the day of surgery. Surgical services are also valued to include typical follow-up care for the presenting problem during a defined global period (eg, 10 or 90 days after the service).

2. *Practice expense:* This component is an estimate of preservice, intraservice, and post-service clinical staff time; medical supplies; and procedure-specific and overhead equipment. Practice expense makes up about 44% of the total RVUs for most services. Practice expense varies by site of service (facility vs non-facility). See the Place of Service Codes section later in this chapter for more information about how place of service affects payment.

3. *Professional liability:* This smallest component (about 4% of the total RVUs) is based on medical malpractice premium data.

Each RVU component may be independently adjusted slightly upward or downward as a function of geographic area. The Centers for Medicare & Medicaid Services (CMS) calculates Medicare payment for a procedure code by multiplying total RVUs by a dollar conversion factor that is set annually. Medicaid fee schedules vary by state and are not consistently related to RVUs or the Medicare Physician Fee Schedule. Commercial payments for many procedure codes are often linked to a percentage of Medicare payment. Alternatively, payers may offer their own fee schedule for a practice's most utilized procedure codes. It is important to obtain the payer's fee schedule for all codes used or likely to be used by a practice and compare these with Medicare and other published fee schedules. Although Medicare assigns a status of "N" ("non-covered") to *Current Procedural Terminology* (*CPT*®) codes **99381–99385** and **99391–99395** in the fee schedule, they do have component RVUs that allow calculation of Medicare equivalent payments. Medicaid and proposed commercial payments for pediatric preventive care can be evaluated in light of the Medicare equivalent payments. Tip: When reviewing a payer's fee schedule, make sure the payer also fully discloses its policies for paying for services that it considers to be *bundled,* ie, payment for 2 or more codes during the same encounter may be less than the sum of the individual payments. If a contract links payment to the Medicare fee schedule, it is important to be specific about which fee schedule is used, as these change annually. Resetting payment based on the Medicare Physician Fee Schedule for the year of service may result in lower payments.

The RBRVS payment methodology may be used with practice- and physician-specific data generated from a practice's accounting and practice management systems to estimate an approximate cost of providing each service. The result should be a list of services each assigned a share of the practice's overhead cost as well as the margin and actual cost of providing the service. From the accounting system, an administrator may calculate the total practice expenses for a period, subtracting billable services that are not paid based on RVUs such as vaccines and medications. From the practice management system, reports may be generated to provide a total of the number of procedures billed by code, RVUs for each service, and total RVUs billed by the practice for the same period. By dividing total practice expenses by total RVUs, an administrator can calculate the practice cost per RVU. Additional calculations may be used to compare payment per RVU or per service among contracted payers. (Calculations should be viewed in context of other factors, such as history of timely and correct payment.)

Such calculations can be used to inform decisions on acceptance of contractual fee schedules, number of services necessary to break even or profit from provision of services, and return on investment potential for new equipment or services. The practice cost for providing a service may also be of significant value when approached by an ACO to participate in a financial agreement in which certain services are paid with a single lump payment that is then distributed among providers of service. A physician will need to know the cost of providing the service to negotiate a fair portion of the lump payment. (See the Accountable Care Organizations [ACOs] section later in this chapter.) More accurate estimates of cost may be determined on an actual cost basis. However, RVU calculations are straightforward and typically provide a reasonably reliable result.

Pediatric physicians can also play a role in recommending values for services to the CMS by participation in American Academy of Pediatrics (AAP) surveys conducted through the American Medical Association/Specialty Society Relative Value Scale Update Committee (RUC). These surveys are conducted to estimate the time and complexity of performing a service in comparison with another service. American Academy of Pediatrics staff sends out requests for participation to AAP section members to allow completion by physicians who most typically perform the service being surveyed. To learn more about participation in RUC surveys, see the "Understanding the RUC Survey Instrument" videos at https://www.aap.org/en-us/professional-resources/practice-transformation/getting-paid/Coding-at-the-AAP/Pages/Code-Valuation-and-PaymentRBRVS.aspx.

> ### ~ More From the AAP ~
>
> For more information on relative value units, see the AAP policy statement, "Application of the Resource-Based Relative Value Scale System to Pediatrics," at http://pediatrics.aappublications.org/content/133/6/1158.full.pdf.

Clean Claims to Correct Payment

An effective charge accumulation system, accurate billing of procedure codes, and an efficient claims filing system are necessary but not sufficient to achieve clean claim submissions. Although the physician is ultimately responsible for the accuracy of codes selected and claims submitted, it typically takes a team effort to create and maintain an effective accounts receivable system, including

- Development and use of management tools.
  - ❖ Incorporation of claims processing tools for analysis of your claims processing procedures. A self-assessment tool for improving claims processing and payment can be found at https://www.aap.org/en-us/Documents/ImprovingClaimsProcessing.pdf.
  - ❖ Electronic health record (EHR) and/or billing systems may include automated tools to help identify errors prior to billing, alert to payments that do not align with contracted fees, and provide data for monitoring the time lapse from provision of service to payment.
- Continuing provider and staff education with constant oversight and communication with staff, payers, and patients.
  - ❖ Policies and procedures that support continuous monitoring of payer communications and disseminate information on benefit policy changes that affect coding and payment.
  - ❖ Assurance that staff assigned with responsibilities related to correct coding and billing have access to authoritative resources on coding and documentation (eg, current Medicaid National Correct Coding Initiative [NCCI] edits and manual). See Chapter 3, Modifiers and Coding Edits, and Chapter 18, Preventing Fraud and Abuse: Compliance, Audits, and Paybacks, for more information on code edits and compliant coding and billing.
- Performance of regular audits to identify potential corrective actions required to be compliant with billing standards, coding guidelines, and federal rules and regulations (eg, Health Insurance Portability and Accountability Act of 1996, Anti-Kickback Statute, False Claims Act). Audits benefit the practice by identifying
  - ❖ The number of timely and correctly submitted claims, resulting in faster and more appropriate payments
  - ❖ The need for physician and staff education on coding and documentation
  - ❖ Inappropriate carrier denials and reductions requiring appeals, thus decreasing practice costs
  - ❖ Issues for payer contract negotiations
  - ❖ Incorrect coding and related potential risk for charges of fraud or abuse
  - ❖ Areas in need of written office policies and procedures (eg, pre-authorizations and referrals processes, claims follow-up processes, control systems)
- Procedures for efficient review of payments. Timely identification of payment errors is necessary to obtain redress because contracts often specify a time limit on appeals.
- Guidance for write-offs and initiation of appeals processes.

The Encounter Form

Designing and Reviewing the Encounter Form

The encounter form, whether computer generated or printed, should be reviewed periodically and updated at the time of the *CPT®*; *International Classification of Diseases, 10th Revision, Clinical Modification (ICD-10-CM)*; and Healthcare Common Procedure Coding System (HCPCS) updates (ie, January, April, July, and October) to be certain it includes most, if not all, of the services and procedures commonly performed in the practice and the codes are accurate.

See the Capturing Charges in the Electronic Health Record section later in this chapter for information on code maintenance and charge capture in an EHR.

Chapter 19: The Business of Medicine: Working With Current and Emerging Payment Systems

Practices Generating Charges From a Printed Encounter Form (Superbill)

When developing the encounter form

- Include all levels of service for each category of E/M services (eg, **99201–99205, 99221–99223**) and ensure time is listed for coding based on time.
- List procedures (eg, laboratory) in alphabetic order within the category of service. For example, group vaccine administration codes and vaccine product codes together.
- Allow space on the printed encounter form to write in specific details of a procedure when required. For example

  Code **120**_____ Laceration repair; loc*_____; size_____ (*location)
- Include the most commonly reported diagnosis codes. Consider grouping diagnosis codes by organ system, and then alphabetically within the system.
- Leave space on the printed form to allow the reporting of the specific diagnosis and full *ICD-10-CM* code. For example

  ICD-10-CM: **M25.0**___ Joint pain; loc _____
- Include the most frequently used modifiers.
- Include add-on codes for prolonged and special services. For example

  99354   Prolonged service in the office or outpatient, first hour

  99058   Services provided on an emergency basis in the office, disrupting other scheduled services
- Develop a separate encounter form for hospital and outpatient hospital services. Make sure it includes all the services most commonly performed in the hospital setting.
- Leave space on the printed form to write in any services or diagnoses that are not included.

> **~ More From the AAP ~**
>
> The AAP Pediatric Office Superbill may be purchased from shopAAP at https://shop.aap.org/pediatric-office-superbill-2018.

Completing the Printed Encounter Form

Every practice should develop a written policy of the requirements needed to complete the form. Some points that should be part of the policy include

- The encounter form is *not* part of the medical record. Information such as the need for follow-up care, diagnostic tests, or referrals must always be documented in the medical record even if written on the encounter form.
- Services must be clearly identified (eg, circle procedure, use check mark).
- The person providing the service (eg, physician, laboratory technologist, medical assistant) should document that service on the encounter form to ensure only the procedures performed are reported. For example, it is common for a physician to mark a urinalysis on the encounter form when he or she orders the test. However, if a specimen could not be obtained, the procedure would have been billed inappropriately. If the nurse (under supervision of the physician) had been responsible for reporting the service when performed, it would not have been reported because the urine was not obtained.
- The physician is ultimately responsible for the services reported and billed.
- The physician should identify the diagnosis as, for example, primary or secondary.
- Diagnoses and services or procedures must be numbered and linked to each other. For example, an E/M service and removal of impacted cerumen from the right ear (**69210**) is performed. The physician reports the primary diagnosis (acute suppurative otitis media without spontaneous rupture of eardrum, right ear [**H66.001**]) (1) and the secondary diagnosis (impacted cerumen, right ear [**H61.21**]) (2). *ICD-10-CM* diagnosis code **H66.001** is linked to the office visit and the secondary diagnosis code is linked to the procedure.

  99213 25 (1)   **H66.001** (1)

  69210 (2)   **H61.21** (2)

⚬ On a paper claim form, the linking of diagnoses to procedures would look like

21. Diagnosis or nature of illness or injury (Relate A–L to service line below 24E) A. **H66.001** B. **H61.21** C. D. E. F. G. H. I. J. K. L.				ICD Ind. 0					
24. A. Dates of service	B. Place of service	C. EMG	D. Procedures, services or supplies CPT/HCPCS	Modifier	E. Diagnosis Pointer	F. Charges	G. Days or units	H. EPSDT	I. ID Qual	J. Rendering Provider #
1/1/2017– 1/1/2017	11		**99213** (E/M)	**25**	A	$$$	1		NPI	123456789
1/1/2017– 1/1/2017	11		**69210** (cerumen removal)		B	$$$	1		NPI	123456789

Abbreviations: CPT, Current Procedural Terminology; *E/M, evaluation and management; EMG, emergency; EPSDT, Early and Periodic Screening, Diagnosis, and Treatment; HCPCS, Healthcare Common Procedure Coding System;* ICD, International Classification of Diseases; *NPI, National Provider Identifier.*

⚬ Procedures or diagnoses must be written, if not preprinted, on the form.
⚬ A billing manager or clerk should only add or change a service or diagnosis with the agreement of the provider of service.
⚬ A system should be instituted to monitor and ensure capture of all of the day's patient encounter forms (eg, cross-reference to the patient sign-in records).

Reviewing the Encounter Form

A staff member who understands correct coding and reporting guidelines should always review the completed encounter form before charges are posted and the claim submitted to ensure that all procedures and services are captured and accurate.

For example, the reviewer should look to see that

⚬ An administration code is reported with vaccines and/or injections.
⚬ A venipuncture or finger stick is reported with a laboratory test.
⚬ A handling fee is reported when the specimen is prepared and sent to an outside laboratory.
⚬ A modifier is appended when appropriate (eg, modifier **76** for repeat procedures or services).
⚬ The office visit is reported using the correct new or established patient category of service. (See Chapter 4, Evaluation and Management Documentation Guidelines, for more information on new and established patient code selection.)
⚬ The diagnoses reported as primary and secondary are appropriate and are linked to the appropriate services or procedures.
⚬ The documentation to support each service has been completed with required dates and signatures.

Capturing Charges in the Electronic Health Record

Many physicians now capture encounter and billing information in the EHR. Compliant documentation and code selection is discussed in Chapter 18, Preventing Fraud and Abuse: Compliance, Audits, and Paybacks. The basics of charge capture in the EHR are accurate listing of diagnoses, selection of complete codes, and procedure code selection based on work performed and documented. While integrating charge capture into the encounter documentation should provide efficiency, there are pitfalls to be avoided.

When using an EHR, make sure that codes in the system are accurate and updated in accordance with code set updates. It is important to verify with your electronic system vendors how code updates are incorporated into the system. This may be via scheduled upgrades that may or may not require system downtime or may occur via automated upgrades during night or weekend hours. Code updates should be based on the effective date of changes (eg, deleted codes may be entered for charges with a date of service prior to the effective date of deletion even after the update has been made). Practice and billing managers must maintain contact with the system vendor's upgrade and support staff and verify what, if any, manual steps are required on the part of the practice in relation to code changes.

It is also important that code descriptors displayed in code selection are adequate for accurate code selection. Truncated descriptors may omit key information that differentiates one code from another (eg, hypertrophy of tonsils should provide options for hypertrophy of tonsils alone or hypertrophy of tonsils and adenoid and prompt reporting of a code for tonsillitis when both tonsillitis and hypertrophy are diagnosed).

Documentation of the diagnoses has been problematic in some EHR systems. As with the paper record, the physician must have the ability to fully describe patient diagnoses (eg, behavioral issues at home and in school, rule out attention-deficit/hyperactivity disorder [ADHD]) for each encounter.

- Systems should not use diagnosis codes for populating the physician's diagnostic statement or assessment. Code descriptors may provide only generalized information and would not capture the physician's differential diagnoses (eg, rule out ADHD is an important indicator of necessary follow-up care but is not captured in diagnosis coding).
- The EHR should not reorder diagnoses entered by the physician. Physicians should list first the diagnosis most responsible for the encounter, followed by additional diagnoses. An EHR that reorders documented diagnoses (eg, alphabetically) results in noncompliance with diagnosis coding guidelines.
- The patient problem list should not be pulled forward as the diagnoses for each encounter. Only those conditions addressed or that affected management or treatment of conditions addressed should be reported for each encounter.

Automated code selection is also problematic. An EHR may be designed to determine the level of E/M service provided based on information documented. However, physicians must make the code determination based on the medically necessary key components or time spent counselling and/or coordinating care. Automatic population of records may result in documentation that overstates the level of work and intensity of the service provided. (See more on compliant EHR documentation in Chapter 18, Preventing Fraud and Abuse: Compliance, Audits, and Paybacks.) Therefore, when EHR functionality includes automated E/M code determinations, physicians must view the EHR code as a suggestion that must be confirmed or rejected based on documentation and medical necessity. Failure to override suggested codes when appropriate may be considered an abusive practice.

Submitting Clean Claims

Many states have enacted laws that require prompt payment of "clean claims." In general, clean claims are those that contain sufficient and correct information for processing without further investigation or development by the payer (definitions may vary by state). Submitted claims must be accurate and in accordance with the process as outlined in the executed carrier or health plan agreement. Knowing a payer's claim requirements will decrease chances of denied claims. Make sure the practice understands payer rules, for example, for billing for nonphysician services and incident-to billing. (See Chapter 4, Evaluation and Management Documentation Guidelines, and Chapter 14, Allied Health and Clinical Staff Services, for more information on billing for nonphysician services.) Be aware of any updates issued by the carrier that affect billing and claims submission. Generally, a clean claim should have the following information:

- Practice information (name, address, phone, National Provider Identifier [NPI], group tax identification number)
- Patient information (patient name, birth date, policyholder, policy number, patient identification number, address)
- Codes (CPT®, ICD-10-CM, HCPCS, place of service), modifiers, and service dates
- Carrier information
- Secondary insurance information
- Referring physician name and NPI, if applicable
- Facility name and address, as appropriate

If additional information is necessary to support a service or explain an unusual circumstance (eg, unlisted procedure code, unusual procedure, complicated procedure)

- Utilize the attachments feature of your claims system, clearinghouse, or other electronic claim attachment procedure as directed by the payer (eg, submission of attachments by fax) or send a hard-copy claim with a cover letter and a narrative report or copy of the appropriate part of the medical record (eg, progress note, procedure note) to facilitate claim processing.

* Any documentation (eg, coordination of benefits information, letter of medical necessity, clinical reports) should include the patient's name, service date, and policy number on each page in case the papers become separated. Documentation submitted electronically may require inclusion of the payer's internal control number (ICN) for the associated claim. The ICN is found on the claim acknowledgment report generated after claim submission.
* Keep a copy of the claim and supporting information for follow-up of payment.
* When filing claims for patients with coordination of benefits, make certain all required information (ie, primary and secondary insurance information) has been obtained from the patient and claims are filed with the supporting information (eg, explanation of benefits [EOB] or electronic remittance advice information), according to plan requirements.

Claims should be submitted for payment as soon as possible and before the deadline specified in the agreement. The optimum time for filing outpatient claims is on the day of or the day following the service but no more than 2 to 3 days from the date of service. Inpatient encounter forms for patients with prolonged hospitalizations may allow codes to be documented for 7 consecutive days; in this case, claims should be filed within 2 to 3 days of the end of the service week. Policy should be adopted requiring completion of medical record documentation within a specified period to support prompt billing of services. Physicians must understand that timely completion of documentation is required for appropriate code selection, claim filing, and, ultimately, prompt payment.

Coding Pearl

Practices should monitor lag time between completion of each service and submission of a claim for the service to identify and correct any cause of delayed submission.

Place of Service Codes

The place of service is indicated on each claim by a place of service code (often integrated into billing systems without need for manual entry with each charge). The place of service may appear evident when reporting codes for services such as inpatient hospital care, but this is not always the case. When providing services in a facility such as a hospital outpatient clinic, it is important to report the correct place of service because differences in practice expense in a facility versus a non-facility setting affect physician payment. For instance, a procedure performed in a surgical center would be paid at a lower fee schedule amount than the same procedure performed in a physician's clinic (not hospital-based) because the fee schedule takes into account the overhead or practice expense of providing, for example, the procedure room, supplies, and clinical staff. If services provided in a facility setting are reported as if provided in a physician's clinic, an overpayment may occur.

Physicians in provider-based practices, those practices owned and operated as a part of a hospital, should be aware that the place of service code is especially important in this setting. Because the physician and practice expense portions of the patient's charges are often billed separately, the same services provided in a provider-based practice are often more costly than those provided in an independent (physician-owned) practice. Facility fees charged by the provider are often significantly higher than the non-facility fees charged in independent practices. The increased number of high-deductible health plans has raised awareness of the greater costs to patients when services are rendered in provider-based facilities and have prompted the Medicare program and some states to take actions to reduce the added costs. Practices should be aware of any such restrictions that apply to billing in their locality and under payer contracts.

Place of service codes that may be reported for pediatric services include

02	Telehealth
03	School
04	Homeless shelter
11	Office
12	Home
13	Assisted living facility
14	Group home
16	Temporary lodging
19	Off campus—outpatient hospital
20	Urgent care facility
21	Inpatient hospital

22	On campus—outpatient hospital
23	Emergency room—hospital
24	Ambulatory surgical center
25	Birthing center
26	Military treatment facility
33	Custodial care facility
71	Public health clinic
72	Rural health clinic

> **~ More From the AAP ~**
>
> For more information about place of service codes, see "Place of Service: Not Always Office" in the April 2015 *AAP Pediatric Coding Newsletter*™ at http://coding.aap.org (subscription required).

Place of service codes are further discussed for certain E/M services in chapters 6 through 12. See a full list of place of service codes at www.cms.gov/Medicare/Coding/place-of-service-codes/Place_of_Service_Code_Set.html.

Special Consideration for Medicare Claims

Many health plans receive Medicare claims automatically when they are the secondary payer. In this case, the explanation of Medicare benefits will indicate that the claim has been automatically crossed over for secondary consideration. Physicians and providers should look for this indication on their EOBs and should not submit a paper claim to the secondary payer.

Monitoring Claim Status

An important aspect of billing operations is prompt and routine claim monitoring. A defined process for verifying that submitted claims were received and accepted by claim clearinghouses and/or payers should be included in the practice's or billing service's written billing procedures. Steps may include (see the last bullet if billing is outsourced or centralized outside the practice)

* Identify each type of report and/or dashboard feature of the practice's billing system for use in verifying claim submission and acceptance for processing, assigning follow-up activities for unpaid claims, and tracking average time from date of service or submission to receipt of payment.
* Assign responsibilities for verifying that electronic claim submissions were received and accepted for processing as soon after transmission as possible.
  * Most clearinghouses will send a report indicating acceptance or rejection of a batch of claims within minutes of transmission and a report with individual claim-level detail within 24 hours of submission.
* Electronic claim submission reports must be promptly reviewed for rejections or denials. All rejected or denied claims must be investigated to determine what corrections or payer contact is necessary to resubmit or return the claim for re-adjudication (eg, when a payer system error is corrected).
* Claims should not be resubmitted without investigation, as resubmission of a claim containing errors is unlikely to result in payment. Resubmission of the claim with errors may reset the aging of the claim in the billing system and result in late follow-up or denial for lack of timely filing.
* Identify staff responsible for claims follow-up and establish standards for timely follow-up on unpaid claims. System-generated reports are useful in identifying the age of claims.
* If centralized billing or an outsourced billing service is used, maintain oversight of performance by reviewing reports that show any lag time between completion of documentation and submission of claims, aging reports that show the average number of days since claim submission for unpaid claims, and reports of amounts adjusted or written off. (Even salaried physicians are affected by lost revenue and should have interest in the effectiveness of the practice's billing processes.)

Monitoring Payments

Develop a process to monitor the timeliness of all payments. Tips for monitoring payments include

* Identify payers who do not pay clean claims within the time frame agreed on in your contract and follow up on all late payments with the payer. Check the provisions of your state prompt pay law and know the provisions for clean claims, timely filing, and penalties. Report the payer's practice of late or delinquent payments to the proper agency because your practice may be entitled to payment plus interest.

Chapter 19: The Business of Medicine: Working With Current and Emerging Payment Systems

- Review each EOB and/or remittance advice (electronic or paper) carefully to determine if the payment is correct. Familiarity with standard claim adjustment reason codes and remittance advice remark codes is essential to identifying denial reasons, such as a non-covered service, bundled payment, or provision of service not typical for physician specialty (not relevant for taxonomy code), and any patient responsibility for denied charges.

- Compare the EOBs and/or remittance advice to a spreadsheet listing your top 40 codes and their allowable payments by carrier to monitor contract compliance. Practice management software may also include the ability to add contractual allowances by payer. Make certain that the payment is consistent with the fee schedule, write-offs, and discounts agreed to by the practice and payer. Follow up with the payer on any discrepancies.

- Identify any discrepancies, such as changes to codes, reduced payment, or denials.

- Review all payer explanations, particularly reasons for denials or downcoding. If the service provided is not a benefit covered by the plan, the patient should be billed directly (may need a signed waiver form).

- Make certain that any denials or reductions in payment are not due to practice billing errors (eg, incorrect modifiers, obsolete codes) or are incorrect applications of an NCCI edit that does not pertain to pediatrics. If so, correct the errors immediately and educate staff members as appropriate to ensure correct future claim submissions.

- One efficiency of many electronic systems is automatic application of payments and adjustments. However, systems may apply incorrect adjustments based on payer remark codes. Staff should monitor all denials and reduced payments as appropriate and appeal incorrect adjustments when applicable.

- Maintain a log of all denials or payment reductions. This can be used as a basis for future negotiations or education of the payer. (Identify one individual who has billing and coding expertise to monitor as well as accept or reject denials.)

- Review your fee schedule to see if your practice is paid at 100% of the billed charges because this is an indication that your fees are below the maximum amount established by the carrier.

- Review your fees annually and understand the Medicare RBRVS, using it to value the services you provide. (For details on using the RBRVS, see "2018 RBRVS: What Is It and How Does It Affect Pediatrics?" at www.aap.org/coding, access code AAPCFP23.)

- Review your payment to make sure it exceeds your cost of providing that service.

> ||||||||| **Coding Pearl** |||||||||
>
> When contracting with payers, be aware of payment options that may be specified (eg, paper checks, electronic fund transfers, virtual credit card payment). It is important to understand the pros and cons of each (eg, credit card processing fees typically apply to card-based payment). Health plans must provide payment in compliance with electronic fund transfer standards of the Health Insurance Portability and Accountability Act rather than virtual card or wire transfer when requested by a physician. Agreements to accept electronic fund transfers should not allow health plans to debit an account without notification and consent. Banks may offer additional protections against unauthorized withdrawals.

> ||||||||| **Coding Pearl** |||||||||
>
> Find claim adjustment reason code and remittance advice remark code descriptions online at www.wpc-edi.com/reference.

Filing Appeals

Do not assume that the carrier's denials or audits are accurate. Be prepared to challenge the carrier. If you are coding correctly and in compliance with coding conventions, you should appeal all inappropriately denied claims and carrier misapplication of *CPT®* coding principles. Develop a system to monitor payer updates and any changes to the provider agreement so you are aware of the current payment policies and coding edits used by the payer.

- By accepting inappropriate claim denials, a practice may be setting itself up to charges of billing fraud.

- If a practice recodes claims as a result of inappropriate carrier denials, the resubmitted claim may not actually reflect the treatment the patient received.

Here is a summary of basic guidelines and tips for appealing payments.

- When in contact with the payer, always document the date, name, and title of the payer representative with whom you have talked and a summary of the details of the conversation. If a payer requests you submit a claim using codes or modifiers that are not consistent with clean coding standards, ask for documentation of the direction in writing.
  - Address issues with the person who has the authority to make decisions to overturn denials or reductions in payment.
  - Keep an updated file with names and contact information of the appropriate personnel with each of your contracted payers.
  - Request an e-mail or letter verifying the information provided and archive written correspondence containing payer representative advice and payer policies. If the carrier does not provide written documentation, prepare a summary and send it to your contact, stating that this will constitute the documentation of the discussion.
- Submit all appeals in writing.
  - Understand the payer's appeal process and appeal within its timeliness guidelines.
  - Format the letter to include the name of the patient, policy number, claim control number, and date of service(s) in question on each page of the letter.
  - The body of the letter should state the reason for the appeal and why you are in disagreement with the payer's adjudication of the claim.
  - Specify a date by which you expect the carrier to respond.
  - Support your case by providing medical justification and referencing *CPT*® coding guidelines. If necessary, consult with the AAP Coding Hotline for clarification of correct coding. It may be helpful to hire a certified coding expert with knowledge in pediatric coding to review your claims. (If hiring a full-time certified coding expert is not practical for a small practice, part-time employment or periodic consultation may be options for access to coding and compliance expertise.)
  - Consider sending correspondence to the carrier by certified mail to verify receipt. Document and retain copies of all communications with the carrier about the appeal.
- Maintain an appeals pending file.
  - If there is no response from the payer within 4 weeks of the date of the letter, send a copy of the appeal letter stamped "Second Request."
  - If there is no response within 2 weeks, or if the matter continues to remain unresolved, contact the state department of insurance (or other appropriate agency in your state) to file a complaint or engage its assistance.
  - Contact your AAP chapter and pediatric council, if your chapter has one, to make them aware of the situation with the payer. American Academy of Pediatrics chapter pediatric councils meet with health plans to discuss carrier policies and practices affecting pediatrics and pediatricians.

The AAP has developed several sample appeal letters that may be used as templates in appealing payer decisions. The appeal letter templates can be found on MyAAP at https://www.aap.org/en-us/professional-resources/practice-transformation/getting-paid/Pages/Private-Payer-Advocacy-Templates-for-Appeal-Letters.aspx. Template topics include

- Bundling of services
- Immunization administration services (**90460**, **90461**; **90471–90474**)
- Inappropriate linking of *CPT* and diagnosis (*ICD-10-CM*) codes
- Modifier **25**
- Vision screen (**99173**)
- Well-child care (**99381–99395**) and sick visit (**99201–99215**) reported on the same calendar day

In addition, the AAP has posted a narrative that explains the appropriateness of reporting certain circumstances based on NCCI edits.

When the AAP recognizes systemic issues with payer policies, it sends letters to payers on specific issues that need resolution or for information. These letters and carrier responses are posted on MyAAP on the Payer Advocacy page (https://www.aap.org/en-us/professional-resources/practice-transformation/getting-paid/Pages/Private-Payer-Advocacy-Letters-to-Carriers.aspx).

Knowing when to appeal a payer denial is just as important as knowing how to properly appeal. Writing an effective appeal letter to payers requires knowledge of *CPT*® guidelines, CMS policy, and payer policy. The AAP Private Payer Advocacy Advisory Committee has developed resources to effectively respond to inappropriate claim denials and handling requests for refunds, managing private payer contracts and denials, and how to respond to payer audits. (See https://www.aap.org/en-us/professional-resources/practice-transformation/getting-paid/pages/Oops-We-Overpaid-You-How-to-Respond-to-Payer-Audits.aspx.)

> ### ~ More From the AAP ~
>
> For more information about resubmissions and appeals, see "Denials to Dollars: Resubmissions and Appeals" in the August 2016 *AAP Pediatric Coding Newsletter*™ at http://coding.aap.org (subscription required).

Negotiating With Payers

Payers need to be made aware and held accountable when their payment policies negatively affect the physician–carrier contractual arrangement. Previous class-action lawsuits against national carriers in response to payers' inappropriate down-coding and bundling of services have strengthened the position of physicians appropriately following *CPT* guidelines.

The following suggestions can facilitate negotiations:

- Know a health plan's policies and procedures and their effect on pediatric services. Develop a system to monitor all updates and changes to the physician contract. Be aware of updates that are provided with periodic e-mail bulletins or information posted on a payer Web site that practices have been instructed to review periodically. Practices must be aware that these alternative ways of disseminating payment information are often considered legal and binding.
- When adding new physicians to your practice, be aware of each payer's fee schedule policies. Do not assume that the same fee schedule will be applied across all physicians in the practice (eg, a payer may assign a reduced fee schedule to new physicians or carry forward a physician's contract from a previous practice).
- Be aware of any accountability (eg, penalties or other effect on shared savings) that a plan attributes to the practice when patients receive care outside their plan's network without referral by physicians within the practice.
- Know *CPT* codes, modifiers, and guidelines for their use.
- Understand how the NCCI adopted by some payers (including Medicaid) may relate to your practice.
- Understand and be able to describe the scope of services provided and the time requirements for the service.
- Be prepared to demonstrate cost savings that may be recognized by the plan as well as the value the practice brings to the plan in terms of savings, quality of care data, and/or patient satisfaction. This is your leverage. Negotiating payment with payers can be more successful if a practice is also prepared to provide quality of care data according to standard quality measures.
- Monitor and know the use (distribution) of codes by each physician and, if in a group practice, for the practice as a whole.
- Identify your payer mix. Know how many patients you have in each plan and what percent of your total patients that represents. In addition, know what percentage of RVUs each payer pays for your most frequently used codes and how they compare in payment with each other. Accurate information on payer mix and potential value/loss to the practice is essential in making participation decisions.
- Know and understand the payment basis and process.
- Have specific codes or issues to discuss, not generalities (agreement with general ideas may not address specific issues).
- Try to negotiate for coverage and payment of services or, if payers refuse to cover services, get your contract amended to state that you can bill the service as non-covered. If the plan will allow for billing the patient for non-covered services, you must then advise your patients of this policy.
- If the plan does agree to provide coverage for a particular service, make certain you understand how the carrier will cover and pay for the service and if there will be any restrictions or limitations.
- Keep notes during the discussion and be certain you understand answers to any of your questions. Any specific agreements should be in writing and signed by both parties.

- Engage parents or employers to work in partnership to help you negotiate with a plan. Encourage parents to work through their human resources department to communicate and appeal with payers. Petition from them can be very effective.

  Many AAP chapters have developed pediatric councils, which meet with payers to address pediatric issues. Advise your chapter pediatric council of specific issues you have experienced and see how it can work with the plan. If your chapter does not have a pediatric council, this may be the right time to work with your chapter to begin developing one. To see if your state has a pediatric council or for more information, visit https://www.aap.org/en-us/professional-resources/practice-transformation/getting-paid/Pages/aap-pediatric-councils.aspx (AAP members only).

- If the insurance company is not addressing your concerns satisfactorily, you should be willing to withdraw from its plan. Inform the payer (a formal notification process may be outlined in your contract), patients' families, and even the state insurance commission why continued participation is impossible. Some reasons for withdrawal might be slow payment, excessive documentation requirements, and substandard payment compared with other plans. Many times, negotiation begins when you walk away from the table.

Documentation and Coding Audits

Medicare, state Medicaid programs, and commercial payers will audit claims as well as monitor E/M coding profiles. Physician practices should also adopt standards for conducting internal audits or reviews. Internal audits provide important information to inform practice policy and procedures, detect missed revenue, protect against erroneous billing, and avoid issues with payers and outside auditors. Some key benefits of internal auditing are

- Identification of negative billing and revenue trends, including
  - ❖ Increased lag time between encounter and billing (eg, delays in finalization of documentation, delayed coding or billing functions, technology issues)
  - ❖ Denial or underpayment of new services or new or revised procedure codes
  - ❖ Significant unexpected increase or decrease in revenue
  - ❖ Inappropriate adjustments or write-offs of unpaid or underpaid claims that should be appealed
- Charge verification (eg, number of charges is equal to or greater than number of encounters, with exception of visits included in a global period)
- Identification of incorrect billing and coding practices
- Identification of payment that does not align with payer contract
- Identification of electronic system or work-flow issues
- Identification of areas where new or additional training is necessary

See Chapter 18, Preventing Fraud and Abuse: Compliance, Audits, and Paybacks, for more detailed information on conducting internal audits.

Tools for the Pediatric Practice

Working with third-party payers on coding and payment issues can be a difficult task because there is little uniformity between carriers and, frequently, great inconsistencies within the same umbrella organization of carriers. The AAP Private Payer Advocacy Advisory Committee is charged with enhancing systems for members and chapters to identify and respond to issues with private carriers.

To assist the pediatric practice, the AAP has several available resources to consider.

- American Academy of Pediatrics staff is available to provide clarification on coding issues. The AAP Coding Hotline can be accessed online through the AAP Web site at www.aap.org/en-us/professional-resources/practice-support/Coding-at-the-AAP/Pages/Coding-Inquiry-Form.aspx (AAP members only) as well as by e-mail at aapcodinghotline@aap.org.

Chapter 19: The Business of Medicine: Working With Current and Emerging Payment Systems

- ☀ Claim processing tools, a collection of template letters practices can use in appealing inappropriate carrier claim denials, and other claims processing tools are available through the AAP Resources for Payment site at https://www.aap.org/en-us/professional-resources/practice-transformation/getting-paid/Pages/resources-for-payment.aspx (AAP members only). Also, the AAP Coding Calculator allows physician practices to compare their actual E/M code use distribution to statistical norms and assess the potential effect on payment. It can be accessed at https://www.aap.org/en-us/professional-resources/practice-transformation/getting-paid/Coding-at-the-AAP/Pages/Coding-Calculator.aspx.

- ☀ Many AAP state chapters have developed pediatric councils to meet regularly with carriers to discuss pediatric issues related to access, coverage, and quality. Pediatric councils have the potential to facilitate better working relationships between pediatricians and carriers by identifying, informing, and educating payers on issues affecting pediatrics and pediatricians. The AAP chapter pediatric councils are not forums for contract negotiation, setting fees, or discussing payments. For information on pediatric councils, go to https://www.aap.org/en-us/professional-resources/practice-transformation/getting-paid/Pages/aap-pediatric-councils.aspx (AAP members only).

- ☀ The AAP has created tools to assist practices with managed care contracting. These resources are available at https://www.aap.org/en-us/professional-resources/practice-transformation/getting-paid/Pages/resources-for-payment.aspx.

- ☀ Members of the AAP are encouraged to access the AAP Hassle Factor Form online to report health plan issues. The information submitted is used to assist the AAP and chapters in identifying issues and facilitating public and private payer advocacy related to health plans, including discussion topics with national carriers and at chapter pediatric council meetings with regional carriers. The Hassle Factor Form can be accessed at https://www.aap.org/en-us/professional-resources/practice-transformation/getting-paid/Pages/Hassle-Factor-Form-Concerns-with-Payers.aspx (AAP members only) and can be submitted electronically.

- ☀ American Academy of Pediatrics members and their staff are encouraged to attend AAP Pediatric Coding Webinars, presented by pediatric coding experts. To obtain a list of scheduled webinars and to register, visit www.aap.org/webinars/coding.

Emerging Payment Methodologies

Payers are beginning to transition from volume-based payments, such as fee for service, to value-based payment models that offer incentive payments to providers based on the quality of care, outcomes, and cost containment attributable to their practice. The intent is to promote patient value and efficiency, but one consequence is that some risk is shifted to physician practices. Under these emerging payment models, practice viability will be dependent on how well quality, cost, and efficiency are managed. Examples of some of these newer payment models include bundled payments, shared savings, and pay for performance. Physician payments may be based on a combination of fee for service and newer payment methodologies. Emerging forms of health care financing and delivery models include ACOs and integrated delivery systems.

- ☀ *Bundled payments:* These are a type of prospective payment in which health care providers (hospitals, physicians, and other health care professionals) share one payment for a specified range of services as opposed to paying each provider individually. The intent of bundled payment is to foster collaboration among multiple providers to coordinate services and control costs, thereby reducing unnecessary utilization.

- ☀ *Shared savings:* Under a shared savings arrangement, providers and payers seek to deliver care at a cost that is below current budgeted amounts, and the resulting savings are shared between the payer(s) and providers. The contractual arrangement between the payer(s) and providers will specify how the savings are calculated and distributed. Shared savings models may include upside reward exclusively or upside reward and downside risk. In an upside-reward–only arrangement, the provider only shares in any savings and is not at risk for a loss. Under reward-and-risk arrangements, the practice shares a reward if costs are less than budgeted but also would share the loss should actual total costs exceed budgeted costs. Shared savings should include an up-front agreement to continue additional payments for ongoing support of infrastructure for future years when the payer may want to cut back on the shared savings margin or reduce as those savings plateau. Quality metrics are typically tied to payment of shared savings, with physicians not meeting established quality benchmarks not receiving a portion of savings. See Chapter 17, Coding to Demonstrate

Quality and Value, for more information on coding to support quality and performance measurement. For more information on shared savings, see https://www.aap.org/en-us/Documents/practicet_gainsharing_and_shared_savings.pdf.

⦿ *Pay for performance:* In this arrangement, physician payments are based on a prospectively determined comparison of the provider's performance against acknowledged benchmarks. If the provider meets or exceeds those benchmarks, an enhanced payment or bonus is provided. Benchmarks are often similar to the National Committee for Quality Assurance Healthcare Effectiveness Data and Information Set quality metrics (discussed in Chapter 17, Coding to Demonstrate Quality and Value). As examples, some of the most common metrics for pediatrics include rates of immunizations; rates of patient adherence to Early and Periodic Screening, Diagnosis, and Treatment visits; and rates of appropriate prescription of asthma medications. Pay for performance arrangements often include the following 4 types of measures:

❖ Structure: Measures use of staff capabilities, policies and procedures, and systems such as EHR and computerized physician order entry.

❖ Process: Determines the extent to which providers consistently give patients specific services that are consistent with recommended guidelines for care.

❖ Outcome: Measures the effects that one or more clinical interventions have had on patients' health, health status, and function.

❖ Patient experience: Measures patient-reported experience of care.

Each type of measure may include additional subtypes, and payers may use composite measures (2 or more measures that result in a single score).

In considering whether to participate in one of these newer payment models, a practice needs to determine expected costs and utilization and assess whether it can deliver services under the projected budget. Using *CPT*® codes and their RVUs will aid in this assessment. Projections can be made using RVUs of the services currently provided and projected to be provided. With these types of data, the practice can assess the effect of new payment methodologies to its bottom line.

Other considerations for pediatricians include

⦿ Depending on how the payment model is set up, managing a healthy population of patients may not result in significant cost savings.

⦿ Ability to access and monitor patient population and performance metric data is important to successful participation in new payment methodologies.

⦿ Physicians need to understand the links between new payment methodologies and data collection to support quality metrics (eg, failure to report codes for screening services performed may result in negative performance measurement and lost opportunity for enhanced payment).

⦿ Physicians should understand how health plans attribute patients to individual physicians and/or groups for purposes of performance measurement and cost of care. Factors such as time of continuous enrollment with the health plan and number of visits to a provider may affect how patients are attributed.

⦿ In states where the Children's Health Insurance Program (CHIP) operates independent of a state Medicaid program, children covered by CHIP may or may not be included in new payment methodologies and/or performance measurement.

See the *AAP News* article, "PPAAC: Chapter pediatric councils work with payers on medical home programs," at www.aappublications.org/news/2016/03/18/PPAAC031816 for examples of how AAP chapters and their pediatric councils advocate for developing adequate financing for pediatric medical homes under value-based payment methodologies.

Accountable Care Organizations (ACOs)

Most of the content about ACOs is adapted with permission from the January 2011 *AAP News.* The information provided herein has been updated since publication of that article.

As defined by the CMS, an ACO is an organization of health care professionals that agrees to be accountable for the quality, cost, and overall care of beneficiaries. In return, the ACO will receive incentive payments based on

> ### ~ More From the AAP ~
>
> For more on value-based payment, alternative payment models, and ACOs, go to https://www.aap.org/en-us/professional-resources/practice-transformation/getting-paid/Pages/value-based-payment.aspx.

quality and cost containment instead of volume and intensity. Eligible providers are likely to be individual and group practices, hospitals, integrated delivery systems, and others who create a legal entity with a management structure able to deliver and report on evidence-based and informed care to a defined population, effectively engage patients, and receive and distribute shared savings.

The Patient Protection and Affordable Care Act of 2010 (PPACA) included a number of provisions that establish ACOs in Medicare, Medicaid, and CHIP. In October 2011, the CMS issued final regulations to assist physicians, hospitals, and other health care professionals in coordinating care through ACOs.

Interest in ACOs is accelerating, and the market continues to witness a growth in their numbers. As of April 2015, the CMS has documented 404 Shared Savings Program ACOs. In addition, there are currently 35 ACOs participating in the Advanced Payment ACO Model, which is designed for physician-based and rural providers who have come together voluntarily to provide coordinated care to the Medicare patients they serve. Participants in this model will receive up-front and monthly payments, which they can use to make critical investments in their care coordination infrastructure. Finally, there are 19 Pioneer ACO Models starting their third year in demonstration. This approach will evaluate the effectiveness of various payment models and how their approach can provide better care, work in conjunction with private payers, and reduce Medicare cost growth.

Beyond the federal government's push toward ACOs, commercial health insurers are also actively exploring the development of ACOs. One of the special features of commercially driven ACOs is their flexibility in implementing accountable care contracts. Many private ACOs emulate the CMS Medicare Shared Savings Program (MSSP) approach; however, the flexibility provided by market-driven ACOs permits them to undertake more creative approaches in modeling payment methodologies. Leavitt Partners, a national health intelligence firm, reported in 2016 that there are 782 public and private ACOs.

Pediatricians must be in a position to assess the ACO transition locally. More importantly, pediatricians need to be actively engaged in this transition to a new care model to ensure it best serves the needs of children and families and the pediatric health care delivery system.

The growing interest in ACOs as a principal driver in the reconfiguration of the US health care delivery system aligns with the Triple Aim espoused by former CMS administrator Don Berwick, MD. In the aggregate, the Triple Aim is designed to improve the individual experience of care, improve the health of populations, and reduce per capita costs of care for populations.

The Pediatric ACO Demonstration Project, legislated as part of the PPACA but unfunded, calls for participating state Medicaid programs to allow pediatric medical professionals to form ACOs and receive incentive payments. The US Department of Health and Human Services will develop quality guidelines that must be met. The applicant state and ACO must meet a certain level of savings or slow the rate of growth in health care costs to receive an incentive payment. However, if funded, it is anticipated the CMS will derive many of the ACO requirements on the basis of its MSSP.

AAP Resources for More Information on ACOs

In response to growing interest in the development of ACOs, in 2011, the AAP ACO Workgroup produced guidance for members on factors to consider in evaluating an opportunity to participate in an ACO (https://www.aap.org/en-us/professional-resources/practice-Transformation/Pages/practice-transformation.aspx). The guidance was reevaluated in 2013 by a group of pediatrician experts in financing and economics and deemed to still be timely.

The AAP has since collaborated with Leavitt Partners, LLC, to carry out a study of pediatric ACOs, including a series of 5 case studies of diverse pediatric models, a scan of Medicaid ACOs, and a summit of leaders in pediatric ACO development. These collaborative activities identified several issues in ACO formation and sustainability in pediatric settings and outlined a number of opportunities for the pediatric community in areas of organization, model change, and market dynamics; payment, financing, and contracting; quality and value; and use of new technologies. More information is available in the January 2017 *Pediatrics* article, "Pediatric Accountable Care Organizations: Insight From Early Adopters" (http://pediatrics.aappublications.org/content/early/2017/01/29/peds.2016-1840).

> **~ More From the AAP ~**
>
> Learn more from webinars on preparing your practice; go to https://www.aap.org/en-us/professional-resources/practice-transformation/getting-paid/Pages/alternative-payment-models.aspx and scroll down to "AAP Webinar Series on Alternative Payment Models."

In addition, the CMS has published fact sheets that provide general information about ACOs and their operational and financial characteristics. They can be accessed at http://innovations.cms.gov/initiatives/ACO/index.html.

Preparing for New Payment Models

The new payment models discussed previously are already in place in some areas and will soon be adopted in others. Whether your practice provides primary or specialty care, there are steps that you should take to prepare for success. When payment is based on the costs of care and patient experience, practices must take responsibility for keeping costs low and quality of care and patient experience high. This includes such activities as

- Learn more about value-based payment options.
- Generate and use reports of your costs, quality measurement, etc.
- Learn who your active patients are and stay up-to-date through routine data analysis.
- Obtain lists of patients attributed to your practice by payers and reconcile to your active patient list.
- Identify and agree on a methodology by which any disputes over attributed patient panels will be reconciled.
- Embrace automation and alternatives to paper handling and traditional office-based care.
- Seek to remove inefficiencies by reviewing routine tasks and patient flow. Provide staff with incentives and an expectation to create consistency and efficiency.
- Learn about the communities of your patients—school and community resources, school schedules, average income and education of caregivers, urgent and emergency care utilization patterns—and use the information in providing care.
- Know the costs of the care you provide and order for your patients. Recognize that every provider within and outside of your practice must contribute to reducing the cost of care to reduce the practice's risk under new payment models.
  - Collaborate with subspecialists to ensure patients receive evidence-based and cost-effective care, including consideration of formulary and total cost of coordinated care.
- Consider options for adding nonphysician health care professionals, such as care coordinators, patient educators, and emotional/behavioral health specialists, to your practice.
- Embed clinical guidelines into care delivery through protocols and reminders.
- Configure and use your EHR and other automated systems to promote efficiency (eg, display generic drugs first when brand name is entered).
- When considering an alternative payment model contract, seek expert consultation to help identify and, as necessary, negotiate points of concern within the contract.

Continuing Education Units (CEUs) for American Academy of Professional Coders

This publication has prior approval of the American Academy of Professional Coders (AAPC) for 4.0 continuing education units (CEUs). Granting of this approval in no way constitutes endorsement by the AAPC of the publication, content, or publication sponsor.

To earn your CEUs, complete the 40-question quiz online (www.aap.org/cfp). Click on "CEU Quiz for Coding for Pediatrics, 2018." A passcode will be required; enter AAPCFP23.

You will only need the current Coding for Pediatrics 2018 publication and Current Procedural Terminology® and International Classification of Diseases, 10th Revision, Clinical Modification manuals to answer the questions. A 70% score or better is required to earn the CEUs. You will be notified by e-mail whether or not you have passed. If you pass the test, you will receive a CEU certificate. If you do not receive a passing score, the test will be returned to you graded. However, it may be resubmitted for possible credit. This quiz will expire on October 1, 2018.

E-mail aapcodinghotline@aap.org if you have any questions.

4.0 Continuing Education Units

1. Under what circumstances can a physician report time-based critical care (**99291**, **99292**) when another physician of a different specialty is providing daily neonatal or pediatric critical care (**99468–99476**)?

   A. Only when the physician reporting **99291** or **99292** is providing critical care prior to hospital admission

   B. When the reporting physician personally performs critical care services while covering for the attending physician, who reports **99468–99476**

   C. When the physician reporting **99291** or **99292** is of a different specialty and different group practice from the physician reporting **99468–99476**

   D. When the physician reporting **99291** or **99292** is of a different specialty and same or different group practice from the physician reporting **99468–99476**

2. What code or codes are appropriate for reporting bone marrow biopsy and aspiration performed at the same session?

   A. **38221, 38220 59**

   B. **38222**

   C. **38220, 38221 58**

   D. **38821** (Aspiration is included in biopsy.)

3. In *Current Procedural Terminology* (*CPT*®) *2018* codes for chest and/or abdominal radiographs are selected based on which of the following characteristics?

   A. The types of views obtained

   B. The type of imaging (film or digital)

   C. The reason chiefly responsible for obtaining the radiographs

   D. The number of views obtained

4. *International Classification of Diseases, 10th Revision, Clinical Modification* (ICD-10-CM) codes in category **Z38** (liveborn infants according to place of birth and type of delivery) are reported for which of the following situations?

   A. All care provided during the perinatal period (birth to 28 days after birth)

   B. All care provided by the attending physician during the birth admission

   C. All care by the attending physician provided in the birth admission and care at a receiving facility when a transfer from the birth facility has occurred

   D. All care provided by the attending physician to the neonate who is not awaiting adoption or mother's discharge

5. Which of the following statements is true regarding reporting of *ICD-10-CM* codes?

   A. Only the code representing the condition carrying the highest risk or that is the main reason for the service is reported on the claim.

   B. Report all conditions and reasons for encounter, but list first any chronic conditions.

   C. The diagnoses may differ for each service on the claim.

   D. A different code is required for each service on the claim.

6. Which of the following reasons (without further justification) *is not* compliant with *CPT* and National Correct Coding Initiative (NCCI) guidelines for appending modifiers?

   A. A service that may be provided for diagnostic or preventive purposes was provided for preventive purposes.

   B. A service provided within the global period of a previous service is unrelated, more extensive, performed on a different body area, or performed at separate encounters.

   C. Two or more services are bundled by NCCI edits and a modifier will override the edits.

   D. The same service was repeated on the same date.

7. When is modifier **22** (increased procedural services) appropriately appended to an evaluation and management (E/M) service?

   A. When a patient is seen by the same physician twice on the same date

   B. When a patient requires intensive but not critical care

   C. When the typical time of the E/M service is exceeded by 15 but not 30 minutes

   D. Never

8. According to Medicare and most private payers, which documentation guidelines may be used by pediatricians providing primary care?
    A. Either the 1995 or 1997 guidelines
    B. Only the 1995 guidelines
    C. Either the 1995 or 1997 guidelines, but medical decision-making must be determined by the points methodology of the Marshfield Clinic tool
    D. Codes must be selected based on time spent in counseling and/or coordinating care.

9. How many systems must be reviewed to support a complete review of systems (ROS)?
    A. All systems related to the presenting problem
    B. 14
    C. At least 10
    D. 2 to 9 systems

10. The key difference between the 1995 and 1997 E/M guidelines is which of the following?
    A. Patient group variations on history and examination are appropriate only in the 1997 guidelines.
    B. The 1997 guidelines were developed specifically for the pediatric patient population.
    C. Guidance for selecting a level of medical decision-making is more comprehensive in the 1995 guidelines.
    D. The 1997 guideline includes specific examination elements for a general multisystem examination and for single-system examinations.

11. Documentation of an established patient office visit includes 20 minutes spent counseling and/or coordinating care and a total face-to-face time of 45 minutes. Which code(s) is appropriately reported for this service per *CPT®* instructions for time-based reporting?
    A. **99215**
    B. The requirements for time-based coding are not met. The service must be reported based on key components.
    C. **99213, 99354**
    D. **99214**

12. Which elements of the history component must be documented by the physician or other qualified health care professional (QHP)?
    A. History of present illness (HPI) and ROS
    B. HPI
    C. HPI, ROS, and past, family, and social history (PFSH)
    D. ROS and PFSH

13. A 12-year-old new patient is seen for a well-child visit and the physician also addresses a new problem of headaches with key components of problem-focused history, expanded problem-focused examination, and low medical decision-making. What codes represent the services provided?
    A. **99384, 99212 25**
    B. **99384, 99201 25**
    C. **99384**; only one E/M service may be reported.
    D. **99384 25, 99201**

14. A comprehensive history in a preventive medicine service contains which elements?
    A. Chief complaint and HPI
    B. Age- and gender-appropriate ROS and past medical history
    C. Age- and gender-appropriate ROS and PFSH
    D. A comprehensive history as defined in the 1995 and 1997 E/M documentation guidelines

15. A QHP provides an E/M service to an established patient of the supervising physician, whose plan of care calls for re-evaluation of asthma control. The QHP also addresses concerns that the patient is constipated. What type of service is this?
    A. Split/shared E/M service
    B. Established patient visit billed under the incident-to guidelines
    C. Established patient visit billed by the QHP in accordance with state regulations and payer specifications
    D. Concurrent care

16. What is required to support examination of the constitutional system under the 1997 E/M documentation guidelines?
    A. Orientation to time, place, and person
    B. Any of 7 vital signs
    C. Height (length), weight, blood pressure, and temperature
    D. Any 3 of 7 vital signs

17. Which of the following services may be separately reported from an office or other outpatient E/M service (**99201–99205, 99211–99215**) per *CPT*®?
    A. Preventive medicine counseling and/or risk-factor reduction
    B. Removal of an earring not requiring an incision
    C. Use of a fluorescein dye and Wood lamp to examine a corneal abrasion
    D. Puncture of an abscess without aspiration

18. Which of the following conditions *may not be used* to support the time spent in chronic care management (CCM) activities reported with code **99490**?
    A. A physician's or QHP's time spent personally performing CCM activities
    B. Time spent by a non-licensed clinical staff member
    C. The individual times of more than one clinical staff member who meet together to discuss the patient's care
    D. Time spent by clinical staff on a date when no face-to-face E/M service takes place

19. A behavioral health care manager, as defined for psychiatric collaborative care management, must have what qualifications?
    A. Master's or doctoral-level education or specialized training in behavioral health
    B. State license to practice psychology
    C. Degree of medical doctor or doctor of osteopathy
    D. Certification as a medical assistant

20. True or false? Psychiatric collaborative care management requires establishment of a care plan for all the patient's health care needs.
    A. True
    B. False

21. Which of the following services may be reported when provided on the same date of service as attendance at delivery (**99464**)?
    A. Initial care of the normal newborn (**99460**)
    B. Initial care of the sick newborn (**99221–99223**)
    C. Initial intensive care of the newborn (**99477**)
    D. All of the above

22. A newborn delivered at 10:45 pm Sunday receives initial care on Monday morning at 6:30 am and is discharged by the same physician at 5:30 pm on Monday. What code(s) does the physician report for these encounters?
    A. **99460, 99462**
    B. **99460, 99238**
    C. **99460**
    D. **99463**

23. A physician spends 30 minutes on the unit or floor providing initial hospital care to a patient with more than half of that time spent in counseling and/or coordination of care. Later the same day, the same physician spends 15 minutes on the phone discussing the patient with nursing staff. Based on this information, what *CPT* code should be reported for this encounter?
    A. **99221**
    B. **99222**
    C. **99223**
    D. **99281, 99222**

Chapter 20: Continuing Education Units (CEUs) for American Academy of Professional Coders

24. A child is admitted to inpatient hospital care on the evening of June 1. The child's attending physician provides initial hospital care at 7:00 am on June 2. What is the date of service for the physician's initial hospital care?
A. June 1
B. June 2
C. The date that the hospital lists as the admission date
D. The physician cannot report initial hospital care because there was no encounter on the date of admission.

25. A 3-year-old child is seen in the emergency department (ED) for fever, vomiting, and lethargy. An ED physician performs an ED visit with an expanded problem-focused history, detailed examination, and moderate medical decision-making. The physician also orders and supervises intravenous hydration over the course of 1 hour. Which *CPT®* code(s) will the pediatrician report for his or her services?
A. 99284
B. 99284 25, 96360
C. 99283
D. 99283 25, 96360

26. Can an ED physician report ED care (**99281–99285**) and hourly critical care services (**99291, 99292**) on the same date?
A. No. The ED visit is always bundled into the critical care.
B. Yes, but only if the services are provided at 2 separate encounters on the same date.
C. Yes, but there must be documentation supporting 2 distinct services.
D. Yes, an ED visit is always billed in addition to critical care.

27. Which of the following services *is not* included in critical care services when performed during the critical period per *CPT*?
A. Thoracentesis (**32554**)
B. Introduction of needle or intra-catheter, vein (**36000**)
C. Nasogastric/orogastric intubation, fluoroscopic guidance (**43752**)
D. Ventilation initiation; inpatient observation, initial day (**94002**)

28. What guidelines apply to reporting of critical care services by a teaching physician?
A. The teaching physician must provide a face-to-face encounter on the same date.
B. The teaching physician must be present for the key portions of the service.
C. The teaching physician cannot report critical care, as only the individual providing hands-on service may report critical care.
D. The teaching physician must be present for the entire period during which critical care services were rendered.

29. A pulmonologist in her office provides a telehealth consultation, including a comprehensive history, detailed examination, and moderate medical decision-making, to a patient in a rural hospital 2 hours away via real-time, interactive audio and video conferencing. The child's attending physician consulted the pulmonologist, who will not assume ongoing care of the patient. What code is appropriate for reporting this service?
A. 99253
B. 99253 95
C. 99243
D. 99243 95

30. A pediatric intensivist provides 45 minutes of critical care to a 3-year-old in a hospital 2 hours away via real-time interactive video conference. What is the *CPT* code for this service?
A. 0188T 95
B. 0188T
C. 99475 95
D. 99291 95

31. Which type of health care professional may obtain a National Provider Identifier?
    A. Only physicians
    B. Physicians and QHPs who may provide E/M services
    C. Any individual who directly provides health care services
    D. Any individual who may provide services without direct physician supervision

32. Which of the following encounters *does not* describe a service that may be reported as incident to (as defined by Medicare) a physician's service?
    A. A QHP provides a sports physical.
    B. A nurse administers immunizations ordered by a physician or QHP.
    C. A nurse provides patient education on diabetes as directed by a physician's plan of care.
    D. A lactation consultant provides counseling in the physician's practice to a new mother as per a physician's order.

33. Which of the following encounters is reported with code **99024**?
    A. An office visit to address an unrelated problem during the global period of a service
    B. A preoperative examination
    C. A postoperative follow-up visit during the global period
    D. Removal of sutures placed by another physician

34. Which of the following statements *is not* true regarding reporting of negative pressure wound therapy?
    A. Negative pressure wound therapy is reported based on the surface area of the wound.
    B. Negative pressure wound therapy is not reported for care of surgical wounds.
    C. Negative pressure wound therapy requires direct physician or QHP contact with the patient.
    D. Negative pressure wound therapy includes application of dressings.

35. Per *CPT®* instruction, what codes are appropriate for reporting a Level III established patient office visit when spirometry is provided followed by an inhalation treatment and repeat spirometry?
    A. **94010, 94640 59, 94010 59**
    B. **99213, 94010, 94640 59, 94010 59**
    C. **99213 25, 94010, 94640 59, 94010 59**
    D. **99213 25, 94060**

36. Which of the following codes is reported for administration of a validated depression screening instrument to the mother of a newborn?
    A. **96110**
    B. **96127**
    C. **96161**
    D. This service is included in a related E/M service per *CPT*.

37. A pediatrician performs a well-child examination on a 13-month-old established patient. As part of the service the physician asks the parent a series of questions about the child's development. What procedure code(s) is assigned for this encounter?
    A. **99392**
    B. **99392 25, 96110**
    C. **99392 25, 96160**
    D. **99392**, the appropriate level of established patient office or outpatient E/M with modifier **25**

38. Which of the following actions *would not* positively affect a physician's Healthcare Effectiveness Data and Information Set (HEDIS) score?
    A. A performance measure for patients 12 years and younger is provided at the first opportunity after the patient's 13th birthday.
    B. Both procedure and diagnosis codes are used to show performance of applicable HEDIS measures.
    C. A physician proactively recommends services that are included in HEDIS measures.
    D. Timely response to a health plan's request for records in relation to HEDIS

39. Which of the following statements supports compliant documentation and coding in an electronic health record (EHR)?
    A. Physicians choose diagnosis codes to populate the physicians' diagnostic statements.
    B. Physicians may cut and paste information from documentation of prior encounters.
    C. The EHR alone determines the level of E/M services.
    D. Physicians are able to enter information in free text format.

40. Typical pay-for-performance methodologies include which of the following characteristics?
    A. Sharing of a single payment by all providers for a specified range of services
    B. Physicians and providers contract to receive a share of health plan savings.
    C. Physicians are provided funds to pay for transitioning to a medical home.
    D. Health plans prospectively determine a physician's performance in meeting specified benchmarks and provide enhanced payment or bonuses for meeting benchmarks.

Appendixes

More coding resources, including online forms for the documents listed herein, can be accessed at www.aap.org/cfp. Use access code AAPCFP23.

I. Sample Assessment/Testing Tools

NOTE: These are provided as examples only; the American Academy of Pediatrics implies no endorsement or restriction of code use to these instruments. If you choose to use an instrument not listed below, be sure it is validated/standardized.

Instrument	Abbreviation	CPT® Code
Ages & Stages Questionnaire—Third Edition	ASQ	96110
Ages & States Questionnaire: Social-Emotional	ASQ:SE	96127
Australian Scale for Asperger's Syndrome	ASAS	96127
Beck Anxiety Inventory	BAI	96127
Beck Depression Inventory	BDI	96127
Beck Youth Inventories—Second Edition	BYI-II	96127
Beery-Buktenica Developmental Test of Visual-Motor Integration—Sixth Edition	BEERY-VMI	96111
Behavior Assessment Scale for Children—Second Edition	BASC-2	96127
Behavioral Rating Inventory of Executive Function	BRIEF	96127
Child Behavior Checklist	CBCL	96127
Children's Depression Inventory	CDI	96127
Clinical Evaluation of Language Fundamentals—Fifth Edition	CELF-5	96111
Clinical Evaluation of Language Fundamentals—Preschool Version-2		96111
Columbia DISC Depression Scale		96127
Comprehensive Test of Nonverbal Intelligence—Second Edition	CTONI-2	96111
Connor's Rating Scale		96127
Developmental Test of Visual Perception—Third Edition	DTVP-3	96111
Hamilton Anxiety Scale		96127
Hamilton Rating Scale for Depression	HRSD	96127
Kaufman Brief Intelligence Test—Second Edition	KBIT-2	96111
Modified Checklist for Autism in Toddlers	M-CHAT	96110
Multidimensional Anxiety Scale for Children	MASC	96127
Parents' Evaluation of Developmental Status	PEDS	96110
Patient Health Questionnaire	PHQ-2 or PHQ-9	96127
Peabody Picture Vocabulary Test—Fourth Edition	PPVT-4	96111
Pediatric Symptom Checklist	PSC/PSC-Y	96127
Screen for Child Anxiety Related Disorders	SCARED	96127
Test of Auditory-Perceptual Skills—Third Edition	TAPS-3	96111
Test of Language Competence—Expanded Edition		96111
Test of Nonverbal Intelligence—Fourth Edition		96111
Test of Problem Solving 3: Elementary Version	TOPS 3: Elementary	96111
Test of Word Knowledge		96111
Vanderbilt Rating Scales		96127
Woodcock-Johnson Test of Cognitive Abilities—Third Edition		96111

Appendixes

II. Vaccine Products: Commonly Administered Pediatric Vaccines

This list was current as of July 1, 2017.

For updates, visit https://www.aap.org/en-us/Documents/coding_vaccine_coding_table.pdf.

CPT® Product Code	Separately report the administration with Current Procedural Terminology (CPT®) codes 90460–90461 or 90471–90474 [Please see Immunization Administration (IA) Codes at bottom of table.]	Manufacturer	Brand	# of Vaccine Components
90620	Meningococcal recombinant protein and outer membrane vesicle vaccine, serogroup B, 2 dose schedule, for IM use	Novartis	Bexsero	1
90621	Meningococcal recombinant lipoprotein vaccine, serogroup B, 3 dose schedule, for IM use	Pfizer	Trumenba	1
90630	Influenza virus vaccine, quadrivalent (IIV4), split virus, preservative free, for intradermal use	Sanofi Pasteur	Fluzone Intradermal Quadrivalent	1
90633	Hepatitis A vaccine (Hep A), pediatric/adolescent dosage, 2 dose, for IM use	GlaxoSmithKline Merck	HAVRIX VAQTA	1
90644	Meningococcal conjugate vaccine, serogroups C & Y and Hemophilus influenza B vaccine (MenCY-Hib), 4-dose schedule, when administered to children 2–15 months of age, for IM use	GlaxoSmithKline	MenHibrix	2
90647	Hemophilus influenza B vaccine (Hib), PRP-OMP conjugate, 3 dose, for IM use	Merck	PedvaxHIB	1
90648	Hemophilus influenza B vaccine (Hib), PRP-T conjugate, 4 dose, for IM use	Sanofi Pasteur GlaxoSmithKline	ActHIB HIBERIX	1
90651	Human Papillomavirus vaccine types 6, 11, 16, 18, 31, 33, 58, nonavalent (HPV), 2 or 3 dose schedule, for IM use	Merck	GARDASIL 9	1
90656	Influenza virus vaccine, trivalent (IIV3), split virus, preservative free, 0.5ml dosage, for IM use	Seqirus Novartis	AFLURIA Fluvirin	
90658	Influenza virus vaccine, trivalent (IIV3), split virus, 0.5ml dosage, for IM use	Seqirus Seqirus	AFLURIA Fluvirin	1
90670	Pneumococcal conjugate vaccine, 13 valent (PCV13), for IM use	Pfizer	PREVNAR 13	1
90674	Influenza virus vaccine, quadrivalent (ccIIV4), derived from cell cultures, subunit, preservative and antibiotic free, 0.5 mL dosage, IM	Seqirus	Flucelvax	1
90680	Rotavirus vaccine, pentavalent (RV5), 3 dose schedule, live, for oral use	Merck	RotaTeq	1
90681	Rotavirus vaccine, human, attenuated (RV1), 2 dose schedule, live, for oral use	GlaxoSmithKline	ROTARIX	1
90685	Influenza virus vaccine, quadrivalent (IIV4), split virus, preservative free, 0.25ml dose, for IM use	Sanofi Pasteur	Fluzone Quadrivalent	1
90686	Influenza virus vaccine, quadrivalent (IIV4), split virus, preservative free, 0.5ml dosage, for IM use	Seqirus Sanofi Pasteur GlaxoSmithKline GlaxoSmithKline	AFLURIA Fluzone Quadrivalent FLUARIX Quadrivalent FLULAVAL	1

CPT® Product Code	Separately report the administration with *Current Procedural Terminology (CPT®) codes* 90460–90461 or 90471–90474 [Please see Immunization Administration (IA) Codes at bottom of table.]	Manufacturer	Brand	# of Vaccine Components
90687	Influenza virus vaccine, quadrivalent (IIV4), split virus, 0.25ml dosage, for IM use	Sanofi Pasteur	Fluzone Quadrivalent	1
90688	Influenza virus vaccine, quadrivalent (IIV4), split virus, 0.5ml dosage, for IM use	Sanofi Pasteur GlaxoSmithKline	Fluzone Quadrivalent FLULAVAL Quadrivalent	1
90696	Diphtheria, tetanus toxoids, and acellular pertussis vaccine and inactivated poliovirus vaccine (DTaP-IPV), when administered to children 4 years through 6 years of age, for IM use	GlaxoSmithKline Sanofi Pasteur	KINRIX Quadracel	4
90697	Diphtheria, tetanus toxoids, acellular pertussis vaccine, inactivated poliovirus vaccine, Haemophilus influenza type b PRP-OMP conjugate vaccine, and hepatitis B vaccine (DTaP-IPV-Hib-HepB), 6 months–4 years of age, for IM use	⚡	⚡	6
90698	Diphtheria, tetanus toxoids, acellular pertussis vaccine, Haemophilus influenza Type B, and inactivated poliovirus vaccine (DTaP -IPV/Hib), for IM use	Sanofi Pasteur	Pentacel	5
90700	Diphtheria, tetanus toxoids, and acellular pertussis vaccine (DTaP), when administered to younger than seven years, for IM use	Sanofi Pasteur GlaxoSmithKline	DAPTACEL INFANRIX	3
90702	Diphtheria and tetanus toxoids (DT), adsorbed when administered to younger than seven years, for IM use	Sanofi Pasteur	Diphtheria and Tetanus Toxoids Adsorbed	2
90707	Measles, mumps, and rubella virus vaccine (MMR), live, for subcutaneous use	Merck	M-M-R II	3
90710	Measles, mumps, rubella, and varicella vaccine (MMRV), live, for subcutaneous use	Merck	ProQuad	4
90713	Poliovirus vaccine (IPV), inactivated, for subcutaneous or IM use	Sanofi Pasteur	IPOL	1
90714	Tetanus and diphtheria toxoids (Td) adsorbed, preservative free, when administered to seven years or older, for IM use	Sanofi Pasteur	TENIVAC	2
90715	Tetanus, diphtheria toxoids and acellular pertussis vaccine (Tdap), when administered to 7 years or older, for IM use	Sanofi Pasteur GlaxoSmithKline	ADACEL BOOSTRIX	3
90716	Varicella virus vaccine (VAR), live, for subcutaneous use	Merck	VARIVAX	1
90723	Diphtheria, tetanus toxoids, acellular pertussis vaccine, Hepatitis B, and inactivated poliovirus vaccine (DTaP-Hep B-IPV), for IM use	GlaxoSmithKline	PEDIARIX	5

Appendixes

CPT® Product Code	Separately report the administration with *Current Procedural Terminology (CPT®)* codes 90460–90461 or 90471–90474 [Please see Immunization Administration (IA) Codes at bottom of table.]	Manufacturer	Brand	# of Vaccine Components
90732	Pneumococcal polysaccharide vaccine, 23-valent (PPSV23), adult or immunosuppressed patient dosage, when administered to 2 years or older, for subcutaneous or IM use	Merck	PNEUMOVAX 23	1
90733	Meningococcal polysaccharide vaccine, sero-groups A, C, Y, W-135, quadrivalent (MenACWY or MPSV4), for subcutaneous use	Sanofi Pasteur	Menomune	1
90734	Meningococcal conjugate vaccine, serogroups A, C, Y and W-135 quadrivalent (MenACWY or MCV4), for IM use	Sanofi Pasteur Novartis	Menactra Menveo	1
90740	Hepatitis B vaccine (HepB), dialysis or immuno-suppressed patient dosage, 3 dose, for IM use	Merck	RECOMBIVAX HB	1
90743	Hepatitis B vaccine (HepB), adolescent, 2 dose, for IM use	Merck	RECOMBIVAX HB	1
90744	Hepatitis B vaccine (HepB), pediatric/adolescent dosage, 3 dose, for IM use	Merck GlaxoSmithKline	RECOMBIVAX HB ENERGIX-B	1
90746	Hepatitis B vaccine (HepB), adult dosage, for IM use	Merck GlaxoSmithKline	RECOMBIVAX HB ENERGIX-B	1
90747	Hepatitis B vaccine (HepB), dialysis or immuno-suppressed patient dosage, 4 dose, for IM use	GlaxoSmithKline	ENERGIX-B	1
90748	Hepatitis B and Hib (Hep B-Hib), for IM use	Merck	COMVAX	2
90749	Unlisted vaccine or toxoid Please See *CPT* Manual			

Immunization Administration (IA) Codes

IA Through Age 18 With Counseling		Immunization Administration	
90460	IA through 18 years of age via any route of administration, with counseling by physician or other qualified health care professional; first or only component of each vaccine or toxoid component administered (Do not report with **90471** or **90473**)	90471	IA, one injection (Do not report with **90460** or **90473**)
		+90472	IA, each additional injection (Report in addition to **90471** or **90473**)
+90461	IA through 18 years of age via any route of administration, with counseling by physician or other qualified health care professional; each additional vaccine or toxoid component administered (Report only with **90460**)	90473	IA by intranasal/oral route; one vaccine (Do not report with **90460** or **90471**)
		+90474	IA by intranasal/oral route; each additional vaccine (Report in addition to **90471** or **90473**)

Abbreviations: CPT, Current Procedural Terminology; FDA, US Food and Drug Administration; ICD-10-CM, International Classification of Diseases, 10th Revision, Clinical Modification; IA, immunization administration; IM, intramuscular.

On October 1, 2015, ICD-10-CM was implemented. Code Z23 is reported for all vaccine-related encounters for all vaccines given. You will link both the CPT vaccine product code and the CPT vaccine administration code to Z23. Remember that Z23 is also reported in addition to any health examination codes.

⚡ Denotes vaccine pending FDA approval (https://www.ama-assn.org/practice-management/cpt-category-i-vaccine-codes).

+ Denotes add-on code.

III. Chronic Care Management Worksheet

Chronic Care Management Worksheet		
Reporting month/year	Patient	
DOB	MR#	Type of residence[a]
Chronic condition(s):		
Other medical conditions:		
Other needs (social, access to care):		
Physician/QHP	Date initial plan of care developed	
Date plan of care provided to patient/caregiver		

Clinical Staff Documentation: In the following table, include date, activity description, time spent, and location of any associated documentation (eg, plan of care, call notes). Activities may include
- Communication (with patient, family members, guardian/caregiver, surrogate decision-makers, or other professionals) about aspects of care
- Communication with home health agencies and other community services used by the patient
- Collection of health outcomes data and registry documentation
- Patient or family/caregiver education to support self-management, independent living, and activities of daily living
- Assessment of and support for treatment regimen adherence and medication management
- Identification of available community and health resources
- Facilitating access to care and services needed by the patient/family
- Management of care transitions not reported as part of transitional care management (99495, 99496)
- Ongoing review of patient status, including review of laboratory and other studies not reported as part of an E/M service
- Development and maintenance of a comprehensive care plan

Date	Activity (include reference to other documentation when indicated)	Time (start and stop)	Total Time	Clinical Staff Signature (legible/ credentials)
		Total Time	min	

____ **99487** first hour of clinical staff time with care plan establishment/substantial revision, per calendar month
____ **99489** each additional 30 minutes of clinical staff time per calendar month (Enter number of units.)
____ **99490** at least 20 minutes of clinical staff time per calendar month

Supervising physician/QHP signature_____

Date_____

Abbreviations: DOB, date of birth; E/M, evaluation and management; MR, medical record; QHP, qualified health care professional.

[a] Specify if patient lives in a private residence, group home, or other type of domiciliary. Do not report chronic care management services for patients residing in a facility that provides more than minimal medical care (eg, nursing facility).

IV. Care Plan Oversight Encounter Worksheet

Care Plan Oversight Encounter Worksheet

See www.aap.org/cfp for an online version of this worksheet (access code AAPCFP23).

Physician: _____ Patient Name: _____

Services Provided:

The letter that corresponds with each service provided should be placed in column #2.

A. Regular physician development and/or revision of care plans
B. Review of subsequent reports of patient status
C. Review of related laboratory or other studies
D. Communication (including telephone calls not separately reported with codes 99441–99443) with other health care professionals involved in patient's care
E. Integration of new information into the medical treatment plan and/or adjustment of medical therapy
F. Other (Attach additional explanatory materials on the services provided.)

Date of Service XX/XX/XXXX	Services Provided	Contact Name and Agency	Start Time	End Time	Total Minutes	Monthly Subtotal

Explanation for additional services provided:

Date:_____/_____

_____

Date:_____/_____

_____

Date:_____/_____

_____

Time Requirements per Calendar Month	Patient in Home, Domiciliary, or Rest Home (eg, assisted living facility)	Patient Under the Care of a Home Health Care Agency	Hospice Patient	Nursing Facility Patient
15–29 min	99339	99374	99377	99379
≥30 min	99340	99375	99378	99380
≥30 min Medicare code		G0181	G0182	

Monthly Total: _____ CPT® Code: _____

V. Global Per Diem Critical Care Codes: Direct Supervision and Reporting Guidelines

Global Per Diem Critical Care Codes: Direct Supervision and Reporting Guidelines
The delivery of neonatal and pediatric critical care has undergone significant changes in the last 2 decades, incorporating expanded technology and services and new patterns of delivery of care. Neonatal intensive care units (NICUs) have grown dramatically as improvements in perinatal care have led to markedly improved survival rates of the small preterm neonate. There has also been a growing national population with major socioeconomic shifts. These changes have led to a large increase in NICU beds. Simultaneous to these demographic and epidemiologic changes, serious Accreditation Council for Graduate Medical Education and Residency Review Committee limitations in resident and fellow work hours and, more specifically, to those hours allocated to clinical care in the NICU have reduced the number of house officers providing neonatal critical care. There has been a rapid expansion of other neonatal providers working as a team in partnership with an attending physician to meet expanding bedside patient care needs. These nonphysician providers (NPPs by Centers for Medicare & Medicaid Services nomenclature) are primarily neonatal nurse practitioners (NNPs). They have assumed a critical role in assisting the attending physician in caring for this expanding population of patients.
Neither NNPs nor residents or fellows are substitutes for the attending physician, who continues to remain fully in charge of these patients and directly supervises NNPs and residents or fellow physicians as well as other ancillary providers (eg, registered nurses, respiratory therapists, nutritionists, social workers, physical therapists, occupational therapists), who all play important contributory roles in the care of these critical patients. Unlike the supervision for residents or fellows enrolled in graduate medical education programs, the attending physician's supervision and documentation of care provided by NNPs is not covered by Physicians at Teaching Hospitals (PATH) guidelines. The attending physician is not "sharing services" with the NNP or resident or fellow. The attending physician (the physician responsible for the patient's care and reporting the service for that date) remains solely responsible for the supervision of the team and development of the patient's plan of care. In developing that plan, the attending physician will use the information acquired by and discussed with other members of the care team, including that of the resident or fellow and NNP.
When supervising residents or fellows, the attending physician will use this collective information as part of his or her own documentation of care. The attending physician must demonstrate in his or her own note that he or she has reviewed this information, performed his or her own focused examination of the patient, documented any additional findings or disagreements with the resident's or fellow's findings, and discussed the plan of care with the resident or fellow to meet PATH guideline requirements. These rules allow the attending physician to use the resident or fellow note as a major component of his or her own note and in determining the level of care the attending physician will report for that patient on that date.
Physicians at Teaching Hospitals guidelines do not apply to patients cared for by NNPs because NNPs are not enrolled in postgraduate education. This is true whether the NNP is employed by the hospital, medical group, or independent contractor. Centers for Medicare & Medicaid Services rules prohibit NPPs (in this case NNPs) and the reporting physician from reporting "shared or split services" when critical care services are provided. The reporting physician may certainly review and use the important information and observation of the NNPs, but the physician also provides his or her own evaluation along with documentation of the services he or she personally provided. Documentation expectations for the reporting physician include review of the notes and observations of other members of the care team; an independent-focused, medically appropriate bedside examination of the patient; and documentation that he or she has directed the plan of care for each patient whose services the physician reports. In many critically ill but stable patients, this requirement can be met by a single daily note. In situations in which the patient is very unstable and dramatic changes and major additional interventions are required to maintain stability, more extensive or frequent documentations are likely and may be entered by any qualified member of the care team.
In some states NNPs, through expanded state licenses, are permitted to independently report their services. If these NNPs are credentialed by the hospital and health plan to provide critical care services and procedures and possess their own National Provider Identifier (NPI), they may independently report the services they provide. In these states they can function as independent contractors or as employees of the hospital or

Global Per Diem Critical Care Codes: Direct Supervision and Reporting Guidelines

a medical group, reporting their services under their own NPI. It is important to emphasize again that the NNP and the physician do not report a shared critical care service. Critical care services are reported under the NNP or physician NPI, dependent on who was primarily providing the patient service and directing the care of the patient. Two providers may not report a global per diem critical care code (eg, **99468**, **99469**) on the same date of service. In most situations the physician is serving as responsible and supervising provider and the NNP (employed by the group or hospital) is acting as a member of the team of providers the physician supervises.

Physician Supervision

Current Procedural Terminology (*CPT®*) states that codes **99468–99476** (initial and subsequent inpatient neonatal and pediatric critical care, per day, for the evaluation and management of a critically ill neonate or child through 5 years of age) are used to report services provided by a physician directing the inpatient care of a critically ill neonate or young child. *Current Procedural Terminology* makes clear that the reporting provider is not required to maintain 24-hour, in-hospital physical presence. *Current Procedural Terminology* notes that the physician or other reporting provider must be physically present and at bedside at some time during the 24-hour period to examine the patient and review and direct the patient's care with the health care team. The physician must be readily available to the health care team if needed but does not have to provide 24-hour, in-house coverage. One provider reports the appropriate code only once per day, even though multiple providers may have interacted with the patient during the 24-hour global period (eg, on-call physician, NNP).

Medical Record Documentation

The medical record serves the dual purpose of communicating the medical status and progress of the patient and documenting the work of the reporting provider.

Based on the information presented previously, it is the suggestion of the American Academy of Pediatrics Committee on Coding and Nomenclature that the medical record documentation by the reporting physician or NPP supporting critical care codes should contain at a minimum

- Documentation of the critical status of the infant or child (This is not to be inferred.)
- Documentation of the *bedside* direction and supervision of all aspects of care
- Review of pertinent historical information and verification of significant physical findings through a medically indicated, focused patient examination
- Documentation of all services provided by members of the care team and discussion and direction of the ongoing therapy and plan of care for the patient
- Additional documentation of any major change in patient course requiring significant hands-on intervention by the reporting provider

The following are *not* required of the reporting physician or NPP:
- Twenty-four–hour presence in the facility or bedside
- Two or more documented notes a day
- Personally ordering all tests, medications, and therapies
- Performing all or any of the bundled procedures
- Documenting a daily comprehensive physical examination
- Documenting stable or unstable status so long as the infant or child meets critical care criteria

Each patient has a different level of illness(es), grouping of diagnoses, and medical and socioeconomic problems. The following are only examples of notes and should not be interpreted as requirements in every note for each patient:

A. The following note represents a sample attestation that could be appended to a resident or fellow's progress note:

"I have reviewed the resident's progress note and the baby has been seen and examined by me. He continues to be critically ill with respiratory failure requiring mechanical ventilation. I concur with the resident's evaluation and findings, though I did not appreciate abdominal tenderness on examination. I have discussed and agreed on a plan of care with the resident."

Global Per Diem Critical Care Codes: Direct Supervision and Reporting Guidelines

B. The following 2 paragraphs represent a single sample documentation that a reporting physician might write when care is delivered by an NNP and physician team. This note could be appended by the reporting physician to the NNP documentation or written as separate physician documentation.

"(Name) has been seen and examined by me on bedside rounds. The interval history, laboratory findings, and physical examination of the patient have been reviewed with members of the neonatal team. The notes have been reviewed. All aspects of care have been discussed, and I have agreed on an assessment and plan for the day with the care team.

"(Name) continues to be critically ill, requiring high-frequency jet ventilation. On examination, her breath sounds are coarse but equal, there is no heart murmur, and the abdomen is soft and non-tender. Her oxygen requirements have been at 100% for the past 12 hours. She remains on antibiotics for *Proteus* sepsis. At the recommendation of infectious disease, we have changed her antibiotic coverage to cefotaxime and gentamicin. Her blood pressure is acceptable today, but her urine output is only at 1 mL/kg/h. We are watching this closely and may need to restart dopamine. She remains NPO and is on total parenteral nutrition."

Approach to Documentation

This information deals largely with neonatal care. However, the same coding and documentation principles apply for critical care services provided to all children through the age of 5 years. The guidelines provided in this statement represent clarification of documentation recommendations for this unique code set. They are intended to create clarity going forward for physicians and other parties as they incorporate this new guidance into their documentation processes. Physicians should structure their documentation such that on review of a medical record representing a physician-rendered per-day neonatal or pediatric critical care service, one should be able to discern the reporting physician's unique documentation in support of the physician's role in that patient's care. It is especially important that an electronic health record used in documenting these services be configured to uniquely identify the author of each entry and allow for timely response to requests for documentation substantiating billed services. It is equally as important to log out of the record when your documentation is complete.

Appendixes

VI. Effective Health Plan Appeals: The Ins and Outs

I.   Know How and Why to Appeal Inappropriate Health Plan Claim Denials

II. Supporting Your Appeals for Payment

III. Elements of an Effective Appeal Letter

IV. Sample Appeal Letter: Well/Sick Same Day

I. Know How and Why to Appeal Inappropriate Health Plan Claim Denials

It is estimated that physicians are losing billions of dollars in revenue each year by not appealing inappropriate claim denials.

There are many reasons why physician practices do not appeal denied claims; the most common is that they believe appealing claims will create an increased administrative burden on the practice. However, not appealing denied or partially paid claims can be quite costly to your practice and can often result in decreased revenue. Since health plans have introduced claims editing software into their claims processing systems, they have generated an increased number of inappropriate claim denials and reductions in payment. An effective way for your practice to combat these erroneous payment reductions and denials is to be diligent in submitting appeals.

Why Appeal?

When your practice increases its appeals for wrongfully underpaid or denied claims, the health plan may correct its claims editing software and processes. This, in turn, may result in improved claim processes and appropriate payment to your practice for the provision of health care services. The 12 steps under How to Simplify the Claim Auditing and Appeals Processes below simplify the claim auditing and appeals processes and can help to reduce your administrative burden. These processes make it easy for your practice to identify and appeal health plan claim denials when the health plan misapplies the American Medical Association *Current Procedural Terminology* (*CPT*®) codes, guidelines, and conventions or the health plan's contracted policies. When a physician performs a procedure or service and then reports according to *CPT* codes, guidelines, and conventions, the health plan should recognize the physician work involved in providing this patient care. To ensure that your work is recognized, your practice should identify all inappropriate claim denials and communicate with the appropriate health plan representatives through each plan's claim appeals processes.

What Is Lost When Your Practice Does Not Appeal?

When your practice does not audit and appeal inappropriately paid or denied health plan claims, you may lose revenue. You also may lose the opportunity to recover overhead expenses by not implementing a claims management process. This process is your practice's internal designated work flow for accurately preparing, submitting, and collecting on claims. When you challenge inappropriate claim payments, you demonstrate that your practice has made an effort to correct the plan's inaccuracy. This could lead to a positive change in the health plan's business practices. Appealing claims that are inappropriately denied by health plans can make a difference in your practice by reducing future denials.

For additional information, there are 2 easy ways to contact the American Academy of Pediatrics (AAP) Private Payer Advocacy Advisory Committee.

1. Go to www.aap.org/en-us/professional-resources/practice-support/financing-and-payment/Pages/Private-Payer-Advocacy.aspx (AAP members only).
2. Contact the AAP Coding Hotline at aapcodinghotline@aap.org.

How to Simplify the Claim Auditing and Appeals Processes

1. Know the health plan's claim appeals processes before you need to submit a claim appeal. Understanding these processes will allow you to acquire the health plan information (eg, supporting documentation, health plan language) required to prepare a claim appeal.
2. Know where to locate the following health plan policies and, if possible, include them in the health plan contract:
   - Claim adjudication procedures (ie, definitions of complete or clean claims and medical necessity)
   - Rates and payment methodology, including a comprehensive fee schedule
   - Claim appeals processes
3. Document, document, document. The supporting documentation of a claim submitted to a health plan must substantiate the performance of a service by the treating physician or health care professional. If a service is not documented, it didn't happen in the eyes of the health plan, and the claim may not be paid.

I. Know How and Why to Appeal Inappropriate Health Plan Claim Denials

4. Review and monitor all claims before submitting them to the health plan to ensure that you are filing complete and accurate claims. One way to avoid a claim denial is to correctly code the original claim. Implement a checks-and-balances system between physicians and the coding and billing professionals in your practice to determine whether claims are being coded appropriately.

5. Maintain a coding reference sheet in your practice with a list of commonly used *International Classification of Diseases, 10th Revision, Clinical Modification* codes and *CPT*® codes, as well as any other commonly reported codes on the standard claim form.

6. Evaluate the health plan's explanation of benefits (EOB) for accuracy (eg, potential processing errors, lack of recognition of a *CPT* modifier, incorrect Physician Fee Schedule).

7. Know your contracted fee schedule rate with each health plan for procedures and services commonly performed in your practice. Review each EOB you receive to ensure the negotiated payment and discount rate with each health plan is calculated appropriately.

8. Maintain a health plan follow-up log that contains the reason that the claim was partially paid, delayed, or denied by the health plan and also the internal follow-up action by practice staff to reduce future health plan underpayments and denials.

9. When submitting a formal claim appeal letter to a health plan, thoroughly explain your rationale for challenging the health plan's claim denial. Additionally, include the appropriate documentation to support your request to reverse the denial.

10. Streamline your practice's claim auditing and appeals processes by maintaining an appeals resource file with appeal template letters, rationales, and supporting documentation of previously submitted claim appeal letters that resulted in overturning the denial.

11. Keep on appealing. It may take more than one appeal to reverse a health plan's incorrect denial. When a procedure or service has been appropriately performed, documented, and reported, be persistent to ensure your practice obtains the proper compensation based on the negotiated health plan contracted rate.

12. If the appeal is not overturned by the health plan after appeals are exhausted, file for an external review if available through the appropriate state or federal regulatory agency.

II. Supporting Your Appeals for Payment

Filing appeals using these suggestions makes the payer aware that the physician is knowledgeable of coding guidelines and adheres to coding conventions.

- Include a quote from the current coding guidelines that is applicable to the billed service. Example: "According to *Current Procedural Terminology* (*CPT*®), modifier **25** is used to identify a 'significant, separately identifiable evaluation and management (E/M) service by the same physician or other qualified health care professional on the same day of the procedure or other service.' See the American Medical Association publication *CPT*®."

- Note where a denial is in conflict with the payer's written policy, quoting from its policies and procedures manual. Example: "According to Section xxx.x of your Professional Services Manual dated July 1, 2016, your policy is to follow National Correct Coding Initiative (NCCI) edits in your claim adjudication process."

- Quote NCCI edits reflecting correct coding and/or use of modifiers. Example: "According to Version xxx of the Centers for Medicare & Medicaid Services NCCI edits, there is no edit that pairs *CPT* code **69210** (removal of cerumen) with an E/M service. The E/M service was necessary to diagnose otitis media, and the removal of cerumen was medically indicated because the patient had impacted cerumen. The reported diagnoses were linked to the appropriate service performed and billed."

- Include as appropriate any operative and/or procedure notes. Highlight the procedures that relate to the codes.

If a problem is recurring, suggest to the insurer ways it can be avoided in the future. Frame the proposed resolution in a way that enhances quality, access, value, and cost-effectiveness to patients, the payer, and the practice.

Appendixes

III. Elements of an Effective Appeal Letter

Generally, an appeal letter should contain the following information:

Date:
Carrier Address:

Address the letter to one having the authority to make a decision on the claim, such as the Carrier Claims Review Department Director or Carrier Medical Director.

Dear:
RE: Claim #:
I am writing regarding the aforementioned claim and (Insurance Carrier Name)'s practice of

List the offending carrier practice (eg, bundling codes, not recognizing codes).

Provide rationale as to why this practice is unacceptable to the pediatrician, the patient, and fair business practice. Reference appropriate *CPT*® guidelines, contract language, fee schedule, and state or federal law.

State how the situation is to be rectified and what you expect the carrier to do. Specify a time frame for a response and how the carrier may reach you should it have any questions.

Enclosed is a copy of the original claim that was submitted with a request that you process payment as indicated on the claim. I look forward to receiving your response by (date).
If you have any questions, please feel free to contact me at _____.

Sincerely,

Also available at www.aap.org/cfp, access code AAPCFP23.

IV. Sample Appeal Letter: Well/Sick Same Day

Date:

Insurance Carrier Claims Review Department and address or
Insurance Carrier Medical Director and address
Dear:

RE: Claim #:

I am writing regarding the aforementioned claim and (Insurance Carrier Name)'s practice of bundling preventive medicine service codes and office/outpatient service codes. *Current Procedural Terminology* (*CPT*®) guidelines indicate that in certain cases, it is appropriate to report a preventive medicine service code (99381–99397) in conjunction with an office/outpatient service code (99201–99215) on the same date of service.

According to American Medical Association *CPT* guidelines, "If an abnormality(ies) is encountered or a preexisting problem is addressed in the process of performing a preventive medicine evaluation and management service, and if the problem/abnormality(ies) is significant enough to require additional work to perform the key components of a problem-oriented service, then the appropriate office/outpatient code should also be reported. Modifier 25 should be added to the office/outpatient code to indicate that a significant, separately identifiable evaluation and management service was provided by the same physician on the same day as the preventive medicine service. The appropriate preventive medicine service is additionally reported." These statements clearly indicate that a "well" and a "sick" visit should be recognized as separate services when reported on the same day.

Unfortunately, many carriers are not familiar with the *CPT* guidelines that allow for the reporting of 2 visits on the same day of service by use of modifier 25. Further, there are no diagnosis (*International Classification of Diseases, 10th Revision, Clinical Modification* [*ICD-10-CM*]) requirements tied to the use of modifier 25. In fact, "The descriptor for modifier 25 was revised to clarify that since the E/M service may be prompted by the symptom or condition for which the procedure and/or service was provided, different diagnoses are not required to report the E/M services on the same date" (*CPT Assistant.* May 2000;10[5]). This basic tenet of *CPT* coding underscores the fact that it is *inherently incorrect for carriers to place restrictions on the number, type, or order of diagnoses associated with the reporting of 2 visits on the same day.*

There are also some carriers that, through failure to recognize all services provided during a single patient session, *potentially increase the number of visits necessary to address a patient's concerns.* If a patient is seen for a preventive medicine visit and the physician discovers that the patient has symptoms of otitis media during the examination, clinical protocol and common sense would dictate that the physician take care of the well-child examination and the treatment of the otitis media during that single patient visit. Unfortunately, the fact that some carriers fail to fairly pay the physician for providing both services will motivate providers to address only the acute problem and have the patient/parent return at a later date for the preventive medicine visit. This situation is frustrating for everyone involved, especially for the insureds.

While there is no legal mandate requiring private carriers to adhere to the aforementioned *CPT* guidelines, it is considered a good-faith gesture for them to do so, given that the guidelines are the current standard within organized medicine. Because providers are clearly instructed that an office/outpatient "sick" visit cannot be reported unless it represents a significant, separately identifiable service beyond the preventive medicine service, carriers should feel confident that the reporting of 2 visits on a single date of service *will not occur unless it is justified.*

Enclosed is a copy of the original claim that was submitted with a request that you process payment as indicated on the claim. I look forward to receiving your response.

If you have any questions, please feel free to contact me at _____.

Sincerely,

VII. Sample Denial Tracking Tool

Codes Paid When Submitted as a Clean Claim	Payer Name	Payer Name	Payer Name	Payer Name	Payer Name	Payer Name	Payer Name	Payer Name
Example: 90460/90461; 90471/90472: Immunization admin codes	Yes							
Example: 992__ with preventive medicine visit (9938_/9939_) on same date of service	No							
Example: Normal newborn care or hospital visits/discharges when billed with circumcision								
Example: 92551: Hearing screen		No, adj off						
Key: Yes = paid; No = no payment, appealed; Varies = payment is specific to employer's benefit plan; No, adj off = billed, denied, NO APPEAL, based on contract, adjust off.								

Appendixes

Subject Index
Code Index

Subject Index

Subject Index

CODE INDEX

References are to pages. **Boldfaced** *page numbers indicate the pages on which the primary code descriptions reside.* Current Procedural Terminology (CPT®) *codes begin on this page;* International Classification of Diseases, 10th Revision, Clinical Modification (ICD-10-CM) *codes begin on page 529; and* Healthcare Common Procedure Coding System (HCPCS) *codes begin on page 531.*

CPT CODES

0000F: 440
00100–01999: 45, 306, 403, 405, 406
00102: 406
0012F: 440
00326: 406
00561: 406
00834: 406
00836: 406
0174T: 13
0175T: 13
01820: 406
0188T: 16, 58, **328**, 344, 345, 346, 348
0189T: 16, 58, **328**, 344, 345, 346
0200T: 11
0201T: 11
0208T: 16
0208T–0212T: 159, 419
0209T: 16
0210T: 16
0211T: 16
0212T: 16
0232T: 11, 12, 412
0333T: 15, 16, **159**, 160
0341T: 16
0359T: 16
0359T–0374T: 373
0360T: 16
0361T: 16
0362T: 16
0363T: 16
0364T: 16
0364T–0367T: 361
0365T: 16
0366T: 16
0367T: 16
0368T: 17, 58
0369T: 17
0370T: 17
0371T: 17
0372T: 17
0373T: 17, 361
0374T: 17, 361
0381T: 17
0382T: 17
0383T: 17
0384T: 17
0385T: 17
0386T: 17
0403T: 17
0446T: 17
0447T: 17
0448T: 17
0464T: 16
0469T: 18, 159, 160

0479T: 16
0480T: 16
0485T: 18, **419**, 420
0486T: 18, **419**, 420
0500F: 440
0505F: 444
0545F: 440, **446**, 447
1000F: 440
10021–69990: 377
1005F: 448
10060: 46, 55, 300
10120: 40, 300, 383, **389**, 390
10121: 383, 389
10160: 301
1026F: 440
1031F: 440, 443
1031F–1033F: 448
1032F: 443
1033F: 443
1038F: 443, 448
1039F: 443
1040F: 446, 447
1050F: 440
11042–11047: 385, 388
1116F: 442, 447
1119F: 445
11200: 382, 383
1121F: 445
11601: 52
11602: 52
11740: 138, 301
11760: 301, 383, **386**
11765: 42
12001: 42, 48, 300, 305, **384**
12001–12018: 383, **384**, 386
12001–13160: 384
12002: 55, 300
1200F: 445
12011: 40, 300, 305, **384**, 385
12013: 300
12031: 48, 301, **385**, 405
12031–12057: 383, **384**, 386
12032: 301, 305, **385**
12041: 301
12042: 301
12051: 301
12052: 301
1205F: 445
13100–13153: 383, 386
13100–13160: 384
16000: 386, 387
16000–16030: 383
16020: 300, **386**, 387
16020–16030: 386
16025: 300, 386
16030: 300, 386
17110: 48, **382**, 383
17111: 382, 383
17250: 10, **382**, 383
20000–69999: 54, 304
2000F: 440
2001F: 441, 443
2010F: 440
2014F: 440
20150: 11
2015F: 442, 448

2016F: 442, 448
2018F: 440
20220: 11
20225: 11
2030F: 180, 440, 443
2031F: 443
2035F: 442
2060F: 446, 447
20936: 11
20938: 11
20939: 11, 12, 412
20999: 11
22319: 11
22510: 11
22511: 11
22512: 11
22513: 11
22514: 11
22515: 11
22532: 11
22533: 11
22534: 11
22548: 11
22548–22558: 11
22551: 11
22552: 11
22554: 11
22556: 11
22558: 11
22590: 11
22590–22612: 11
22595: 11
22600: 11
22610: 11
22612: 11
22630: 11
22633: 11
22634: 11
22800: 11
22800–22812: 11
22802: 11
22804: 11
22808: 11
22810: 11
22812: 11
23500: 300, 304, **391**
23650: 300
24200: 61, 389
24201: 61, 389
24515: 56
24640: 301, **391**, 392
25111: 46
25500: 391
25600: 391, 392
25605: 307
26011: 300
26720: 300, 391
26750: 300, 391
26990: 56
27603: 50, 51
28190: 48, 383, **389**
28192: 383, 389
28470: 51, 391
28490: 391
28510: 391
28820: 59

Code Index

New 2018 pediatric-specific coding resources
from the AAP!

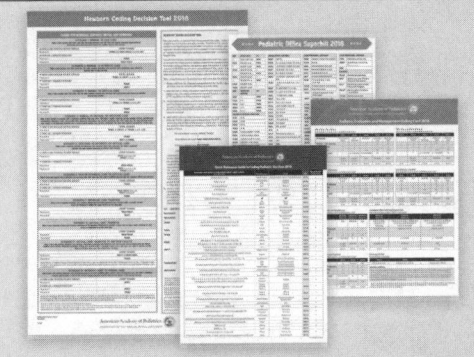

Coding for Pediatrics 2018, 23rd Edition
A Manual for Pediatric Documentation and Payment

This year's completely updated edition features all changes in *CPT®* codes for 2018, plus expert guidance for their application. New chapters have been added, and clinical vignettes and examples are also highlighted.

Spiral-bound, 2017—552 pages • MA0832 • Price: $134.95 • *Member Price: $107.95*
Book ISBN 978-1-61002-102-9 • eBook ISBN 978-1-61002-108-1

Pediatric ICD-10-CM 2018
A Manual for Provider-Based Coding, 3rd Edition

This purpose-built tool streamlines the coding process by condensing the vast *ICD-10-CM* code set to only pediatric-centered guidelines and codes. Completely updated for 2018.

Spiral-bound, 2017—568 pages • MA0831 • Price: $114.95 • *Member Price: $91.95*
Book ISBN 978-1-61002-101-2 • eBook ISBN 978-1-61002-107-4

Quick Reference Coding Tools

Pediatric Evaluation and Management Coding Card 2018
MA0834 • Price: $21.95 • *Member Price: $16.95*
ISBN 978-1-61002-104-3

Quick Reference Guide to Coding Pediatric Vaccines 2018
MA0833 • Price: $21.95 • *Member Price: $16.95*
ISBN 978-1-61002-103-6

Newborn Coding Decision Tool 2018
MA0835 • Price: $21.95 • *Member Price: $16.95*
ISBN 978-1-61002-105-0

Pediatric Office Superbill 2018
MA0836 • Price: $21.95 • *Member Price: $16.95*
ISBN 978-1-61002-106-7

AAP Pediatric Coding Webinars
presented by the American Academy of Pediatrics
DEDICATED TO THE HEALTH OF ALL CHILDREN®

New coding webinars coming soon!
- Coding with Modifiers
- Coding for Non–Face-to-Face-Services (part 1)
- Coding for Non–Face-to-Face Services (part 2)
- Importance of Understanding the Role of Time in Coding

aap.org/webinars/coding.

AAP Pediatric Coding Newsletter™

This information-packed monthly publication brings you proven coding strategies, tips, and techniques you won't see on any other periodical.

SUB1005 1-YEAR SUBSCRIPTION
Price: $235 • *Member Price: $200*

Subscribe for 2 years and SAVE!
Price: $423 • *Member Price: $360*

shop.aap.org

American Academy of Pediatrics
DEDICATED TO THE HEALTH OF ALL CHILDREN®

ORDER TODAY! **Online** at shop.aap.org/books • **Phone** at **888/227-1770** toll-free from 7:30 am to 5:00 pm CST

AD334REV2 0917

19. Confirm initial screen was accomplished, verify results, and follow up, as appropriate. The Recommended Uniform Newborn Screening Panel (http://www.hrsa.gov/advisorycommittees/mchbadvisory/heritabledisorders/recommendedpanel/uniformscreeningpanel.pdf), as determined by The Secretary's Advisory Committee on Heritable Disorders in Newborns and Children, and state newborn screening laws/regulations (http://genes-r-us.uthscsa.edu/sites/genes-r-us/files/nbsdisorders.pdf) establish the criteria for and coverage of newborn screening procedures and programs.

20. Verify results as soon as possible, and follow up, as appropriate.

21. Confirm initial screening was accomplished, verify results, and follow up, as appropriate. See "Hyperbilirubinemia in the Newborn Infant ≥35 Weeks' Gestation: An Update With Clarifications" (http://pediatrics.aappublications.org/content/124/4/1193).

22. Screening for critical congenital heart disease using pulse oximetry should be performed in newborns, after 24 hours of age, before discharge from the hospital, per "Endorsement of Health and Human Services Recommendation for Pulse Oximetry Screening for Critical Congenital Heart Disease" (http://pediatrics.aappublications.org/content/129/1/190.full).

23. Schedules, per the AAP Committee on Infectious Diseases, are available at http://redbook.solutions.aap.org/SS/Immunization_Schedules.aspx. Every visit should be an opportunity to update and complete a child's immunizations.

24. See "Diagnosis and Prevention of Iron Deficiency and Iron-Deficiency Anemia in Infants and Young Children (0–3 Years of Age)" (http://pediatrics.aappublications.org/content/126/5/1040.full).

25. For children at risk of lead exposure, see "Low Level Lead Exposure Harms Children: A Renewed Call for Primary Prevention" (http://www.cdc.gov/nceh/lead/ACCLPP/Final_Document_030712.pdf).

26. Perform risk assessments or screenings as appropriate, based on universal screening requirements for patients with Medicaid or in high prevalence areas.

27. Tuberculosis testing per recommendations of the AAP Committee on Infectious Diseases, published in the current edition of the AAP *Red Book: Report of the Committee on Infectious Diseases*. Testing should be performed on recognition of high-risk factors.

28. See "Integrated Guidelines for Cardiovascular Health and Risk Reduction in Children and Adolescents" (http://www.nhlbi.nih.gov/guidelines/cvd_ped/index.htm).

29. Adolescents should be screened for sexually transmitted infections (STIs) per recommendations in the current edition of the AAP *Red Book: Report of the Committee on Infectious Diseases*.

30. Adolescents should be screened for HIV according to the USPSTF recommendations (http://www.uspreventiveservicestaskforce.org/uspstf/uspshivi.htm) once between the ages of 15 and 18, making every effort to preserve confidentiality of the adolescent. Those at increased risk of HIV infection, including those who are sexually active, participate in injection drug use, or are being tested for other STIs, should be tested for HIV and reassessed annually.

31. See USPSTF recommendations (http://www.uspreventiveservicestaskforce.org/uspstf/uspscerv.htm). Indications for pelvic examinations prior to age 21 are noted in "Gynecologic Examination for Adolescents in the Pediatric Office Setting" (http://pediatrics.aappublications.org/content/126/3/583.full).

32. Assess whether the child has a dental home. If no dental home is identified, perform a risk assessment (http://www2.aap.org/oralhealth/docs/RiskAssessmentTool.pdf) and refer to a dental home. Recommend brushing with fluoride toothpaste in the proper dosage for age. See "Maintaining and Improving the Oral Health of Young Children" (http://pediatrics.aappublications.org/content/134/6/1224).

33. Perform a risk assessment (http://www2.aap.org/oralhealth/docs/RiskAssessmentTool.pdf). See "Maintaining and Improving the Oral Health of Young Children" (http://pediatrics.aappublications.org/content/134/6/1224).

34. See USPSTF recommendations (http://www.uspreventiveservicestaskforce.org/uspstf/uspsdnch.htm). Once teeth are present, fluoride varnish may be applied to all children every 3–6 months in the primary care or dental office. Indications for fluoride use are noted in "Fluoride Use in Caries Prevention in the Primary Care Setting" (http://pediatrics.aappublications.org/content/134/3/626).

35. If primary water source is deficient in fluoride, consider oral fluoride supplementation. See "Fluoride Use in Caries Prevention in the Primary Care Setting" (http://pediatrics.aappublications.org/content/134/3/626).

Summary of Changes Made to the
Bright Futures/AAP Recommendations for Preventive Pediatric Health Care
(Periodicity Schedule)

This schedule reflects changes approved in February 2017 and published in April 2017.
For updates, visit www.aap.org/periodicityschedule.
For further information, see the *Bright Futures Guidelines*, 4th Edition, *Evidence and Rationale chapter* (https://brightfutures.aap.org/Bright%20Futures%20Documents/BF4_Evidence_Rationale.pdf).

CHANGES MADE IN FEBRUARY 2017

HEARING

- Timing and follow-up of the screening recommendations for hearing during the infancy visits have been delineated. Adolescent risk assessment has changed to screening once during each time period.

- Footnote 8 has been updated to read as follows: "Confirm initial screen was completed, verify results, and follow up, as appropriate. Newborns should be screened, per 'Year 2007 Position Statement: Principles and Guidelines for Early Hearing Detection and Intervention Programs' (http://pediatrics.aappublications.org/content/120/4/898.full)."

- Footnote 9 has been added to read as follows: "Verify results as soon as possible, and follow up, as appropriate."

- Footnote 10 has been added to read as follows: "Screen with audiometry including 6,000 and 8,000 Hz high frequencies once between 11 and 14 years, once between 15 and 17 years, and once between 18 and 21 years. See 'The Sensitivity of Adolescent Hearing Screens Significantly Improves by Adding High Frequencies' (http://www.jahonline.org/article/S1054-139X(16)00048-3/fulltext)."

PSYCHOSOCIAL/BEHAVIORAL ASSESSMENT

- Footnote 13 has been added to read as follows: "This assessment should be family centered and may include an assessment of child social-emotional health, caregiver depression, and social determinants of health. See 'Promoting Optimal Development: Screening for Behavioral and Emotional Problems' (http://pediatrics.aappublications.org/content/135/2/384) and 'Poverty and Child Health in the United States' (http://pediatrics.aappublications.org/content/137/4/e20160339)."

TOBACCO, ALCOHOL, OR DRUG USE ASSESSMENT

- The header was updated to be consistent with recommendations.

DEPRESSION SCREENING

- Adolescent depression screening begins routinely at 12 years of age (to be consistent with recommendations of the US Preventive Services Task Force [USPSTF]).

MATERNAL DEPRESSION SCREENING

- Screening for maternal depression at 1-, 2-, 4-, and 6-month visits has been added.

- Footnote 16 was added to read as follows: "Screening should occur per 'Incorporating Recognition and Management of Perinatal and Postpartum Depression Into Pediatric Practice' (http://pediatrics.aappublications.org/content/126/5/1032)."

NEWBORN BLOOD

- Timing and follow-up of the newborn blood screening recommendations have been delineated.

- Footnote 19 has been updated to read as follows: "Confirm initial screen was accomplished, verify results, and follow up, as appropriate. The Recommended Uniform Newborn Screening Panel (http://www.hrsa.gov/advisorycommittees/mchbadvisory/heritabledisorders/recommendedpanel/uniformscreeningpanel.pdf), as determined by The Secretary's Advisory Committee on Heritable Disorders in Newborns and Children, and state newborn screening laws/regulations (http://genes-r-us.uthscsa.edu/sites/genes-r-us/files/nbsdisorders.pdf) establish the criteria for and coverage of newborn screening procedures and programs."

- Footnote 20 has been added to read as follows: "Verify results as soon as possible, and follow up, as appropriate."

NEWBORN BILIRUBIN

- Screening for bilirubin concentration at the newborn visit has been added.

- Footnote 21 has been added to read as follows: "Confirm initial screening was accomplished, verify results, and follow up, as appropriate. See 'Hyperbilirubinemia in the Newborn Infant ≥35 Weeks' Gestation: An Update With Clarifications' (http://pediatrics.aappublications.org/content/124/4/1193)."

DYSLIPIDEMIA

- Screening for dyslipidemia has been updated to occur once between 9 and 11 years of age, and once between 17 and 21 years of age (to be consistent with guidelines of the National Heart, Lung, and Blood Institute).

SEXUALLY TRANSMITTED INFECTIONS

- Footnote 29 has been updated to read as follows: "Adolescents should be screened for sexually transmitted infections (STIs) per recommendations in the current edition of the AAP *Red Book: Report of the Committee on Infectious Diseases*."

HIV

- A subheading has been added for the HIV universal recommendation to avoid confusion with STIs selective screening recommendation.

- Screening for HIV has been updated to occur once between 15 and 18 years of age (to be consistent with recommendations of the USPSTF).

- Footnote 30 has been added to read as follows: "Adolescents should be screened for HIV according to the USPSTF recommendations (http://www.uspreventiveservicestaskforce.org/uspstf/uspshivi.htm) once between the ages of 15 and 18, making every effort to preserve confidentiality of the adolescent. Those at increased risk of HIV infection, including those who are sexually active, participate in injection drug use, or are being tested for other STIs, should be tested for HIV and reassessed annually."

ORAL HEALTH

- Assessing for a dental home has been updated to occur at the 12-month and 18-month through 6-year visits. A subheading has been added for fluoride supplementation, with a recommendation from the 6-month through 12-month and 18-month through 16-year visits.

- Footnote 32 has been updated to read as follows: "Assess whether the child has a dental home. If no dental home is identified, perform a risk assessment (http://www2.aap.org/oralhealth/docs/RiskAssessmentTool.pdf) and refer to a dental home. Recommend brushing with fluoride toothpaste in the proper dosage for age. See 'Maintaining and Improving the Oral Health of Young Children' (http://pediatrics.aappublications.org/content/134/6/1224)."

- Footnote 33 has been updated to read as follows: "Perform a risk assessment (http://www2.aap.org/oralhealth/docs/RiskAssessmentTool.pdf). See 'Maintaining and Improving the Oral Health of Young Children' (http://pediatrics.aappublications.org/content/134/6/1224)."

- Footnote 35 has been added to read as follows: "If primary water source is deficient in fluoride, consider oral fluoride supplementation. See 'Fluoride Use in Caries Prevention in the Primary Care Setting' (http://pediatrics.aappublications.org/content/134/3/626)."